# Lippincott's CRNE Prep Guide

# Lippincott's CRNE Prep Guide

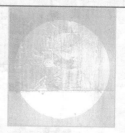

**Elaine Schow, RN, BScN, MN**
Faculty, School of Nursing
Mount Royal College
Calgary, Alberta

**Christina Murray, BA, BScN, RN, MN**
Faculty, School of Nursing
Mount Royal College
Calgary, Alberta

Wolters Kluwer | Lippincott Williams & Wilkins
Health

Philadelphia · Baltimore · New York · London
Buenos Aires · Hong Kong · Sydney · Tokyo

*Executive Acquisitions Editor:* Elizabeth Nieginski
*Senior Managing Editor:* Helen Kogut
*Editorial Assistant:* Laura Scott
*Production Project Manager:* Cynthia Rudy
*Director of Nursing Production:* Helen Ewan
*Senior Managing Editor / Production:* Erika Kors
*Senior Designer:* Joan Wendt
*Manufacturing Coordinator:* Karin Duffield
*Production Services / Compositor:* Aptara, Inc.

9 8 7 6 5 4

Printed in the United States of America

**Library of Congress Cataloging-in-Publication Data**

Lippincott's CRNE prep guide / [edited by] Elaine Schow, Christina Murray.
  p. ; cm.
  Includes bibliographical references.
  ISBN 978-0-7817-7907-4
  1.  Nursing—Canada—Examinations, questions, etc.   I.  Schow, Elaine.
II.  Murray, Christina.  III.  Title: CRNE prep guide.
  [DNLM: 1.  Nursing Care—methods—Canada—Examination Questions.
WY 18.2 L7645 2009]
  RT55.L55 2009
  610.73076—dc22

                                                        2008029031

Care has been taken to confirm the accuracy of the information presented and to describe generally accepted practices. However, the authors, editors, and publisher are not responsible for errors or omissions or for any consequences from application of the information in this book and make no warranty, expressed or implied, with respect to the currency, completeness, or accuracy of the contents of the publication. Application of this information in a particular situation remains the professional responsibility of the practitioner; the clinical treatments described and recommended may not be considered absolute and universal recommendations.

The authors, editors, and publisher have exerted every effort to ensure that drug selection and dosage set forth in this text are in accordance with the current recommendations and practice at the time of publication. However, in view of ongoing research, changes in government regulations, and the constant flow of information relating to drug therapy and drug reactions, the reader is urged to check the package insert for each drug for any change in indications and dosage and for added warnings and precautions. This is particularly important when the recommended agent is a new or infrequently employed drug.

Some drugs and medical devices presented in this publication have Food and Drug Administration (FDA) clearance for limited use in restricted research settings. It is the responsibility of the health care provider to ascertain the FDA status of each drug or device planned for use in his or her clinical practice.

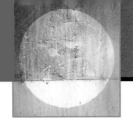

# Contributors

**Susan Ruth Beischel, RN, CNM, MN**
Program Coordinator/Instructor
Maternal Infant Child Healthcare Program
Department of Advanced Specialty Health Program
Mount Royal College
Calgary, Alberta
*Chapter 6*

**Eleanor Benterud, RN, MN**
Population Health Nurse Specialist
Calgary Health Region
Calgary, Alberta
*Chapter 4*

**Christine Boyle, RN, BScN, MA**
Faculty, School of Nursing
Mount Royal College
Calgary, Alberta
*Chapter 4*

**Nancy J. Cochrane, RN, PhD, MCPA**
Psychological and Educational Consultant
Dr. N. J. Cochrane & Associates, Inc.
Richmond, British Columbia
*Chapter 1*

**Sonya L. Jakubec, RN, RHScN, MN, PhD(c)**
Faculty, School of Nursing
Mount Royal College
Calgary, Alberta
*Chapter 7*

**Elizabeth Matthewson, RN, BScN, MPH, COHN(c), CRSP**
Nursing Professor
Sir Sandford Fleming College
Peterborough, Ontario
*Chapter 3*

**Linda Poirier, RN, BScN, MHS**
Nursing Professor
Sir Sandford Fleming College
Peterborough, Ontario
*Chapter 5*

**Pattie Pryma, RN, BScN, MEd**
Faculty, School of Nursing
Mount Royal College
Calgary, Alberta
*Chapter 7*

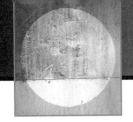

# Reviewers

**Dorothy Andrews, RN, BN, MN**
Part Time Clinical Nursing Instructor
Western Regional School of Nursing and College of
the North Atlantic
Corner Brook, Newfoundland and Labrador

**Tanya Baldwin, BSN**
Registered Nurse
Peterborough Regional Health Centre
Peterborough, Ontario

**Angela Carlson**
Nursing Student
University of Lethbridge
Lethbridge, Alberta

**Rachel Childs**
Nursing Student
Dalhousie University
Halifax, Nova Scotia

**Joanna Cox**
Nursing Student
Dalhousie University
Halifax, Nova Scotia

**Isabelle Cyr, RN, MEd, CNCC(c)**
Part-time Professor
University of Ottawa School of Nursing
Ottawa, Ontario

**Penny Davis, BScN, MEd**
Instructor
University of Manitoba
Winnipeg, Manitoba

**Kimberly Foxworthy, RN, BN**
NICU Nurse
Children's Hospital
Winnipeg, Manitoba

**Donald Froese, RPN, BA, BTh, Ed. Cert.**
Nursing Instructor and Psychiatric Nursing
Coordinator
Nursing Education Program of Saskatchewan
Saskatoon, Saskatchewan

**Elizabeth E. Harris, RN, BScN, MEd**
Professor of Nursing
University of Ottawa/Algonquin College
Collaborative BScN Program
Algonquin College
Ottawa, Ontario

**Kelly Kidd, RN, BScN, MN**
Coordinator, Practical Nursing Program
Algonquin College
Pembroke, Ontario

**Sandy Klein, RPN**
Staff Psychiatric Nurse, Dual Diagnosis Recovery
Program
Centennial Centre for Mental Illness and Brain Injury
Ponoka, Alberta

**Roxanne R. Laforge, RN, BSN, BA, MS**
Lecturer and Clinical Instructor, College of Nursing
Coordinator, Perinatal Education Program
College of Nursing and College of Medicine
University of Saskatchewan
Saskatoon, Saskatchewan

**Gemma Langor, MEd, BN, RN**
Nurse Educator, BN Collaborative Program
Centre for Nursing Studies
St. John's, Newfoundland and Labrador

**Robert Lockhart, Dip.SW, RPN, RN, BScN, MA**
Faculty/Site Coordinator
Psychiatric Nursing Program, School of Nursing
Grant MacEwan College
Edmonton and Ponoka, Alberta

**Nancy C. Logue, RN, MN**
Senior Teaching Associate
Department of Nursing
University of New Brunswick–Saint John
Saint John, New Brunswick

**Katie Lum, BScN, RN, ICU**
Peterborough Regional Health Center
Peterborough, Ontario

**Judy McAulay, RN, BN, MEd**
Associate Professor
University of British Columbia–Okanagan
Kelowna, British Columbia

**Wendy McMillan, RN, BSCN, MN**
Nursing Instructor
Grande Prairie Regional College
Grande Prairie, Alberta

**Jeanette Murray, RN, BScN, MA**
Chairperson, School of Nursing
Thompson Rivers University
Kamloops, British Columbia

**Valerie Needham, RN, BScN, MA**
Professor
Algonquin College
Ottawa, Ontario

**Tia Louise Nymark, RN, BScN**
Faculty of Nursing
John Abbott College
Montreal, Quebec

**Norma Poirier, MN, PhD**
Professor, Health Services
Université de Moncton
Moncton, New Brunswick

**Judy Sabiston, MS, MEd**
Nursing Teacher
John Abbott College
Ste. Anne de Bellevue, Quebec

**Janice Sadownyk, RN, BScN, MEd**
Chair, Baccalaureate Nursing Program
School of Nursing, Faculty of Health
    and Community Studies
Grant MacEwan College
Edmonton, Alberta

**Pamela Shpak**
Nursing Student
University of Manitoba
Winnipeg, Manitoba

**Debbie Styles, RN, BScN, MEd**
Faculty, School of Nursing
Grant MacEwan College
Edmonton, Alberta

**Dale Wagner, RN, BSN, MS**
Lecturer
Thompson Rivers University
Kamloops, British Columbia

**Yim Warrington, RN, BScNEd, MEd**
Professor, Faculty of Health, Public Safety,
    and Community Studies
Algonquin College of Applied Arts and Technology
Nepean, Ontario

**Bernadine Wojtowicz, RN, BN**
Academic Assistant/Clinical Instructor
University of Lethbridge
Lethbridge, Alberta

# Preface

All graduate nurses entering practice in Canada must demonstrate competence in several areas of professional practice. *Lippincott's CRNE Prep Guide* was designed to provide a comprehensive product for students to use in preparation for successfully writing the Canadian Registered Nurse Exam (CRNE), which is "administered by all provincial and territorial regulatory authorities, except in Quebec" (Canadian Nurses Association, 2005). In June, 2005, the CNA adopted a new style of testing that uses two types of questions: short-answer questions and multiple-choice questions that are either case-based or independent, and that are organized according to competency categories rather than core content areas (this may be adapted in the future).

This guide can benefit you in many ways as you study for the CRNE.

## BENEFITS OF REVIEWING WITH *LIPPINCOTT'S CRNE PREP GUIDE*

1. Chapter 1 provides a comprehensive overview of the format of the CRNE to help you understand the knowledge and skill sets required to be successful when you write the exam. The chapter also includes detailed study plans and CRNE preparation strategies. It is important that you carefully read these strategies and consider how you can use them to strengthen your test-taking skills. Your overall exam score is likely to increase if you understand how to write the exam, are physically and psychologically prepared to write the exam, and are confident in your level of preparation and knowledge base. This text can assist you in all of these important areas.

2. *Lippincott's CRNE Prep Guide* contains review chapters that provide multiple-choice and short-answer questions in each of the nursing specialty areas: maternal–child health, mental health, child health, and adult and older adult health. Additionally, an entire chapter has been developed on the competency area of Professional Practice. We recognize that this area may require extra study time, so the chapter integrates all the nursing specialty areas with a focus on Professional Practice questions.

3. Each review chapter is written in the CRNE format to test your knowledge of each competency group, structural variable, and contextual variable used in the CRNE. You will have the opportunity to answer questions from various practice perspectives and settings. This allows you to test your knowledge base, apply your knowledge, and evaluate your critical thinking skills. It also provides a great deal of practice in transferring these skill sets to different nursing specialty areas within a variety of health care settings.

4. The final chapter of *Lippincott's CRNE Prep Guide* provides two comprehensive practice exams. They allow you to determine your knowledge base, depth of application, and critical thinking skills, and to judge how well you manage your test-writing time. The tests are written in the same format as the CRNE and are similar to it in length, to give you "real-life" practice writing the exam.

## ORGANIZATION OF *LIPPINCOTT'S CRNE PREP GUIDE*

*Lippincott's CRNE Prep Guide* is organized according to the professional competencies that Canadian nurses are expected to be able to demonstrate in the day-long exam. It comprises two basic sections:

1. *An overview of test-taking skills and strategies* that will increase the comfort level of the user who is preparing to take the exam.

2. The actual *review practice section* that is organized around the framework upon which the CRNE is based. This framework includes Professional Practice (44 competencies); Nurse–Person Relationship (21 competencies); Nursing Practice: Health & Wellness (46 competencies); and Nursing Practice: Alterations in Health (83 competencies). Within each framework category, questions are presented to reflect the overall "weight" of the CRNE.

The student is also expected to demonstrate competence and awareness of areas including culture (awareness, sensitivity, and respect for individual belief systems and practices different from one's own); health situation (a holistic view of patients); and health care environment (institutions, homes, clinics, communities). Therefore, these areas are also incorporated into the variety of questions included in this review book.

## LOOKING FORWARD

*Lippincott's CRNE Prep Guide* offers a way to test and analyze your knowledge base. It will help you review each nursing competency and practice specialty area, and provide you with a good understanding of what you know and in which content areas you need to improve. It is important to begin your exam preparation early, to maximize the benefits of *Lippincott's CRNE Prep Guide*. We wish you a productive and successful study time!

ELAINE SCHOW
CHRISTINA MURRAY

*Reference*
Canadian Nurses Association (2005). *Canadian Registered Nurse Prep Guide* (4th edition). Ottawa: Author.

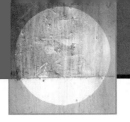

# Acknowledgments

In nursing and nursing education, you are touched and shaped by everyone you work with. Students, mentors, international nurses, and colleagues have all taught me that life is about relationships and caring. Nursing and nursing education have long been passions for me.

Co-editing this book has been a wonderful opportunity to combine both of these passions. Working with Christina Murray has been effortless and rewarding. I would like to acknowledge her insights, her editing ability, and most important, her teamwork approach that made this project come together so easily. I would also like to thank Corey Wolfe, Margaret Zuccarini, and Sheba Jalaluddin for their direction and guidance throughout the project. I would especially like to thank our contributors and reviewers for their quality of work, attention to timelines, and expertise in nursing practice.

On a personal level, I would like to thank my husband Richard. His constant support and love provide me with balance and joy. Finally, I would like to dedicate this book to my mother, Anne, who long ago passed on to her daughter her dream of becoming a nurse, and who taught me the value of caring.

Elaine Schow

This project has been a journey, and along the journey many people have contributed to its development. To begin, I would like to thank my co-editor, Elaine Schow. What began as a discussion and an idea drafted on paper is now a reality. To Corey Wolfe, Margaret Zuccarini, and Sheba Jalaluddin, thanks for your direction and guidance throughout the project. To our contributors and reviewers, a huge thank-you for all of your work. It has been greatly appreciated.

Personally, I would like to thank my husband, Gilles; parents, Faye and Whitney; and sisters, Charlotte, Rachel, and Sarah, for their tremendous love and support; and my daughter, Mairin, who has taught me the meaning of joy, and the importance of striving for balance. Finally I would like to thank Dr. Sandra Tenove, who believed in my abilities as a nurse educator before I even knew they existed. Through your guidance, mentoring, and encouragement, you taught me what it means to a teacher.

This book is dedicated to my nursing students, both past and future. May you find your passion in nursing, and flourish.

Christina Murray

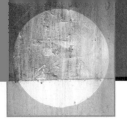

# Contents

*Chapter 1:*  **The CRNE: Content, Process, and Strategies**  1

*Chapter 2:*  **Effective Use of** *Lippincott's CRNE Prep Guide*  12

*Chapter 3:*  **Professional Practice**  16

*Chapter 4:*  **Care of Adults and Older Adults**  77

*Chapter 5:*  **Child Health Nursing**  171

*Chapter 6:*  **Maternal–Child Health Nursing**  222

*Chapter 7:*  **Mental Health Nursing**  276

*Chapter 8:*  **Comprehensive Practice Exams I & II**  336

## A Note on Question Types

Currently, the CRNE does not include "short-answer questions." However, in this reference, a small number of short-answer questions appear at the end of each chapter. While not on the exam itself, practice with this type of question will help develop the critical thinking skills needed for success on CRNE.

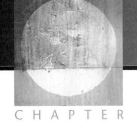

# 1  The CRNE: Content, Process, and Strategies

This chapter contains strategies and tools to help you prepare for the Canadian Registered Nurse Examination (CRNE). The chapter provides an in-depth look at the type of material covered, the structure of the exam, and various test-taking strategies. It is designed to give you a better understanding of the exam, as well as its framework, so that you will write it successfully.

## PREPARING FOR THE CANADIAN REGISTERED NURSE EXAMINATION

Eligibility criteria to write the CRNE are dictated and controlled by each provincial regulatory body. Candidates must first select where they will practice nursing because each province governs the practice of its registrants. Applicants arrange to write the CRNE by contacting the RN regulatory authority in the province or territory where it will be written. The staff will inform the candidate of the required documentation that must be provided to register for the exam, as well as the fee required. Persons with disabilities are accommodated during exam administration procedures provided that the regulatory body knows in advance of the accommodations required. The CRNE cannot be completed online. The exam can only be completed onsite after obtaining written approval from the regulatory bodies.

In Canada, the exam is invigilated in each province on the same scheduled dates. Candidates must have received a letter from their provincial regulatory body indicating that they have fulfilled all registration requirements and have permission to write the exam. Before receiving permission to write the CRNE, a candidate must have submitted academic transcripts for review by the provincial body. If necessary, the candidate must have successfully completed an approved RN qualifying program in one or more clinical areas to meet the requirements to write the CRNE. An additional step required for registration of internationally educated nurse applicants (IENs) is that they must have passed a test of oral and written English proficiency.

A candidate can attempt to write the CRNE three times. After three failed attempts, the candidate is requested to upgrade his or her competencies or English literacy, as specified by the regulatory authority.

After candidates successfully write the CRNE, they are issued an interim permit to practice nursing until the exam results are released. These same procedures apply to international nurses, who may practice nursing with an interim permit while awaiting test results.

## CONSTRUCTION AND DESIGN OF THE CANADIAN REGISTERED NURSE EXAMINATION

### Structure

Let's examine the structure of the exam. The exam consists of multiple-choice questions, which require you to assess the information given to you, identify what is being asked, review the possible options, and choose the most correct response. In other words, the exam requires you to proceed through the nursing process of assessing, diagnosing, planning, implementing, and evaluating! Each question on the exam is designed to test your applied knowledge of a specific competency at the entry level of practice.

Multiple-choice questions are related to a problem or case study. The questions contain a stem situation with four options or responses from which to select the correct response. The stem situation typically consists of one to three sentences that provide the necessary and relevant information and the specific question that is being asked. You must select only one response. If you select two responses, you will receive no credit for that question.

*Please note that in this type of exam, there are sometimes several correct responses, but there is only one response that is the most suitable or appropriate for the given situation.* Be careful that you are not impulsive in choosing the first correct response because it may be followed by a more suitable response.

The CRNE often includes experimental questions that are being pilot tested to determine if they are suitable for future exams. Your answers to these experimental questions do not count, but you will not know which questions are experimental. You must answer all questions asked on the exam.

The "client" (who is often referred to as the "patient") is identified as the individual, family, group, population, or community that accesses the services of entry-level nurses (Canadian Nurses Association, 2000). The information includes the age and gender of the client, but the diagnosis is not always given. Client age classifications are as follows: infant, birth to 1 year; child and adolescent, 1 to 18 years; adult, 19 to 64 years; older adult, 65 to 79 years; and adults of advanced age, 80+ years.

The clinical site for each exam question may pertain to (but not specify) the following settings: hospitals, institutions, clinics, homes, or communities. For the purpose of the exam, the health care setting is specified only when it is required to provide guidance to the candidate in understanding the question.

Cultural issues are imbedded in the questions pertaining mostly to nurse–client relationships, health promotion, supportive care, and professional practice. Questions are included to evaluate your awareness, sensitivity, and respect for different cultural values, beliefs, and practices, sometimes without introducing specific cultural types or nations. In these situations, you will be required to consider nursing management that is culturally sensitive and safe.

The exam is written in two parts, or in two books, on the same day. On the day of the exam, you will complete Book I in the morning and Book II in the afternoon. You will have 3.5 hours to write each exam book, and you will be permitted to have a lunch break between them. It is important to be rested and alert before writing each exam section.

### Standards of Nursing Practice in Canada

Because it is expected that the role of the nurse will be defined within each provincial health act, you will need to review the Health Authorities and scope of practice (especially for RN and nurse practitioner roles) in the province where you will be writing your exam. Ethics, responsibility, and accountability of nurses in Canada are different from those in other countries, and educational programs differ regarding the standards and scope that are expected for nursing practice. The six standards of nursing practice in each province are drawn from the Canadian Nurses Association (CNA) standards of practice:

Standard 1: Responsibility and Accountability
Standard 2: Specialized Body of Knowledge
Standard 3: Competent Application of Knowledge
Standard 4: Code of Ethics
Standard 5: Provision of Service in the Public Interest
Standard 6: Self-Regulation

It is the responsibility of all members to understand the standards and apply them to their nursing practice regardless of their role or context of practice (Canadian Nurses Association, 2000).

## REQUIRED COMPETENCIES OF NEW GRADUATES

In *Competencies Required of a New Graduate* (Sections One and Two, Canadian Nurses Association, 1999), the CNA published a set of competencies expected of new registered nurse graduates. These competencies became effective on December 1, 2000, for the purposes of basic and refresher nursing education programs. Together with the Standards of Nursing Practice, the competencies required of new graduates constitute the professional practice requirements used in the nursing education program approval process as set out in the *Nurses (Registered) Act Rules, Part 3: Approval of Schools of Nursing.* The competencies may be viewed as indicators of the standards of practice in each province for entry-level practice in nursing. Thus, only graduates of approved programs and curricula of study are eligible to write the CRNE.

If you understand the RN entry-level competencies, you will be well prepared to write the RN examination. Take time to review the categories of nursing competencies and what is expected of new graduate nurses. You need not commit to memory the specific wording of these competencies; instead, remember the categories and understand and apply them to nursing practice in the questions found in this book.

### Categories of Competencies

The RN level competencies are organized into different section headings:

1. Professional Practice
2. Nurse–Person Relationship
3. Nursing Practice: Health and Wellness
4. Nursing Practice: Alterations in Health

The CNA has released the list of competencies associated with these categories for the 2005–2009 CRNE. These competencies formed the basis for the updated CRNE that was introduced in June 2005. You can access them on the CNA's web site at http://www.cna-nurses.ca/CNA/nursing/rnexam/competencies/default_e.aspx

## Competency Framework

A framework was developed by Canadian nurses to identify and organize the competencies that the CRNE should assess. The framework and description of the four categories are presented in the following sections. Additionally, each competency within the category has been grouped according to its relative importance for safe and effective practice. Group 1 contains the competencies identified as *very important* for the safe and effective practice of entry-level registered nurses; group 2 has been identified as *important* for the safe and effective practice of entry-level registered nurses.

### Professional Practice

All nurses are accountable for safe, competent, and ethical nursing practice. Professional practice occurs within the context of the CNA Code of Ethics (2002), provincial and territorial standards of practice, and legislation. Nurses are expected to demonstrate professional conduct as reflected by attitudes, beliefs, and values espoused in the CNA Code of Ethics (Canadian Nurses Association, 2008). Thus, in your decision-making processes, it is prudent to keep in mind what would be the most ethical and safe practice and to use a clinical pathway that would apply to each test question. The *clinical pathway* refers to your problem solving or the decisions you make in nursing practice when a clinical situation is presented to you.

Professional practice in nursing involves the demonstration of teamwork, leadership attributes, basic management skills, consultation, advocacy, and political awareness. Leadership attributes, such as good judgment and decision making, vision, knowledge, initiative, integrity of ethics, confidence, communication, and innovation, are necessary (Canadian Nurses Association, 2008). Entry-level management skills involve the ability to work within an organization using appropriate resources to achieve the organization's mission and vision and to work within your scope of practice, as defined by the RN competencies.

Professional practice includes awareness of the need for and the ability to ensure continued professional development. This involves the capacity to perform self-assessments, seek feedback, and plan self-directed learning activities that ensure professional growth. Nurses are expected to know how to locate and critically appraise evidence and apply research findings to inform and build an evidence-based practice (Canadian Nurses Association, 2008). To do this, they must be able to appraise the information given to them, determine the quality of evidence of symptoms and causation of disease, and select the protocols for best practice.

### Nurse–Person Relationship

The nurse–person relationship is a therapeutic partnership established to promote the health of the client. (In this text, a client or patient is defined as the individual, family, group, population, or community that accesses the services of entry-level registered nurses.) This relationship is based on trust, respect, and sensitivity to cultural and socioeconomic diversity. An essential element involves gathering information that reflects the uniqueness of the client. It involves therapeutic use of self, communication skills, nursing knowledge, and the facilitation of empowerment to achieve collaboratively identified health goals (Canadian Nurses Association, 2008). From a legal standpoint, the nurse must be accountable for all actions and decisions made in the nurse–person relationship.

### Nursing Practice: Health and Wellness

Nursing competencies in this category focus on recognizing and valuing health and wellness. These competencies encompass health promotion, illness and injury prevention, and implementation of community-based and participatory approaches. Practice is guided by the principles of primary health care. Nurses work in partnership with communities to influence the determinants of health of populations and individuals with the goal of enabling people to increase control over and improve their health status. Nurses partner with clients to develop personal skills, create supportive environments for health, strengthen community action, reorient health services, and build healthy public policy (Canadian Nurses Association, 2008). Your response to the CRNE test items should reflect your understanding of the principles of population health.

RN practice reflects changes in cultural composition, demographics, population health trends, and economic factors (e.g., aging population, globalization). *Thus, your nursing approach should vary depending on the age, cultural status, available resources, presenting symptoms, and strengths and weaknesses of each client in a person–situation–environment.* For example, an Aboriginal youth who presents with symptoms of depression and suicide ideation must be assessed and assisted with the resources available in the community; the multidisciplinary practice team (if it exists); and your ability to recognize the level of client risk factors, community resources, and coping and problem-solving skills of the client at risk (Cochrane, 2006). If you are a nurse working in a predominantly Aboriginal community, you will need to adopt a community-based and culturally informed practice of care (Cochrane et al, 2006).

### Nursing Practice: Alterations in Health

Nursing competencies in this category involve care across the lifespan for the client experiencing alterations in health that require acute, chronic, rehabilitative, or palliative care. Such care may be delivered across a range of institutional and community settings. Essential aspects of nursing involve critical thinking, problem solving, and decision making in providing care. Using current knowledge, nurses collaborate with clients and other health professionals to identify health priorities. In responding to and managing health issues within their scope of practice, nurses aim to promote maximal independence and to help their clients maintain an optimal quality of life or a peaceful death (Canadian Nurses Association, 2008).

## THE DOMAINS OF TESTING IN THE CANADIAN REGISTERED NURSE EXAMINATION

In addition to testing your nursing competencies, the CRNE measures your knowledge and application according to learning competencies. Bloom (1956) created a taxonomy for categorizing levels of abstraction of questions that commonly occur in educational settings and test situations. You will need to apply various learning processes and skills in writing for the CRNE. It is important to identify the competency or skill that is required of you when you read each test question on the CRNE. The following types of questions based on Bloom's taxonomy of learning achievements and competencies may be asked: knowledge, comprehension, application, analysis, synthesis, and evaluation (Bloom, 1956).

The CRNE addresses several domains of your learning function. Bloom (1956) identified three domains of educational activities: the cognitive, affective, and psychomotor domains.

- **Cognitive:** Mental skills (*knowledge*)
- **Affective:** Growth in feelings or emotional areas (*attitude*)
- **Psychomotor:** Manual or physical skills (*skills*)

The cognitive domain includes knowledge, recall of information or data, and critical thinking. When you engage in critical thinking, you critically appraise the information given to you and select the most important and relevant issues to address. This critical thinking skill is used repeatedly when you take the CRNE. The cognitive domain requires you to attend to information (i.e., the test case study or short answer question), process the information (i.e., comprehend the case and the clinical situation), store it in working memory (i.e., reflect upon it), and then retrieve the information so you can select the best choice or response to the test question. Each step in the cognitive process requires sustained attention, comprehension, critical appraisal of the options, and memory skills. The CRNE evaluates your cognitive skills by engaging you in a problem-solving process.

The affective domain refers to the use of your emotions, values, and reactions to a clinical situation. According to Bloom (1956), this domain refers to receiving phenomena, which involves awareness, a willingness to hear, and selective attention. Thus, it is not so much an affective domain (which refers to affect or mood) as it is a skill that involves your perception and judgment.

Be aware that in the CRNE, you will *not* be tested on definitions of the various learning competencies, such as the cognitive and affective domains. Do not waste time during the exam trying to guess which domain is being tested; instead, try to determine which *competency* is required of you according to Bloom's taxonomy of learning competencies (e.g., knowledge, application, critical thinking). You will see these competencies listed as taxonomy levels in the Answers and Rationales sections at the end of each chapter. In time, this decision-making process will become automatic to you, requiring very little time, but it is important for you to practice the process.

## TEST-TAKING STRATEGIES

It is important to note that the critical thinking skills that you need to be successful in taking the CRNE are similar to the skills you use in applying the nursing process. The nursing process involves the following stages of problem solving: assessment, diagnosis, planning, implementation, and evaluation. The second step, diagnosis, involves the judgment that the nurse makes about the assessment of data. The judgment can be a problem, risk for a problem, or strength (Carpenito-Moyet, 2006).

Critical thinking is required in all steps of the nursing process, especially in assessment (diagnostic) and management. The ability to solve problems is critical to success in any career; in nursing, this problem-solving process is called the "nursing process." The process is important because it involves identifying the right problem based on knowing the possible causes of the problem. With these possible causes in mind, the nurse then asks questions to prove or rule out each potential cause. This process is also referred to as concept mapping (Carpenito-Moyet, 2006), and it is a required skill for correctly answering many of the CRNE questions. Let's examine a list of possible questions that are involved in the process.

You need to be aware of the nursing competencies that were previously discussed in order to selectively respond to these questions:

- What physical symptoms does the client exhibit? What are the possible causes of the symptoms, according to pain and the disease or stress process? What does your symptom analysis suggest in terms of the possible causes of the client's condition? List some possible causes (e.g., diseases, disorders, or conditions) that may account for the client's symptoms.

- What are the significant findings from the client's history, physical examination, symptom analysis, and diagnostic tests?

- What, if any, are the compounding stressors in the client's life, and what support system or resources does the client have that could ameliorate or exacerbate the presenting problems?

- Is the client physically and mentally stable or unstable? What is the evidence? Consider your need to conduct a consultation with a nurse practitioner or physician based on the stability of the client and your scope of practice.

- What is the quality of the client's support system (family, partner, friends, community resources, economic status), and how does the client rely on the support system? How would you assess the client's support system?

- What is your nursing diagnosis? In making a diagnosis, make sure to consider the cause of the patient's symptoms; how stable or unstable the condition is; whether the patient is coping effectively or ineffectively; what the patient's resources and support systems are; and what the patient's specific health needs are at the present time, including how these needs will be managed immediately or in the short or long terms.

- What is the level of acuity (critical, acute, subacute) of this client? Determine your scope of practice to stabilize and transfer or stabilize and manage the client.

Now take some time to practice applying the nursing diagnostic process using the following case study.

***Case Study 1.1:*** *Mary is a 16-year-old Aboriginal Canadian living on reserve lands. She has just discovered that she is pregnant and is neither accepting nor receptive to this news. This is Mary's second pregnancy. Her first pregnancy was terminated by a therapeutic abortion. She is in an acute state of crisis and has a very poor support system. Mary is living with her boyfriend's family because of conflict with her parents. Furthermore, the last time Mary discovered that she was pregnant, she attempted suicide. Mary appears to be very distressed, panicked, and depressed. A review of medical records indicates that Mary has been known to be impulsive.*

Based on this case information, develop a nursing diagnosis. You may complete the following table using the information in the case study to help you formulate your diagnosis. Document your assessment and plans for managing Mary's care based on your scope of practice as an entry-level RN.

| NURSING DIAGNOSIS FOR MARY | |
|---|---|
| **Client and Date** | |
| **Health Condition** | |
| **Symptoms** | |
| **Test Findings** | |
| **Stressors** | |
| **Stable or Unstable Condition** | |
| **Support System** | |

After completing this table, what is your nursing diagnosis? What steps did you work through in determining your diagnosis and plan of care? These are the same skills that you will use when writing the CRNE.

## Test-Taking Tips and Guidelines

The following sections offer additional ways to help you in answering questions for the CRNE.

### Reading and Assessing the Question

Begin by reading each question carefully. First, concentrate on the information that is given and then on what is being asked in the question. Alternatively, you may find it helpful to read the question first and then relate it to the information given. Try both methods to see which one works best for you in terms of aiding your comprehension and efficiency. Read the question at least twice to make sure that you read it correctly.

After you carefully read the question at least twice, try to understand the client's situation or problem and decide the most appropriate nursing response to that situation. Make sure you understand the question before you select an answer. First, eliminate the options that are obviously irrelevant and unrelated to the question, and then from the relevant answers, try to select the correct response. *Focus on the key idea in the information given to you, as well as in the question.*

### Recognizing Common Questions and Key Words

Pick out important or key words in the question. Review questions in the practice exam, as well as in the following list, to help prepare you to recognize key words and questions that often appear in the exam.

- What should the nurse's intervention be?
- When assessing the client, what sources of information would you use?
- Which of the following sources of information would best assist the nurse to plan and manage the care for the client?
- What should the nurse recommend to the client or family?
- Which of the following complications in the client's condition should the nurse anticipate?
- Which of the following interventions should be given priority in caring for this client?
- Which of the following goals should be a priority in the treatment of this client?
- Which of the following questions should the nurse ask to obtain the most significant information about the client?
- What should the nurse do?
- What should the nurse's response be?
- What priority action should the nurse take?
- Which of the following interventions should the nurse implement to address the client's concerns?
- What would indicate that the patient requires further teaching?
- To minimize the client's discomfort, what should the nurse do?
- What should the nurse document in this situation?

- Which one of the following nursing interventions is most appropriate to facilitate the client's learning?
- Which one of the following assessment tools would be most appropriate for the nurse to use to evaluate the client's condition?
- Which of the following behaviours by the nurse would best demonstrate a caring attitude toward the client or the client's family?
- Which one of the following responses by the nurse would be the most appropriate?
- Which one of the following conditions, diseases, or disorders (i.e., nursing diagnosis) is most likely indicated by these findings?
- When interviewing the client, how should the nurse conduct a comprehensive history?
- Which of the following ordered medical treatments should the nurse initiate first?
- Which of the following positions should the client be placed in during this procedure?
- What should the nurse do initially when he or she reads this order?
- What information should the nurse first obtain before providing analgesia?

### Responding to Questions You Do Not Know How to Answer

If you are confused about a question or you do not know the answer, mark it with a check to the left of the question and return to it at the end of the exam. *Do not let confusing or difficult questions slow you down and increase your anxiety. Use your time well. Maintain your confidence by responding to questions that you can answer quickly and accurately.*

### Changing Your Answer

If you change your mind about an answer, *make sure your first response is completely erased.* You will not receive credit for a question if you select two responses.

### Choosing the Right Answer Among Correct Responses

Sometimes the correct answer is found among two or more similar responses. *Responses that do not relate to the question asked can be eliminated first.* To find the most correct answer from among the correct responses, relate each answer back to the question. Make sure you answer the question without reading too much into it! Simple and direct responding is often best.

## Guessing

After you've answered all the questions you're sure of, go back and guess at the ones you marked with a check. *You will not be penalized for guessing, and you have a one in four chance of getting a guessed answer correct.*

## Determining Whether the Question Focuses on the Client or on the Nurse

A nurse's open-ended questions to the client are generally more appropriate than questions that generate a yes/no response from the client. Open-ended questions stimulate discussion and reflection by the client, and they seek to develop the nurse–client relationship. An example of an open-ended question is: "What do you think of this situation, Mr Smith?"

*Open-ended questions encourage clients to begin talking about how they feel concerning their health situations.* Thus, open-ended questions and responses are often the most appropriate answer to questions on the CRNE that involve nurse–client relationships and communication.

Knowledge of common questions or key words will assist you in adopting pattern recognition and understanding the exam question being asked. *Focusing on stem words or key words in the exam questions helps you attend to the main idea of the question.* Stem words or key words quickly direct you to the correct response. When you do not understand every word in the question, you can often grasp the general meaning of the question through identifying and understanding its key words. Persons with language difficulties may find this tip very useful.

*One way to feel familiar with the examination structure is to practice samples of examination questions.* Using this prep guide is an excellent way to do this. Practicing examples of examination questions will help reduce your anxiety and make you familiar with the types of questions you will encounter on the exam. Practicing can also enable you to recognize areas where improvement is needed specific to your test reactions and test responses.

## Common Abbreviations Used in the CRNE

Try to memorize the following abbreviations before taking the CRNE. *These abbreviations are very important because you are expected to know and use them in your daily nursing practice.*

**b.i.d.:** twice daily
**BP:** blood pressure
**°C:** degrees Celsius
**cm:** centimeter(s)
**g:** gram
**gtt:** drops
**h:** hour
**IM:** intramuscular

**IV:** intravenous
**kg:** kilogram(s)
**L:** litre(s)
**mEq:** milliequivalent
**mg:** milligram(s)
**mL:** milliliter(s)
**mm Hg:** millimeters mercury
**min:** minute(s)
**P:** pulse
**p.o.:** orally
**p.r.n.:** as needed
**q.i.d.:** 4 times daily
**q.8h:** every 8 hours
**R:** respiration(s)
**stat:** immediately
**T:** temperature
**t.i.d.:** 3 times daily

## EVALUATING YOUR RESULTS AFTER TAKING A PRACTICE EXAM

### Common Test-Taking Errors

Many individuals who do poorly on the CRNE may have very good knowledge and skills, but they are not accustomed to the exam's duration or used to writing this type of exam within the Canadian cultural context. *People who take tests occasionally make errors in processing facts and information in the question or case study.* Common technical and perceptual errors of writing tests are listed below:

- Missing important information in the question or case study as a result of not paying close attention to each word
- Misreading the question and misunderstanding its meaning
- Failing to extract important or key words in the question
- Making assumptions in the case study or question by implying information that was not there
- Focusing on insignificant details and missing key issues
- Selecting more than one answer or failing to mark the answer in the proper place
- Incorrectly transferring an answer from selection in the exam book to the computer answer sheet
- Switching the answer from the first response, which was correct, to a second response that is incorrect
- Rushing through the questions as a result of test anxiety

- Failing to check answers at the end of the test and to check the answer sheet to see that each answer corresponds to the right question
- Being impulsive in reading the selection of responses and answers without thinking the question through
- Misperceiving the intent of the question
- Not understanding one or several key words and failing to understand the context of the question
- Making an error in recalling a response from the practice exams to the actual exam rather than solving the problem
- Jumping to conclusions about what the answer is before looking at the options
- Misunderstanding the cultural context of the nurse's role and the nurse–patient relationship
- Using weak deductive reasoning skill
- Lacking experience writing multiple-choice exams
- Feeling tired and ill going into the exam
- Getting insufficient sleep the night before the exam
- Experiencing stressful recent life events that cause preoccupation with other issues
- Becoming distracted by events going on in the testing room, such as someone sitting close by who continues to tap her or his foot
- Not focusing on the test items and being apprehensive about doing well (e.g., making assumptions that a question is too difficult and thus abandoning it or not attempting to make an educated guess)
- Running out of time as a result of poor time management skills (e.g., spending too much time on some questions that are perplexing or difficult)
- Using poor judgment concerning the appropriate nursing actions
- Misinterpreting what a case study is about
- Being confused about the focus (either the client or nurse is the focus, but not usually both)
- Having previous negative test experiences, resulting in excessive test anxiety
- Having a very short attention span
- Having recent trauma or head injury that compromises cognitive functions
- Having recent emotional trauma that compromises attention and concentration

- Not preparing for the exam and not knowing what to expect
- Lacking knowledge of one or more clinical areas
- Possessing outdated knowledge and lacking refresher or continuing education in nursing science
- Having very low self-confidence
- Having a low academic standing in previous nursing education

## Preventing Test-Taking Errors

Now take the time to classify some of the above errors as resulting from insufficient knowledge or technical errors (e.g., misreading the question, giving two answers), transfer errors (e.g., transferring answer to wrong space on answer sheet) or errors created by language and vocabulary problems. In the table below, record the types of test errors you have experienced in the past and the types of test-taking errors you might anticipate when writing the CRNE. As you identify these test errors, also brainstorm ways you will try to prevent yourself from making these errors in the future.

| TYPES OF TEST ERRORS | WAYS OF PREVENTING ERRORS |
|---|---|
|  |  |
|  |  |
|  |  |
|  |  |
|  |  |
|  |  |
|  |  |
|  |  |
|  |  |

Review your completed table, which identifies test errors and ways you plan to prevent these errors in the future. This exercise can be difficult because you must first summarize the types of errors and then recognize patterns of test responses and your specific difficulties. If you can think of ways to prevent these errors, it demonstrates an awareness and understanding of the problem. This puts you in a driving or power position for gaining confidence to improve your test-taking abilities. If you do not do the work on the self-analysis of test results, you cannot complete this table. The more work you can put into completing this chart accurately, the more effective your study time will be in preparation for the CRNE. Chapter 2 provides you with instructions on how to use this text more effectively and how to analyze your knowledge base of each nursing specialty area and each competency area. You will be able to identify which domains of knowledge you have difficulty with, and you can then determine strategies to address these areas.

## PREPARING PSYCHOLOGICALLY AND PHYSICALLY

### Understanding the Causes of Exam Anxiety

In their textbook titled *Psychology, The Adaptive Mind*, Nairne, Smith, and Lindsay (2001) write: "Organisms notice sudden changes in the environment, but they learn to ignore them if they occur repeatedly. For an eating cat, a novel sound leads initially to panic and escape, but if the sound is repeated over days, the cat habituates and continues eating without the slightest reaction" (p. 225).

The authors explain that as adaptive organisms, humans rely on simple learning processes, such as habituation, to help conserve our limited resources. Human beings notice novelty, and when something new happens, we pay close attention. We produce an "orienting response," which involves an automatic shift of attention toward the new event. When writing this exam, you may experience an orienting response. You may pay attention to it with some anxiety because it is a novel or foreign experience.

In the presence of learning a new event, your behaviour will change and improve with repeated experience, which is a result of repetition learning. When you respond in the same way to an event that has become familiar through repeated presentation, you are demonstrating "habituation." Sensitization, however, occurs when responsiveness to an event increases with repeated exposure (Nairne, Smith, Lindsay, 2001).

Generally, whereas the effects of sensitization are short lived, the effects of habituation are short or long term (Domjan, 1998). Coping is defined as "efforts to manage or master conditions of threat or demand that tax one's resources" (Nairne, Smith, and Lindsay, 2001).

*The truth about exams is that we fear them because we don't get enough of them!* You may say this is absurd, but we adapt marvellously to situations to which we are repeatedly exposed. When we receive reinforcement, which occurs when we do well on an exam (even though we feared it in the first place), this strengthens our positive experience about exams, and we become less fearful of them in the future. If you have a few bad experiences with exams (e.g., through achieving poor scores), then it makes sense that you have become conditioned to avoid and resist the feared experience. The difficulty is that the more you avoid the feared stimulus, the worse the problem becomes because your fear overtakes you instead of you overtaking the fear.

*Prepare physically for the CRNE by balancing a healthy mind with a healthy body.* Your body needs physical exercise when you are taxing your brain, especially in preparation for an exam. Stress reduction works best when you have a physical release of tension.

### Dealing With Test Anxiety and Fear

The best antidote or remedy for a fear of any kind is to confront it and expose yourself to the feared object slowly, gradually, persistently, and repeatedly. After an aversive event or disaffirming experience, some adults withdraw from the aversive stimulus until they can find a reaffirming experience from the event (Cochrane, 1981). In other words, persons who have had disaffirming or negative experiences from writing tests are likely to withdraw from or avoid experiences that resemble the experience or event.

Most people will tell you that they would prefer *not* to write an exam, and it is often because of their negative associations with past experiences during exams. Negative appraisal is often the aversive or negative experience that occurs because of a poor test result. People tend to prefer events and experiences that positively reinforce or praise them. Because a low test score is not affirming, it contributes to a negative association with exams or tests in general.

Some of the most easily treated psychological problems are phobias and withdrawal from aversive experiences (Cochrane, 1981; Sakinofsky and Cochrane, 1986). One of the reasons for this is that when a person fears an object, person, or experience, the person tends to avoid or withdraw from the feared object (Crain, 2004). This prevents the person from confronting and dealing with it. *If a person manages to confront or face the feared object with a new experience, the fear often resolves and is changed into a different emotion.*

Classical conditioning shapes behaviour, and the strongest conditioning occurs when an intermittent reinforcement (negative or positive) is contingent on a specific behaviour (Wolfgang, 2002). A conditioned response occurs after a stimulus (in this case, a test) is administered over and over again with the same result (poor test score), and we may begin to fear tests as a consequence. However, when we pair the same stimulus (test) with a positive reinforcement (good test result), we begin to feel favourably toward it. Sometimes dysfunctional behaviour involves habituation to negative appraisal and negative reinforcement. In short, we become accustomed to whatever we are exposed to and what is reinforced over time. Likewise, if we have had bad experiences with testing and evaluation situations, we often expect these experiences to continue to be punitive or unfavourable; thus, past results tends to shape our perspective until we gain new experiences. If you practice the RN exam with increasingly positive results, you will gain confidence in your improved strategies and will apply these strategies to the real testing situation when you need them during the actual writing of the CRNE.

## Using Practice Exams to Reduce Test Anxiety

The reason we recommend completing the practice questions and taking the practice exams in this book is to condition your experiences and behaviour to constructive experiences of this activity through exposure to the questions, practice exams, and improved results. Gradual exposure is similar to successive approximations toward the goal. When you set the goal to excel in the CRNE, you must achieve it with practice, and you must experience positive results. Otherwise your situation would be like that of a person aspiring to become an Olympic gymnast without ever learning gymnastic techniques or practicing them! *Writing exams is a practiced activity, and your ability in writing multiple-choice exams improves with practice.*

As you finish the practice questions and practice exams, you will complete self-assessments of your test-taking strengths and weaknesses. In doing so, you will have been exposed to the exam "stimulus" and increased your knowledge of the process, in turn reducing your test anxiety.

You have already begun to condition yourself to manage your anxiety, and this is half the battle. The more you learn how to apply your knowledge to multiple-choice exams with good results, the more improvement in self-confidence you will have. *Self-confidence reduces anxiety.* Now that you have already reduced your test anxiety and increased your self-confidence, you are on the way to using other effective stress management techniques.

Some other techniques that work well are listed below. However, these techniques do not work as well as conditioning yourself by writing RN practice exams.

## Additional Strategies to Reduce Test Anxiety

1. Nurses teach pregnant women to use Lamaze breathing techniques to increase oxygen flow through the body and induce relaxation in the muscles. Similarly, you can learn to breathe slowly and deeply when you feel anxious. Become aware of your breathing as you are taking the two practice exams. Deep breathing increases oxygen flow to the brain and relaxes smooth muscle. When you are tense and anxious, the oxygen supply to your muscles is reduced, resulting in a feedback loop of increasing anxiety. *The best way to relax is to breathe deeply and get oxygen into circulation to your brain and muscles.*

2. Repeated exposure to the feared stimulus means that the more you practice answering RN exam questions, the less you will fear the RN exam and the more confidence you will have in successfully writing it. Then you can actually look forward to writing it!

3. Gaining insight and understanding about your past test and learning experiences will enable you to realize what has contributed to or caused your previous test reactions to be either positive or negative.

4. Reflecting on your learning experiences will enable you to gain new knowledge about yourself and your study habits, which can be applied to the CRNE.

5. Preparing yourself cognitively, physically, and emotionally to write the CRNE is a result of practicing the balance of all three of these activities in your preparation phase for writing the CRNE. If you balance your needs, you will be holistically prepared to do the best job. *If you attend to your cognitive needs (i.e., your need for knowledge) while ignoring your need for rest and exercise, your preparation will be in imbalance or disharmony.*

6. Studying with a partner or group assists you in reviewing and clarifying material, especially if you are unfamiliar with English language terms in nursing.

7. Use the performance appraisal tool from Chapter 2 to review your areas of weakness and focus on improving those areas in as much detail as you can before writing the RN exam.

8. Rewarding yourself for good study efforts and learning achievements is important in conditioning yourself to feel a sense of accomplishment and high self-esteem. Rewards are treats that you like, such as favourite foods or activities. All work and no play may eventually cause you to lack the motivation to go on. *Motivation is enhanced by rewarding yourself, so be sure to include rewards in your study schedule and write them in your learning log.*

## Learning Activity: Managing Test Anxiety

- Write down one of your worst and one of your best test experiences.
- List any fears you may have about writing the RN exam.
- Discuss how you can reduce your anxiety and concern about the RN exam.
- Explain what specifically affects your anxiety.
- Explore your methods for reducing anxiety about tests or any other stressful life events (e.g., taking a hot bath, watching a movie, going for a walk, jog, listening to favourite music, reading a book, seeing a friend, going out for dinner).
- Which of the above methods of stress management seems to work best for you? How do you know what works best?
- Identify how you can better manage your test anxiety now that you have reflected about it.

## SUMMARY

The better prepared you are for the CRNE, the better you will perform. This chapter has discussed the strategies and tools to help you be successful. If you are familiar with the exam format, you can prepare yourself with the knowledge base required. Exam anxiety, or lack of feeling confident about your knowledge base, strongly influences your success. We encourage you to use all the strategies, study components, and opportunities this book offers as you prepare for the CRNE.

## SUPPLEMENTAL RESOURCES

Bloom, B.S. (1956). *Taxonomy of educational objectives, handbook I: The cognitive domain.* New York: David McKay Co., Inc.

Canadian Nurses Association. (1999). *Blueprint for the Canadian Registered Nurse Examination.* Ottawa: Author.

Canadian Nurses Association. (2000). *The Canadian RN Exam prep guide.* Ottawa: Author.

Canadian Nurses Association. (2002). *Code of ethics for registered nurses.* Ottawa: Author.

Canadian Nurses Association. (2008). *Competencies.* Available at http://www.cna-nurses.ca/CNA/nursing/rnexam/competencies/default_e.aspx; accessed March 27, 2008.

Cochrane, N.J. (1981). *The meanings that some adults derive from their personal withdrawal experiences: A dialogical inquiry.* Toronto: University of Toronto.

Cochrane, N.J. (2006). Identifying high risk indicators for suicide using the problem solving inventory: A comparison of Aboriginal and non-Aboriginal populations. *The Monitor* v. 4 (August). Available at http://www.cnpr.ca; accessed March 27, 2008.

Cochrane, N., Ogen, K., Cochrane, K., & Caillier, L. (2006). Building community support for the prevention of youth suicide and personal injury: Response to the Youth Bridging Project Survey. *The Monitor* 3:1–25. Available at http://www.cnpr.ca; accessed March 27, 2008.

Carpenito-Moyet, L.J. (2006). *Understanding the nursing process: Concept mapping and care planning for students.* Philadelphia: Lippincott Williams & Wilkins.

Crain, W. (2004). *Theories of development: Concepts and applications* (5th ed.). Upper Saddle River: Pearson Education.

Domjan, M. (1998). *The principles of learning and behavior* (4th ed.). Pacific Grove, CA: Brooks/Cole.

Learning Skills Program (2006). *Bloom's taxonomy.* Victoria: University of Victoria.

Nairne, J.S., Smith, M.S., & Lindsay, D.S. (2001). *Psychology: The adaptive mind.* Scarborough, ON: Nelson Thomson Learning.

Sakinofsky, I., & Cochrane, N.J. (1986). A study of coping strategies in parasuicides and controls and a program designed to increase their social competence [abstract]. *Canada's Mental Health,* 34(3), 23.

Wolfgang, C. (2002). *Solving discipline and classroom management problems: Methods and models for today's teachers.* New York: John Wiley & Sons, Inc.

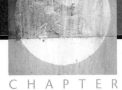

# Effective Use of *Lippincott's CRNE Prep Guide*

This chapter will help you use *Lippincott's CRNE Prep Guide* effectively and to its fullest capacity. The strategies discussed will help you understand how you perform within each Canadian Nurses Association (CNA) competency, domain of learning, and nursing specialty area. It also provides strategies for reviewing nursing content you are not as familiar with to help expand your nursing knowledge.

## USING *LIPPINCOTT'S CRNE PREP GUIDE*

1. This review book is not intended to teach you content; rather, it offers a way to test and analyze your knowledge base. *Lippincott's CRNE Prep Guide* should not replace a review of each specialty area. It will, however, provide you with a good understanding of what you know and which content areas you need to improve. To maximize the benefits of this guide, you need to start your exam preparation early.

2. Begin with one chapter and one practice specialty. Complete all of the study questions without looking up any content or answers. Write your answers on a separate sheet of paper rather than in the book so you can go back and repeat the exam if you think additional practice would be helpful. This will give you a realistic perspective on how well you know the content. If you guess at any questions, indicate it on the answer sheet so you can see how many you needed to guess at and how accurate your guesses were. After you have completed the practice questions, check your answers against the Answers and Rationales at the end of each chapter.

3. It is important to focus on how well you score within each competency area and domain of learning, not solely on your overall grade. As recommended in Chapter 1, look for patterns in how you perform. What strengths do you see? What areas do you have the most difficulty with? If you are not performing well or if you see patterns emerging, you should analyze why you are making these mistakes and identify strategies to help you address these issues.

4. If you determine that you need content review, study current Canadian textbooks. Although it is helpful to just look up the answers to questions you answered incorrectly, you need to have a good overall knowledge base in each specialty area. After you think you have had a thorough content review, you can return to the *Prep Guide* chapter and retake the questions to see if your knowledge has improved.

5. When reviewing your answers, carefully examine the rationales provided for the correct answers. Then return to all of your incorrect answer choices and consider why each of them was incorrect. Ask yourself why you chose the answer you did and think about how it differs from the correct answer. Using this strategy will help you "train your brain" to think critically about the answers and rationales.

6. It is also important to consider how you scored within each of the competency areas. If you are having difficulty with one competency more than others, take the time to review the CNA competencies on the CNA's web site at http://www.cna-nurses.ca/CNA/nursing/rnexam/competencies/default_e.aspx.

7. If you are having difficulty with the higher domains of learning, such as the application and critical thinking questions, you may

need to use additional case study review textbooks to help you develop skills in this area.

8. After you have completed each practice chapter in *Lippincott's CRNE Prep Guide,* set aside a full day to take both of the comprehensive practice exams in Chapter 8. After completing all of the questions, review each answer using the performance appraisal tool shown below. It will help you understand your overall score as well as how you performed in each competency and domain level. You can also use this template to assess your performance in each practice chapter.

## SUMMARY

This chapter has provided a comprehensive overview of *Lippincott's CRNE Prep Guide.* We encourage you to review this chapter before you begin working on the practice questions in Chapters 3 to 8 to ensure that you are using the text and your study time most effectively. The performance appraisal tools provided on pages 14 and 15 will help you assess the strengths and weaknesses in your knowledge base and areas where you require additional review. If you need more content review, choose a resource from the comprehensive bibliography at the end of each chapter. We wish you successful studying!

## PERFORMANCE APPRAISAL TOOL FOR *LIPPINCOTT'S CRNE PREP GUIDE*

This book provides an opportunity to assess your performance in all the practice specialty areas (i.e., adult and older adult, maternal–child, pediatric, and mental health) and to assess your ability to answer questions within each of the nursing competency areas and domains of learning. The following example demonstrates how to use the performance appraisal tool. This tool should be used as you work through the *Prep Guide*. A blank one is provided on page 15 and on the CD-ROM that accompanies this book.

### Using the Performance Appraisal Tool

- Count and record the total number of questions for each competency category on the grid. For example, if the review chapter has 26 questions with the competency category of Professional Practice, write this number in the "No. of questions" box.

- Count and record the number of competency questions you answered incorrectly. If you had six incorrect answers, write "6" in the "No. of Incorrect Answers" box.
- Calculate your score by subtracting the number of incorrect answers from the total number of questions (e.g., 26 − 6 = 20).
- Calculate the percentage of your correct answers (e.g., 20 ÷ 26 = 0.076 = 76%).
- Record your total percentage score for that category.
- Follow this procedure for each category.
- Calculate your overall exam score on both the multiple-choice and short answer questions and record your findings.
- Count and calculate your scores within the three domains of learning.
- Compare all of the scores to gain an understanding of your areas of strength as well as the areas in which you need to improve.

### PERFORMANCE APPRAISAL TOOL—COMPETENCY CATEGORIES

| COMPETENCY | NO. OF QUESTIONS | NO. OF INCORRECT ANSWERS | CALCULATED % | TOTAL SCORE |
|---|---|---|---|---|
| **Professional Practice** | 26 | 6 | 26 − 6= 20<br>20 ÷ 26 = 76% | 76% |
| **Nurse–Person Relationship** | | | | |
| **Nursing Practice: Health and Wellness** | | | | |
| **Nursing Practice: Alterations in Health** | | | | |
| **Total number of questions in chapter or in comprehensive practice exam** | 200 multiple choice<br>50 short answer | 20<br>6 | 200 − 20 = 180<br>180 ÷ 200 = .9<br>50 − 6 = 44<br>44 ÷ 50 = .88 | 90% on multiple choice<br>88% on short answer |

### PERFORMANCE APPRAISAL TOOL—DOMAINS OF LEARNING

| COMPETENCY | NO. OF QUESTIONS | NO. OF INCORRECT ANSWERS | CALCULATED % | TOTAL SCORE |
|---|---|---|---|---|
| **Knowledge/Comprehension** | | | | |
| **Application** | | | | |
| **Critical Thinking** | | | | |

## Instructions

- Count and record the total number of questions for each competency category on the grid.
- Count and record the number of competency questions you answered incorrectly.
- Calculate your score for each category.
- Calculate and record your total percentage of correct answers for each category.
- Calculate and record your overall exam score on both the multiple-choice and short answer questions.
- Count and calculate your scores within the three domains of learning.
- Compare all of your scores to gain an understanding of your areas of strength as well as the areas in which you need to improve.

| PERFORMANCE APPRAISAL TOOL—COMPETENCY CATEGORIES | | | | |
|---|---|---|---|---|
| COMPETENCY | NO. OF QUESTIONS | NO. OF INCORRECT ANSWERS | CALCULATED % | TOTAL SCORE |
| **Professional Practice** | | | | |
| **Nurse–Person Relationship** | | | | |
| **Nursing Practice: Health and Wellness** | | | | |
| **Nursing Practice: Alterations in Health** | | | | |
| **Total number of questions in chapter or in comprehensive practice exam** | | | | |

| PERFORMANCE APPRAISAL TOOL—DOMAINS OF LEARNING | | | | |
|---|---|---|---|---|
| COMPETENCY | NO. OF QUESTIONS | NO. OF INCORRECT ANSWERS | CALCULATED % | TOTAL SCORE |
| **Knowledge/ Comprehension** | | | | |
| **Application** | | | | |
| **Critical Thinking** | | | | |

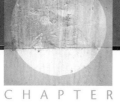

# 3 Professional Practice

**Directions:** Below are 200 multiple-choice and short answer questions totalling 261 points. These questions will test your knowledge of professional practice. These questions offer a wide array of case-based and stand-alone questions representing critical thinking, application, and knowledge/comprehension taxonomies. Also reflected in these questions are various nursing practice competencies. After completing these multiple-choice and short answer questions, compare your work with the Answers and Rationales provided at the end of the chapter. Please make note of the questions you found difficult and develop a plan to help increase your knowledge of these areas.

## ▶ Multiple-Choice Questions

1. A nurse tells a client that she will come back to assess the client's pain in 10 minutes. When the nurse returns in 10 minutes, which aspect of the therapeutic relationship is the nurse developing?

   A. Empathy.
   B. Sympathy.
   C. Trust.
   D. Closure.

2. An individual has been advised to stop smoking. Which of the following statements by the nurse is considered therapeutic?

   A. "I know how you feel; I had to stop smoking when I was pregnant."
   B. "Stopping 'cold turkey' will give you the best chance for success."
   C. "I can offer you some information outlining a variety of ways to stop smoking."
   D. "The most effective way to stop smoking is the nicotine patch; let me ask the doctor to order it for you."

3. A nurse is working in an occupational health clinic within a manufacturing company. When asked by the human resources manager for the names of employees who visited the nurse in the past 24 hours, the nurse should do which of the following?

   A. Refer the human resources manager to the occupational health manager.
   B. Refuse and remind the manager that he or she is bound by confidentiality.
   C. Give the names to the manager because he is the nurse's superior.
   D. Provide the names because this is a normal practice for this organization.

---

*Case Study:* Jessica Smith is 20 years old and has been diagnosed with depression. She is admitted to the mental health unit, where she is encouraged to participate in group sessions. Questions 4 to 6 relate to this scenario.

4. John Stewart, RN, is assigned to work with Jessica. Jessica asks John if he is married or has a girlfriend. John responds by saying, "I am curious what made you ask this question; however, what is important is how you are feeling today." John's response would be considered which of the following?

   A. Inappropriate because Jessica was just interested in John's personal situation.
   B. Inappropriate because John should have answered to establish a therapeutic relationship.
   C. Appropriate because John is neither married nor has a girlfriend.
   D. Appropriate because the focus of a therapeutic relationship is on the client.

5. During the night shift, Jessica tells a nurse that she is going to kill herself, and she is placed on

constant observation. When she asks to use the toilet, the nurse follows her into the bathroom. Jessica says, "I don't need you to follow me into the bathroom. Give me some space." Which of the following statements by the nurse would be considered the most appropriate?

A. "You are right. I don't need to come into the bathroom with you. I will wait outside the door."

B. "I must stay with you until we are sure you are not going to hurt yourself."

C. "If you think you are going to be alright, I will check on you in 5 minutes."

D. "I can't imagine there is anything dangerous in the bathroom, so go ahead, and I will wait for you in the hallway."

6. Jessica is ready to be discharged and tells the nurse, "It would be really good for me if we could meet for coffee if I am feeling depressed again." Which of the following statements indicates that the nurse understands the boundaries of the therapeutic relationship?

A. "That would be okay as long as we go to a public place. Where would you like to meet?"

B. "Before you leave the hospital, I will make sure you have the information about the crisis centre."

C. "We could go to the gym together. Exercise can be very therapeutic for patients experiencing depression."

D. "I often meet with people after they are discharged. Sometimes it is difficult to deal with situations after you leave the hospital."

7. Carol is an RN working an evening shift on an intake unit of a long-term care facility. She must ask one of the unregulated health care workers (UHCWs) to perform a treatment on a resident. What must the RN ensure before delegating a task to a UHCW?

A. The worker has the appropriate knowledge and skills.

B. The worker has practiced the task previously.

C. The worker is supervised during the performance of the task.

D. The worker will be guided through the task by another nurse.

8. Angela, an RN, overhears another RN, Carol, making plans to meet a hospitalized client "for a drink" after the client has been discharged. What should Angela do?

A. Tell the client that he should not meet the nurse socially.

B. Report the conversation to the nurse manager of your unit.

C. Encourage interaction with the client after discharge.

D. Discuss the overheard conversation directly with Carol.

9. Professional regulations and laws that govern nursing practice are in place for which of the following reasons?

A. To limit the number of nurses in practice.

B. To ensure that nurses are in good moral standing.

C. To protect the safety of the public.

D. To ensure that enough new nurses are available.

10. After the death of a patient, the nurse needs to shroud the body. Which of the following reflects the most appropriate time to do this?

A. Before the family enters the room and sees the body.

B. After the family has had time with the body.

C. After the body has been transferred to the morgue.

D. As quickly as possible to accommodate the next admission.

11. A nurse offers to gather a basin of warm water for Mrs. Jones' morning wash. Mrs. Jones refuses and states that she usually prefers to shower in the evening. Which of the following is the nurse's best response?

A. "I will make sure this is noted on your chart to alert the evening staff."

B. "It is hospital policy that all patients bathe in the morning."

C. "It is unlikely that the nurses will have time to help you shower tonight."

D. "I am sure you will feel better if you have a bath now."

12. A nurse enters information on a client's chart but then realizes that a mistake has been made. The appropriate steps in correcting the entry error would be which of the following?

A. Use correction fluid to cover the mistake and write the correct information over top.

B. Erase the entry and write the correct information in the appropriate place.

C. Blacken out the entry with a marker and add the correct data after it.

D. Draw a line through the incorrect entry, date and initial it, and follow it with the correct data.

13. A nurse is caring for a client who refuses further palliative surgery. The nurse understands which of the following?
    A. The client has a right to make this choice about his or her treatment.
    B. The family should be encouraged to make the decision for the client.
    C. The nurse should discuss with the client why the surgery is necessary.
    D. The physician should make this decision on behalf of the client.

14. A nurse is working in a community clinic and is required to administer a medication to a patient. The nurse is not familiar with the medication because she has never administered it before. What is the best step for the nurse to take before giving this medication to the patient?
    A. Administer the medication.
    B. Ask the other nurse in the clinic for some information about the drug.
    C. Consult the Compendium of Pharmaceuticals and Specialties (CPS) or another credible pharmacology resource.
    D. Ask another nurse to administer the medication.

15. An RN is working in the "float pool" at a local hospital. The nurse is assigned to the surgical unit and is assigned to look after an individual with a gastrostomy tube in place. The nurse has not administered medication into a gastrostomy tube before. What should the nurse do?
    A. Refuse the assignment of caring for this individual.
    B. Contact the nurse educator for an inservice and support.
    C. Ask another nurse to administer the medication for this shift.
    D. Give the medication by mouth to avoid using the tube.

16. Abby Jones, RN, has been reviewing research focusing on the benefits of hand washing in preventing the spread of microorganisms. Abby also observes a number of health care workers who are not washing their hands between patient contact. Abby wants to initiate a change in practice. Which of the following should she do?
    A. Develop a poster and pamphlet to be used at the sinks on each unit to promote hand washing.
    B. Report the lack of hand washing to the local Medical Officer of Health for further follow-up.

C. Have a discussion about hand washing with fellow nurses during the morning coffee break.
D. Monitor to ensure that all staff consistently wash their hands between each patient contact.

*Case Study:* *The nurse manager on a surgical unit is holding a meeting with the nursing team to discuss management's decision to reduce staffing on the unit. During the discussion, one of the staff nurses stands up and yells at the nurse manager, using profanity and threatening "to take this decision further." Questions 17 to 19 relate to this scenario.*

17. To defuse this situation, which of the following would be the best step for the nurse manager to take?
    A. Tell the nurse that she is suspended for her behaviour.
    B. Call a break in the meeting and talk to the nurse privately.
    C. Ask the rest of the staff if they are also feeling the same way.
    D. Try to defuse the situation by telling the nurse to act professionally.

18. The nurse manager speaks to the nurse privately in her office. The nurse is still speaking to the manager with a raised voice. The manager realizes she must set some limits on this nurse's behaviour. Which of the following statements would indicate that the manager can effectively set limits?
    A. "Settle down or I will call someone in and take you out of the office."
    B. "Start acting professionally or things will be a lot worse for you."
    C. "That is enough or I will have you escorted out of the building."
    D. "Please lower your voice or you will not be able to return to the meeting."

19. The nurse manager knows that setting limits on unacceptable behaviour should include consequences that are appropriate, enforceable, and which of the following?
    A. Consistent.
    B. Courteous.
    C. Concurrent.
    D. Consensual.

20. Emily and Irene are both RNs working the night shift on a medical unit. Emily completes her initial shift assessment on the patients assigned to

her care. An hour later, Irene finds Emily asleep in the lounge. Emily remains asleep for the next 4 hours and then wakes up to do her patient rounds. What should Irene do in this situation?

A. Cover for Emily by assessing her patients on an hourly basis.
B. Nothing; Emily's patients were asleep and did not call for assistance.
C. Discuss the situation with Emily, including the safety implications of her sleeping.
D. Ask the nurse on the day shift to report the situation to the nurse manager.

21. Andrew, an RN, is employed by a community nursing service and is scheduled for a daily visit to Mr. H. for a blood pressure check. Andrew is very busy and is running late, so he decides to skip the visit to Mr. H. He bases this decision on the rationale that the patient's blood pressure was normal the previous day. Which of the following best describes Andrew's decision?

A. Inappropriate because it would be considered neglect of duty.
B. Appropriate because it would be considered a knowledgeable assessment of the client's situation.
C. Inappropriate because it would be considered client abuse.
D. Appropriate because it would be considered effective prioritizing of his workload for the day.

22. Sylvia, RN, and Ralph, RPN (Registered Practical Nurse), are team nursing on a surgical unit. While Ralph is on supper break, Sylvia is called by one of his patients. The patient is complaining of incisional pain that is rated as 8 out of 10 on the pain scale. Sylvia checks the client's chart and notes that Ralph recorded giving the client morphine 1 hour earlier. This same scenario has occurred four times over the past three shifts that Sylvia has worked with Ralph. What should Sylvia do first in this situation?

A. Report the situation to the immediate supervisor.
B. Check the records of other patients Ralph has looked after.
C. Wait and see if it happens again.
D. Notify the provincial regulating body for RPNs.

23. Roger is an RN working in the emergency department. As per hospital policy, all staff members in the department are encouraged to wear uniforms provided by the hospital, which are referred to as "greens." Roger is often addressed by patients as "doctor." Roger does not correct this misperception. What should Roger's response be to being called "doctor" by the patients?

A. Nothing; he still provides excellent nursing care.
B. Nothing; patients just get confused when they see different caregivers.
C. He should wear a name tag to correct the misperception.
D. He should ask the patients to refer to him as Roger.

24. When assessing if a procedural risk to a client is justified, the ethical principle underlying the dilemma is known as which of the following?

A. Nonmaleficence.
B. Informed consent.
C. Self-determination.
D. Pro-choice.

25. Two nurses are talking about a specific client in the hospital cafeteria. These nurses are at risk of being accused of all of the following *except*:

A. Breach of confidentiality.
B. Gross incompetence.
C. Professional misconduct.
D. Behaviour unbecoming of the profession.

26. On a busy evening shift, the nurse manager of the trauma unit is short staffed and must triage between two people involved in a motor vehicle accident. One is a young mother, and the other is the driver, who was reportedly drunk and hit the other patient. Which of the following is an accurate reflection of this scenario?

A. The driver should be treated first to confirm intoxication.
B. Drunk drivers who cause an accident should wait until the people they hurt are treated.
C. The nurse must treat each client equally without prejudice.
D. The woman was not drinking, so she should be treated first.

27. A visitor who is visiting her husband on your nursing unit asks the nurse about another patient on the unit, who happens to be her friend. The visitor states that she saw this patient's name on the computer screen that another nurse was using at the desk. What should you do?

A. Tell the visitor that the friend is a patient on the unit but do not disclose any further information.

B. Discuss the matter with the other nurse, reminding him or her not to leave client information in view of visitors.

C. Tell the visitor that she should not read information that is confidential and then notify security.

D. Ask the friend to come to the client's room to meet with the wife after you are finished administering medications.

28. A nurse's niece is unexpectedly admitted to the pediatric unit of the hospital where the nurse works. The nurse is working in the emergency department and accesses her niece's computer chart. When telling a coworker what she is doing, the coworker's best response would be?

A. "That is very caring of you to follow up on your niece's treatment."

B. "Did you realize that accessing her chart is a breach of confidentiality?"

C. "I have a pediatric background; I can tell you more about her diagnosis."

D. "I would be interested in hearing how her treatment progresses because her condition is unique."

29. Cameron has been admitted to the intensive care unit after decompression of a cervical fracture. The nurses are concerned that as Cameron begins to wake up, he may try to pull out his endotracheal tube. The nurses decide to apply wrist restraints to Cameron's hands until he is alert and the tube is removed. What must the nurses do before applying the wrist restraints?

A. Obtain consent from Cameron's next of kin.

B. Nothing; this is a nursing decision.

C. Try using elbow restraints because they are more effective.

D. Discuss the decision with the physiotherapist.

30. Mrs. Brown is living in a long-term care facility. Over the past few weeks, she has become increasingly unsteady on her feet. The nurses are worried that Mrs. Brown is going to climb out of bed and fall. Which of the following DO NOT comply with a least restraint policy?

A. Placing Mrs. Brown in a bed with a bed alarm.

B. Providing a bed that is low to the floor.

C. Raising one bed rail to offer stabilization when standing.

D. Raising all side rails while Mrs. Brown is in bed.

31. John, RN, is a visiting home nurse. He has been asked to transfer the care of his client with a tracheotomy to an unregulated health care worker (UHCW). What should John do before transferring the care?

A. Ensure that the UHCW has the knowledge to care for the client.

B. Nothing; the UHCW should know what to do.

C. Ask the client if he or she is comfortable with the transfer of care to the UHCW.

D. Contact the physician and clarify the orders written for this client.

32. An RN working nights with another nurse notices that the other nurse is charting vital signs that she did not actually take on her patients. What should the nurse observing this situation do first?

A. Discuss the observations with the other nurse.

B. Nothing; it is not her place to report this behaviour

C. Notify the union steward representing the nursing employees.

D. Obtain the patients' vital signs for the other nurse.

---

***Case Study:*** *Mr. Edwards lives in a long-term care facility and has signed a form stating that he does not want to be resuscitated. During the winter, he develops an upper respiratory infection that progresses to pneumonia. His health has rapidly deteriorated, and he is no longer competent. His family states that they want everything possible done for Mr. Edwards. Questions 33 and 34 relate to this scenario.*

33. Which of the following should happen in this case?

A. The patient should be resuscitated if he has a respiratory arrest.

B. The patient should be treated with antibiotics for his pneumonia.

C. The wishes of his family should be followed.

D. Pharmacologic intervention should not be initiated.

34. On morning rounds, the nurse finds Mr. Edwards without vital signs. What should the nurse do?

A. Notify the physician that the patient has no vital signs.

B. Begin CPR and call for an ambulance.

C. Call the supervisor for further directions.

D. Go to the desk and review the patient's chart to determine his resuscitation status.

35. An RN gives a client 0.25 mg of digoxin instead of the prescribed dose of 0.125 mg. What should she do?

A. Give the other 0.125 mg as soon as possible.

B. Nothing; the dose will not make a significant difference.

C. Assess the patient and notify the doctor.

D. Hold the next dose to make sure the amount balances.

36. An RN conducting her first shift assessment notes that the patient has D5W hanging in the IV bag instead of 0.9% saline, which was ordered by the physician. What should the RN do first?

A. Slow the D5W to KVO (keep vein open) and call the physician.

B. Remove the D5W and hang 0.9% saline only.

C. Leave the D5W running because it is similar to 0.9% saline.

D. Report error to physician and clarify IV solution ordered.

37. Mr. Ralph has been prescribed a narcotic analgesic to be given around the clock for his cancer-related pain. He is competent and has actively been involved in decisions regarding his care. What should the nurse do when Mr. Ralph refuses his next dose?

A. Try to persuade him to take the medication as ordered by the doctor.

B. Ensure that he understands the rationale for taking the medication as ordered.

C. Ask his wife to hold his hands while you put the pill under his tongue.

D. Document his choice and reassess his pain in 1 hour.

38. Mr. Green is discharged after a brief stay on the surgical unit. He hands his nurse a box of chocolates and says, "These are for you." Which statement demonstrates the nurse's understanding of accepting gifts from a client?

A. "Thank you. I will enjoy these with my husband when I get home."

B. "Thank you. I will take them to the lounge to share with all the staff."

C. "Although I would enjoy them, I cannot accept any gifts from patients."

D. "We ask our client for cookies rather than chocolates because they last longer."

39. A nurse working on a medical floor observes another nurse crushing her patient's pills and mixing them in food that is going to be fed to her patient by a nursing student. What should the nurse do?

A. Congratulate the nurse for being so innovative in medication administration.

B. Discuss with the nurse that she needs to observe her patients taking their medications.

C. Discuss with the student that he should be signing for the medications given.

D. Nothing; this is routine practice for patients who have difficulty swallowing pills.

40. A 70-year-old man is admitted unconscious to the emergency department with a ruptured abdominal aortic aneurysm. No family members are present, and the surgeon instructs the staff to take the client directly to the operating room for life saving surgery. Which of the following actions should the nurse take regarding informed consent?

A. Take the client to the operating room for surgery without informed consent.

B. Keep the patient in the emergency department until the family is contacted.

C. Call the nursing supervisor and ask that the hospital lawyer be contacted.

D. Contact the hospital chaplain so he can sign the consent on the client's behalf.

41. The doctor orders a medication for which the patient is allergic. The nurse places a call to the physician, but the call is not returned before the first dose is due. Which of the following is the appropriate next step the nurse should take in this situation?

A. Notify the nursing supervisor of the situation.

B. Give the medication as ordered by the doctor.

C. Hold the medication and wait to speak to the physician.

D. Call the pharmacist and discuss the patient's allergies.

42. The RN team leader observes a nurse administering a dose of dimenhydrinate (Gravol) IM to another nurse. The medication is stocked on the medication cart. What is the team leader's best first response to this situation?

A. Notify the nurse manager of their observation.

B. Nothing; dimenhydrinate is a stock medication.

C. Approach the nurses individually before going to the manager.

D. Suggest they self-administer dimenhydrinate when feeling nauseated.

43. Roger is a nurse working on a surgical unit and is stuck with a used hypodermic needle while he is walking to the sharps container located in the medication room. This unit has a higher incidence of needlestick injuries than other units

within the agency. Which of the following actions by the nursing manager would demonstrate advocacy for a quality practice environment?

A. Have a meeting with staff to see how they can improve on methods to decrease needlestick injuries.
B. Have an inservice and demonstrate how to use retractable needles.
C. Conduct thorough tracking and verbally reprimanding nurses who have experienced needlestick injuries.
D. Instituting a "zero tolerance" policy regarding needlestick injuries.

---

**Case Study:** *Angela, a Public Health Nurse, is asked to create a teaching tool that focuses on diabetes management for clients who often eat meals outside of the home in restaurants. Questions 44 to 46 relate to this scenario.*

44. Angela understands that before clients can learn, they must believe that they need to learn the information. This is an example of which learning principle?

A. Maturation.
B. Relevance.
C. Initiative.
D. Motivation.

45. Angela is concerned about a client's ability to retain the information she is presenting. Which of the following techniques would enhance the retention of the material in the presentation?

A. Including a bibliography.
B. Using a lecture format.
C. Speaking very softly.
D. Using repetition.

46. Angela invites a group of diabetic clients to her workshop and realizes that the majority of participants are visual learners. Based on this assessment, Angela should use which of the following teaching techniques or tools to best assist this group of learners?

A. Handouts.
B. Lectures.
C. Discussion groups.
D. Question and answer time.

47. Monica, a nurse educator, is speaking to a group of nursing students about effective communication techniques. Which of the following would Monica state is the goal of therapeutic communication?

A. Obtaining information, developing trust, and showing caring.
B. Giving advice, data collecting, and developing a communication style.
C. Self-disclosure, sympathy, and obtaining information.
D. Validation, sympathy, and developing trust.

48. Margaret, the nursing team leader, overhears comments made between two nurses. Gilles, an RN, repeatedly makes remarks that are focused on Stephen's skin color and race. Stephen is observably offended. Which of the following actions by Margaret would demonstrate an understanding of promoting a quality practice environment?

A. Speak to Gilles directly, pointing out that he is harassing Stephen and that it will not be tolerated.
B. In Gilles' mailbox, leave a pamphlet that addresses how to deal with harassment and discrimination.
C. Seek out some posters for the unit that reflect racial diversity and post them at a time when Stephen is not working.
D. Nothing; Stephen must submit a formal complaint to the human rights department before anything will be done.

49. An RN on a surgical unit learns that a group of nursing students will be coming on the unit for 7 weeks with an instructor. The nurse tells the manager that she "wants nothing to do with those students" and tells the manager not to assign a student to her patients. Which of the following is the most appropriate response by the manager to this request?

A. "I understand how time consuming it can be to have a student. I will ask someone else."
B. "The choice is yours. You are under no obligation to work with nursing students."
C. "Most nurses like working with students. I thought you would like to as well"
D. "As a nurse, you have a professional obligation to share your knowledge with students."

50. Linda is a staff nurse who suspects that one of her coworkers is self-administering illegal drugs during work hours. Which of the following is Linda's first priority action?

A. Notify the nurse manager and document the situation.
B. Determine if this is a breach of hospital policy.
C. Report the nurse to the provincial or territorial governing body.
D. Discuss the concerns with one of the doctors.

**51.** A client admitted to the mental health unit has exhibited physical behaviours that put him and others at risk. The nurse applies four-point restraints on the client without obtaining a physician's order or consent. The nurse is at risk of being accused of which of the following?

A. False imprisonment.
B. Negligence.
C. Battery.
D. Malpractice.

**52.** A nurse is caring for a client with a fresh postoperative wound after a femoral–popliteal revascularization procedure. The nurse fails to routinely assess the pedal pulses on the affected leg, and the blood vessel becomes occluded. The nurse is at risk for being accused of which of the following?

A. Malpractice.
B. Negligence.
C. Refusal of treatment.
D. Forgetfulness.

**53.** A nurse is working in the postanesthesia care unit (PACU) when a patient's airway becomes obstructed. The anesthetist is not immediately accessible, so the nurse reintubates the patient with an endotracheal tube and causes trauma to the vocal cords. The nurse is at risk of being accused of which of the following?

A. Malpractice.
B. Negligence.
C. Invasion of privacy.
D. Taking initiative.

**54.** A patient on a surgical unit asks the nurse her opinion of her surgeon. The nurse replies, "He is a rude man, and his patients always end up with infections." The nurse is at risk of being accused of which of the following?

A. Libel.
B. Slander.
C. Negligence.
D. Assault.

**55.** A nurse on a medical unit charts in the patient's medical records that the "doctor was tardy and negligent in his follow-up care" related to the care of his patient. The nurse is at risk of being accused of which of the following?

A. Negligence.
B. Slander.
C. Ignorance.
D. Libel.

**56.** A nurse reports to a physician that the client receiving a blood transfusion has a temperature that is 1°C greater than his baseline and is complaining of a headache. The doctor states to continue the blood infusion. By following the order, the nurse is at risk of being accused of which of the following?

A. Negligence.
B. Assault.
C. Unethical conduct.
D. Malpractice.

**57.** During a clinical experience, the preceptor needs to provide students with feedback on their performance. The nurse knows that all of the following are effective qualities of providing feedback *except*:

A. The feedback is immediate.
B. The feedback is frequent.
C. The feedback is specific.
D. The feedback is provided in front of the client.

**58.** A nurse tells her client that if he does not behave, she is going to give him an injection "with the biggest, dullest needle she can find." The nurse has committed which of the following?

A. Assault.
B. Battery.
C. Insult.
D. Confinement.

**59.** A nurse gets frustrated with the behaviour of a client who is acting out. The nurse slaps the client in an effort to control the client's behaviour. The nurse has committed which of the following?

A. Assault.
B. Battery.
C. Negligence.
D. Abandonment.

**60.** A nurse educator is preparing a workshop regarding cultural influences on health care. The session begins with a definition of "culture." Which of the following should be included in the definition?

A. Culture is a shared system of beliefs, values, and behaviours.
B. Culture is the common understanding of a community.
C. Culture is based on the physical characteristics of the environment.
D. Culture is based on the majority of the dominant religious beliefs.

**61.** Abigail, a nurse in a public health unit, does not smoke, drinks no more than 2 alcoholic beverages per day, and exercises three times a week. How does Abigail's lifestyle promote a healthy lifestyle in others?

   A. Abigail is a role model for healthy lifestyle choices.
   B. Abigail is not wasting health care resources.
   C. Abigail is not accessing her benefit plan at work.
   D. Abigail is not infecting others with an illness.

**62.** Amy, a new home care nurse, asks the nurse manager how frequently she should chart on each client. The manager answers correctly when she states which of the following?

   A. "Only if you provide treatment."
   B. "After each client visit."
   C. "Once a week."
   D. "On the first and the last visit."

**63.** Which of the following would not be a characteristic of patient advocacy?

   A. Believing "the patient comes first."
   B. Promoting the patient's rights and interests.
   C. Providing paternalistic care.
   D. Protecting the interests and rights of the patient.

**64.** Because of staffing shortages, Gary, a nurse from the surgical unit, is asked to work on the pediatric unit. Gary has not worked in a pediatric unit for 10 years. He is not familiar with the pediatric unit in this particular hospital and approaches the nurse manager, telling her that he does not feel competent to work on this unit. What should the nursing manager do?

   A. Find another nurse to cover this unit and send the nurse back to the surgery unit.
   B. Tell the nurse to buddy up with someone else and do the best he can.
   C. Tell the nurse that as an RN, he should be competent to work in any area.
   D. Give the nurse the lightest workload.

**65.** The nursing manager asks one of the RNs to be a preceptor for a new staff member. Which of the following statements by the RN requires follow-up and role clarification by the nurse manager?

   A. "I would benefit from that; it is part of my learning plan for this year."
   B. "I have 4 weeks of vacation starting next week; could you ask another RN?"
   C. "No, but thanks for asking. I don't like being a preceptor."

   D. "Certainly; it is part of my responsibility as an RN."

**66.** James is 16 years old and has been treated for leukemia since he was 8 years old. He is in the hospital and requires chemotherapy. His parents support the physician's recommendation, but James is refusing the treatment. What is the nurse's role in this situation?

   A. Advise James that he should take the treatment because his physician knows best.
   B. Advise James that if his parents agree with the treatment plan, their consent will be honored.
   C. Act as an advocate for James and request that the physician thoroughly explain the benefits and consequences of treatment.
   D. Support James' parents and give advice as to the best method of convincing James to take the treatment.

**67.** Theresa, a nurse educator in the blood conservation nurse program, has discussed with her client that treatment with iron supplements and Eprex will be of equal benefit to treat the client's decrease in hemoglobin as a unit of packed cells would be but without the potential side effects. Linda, a nurse caring for the client, also discusses the treatment with the client. Which of the following statements by Linda should be explored further from a professional or ethical prospective?

   A. "I would take the unit of blood if I were you. It will help you feel better."
   B. "Do you think you have all the answers you need to give informed consent?"
   C. "Have you had an opportunity to ask all the questions you have?"
   D. "Tell me in your own words how the nurse educator explained the procedure."

**68.** A nurse working in the operating room is assigned to the suite where therapeutic abortions are to be performed throughout the day. The nurse believes that she cannot participate in these procedures because it is against her religious beliefs. What should she do after she notifies the operating room supervisor?

   A. Continue working in the suite because it is where she was assigned for the shift.
   B. Complete a work refusal form and leave the surgical suite immediately.
   C. Contact the local right to life association and inform them of the procedures.
   D. Remain in the operating room suite until another nurse arrives to relieve her.

**69.** Michelle is a public health nurse responsible for contact tracing of individuals identified in confirmed cases of sexually transmitted infections. Michelle telephones an individual named by an infected client. The caller demands to be told the name of the person who identified him as a contact. Which of the following is the appropriate response from Michelle?

    A. "Just as I will protect your privacy, I must protect the privacy of the other people involved."

    B. "If you tell me the name of the person you have had sex with, I will tell you if it is the same person who identified you."

    C. "I can only disclose the name if you consent to treatment."

    D. "The individual who named you asked for anonymity or confidentiality."

**70.** The nurse manager of a federally regulated health care agency is interviewing candidates for a full-time nurse position. Which of the following questions would be considered a violation of the Canadian Human Rights Act?

    A. "Can you tell me where you went to college or university?"

    B. "Where have you worked within a team setting?"

    C. "How do you deal with conflict?"

    D. "Do you have a physical disability?"

**71.** Patricia, a nurse within the public health unit, applies for a position in another department. The manager screens the applications and does not interview Patricia. Which of the following are legitimate grounds for not interviewing Patricia?

    A. She is currently pregnant and will soon be going on maternity leave.

    B. She is in a same-sex partnership, and this position is in the sexual health clinic.

    C. She requires a workplace accommodation because she uses a wheelchair.

    D. She does not have the credentials required of the position.

**72.** Kathryn, a 16-year-old young woman, approaches a nurse and discloses that she is pregnant. Kathryn asks the nurse how she can obtain a therapeutic abortion. The nurse responds by stating, "You can't do that. It is immoral, and you will regret that decision for the rest of your life." The nurse is demonstrating which the following?

    A. Client-focused care.

    B. Leadership.

    C. Abuse.

    D. Advocacy.

**73.** Mr. Brown uses a wheelchair because of mobility limitations. On one occasion, he is unable to call the nurse to assist him to the toilet. He urinates in his wheelchair. His nurse scolds him in front of other residents for his "accident." The nurse has demonstrated which of the following?

    A. Verbal abuse.

    B. Incompetence.

    C. Reinforcement.

    D. Negligence.

**74.** John is a resident in a long-term care facility. He is scheduled to have his bath, and the nurse takes him to the tub room. He states he does not want a bath, but the nurse begins to undress him and restrains his arms to get him into the tub. The nurse is guilty of which of the following?

    A. Emotional abuse.

    B. Physical abuse.

    C. Neglect.

    D. Frustration.

---

***Case Study:*** *The school nurse is discussing healthy eating strategies with a group of 8-year-old students. One student repeatedly makes comments of a sexual nature. The student seems to be preoccupied with sexual comments and is knowledgeable regarding a variety of sexual activities. Questions 75 and 76 relate to this scenario.*

**75.** What might this behaviour indicate to the nurse?

    A. The student is age appropriate.

    B. The student may have been sexually abused.

    C. The student has seen a movie with sexual content.

    D. The student is mimicking a younger sibling.

**76.** What is the nurse's best response to this observation?

    A. Notify local Child Protective Services.

    B. Nothing; this is normal for the child's age.

    C. Advise the parents to monitor what the child is watching.

    D. Advise the student not to copy his or her sibling.

**77.** A client is admitted to the mental health unit in the manic phase of bipolar disorder. He refuses to take his medication. What would be the most appropriate action by the nurse?

    A. Call security to assist with administering the medication.

    B. Ask the patient why he doesn't want to take the medication.

C. Put the medication in the client's coffee.

D. Administer the medication by the parenteral route to ensure that it is taken.

78. After the discharge of a client from a surgical unit, the housekeeper brings a blue pill to the nurse. This pill was found in the sheets when the linens were removed from the client's bed. The nurse reviews the client's medication administration record, which shows that the client received this medication at 0800 hrs. What would be the nurse's priority action?

A. Complete an incident form and notify the doctor.

B. Don't do anything because the patient was discharged.

C. Tell the housekeeper not to worry if this happens in the future.

D. Advise the housekeeper to throw the pill in the garbage

79. Maureen, a nurse working on a medical unit, is caring for Sally, a client with anemia. Maureen has a part-time business selling vitamins and supplements and approaches Sally offering to sell her vitamins to help "improve her blood." When another nurse overhears this conversation, he should discuss which of the following with Maureen?

A. How he can also start selling the vitamins and supplements.

B. How impressed he is with the initiative Maureen has taken.

C. That Maureen has a conflict of interest.

D. The cost of the supplements she is selling.

80. An elderly client asks her long-time nurse to become her power of attorney. What should the nurse say in response to this request?

A. "I cannot do this, but I can help you get in contact with a lawyer."

B. "Thank you. I will take the responsibility very seriously."

C. "That is a good idea because you have become forgetful lately."

D. "I am sure your son will be pleased not to have to carry that burden."

81. A nurse working in physician's office observes a doctor sneeze into his hand as he is walking from one examination room to another. He does not wash his hands before he enters the room to examine the next patient. What is the nurse's first priority?

A. Tell the doctor to wash his hands.

B. Nothing because he may fire her for this.

C. Spray the hallway with a bactericidal spray.

D. Tell the patient to come back if he or she begins to sneeze.

82. After surgery, the surgeon writes "resume pre-op meds" as an order on a patient's chart. What should the nurse do with this order?

A. Contact the surgeon for clarification because this is not a complete order.

B. Transcribe the preoperative medication orders the surgeon has ordered.

C. Ask the pharmacist for a list of preoperative medications for this client.

D. Ask the anesthetist to clarify the order.

83. A client has not had a bowel movement for 2 days and is feeling uncomfortable. The physician writes an order that states "laxative of choice." How should the nurse proceed with this order?

A. Ask the patient what type of laxative he or she would like to have to relieve the constipation.

B. Advise the doctor that this is not a complete order and ask for a specific laxative to be ordered.

C. Give mineral oil because it is an effective laxative and does not require a doctor's order.

D. Ask the client if he or she would prefer to have a laxative or an enema administered.

84. A family member of a resident of a long-term care facility reports to the RN that her mother's diamond ring has gone missing. The day before, another resident reported that she could not find a twenty-dollar bill that she thought was in her night table. What should the nurse do in this situation?

A. Report the incident to the facility's lawyer.

B. Nothing; family members and residents should not leave valuables unattended.

C. Pass the information on to the doctor and the next shift staff.

D. Notify the supervisor and call the police.

85. An individual returns to the nursing unit after being discharged demanding Tylenol #3's. He is advised that he is no longer a patient on the unit and this medication cannot be administered. He states that everyone is incompetent and says, "I know where you park your cars, and you had better watch out when you leave here tonight." What is the appropriate next step the nurse should take?

A. Bring the client into the emergency room immediately.

B. Call the police and report the incident.

C. Administer 2 Tylenol #3's immediately.

D. Nothing; the client is just expressing his frustration

86. An elderly man is admitted with a self-inflicted gun shot wound to his abdomen. The wound is deep with minimal bleeding, and it has been determined that it is not life threatening. The patient is alert and oriented. He refuses any medical treatment other than medication for pain medication. Based on this information, what would be the nurse's priority action?

A. Encourage the family to declare the client mentally incompetent.

B. Consider this an emergency and allow the surgeon to operate.

C. Provide medication for pain relief as ordered by the physician.

D. Call the hospital lawyer to obtain power of attorney.

87. The team leader enters a patient's room and observes the physician instructing a nurse on how to insert an arterial line. The nurse is actually holding the cannula and inserting the line. What would be the appropriate response by the team leader?

A. Inform the nurse that he or she is practicing outside of a nurse's legal scope of practice.

B. Nothing; the nurse is performing this act under the direct supervision of the physician.

C. Tell the physician that he or she should allow all of the nurses on the unit to have the same opportunity.

D. Ensure the nurse has ample opportunity to maintain this new skill.

88. A nurse is assisting an anesthetist during the intubation of a patient. The anesthetist visualizes the vocal cords with the laryngoscope and says to the nurse, "This is an easy one. Why don't you give it a try?" indicating that the nurse should insert the endotracheal tube. What would be the most appropriate response by the nurse?

A. "As long as you watch, I will do it."

B. "It would be a good experienced for me in case I need to do it in an emergency."

C. "I have done it before, so it would be good for me to do it again."

D. "No. It is not within my scope of practice."

89. An inmate from a maximum security correctional facility is admitted to a medical unit with pneumonia and is handcuffed. The nurse caring for the patient needs to provide morning care and notices the two correctional officers socializing with the nursing staff at the desk. What should the nurse do?

A. Do the morning care with the client while he is handcuffed.

B. Insist that the officers stay in the inmate's room at all times.

C. Ask another nurse to accompany her into the room.

D. Nothing; the client should not have the officers in the room during morning care.

90. A nurse is caring for a patient who is vomiting. The physician has ordered oral Gravol (dimenhydrinate). The nurse decides to give the antiemetic intravenously instead because of the vomiting. What would this action be considered?

A. Practicing outside of the scope of practice of nursing.

B. Demonstrating initiative to assist the client.

C. Within the scope of nursing practice.

D. Putting the needs of the client ahead of policy.

91. A patient had esophagogastrectomy performed 12 hours ago. The nasogastric (NG) tube was pulled out by the client during a period of confusion. The nurse reinserts the NG tube. This action would be considered which of the following?

A. Unsafe because of the nature of the surgery.

B. Appropriate because the client requires the NG tube.

C. An indication of initiative and advocacy.

D. Appropriate because this was an emergency situation.

92. A nurse in a long-term care facility is always complaining of running behind in her duties during her shift. She consistently gives medications 60 to 90 minutes after the scheduled administration time. She also leaves treatment procedures that are scheduled for her shift for nurses who will be working the next shift to complete. What would be an appropriate strategy for this nurse to pursue?

A. Reschedule all treatment procedures for the next shift.

B. Call in sick for a few days to recuperate and think about her practice.

C. Pre-pour all her medications for the shift to expedite the process.

D. Seek input and direction on time management and priority setting.

**93.** A client on the medical unit has an order for Lasix (furosemide) 20 mg orally at 0800 hrs. The nurse administers the medication at 0830 hrs. What would this action be considered?

   A. A medication error because it was scheduled to be given at 0800 hrs and it is now late.

   B. Appropriate; the nurse has 1 hour before and 1 hour after the established time to give a routine medication.

   C. An indication that the nurse has poor time management abilities.

   D. Appropriate because furosemide should be given at H.S (hour of sleep) only.

**94.** A nurse attends a Halloween party dressed in a white nurse's uniform, including a nursing cap. The nurse becomes intoxicated and begins talking about her peers in a demeaning manner. For which of the following would this nurse be considered?

   A. Not presenting a positive or professional image of nursing.

   B. Appropriate for the situation; it was a private party.

   C. Presenting an antiquated image of nursing.

   D. Someone who has a right to vent regarding her peers' behaviour.

**95.** A nurse is transcribing handwritten physician orders and is having difficulty reading a particular drug name. The nurse knows the client has congestive heart failure and assumes the drug is Lasix. The drug is actually Losec. The nurse gives one dose of Lasix before the pharmacist corrects the error. Who is responsible for the medication error?

   A. The doctor and the nurse.

   B. The doctor.

   C. The pharmacist.

   D. The nurse.

**96.** The nurse provides health teaching regarding postoperative wound care to a client being discharged from a surgical unit. Which of the following statements in the nurse's notes would substantiate that appropriate instruction was provided?

   A. "Client told to come back to the hospital if wound is warm, red, and draining"

   B. "Client advised to call the surgeon's office if pain increases beyond a level of 4 out of 10."

   C. "Client demonstrated, by repeating back to the nurse, steps to follow if wound becomes red and warm."

   D. "Client given written instructions regarding wound care and management."

**97.** After an infant in the newborn baby nursery has a cardiac arrest, the crash cart is placed in the hallway to be restocked by RNs according to the hospital policy. One hour later, the baby arrests again and needs to be resuscitated. The cart has not been restocked, and critical supplies are missing. The baby sustains brain damage because of the delay in obtaining the correct size of endotracheal tube. Which of the following is an accurate statement regarding this situation?

   A. The nurses are responsible because hospital procedure was not followed.

   B. The doctor is liable because he or she was not able to use the available equipment.

   C. The nurses are not responsible for ensuring the supplies were on the crash cart.

   D. No one would be legally responsible because this was a weekend and no one could restock the cart anyway.

**98.** A nurse receives a fax from a physician's office containing confidential information about a client the nurse does not know. What should the nurse do in this situation?

   A. Recognizing the error, dispose of the document in the shredding box immediately.

   B. Contact the physician's office to notify them of the error and shred the document as appropriate.

   C. Fax the information back to the doctor's office using the fax number on the cover sheet.

   D. Inform the police department of the receipt of the fax from the physician's office.

**99.** A mental health nurse is accompanying a client to the mall to do some shopping. A neighbor of the nurse approaches her. What would be the most appropriate response by the nurse to her neighbor?

   A. "Hi. Let me introduce my client, Mr. Green. We are shopping together."

   B. "Now is not a good time to talk. I will telephone you later."

   C. "I am working at the moment. I will telephone you later."

   D. "My client and I are shopping. Would you like to join us?"

**100.** Mary Smith, age 49 years, had a total abdominal hysterectomy 1 day ago. Her nurse has assessed Mary's vital signs and is assisting her to ambulate. The nurse asks Mary if she is experiencing dizziness or nausea, to which she replies, "No." While Mary is walking in the hall with the assistance of her nurse, she falls and injures her hip. Which of the following statements is correct?

A. The nurse would be found negligent because she accompanied the client to ambulate.
B. The nurse was diligent in assessing the client before ambulating and is not negligent.
C. The client should stay in bed for at least 48 hours after surgery so she does not fall.
D. The client should have refused to get out of bed and walk in the hallway.

101. A physician writes an order for the nurse to administer an intravenous medication STAT, which according to the hospital policy, can only be given by a physician. The nurse informs the physician that she cannot administer the medication. The physician tells her, "Give it, and I will cover you." What should the nurse do in this situation?

A. Administer the medication as ordered.
B. Refuse to administer the medication.
C. Call another nurse to see if he or she would give it.
D. Give the medication but have the physician sign for it.

102. A manager needs to address with a new nurse the fact that she wears hoop earrings while working on a complex continuing care unit. Which of the following statements by the manager would be appropriate in this situation?

A. "Hoop earrings are not allowed because they present a safety issue for you and your clients."
B. "I do not allow hoop earring on this unit because I do not believe they are appropriate."
C. "If I allow you to wear hoop earrings, the next thing will be an eyebrow ring."
D. "Hoop earrings worn with a nursing uniform make you look cheap. Please remove them."

103. A client asks the nurse for the results of his recent blood work. Which of the following statements made by the nurse is the most appropriate?

A. "Let me go and get your chart. I will give you the results in a few minutes."
B. "I understand your concern. Let me call the physician so she can review the results with you."
C. "Don't worry about the results. If there were anything wrong, the physician would have told you."
D. "I can't tell you the results, but I would not worry if I were you. I have seen the results, and they are okay."

104. The physician orders calcitonin salmon nasal spray (Miacalcin 200 IU), one spray every day, which is to be administered to a postmenopausal woman. What omission in this mediation order could lead to a medication error?

A. The spray should only be given in one nostril per day.
B. It is not a nasally applied medication.
C. It should not be given to postmenopausal women.
D. It does not need a physicians order.

105. Gail, a nurse working in the emergency department, enters the room of a 40-year-old male patient. The patient is agitated and swears at Gail. He stands up and moves toward Gail in an aggressive fashion. Gail moves toward the door and leaves to call the crisis response team. Which of the following *best* describes the situation?

A. Gail has abandoned the patient.
B. Gail acted appropriately.
C. Gail is liable if the patient becomes agitated.
D. Gail acted in a negligent manner.

106. Mary, an RN, is caring for a client with hypertension. The client's physician has advised the client to decrease the sodium in her diet. The client has expressed frustration because she cooks with large quantities of salt and consumes processed foods. Which of the following would be considered a therapeutic response by Mary?

A. "You do not really need to follow those instructions completely."
B. "Cutting out salt is not hard. I had some health problems and did it myself last year."
C. "You must follow this advice, or your blood pressure will become dangerously high."
D. "Making changes can be difficult. Would you like to make a shopping list?"

107. A clergy person approaches a nurse who is caring for one the members of his congregation. He inquires as to whether the patient has been made aware of her diagnosis. Which of the following would be the best response by the nurse?

A. "Yes, the patient is aware and is taking it quite well."
B. "I saw the physician this morning, so I imagine he has told the patient."
C. "I understand your concern. Have you asked the patient if she knows?
D. "I don't think that the patient's diagnosis should be your concern."

108. A client continually complains of pain after the administration of an oral analgesic. The doctor writes an order for the nurse to administer a placebo to the client the next time he complains of pain. The doctor states, "Tell the client it is a stronger analgesic." What would be the appropriate action by the nurse?

    A. Give the placebo as ordered by the physician.
    B. Give the placebo as ordered but do not tell the client it is a stronger medication.
    C. Refuse to administer the placebo to the client.
    D. Consult with the pharmacist to discuss dosing of the placebo.

109. A police officer arrives on the surgical unit requesting a copy of the results of a blood alcohol level drawn on a patient while he was in the emergency department. What is the most appropriate statement by the nurse?

    A. "I can't give you a copy, but I can tell you the result."
    B. "That information can only be released with a warrant."
    C. "Certainly. Here is a copy of the blood alcohol levels."
    D. "The results are not back yet, but I will send a copy as soon as they are."

---

**Case Study:** *Mildred, an RN, is preparing an educational session for her peers regarding infection control. Questions 110 and 111 relate to this scenario.*

110. Mildred begins the session by asking the group the following question: "What is the single most important infection prevention and control practice?" Which of the following is the correct answer?

    A. Using personal protective equipment.
    B. Hand washing or "hand hygiene."
    C. Sterilizing equipment.
    D. Prophylactic antibiotic use.

111. Mildred continues with her educational session on infection control and begins to discuss personal protective equipment. A nurse asks, "In what situations should personal protective equipment be used?" Mildred would answer correctly by stating what?

    A. "Personal protective equipment should be used when the potential exists for blood or other bodily fluids to come in contact with skin or mucous membranes."
    B. "Personal protective equipment should be used when the doctor caring for the client orders it."

    C. "Personal protective equipment should be used when caring for a client in the hospital setting only."
    D. "Personal protective equipment should always be used."

112. A client on the mental health unit is granted a weekend pass. The physician writes an order for the nurse to provide the patient with enough medication to cover the pass. What would be the most appropriate action by the nurse?

    A. Send the order to the pharmacy for processing of weekend medications only.
    B. Prepare labeled containers with medication taken from the patient's existing medication container.
    C. Refuse to comply with this order because it is considered "dispensing," which this is a pharmacist's responsibility.
    D. Instruct the physician to prepare the weekend medication as ordered for the patient.

---

**Case Study:** *Elizabeth, an RN, is preparing an educational session for her nursing team on the topic of pain. Questions 113 and 114 relate to this scenario.*

113. Elizabeth decides to assess her peers' prior knowledge of pain and asks them which of the following will most influence their client's perceptions of pain.

    A. Cultural background.
    B. The family's response to pain.
    C. The weather.
    D. The physician's response.

114. Elizabeth wants to determine her peers' understanding of how to assess pain in a 5-year-old child. When she asks them which method they would use for this developmental level, she would expect them to correctly say which of the following?

    A. Visual analog scale.
    B. Verbal descriptor scale.
    C. Faces pain intensity rating scale.
    D. Numeric pain intensity rating scale.

115. Allen is an RN mentoring a new graduate on the surgical unit. The new nurse asks Allen how often she should change the IV solution on her client to prevent infection. Allen would be correct if he answers which of the following?

    A. "It is not up to me to tell you something you should already know."
    B. "Every 24 hours."

C. "Whenever you see pus in the tubing."
D. "Every shift or whenever you feel it is necessary."

**116.** To ensure patient safety and that no injury will be sustained during the insertion of an IV line, the nurse would avoid which of the following when selecting a peripheral site?

A. The unaffected arm of a woman who has had a radical mastectomy.
B. A sunburned arm of a teenager admitted for hydration therapy.
C. A tattooed arm of a motorcycle rider diagnosed with renal failure.
D. The arm where an arteriovenous shunt has been inserted.

**117.** At the end of a busy 12-hour shift, Michael, an RN, is ready to go home. He asks Maria, the oncoming nurse, to leave a space in the nurse's notes so he can complete his charting when he returns to work tomorrow. Leaving a space in the nurse's notes would do which of the following?

A. Raise suspicion as to why the documentation was not completed.
B. Be considered an efficient way of catching up within 24 hours.
C. Be considered an efficient way of ensuring the documentation is accurate.
D. Be looked upon as a normal practice in most agencies.

**118.** A new graduate nurse asks her mentor which of the following situations would be considered a medication error. The mentor answers correctly if he states all of them would be considered a medication error *except*:

A. Following an incorrect order.
B. Questioning an incorrect order.
C. Not following a medication order.
D. Not documenting the administration of a medication.

**119.** Angela, a 29-year-old patient, is anxious after hearing the news that she is pregnant. The nurse caring for Angela states, "Don't worry; everything will be alright. Just be positive." The statement by the nurse is not consistent with therapeutic communication because:

A. The nurse is agreeing with the patient.
B. The nurse is reassuring the client by using a cliché.
C. The nurse comes across as disapproving of the patient.
D. The nurse is focusing on the issue but should be changing the subject.

**120.** Jane, an RN, is caring for a 16-year-old client admitted with anorexia nervosa. During the initial nursing assessment, the client tells Jane that she thinks she is an "idiot and all the rest of the nurses are jerks, too." Jane realizes that she needs to establish some limits on the client's verbal behaviour. Which of the following statements by Jane would be considered therapeutic?

A. "No one here is a jerk or an idiot, so please do not say that again."
B. "I would like to help. Why are you angry?"
C. "I agree that some of the older nurses are not very smart, but I can help."
D. "Are you always this rude to people who want to help you?"

**121.** Aiden is a 38-year-old lawyer admitted on a psychiatric unit for assessment. He is angry that he is not allowed to go off the unit. He yells at his nurse, "I have rights, and you must let me go outside. You are not allowed to keep me hostage here." Which of the following would be the most therapeutic response by his nurse?

A. "Going outside at this point in time is not one of your rights."
B. "Why are you getting so angry about not being able to leave?"
C. "Your rights have been terminated while admitted to this unit."
D. "You are right, you do have rights. Let's sit down and discuss them."

**122.** A nurse manager overhears a nurse who is caring for a client with an IV make the following statement: "If you don't stop playing with your IV, I will tie your hand to the side rail." The nurse manager knows she must speak to the nurse immediately because the nurse is exhibiting which of the following?

A. Behaviour that is within the definition of assault.
B. An intervention that should be done before the client plays with the IV again.
C. Excellent role modeling for other staff nurses.
D. Good insight in identifying a risk and taking appropriate action.

**123.** A client is being treated for injuries sustained in a motor vehicle accident that has been well publicized in the media. He caused the accident, which resulted in the death of two children. The client does not want to ambulate in the hallway because he thinks that all the nurses will look at him and judge him for what he has done. What is the most appropriate response by the nurse providing his care?

- A. "I doubt anyone will recognize you with the bruises on your face."
- B. "Don't worry; I am sure it will be okay. Stay positive."
- C. "You are going to have to face the public soon, so it might as well be now."
- D. "You are here for treatment of your injuries, not to be judged."

**124.** During a surgical dressing change, the nurse touches a sterile gauze on the outside of the dressing tray, resulting in the contamination of the gauze. What would be the most appropriate action of the nurse?

- A. Discard the gauze and use another sterile piece.
- B. Nothing; the dressing change is almost finished.
- C. Use the gauze anyway because the wound already has some redness.
- D. Nothing; the outside of the tray is considered sterile.

**125.** Roger, an RN, is a practicing Jehovah's Witness. His patient asks him whether she should have a blood transfusion. Which of the following would be the appropriate response by Roger in this situation?

- A. "You should not have a blood transfusion. I can share with you why I am against them."
- B. "It is your opinion that is important. How do you feel about the transfusion?"
- C. "I can't answer anything about blood transfusions, so I will ask another nurse to speak to you."
- D. "It is not part of my job to discuss blood transfusions. I will call your doctor."

**126.** Marilyn is an RN caring for a client with a PICC line that requires flushing. This is a skill that she has not done previously. To ensure safe, professional care, what should Marilyn do?

- A. Contact the nurse educator for the unit to provide a bedside educational session for her.
- B. Attempt to flush the PICC line in the same fashion as she would do with a peripheral line.
- C. Request a different client assignment and arrange with the nurse educator a session on the care of a PICC line.
- D. Defer the flushing to the oncoming shift.

**127.** An RN, Sarah, notices that a number of medication errors have occurred on the unit. Lasix has

mistakenly been given instead of Losec. What would be an appropriate nursing action for Sarah?

- A. Vary the layout of the medications on the shelves so that medications are not always in alphabetical order.
- B. Develop a system in which the names of nurses making medication errors are posted on a board.
- C. Ask pharmacy not to fill orders for Lasix with Losec for this unit.
- D. Remove all Losec and Lasix from the medication room.

**128.** Stephanie records her client's fingerstick blood glucose level as 8 and gives 2 units of regular insulin as ordered. At the next scheduled blood glucose assessment time, Stephanie realizes that she previously tested and administered the insulin to the wrong client. Recognizing this error, what would Stephanie's next priority action be?

- A. Nothing; the client needed the insulin anyway and looks to be doing fine.
- B. Assess both of the clients and then call the clients' physicians to notify them of the error.
- C. Check current blood glucose levels, and based on the results, determine if the physician needs to be notified.
- D. Only document that the client did not receive the prescribed insulin as ordered.

**129.** Andrew, an RN, inadvertently transcribes a medication order that was written as "Ampicillin 250 mg qid" as Ampicillin 2500 mg qid. Andrew gives two doses as transcribed, and Sylvia, the next nurse, gives one dose before the pharmacist questions the reorder of the medication. What should Andrew and Sylvia do in this situation?

- A. Both nurses must admit to making the medication error.
- B. Tell the pharmacist that the quantity of medication sent to the unit was "spoiled."
- C. Adjust the medication administration record to reflect the correct dose only.
- D. Only Andrew should be accountable for the error.

**130.** Monica is an RN caring for a client before surgery. The client states that she is glad that she will not be going through menopause as a result of her surgery and is only having her uterus removed. Monica reviews the consent form and notes that the surgery is for a total abdominal hysterectomy. What should Monica do in this situation?

A. Nothing; the client is likely correct and knows what the surgery entails.

B. Inform the client that she will go through menopause because she will also be having her ovaries removed.

C. Contact the surgeon and inform him or her that the patient needs further clarification regarding her surgery.

D. Place a note on the front of the chart informing the surgeon to speak with the client.

131. Mr. Brown has had a transurethral resection of his prostate. Before having his Foley catheter removed, he overhears his nurse speaking in the hall about removing his catheter and hears her laughing. How might this nurse's behaviour affect the nurse–client relationship?

A. Mr. Brown will be reluctant to trust the nurse.

B. Mr. Brown will understand that the nurse has a good sense of humor.

C. Mr. Brown's opinion of the nurse will not change.

D. Mr. Brown will understand that the nurse has his best interests in mind.

132. Angela is the mother of a 4-year-old patient who has leukemia. Whenever the nurse approaches Angela to discuss her son's care when he goes home, she states, "Now is not a good time." What would be the best response from the nurse?

A. "You always say that, but we need to talk about this seriously."

B. "Talking about your son is important. When would be a good time?"

C. "Not talking is not healthy. I insist that we must talk about your son now."

D. "We can talk now or tomorrow. What is your choice?"

133. A nurse is examining the Foley catheter of a client who is in a four-bed ward of the surgical unit. The nurse does not pull the curtains and does not cover the client while performing this assessment. Which of the following qualities of ethical care is the nurse violating?

A. Dignity.

B. Confidentiality.

C. Justice.

D. Choice.

134. Dana is a nurse working in the health services department of a community college. She is asked by a student to write a note for her teacher because she missed an exam because of a bladder infection. Which of the following statements by Dana would be appropriate in the note?

A. "The student missed the exam because of cystitis."

B. "The student should be allowed to attempt the exam because she was unable to sit and write the exam because of cystitis."

C. "The student was absent from her exam because of medical reasons."

D. "The student should be allowed to write the exam."

135. Arnold is an RN on the crisis team in the emergency department. His client is angry and is experiencing delusional episodes. He discloses to Arnold that he "is going to kill his wife and chop her up to get rid of her." What is Arnold's priority action?

A. Note it on the mental status form only.

B. Notify the wife that she may be in danger.

C. Include "risk for injury" on his care plan.

D. Nothing; the client is delusional.

136. Shannon is an RN caring for a client requiring a soap suds enema. During the procedure, the client complains of discomfort. Shannon would be practicing safe and competent care if she did which of the following first?

A. Raise the bag containing the fluid.

B. Tell the client to tolerate the discomfort for 5 more minutes.

C. Lower the bag of fluid.

D. Remove the tube from the rectum.

---

***Case Study:*** *A client has had orthopeadic surgery that involved a lengthy general anesthetic. Four days after surgery, the client begins vomiting fecal-smelling emesis. Questions 137 to 139 relate to this scenario.*

137. In reviewing the nurse's assessment notes, which of the following, if omitted, would result in the client's developing fecal-smelling emesis?

A. Assessment of pedal pulses.

B. Assessment of the operative site.

C. Assessment of chest sounds.

D. Assessment of the bowel sounds.

138. The client develops peritonitis because of a distended bowel. The nurses who did not assess the client appropriately would be accused of:

A. Assault.

B. Malpractice.

C. Undignified care.

D. Negligence.

139. The nurse who had worked with this client is required to attend a refresher course on postoperative assessment and the risks of immobility in orthopeadic clients. In the session, the nurse educator would include the risks for increased serum calcium levels, hypotension, and which of the following as risk factors?

A. Paralytic ileus.

B. Increase in caloric intake.

C. Increased preload.

D. Hirsutism.

140. Madeline, an RN employed on a surgical unit, has been diagnosed with type 1 diabetes. She is having difficulty regulating her blood glucose level while working rotating shifts. The nurse manager would be providing appropriate accommodation for Madeline if she did which of the following?

A. Ask Madeline to take sick days until her blood glucose level is stable.

B. Schedule Madeline on day shift until her blood glucose level has stabilized.

C. Have Madeline reassigned to the complex continuing care unit for 1 month.

D. Encourage Madeline to use the employee assistance program.

141. Shelly, RN, is returning to work after treatment for drug addiction. She is restricted from administering or having access to narcotics. Which of the following would be an appropriate accommodation for Shelly?

A. Tell all the nurses on the unit to "keep an eye on Shelley because of her history of drug addiction."

B. Put her in a role in which she is not dispensing narcotics until the restriction is lifted.

C. Put her on unpaid leave of absence until the narcotic administration restriction is lifted.

D. Allow her to give intravenous narcotics only but limit access to oral medications.

142. Stella, an occupational health nurse at a long-term-care facility, performed routine Mantoux testing on nursing staff, and one nurse has a positive test result. Stella overhears a conversation during which a staff member states, "One of the nurses has TB." What would Stella's best response be to this statement?

A. "You are right. One of the nurses has TB, but it is not contagious."

B. "A positive Mantoux test result is not definitive for a diagnosis of TB."

C. "I have contacted the public health unit, and we will have more information for you."

D. "It is not unusual for someone to develop TB, but they caught it outside of work."

143. A student entering a nursing program tests positive on his two-step Mantoux skin test. He approaches the health nurse with concerns that he will not be allowed to enter the nursing program. What would be the best response by the nurse?

A. "A positive test indicates exposure to tuberculosis. Now we will rule out active TB and treat you if needed."

B. "You are correct. A positive Mantoux means you cannot enter the nursing program."

C. "It is better to know now that you will not be employed in health care before you invest in the tuition."

D. "I would not worry. I am sure you will be fine in the program."

144. During orientation for a student nurse, a clinic nurse points out the medication room that houses a refrigerator for vaccine storage. The clinic nurse notices later in the day that the student nurse put her lunch in the refrigerator that houses the vaccines. What would be an appropriate statement by the clinic nurse to the student?

A. "I understand that you want to put your lunch in the fridge, but it must not go in the drug fridge because of cross-contamination reasons."

B. "Why would you use that fridge for your food? Do they not teach you anything at the school you came from?"

C. "That is a good idea. Leave room for other people's lunches, too. There are five other nurses who put there lunches in there."

D. "Can't you read? It says 'NO FOOD' on the outside of the fridge. Maybe you would benefit from another orientation."

145. Roseanne, RN, is working on a rehabilitation unit. She is caring for a client who has just been admitted after a right below-knee amputation. He expresses some frustration with the use of his prosthesis. Roseanne responds by saying, "You will be fine. Just put your mind to it and think positive." Roseanne's response reflects which ineffective communication technique?

A. Arguing with the patient.

B. Passive communication.

C. Offering false reassurance.

D. Changing the subject.

146. Reg is caring for a client who is learning to use a walker after a total knee replacement. The client states, "I hate this stupid thing. Everything is going wrong. I wish you would leave me alone." Reg responds by saying, "You sound frustrated. This surgery has impacted on your ability to be active, and that must be difficult for you." Reg is demonstrating which therapeutic communication technique?

A. Paraphrasing.

B. Sharing of feelings.

C. Asking relevant questions.

D. Empathy and observation.

147. Mary is a nurse working in a school with eighth grade students. One of the students has just returned to school after the death of her grandmother. Mary approaches the student and states, "When I lost my grandmother, I felt very sad. Is that how you are feeling?" Mary is demonstrating which of the following therapeutic communication techniques?

A. Summarizing.

B. Active listening.

C. Self-disclosure.

D. Using silence.

148. Karen is the team leader on a unit where the nursing staff is experiencing conflict. Karen asks one of the nurses to tell her what is taking place among the staff. The nurse gives her some details, and Karen responds by stating, "What I hear you saying is that some nurses feel the holiday schedule is unfair." Karen is using which of the following effective communication techniques?

A. Empathy.

B. Summarizing.

C. Confronting.

D. Providing information.

149. During a taped shift report, the evening nurse reports that Mrs. Myers has been "annoying all evening; she was demanding and on the call bell constantly." The nursing supervisor provides which of the following as feedback to the nurse.

A. "Your report was informative and constructive. I have heard the same from other nurses."

B. "Your report was subjective and not reflective of the cause of the behaviour."

C. "Your report was objective but did not reflect the cause of the behaviour you described."

D. "Your report was too long and not subjective. You need to reflect on this feedback."

150. All of the IV regulating pumps on a surgical unit have been recalled by the manufacturer because of a faulty mechanism. The nurses on the unit must regulate the IV lines by gravity flow. Which of the following is an accurate formula for calculating drip factors?

A. Volume per hour divided by infusion time in minutes multiplied by the drip factor of the tubing.

B. 60 divided by the volume per hour multiplied by the drip factor of the tubing.

C. Drip factor of the tubing multiplied by 60 divided by volume per hour.

D. Volume per hour divided by drip factor of the tubing multiplied by 60.

---

*Case Study:* Robert, a nurse educator, is required to provide his staff with an educational session on Mantoux skin testing. Questions 151 and 152 relate to this scenario.

151. One of the staff nurses asks Robert what he means by a "two-step test." Robert would be correct if he answered with which of the following responses?.

A. "A two-step test involves an injection given on day one and a second test given 48 to 72 hours later."

B. "A two-step test involves an injection given on day one, and if the test result is negative, a second test given 1 to 4 weeks later."

C. "A two-step test involves an injection given on day one; the second step is the nurse or physician assessing the injection site 48 to 72 hours later.

D. "A two-step test involves the administration of a test on day one, and if the test result is negative, a double dose of the test solution injected 1 to 4 weeks later."

152. Robert describes to the nurses how to identify a positive Mantoux skin test result. He would be providing correct information if he stated which of the following?

A. A positive test result consists of greater than 15 mm of induration.

B. A positive test result consists of greater than 10 mm of redness.

C. A positive test result consists of greater than 15 mm of redness.

D. A positive test result consists of greater than 10 mm of induration.

153. Rachel, an RN working in the emergency department, receives an order from an orthopeadic surgeon to get written consent signed from a client for the surgical repair of a fractured forearm. The surgeon has not seen the client but has reviewed the radiographs in the operating room between cases. Which of the following would be the most appropriate response by the nurse to the surgeon?

    A. "It is your responsibility to obtain informed consent from the client."
    B. "I will get that consent signed and attach it to the chart."
    C. "I will get the consent signed, but you must explain the procedure to the client in the operating room."
    D. "I can explain the procedure and have the consent signed all at one time."

154. A client scheduled for the insertion of a percutaneous gastric feeding tube receives morphine 10 mg before the procedure. Upon review of the client's chart, the nurse notices that the client has not signed the consent form. Which of the following is the nurse's priority action?

    A. Get the client to sign the consent before he or she leaves the unit for the procedure.
    B. Send the client for the procedure anyway because you know he or she gave verbal consent.
    C. Inform the surgeon that the consent is not signed and the client has received morphine.
    D. Sign the consent on the client's behalf because you know he is aware of the procedure.

155. A client requires an appendectomy. The surgeon explains the procedure to the client and asks the client to sign the consent for the surgery. The client is Chinese and does not speak fluent English. Which step, taken by the nurse, would demonstrate an understanding of patient advocacy?

    A. Suggest that the physician have a hospital interpreter explain the procedure to the client before the client signs the consent form.
    B. Draw a picture for the client to indicate the location of surgery and where the incision will be made.
    C. Have the client's wife explain the procedure to the client in Chinese.
    D. Nothing; the doctor is responsible for obtaining informed consent

156. After a performance appraisal meeting, the nurse manager asks the nurse to sign the appraisal. The nurse asks why she needs to sign the document. The nurse manager would be correct if she stated which of the following?

    A. "Signing the appraisal indicates that the meeting took place and you received the information."
    B. "We always ask the staff to sign the appraisal. It is just what we do."
    C. "It indicates that you agree with the performance appraisal and have heard what I had to say."
    D. "It is a condition of employment that you sign the document, so it is just a formality."

---

*Case Study:* The nursing staff on a surgical unit has asked a nurse educator to provide a refresher program on blood transfusion, blood alternatives, and transfusion reactions. Questions 157 and 158 relate to this scenario.

157. Based on the principles of adult education, the nurse educator understands that the nursing staff will find the session more meaningful if the learning design includes all of the following *except*:

    A. Specific content identified by the staff.
    B. Information that is relevant to staff practice.
    C. An opportunity to share previous knowledge and experience.
    D. A strict lecture format.

158. One of the nurses asks which agency is responsible for the actual collecting of blood at blood donor clinics in Canada. The educator would be correct if she answered which of the following?

    A. Canadian Blood Services except in the province of Quebec (Hema-Quebec collects it there).
    B. Red Cross Society in all provinces except Ontario.
    C. Canadian Blood Services in Alberta, British Columbia, and the Maritimes.
    D. Hospital blood services in all provinces and territories.

159. Which of the following is the major cause of acute hemolytic transfusion reaction in transfusion recipients?

    A. Administering the blood too quickly.
    B. Laboratory error during the type and screen test.
    C. Having a volunteer pick up the blood at the blood bank.

D. Failure to verify the client's identification before transfusion.

160. A client is to receive 2 units of packed blood cells. All of the following demonstrate that the nurse understands the guidelines for safe administration of blood *except*:
A. Both units should be given at the same time in two separate sites.
B. Each unit should be initiated within 30 minutes of obtaining them from the blood bank.
C. The transfusion should run no faster than 50 mL/hr during the first 15 minutes.
D. Red blood cells should only be transfused with 0.9% normal saline.

161. A nursing student is preparing to dispense a medication to her client and notes that a medication is ordered to be given "p.c." When she asks her preceptor what this abbreviation means, the preceptor would be correct if he states which of the following?
A. Per cup.
B. Before meals.
C. In the afternoon.
D. After meals.

162. A nurse is preparing to administer an antibiotic by the IV route. To administer the medication, she must add the drug to the primary IV tubing in the form of a piggyback infusion. Which of the following would be an appropriate way to hang the infusions?
A. Hang the primary infusion higher than the piggyback infusion.
B. Hang the piggyback infusion higher than the primary infusion.
C. Hang both the primary and piggyback infusions at the same level.
D. It does not matter where the infusions are positioned.

163. A nurse is preparing to administer medication through the client's nasogastric tube. Which of the following cannot be administered through the tube?
A. A liquid medication.
B. A crushed tablet.
C. A crushed enteric-coated tablet.
D. An emptied capsule mixed with 30 mL of water.

164. A nurse is preparing to administer a subcutaneous injection to her client. She recalls that aspiration before injecting the solution is sometimes required. Which of the following

medications require the nurse to aspirate before administration?
A. Heparin.
B. Insulin.
C. Mantoux skin test.
D. Allergy serum.

165. A client with a pulmonary embolus is receiving heparin intravenously. For the nurse to be prepared to intervene in the event of an overdose, he or she should ensure that an adequate supply of reversal agent is available on the unit. Which of the following is the reversal agent for heparin?
A. Protamine sulfate.
B. Vitamin K.
C. Vitamin B12.
D. Enoxaparin.

166. A nursing supervisor telephones the constant observation unit to give the RN report on a new admission. The client has an INR (International Normalizing Ratio) of 12. Which medication should the RN ensure is available in anticipation for treating this client?
A. Protamine sulfate.
B. Vitamin K.
C. Vitamin B12.
D. ASA.

167. A client has an IV infusing to KVO (keep vein open). How long should the IV fluid hang before the bag is replaced?
A. 12 hours.
B. 24 hours.
C. Until it is empty.
D. 72 hours.

168. A nurse is caring for a client with an IV line. When would the nurse not be required to wear protective gloves during the care of the intravenous?
A. When inserting the IV.
B. When discontinuing the IV.
C. When changing the IV site.
D. When spiking a new IV bag.

169. Abby, a newly graduated RN, is working on a unit with senior staff. She has noticed on a number of occasions that some of the nurses seem to "cut corners" when dispensing medications. Abby observes "pre-pouring" and signing off of medication for the entire shift in the morning. Which of the following would be the appropriate step for Abby to take in addressing her observations?

A. Ignore the observations because these nurses have been working for years.
B. Discuss her concerns with the nursing manager and ask for advice.
C. Do as the others do because this is the established norm for this unit.
D. Place a compliant with the union steward to protect herself.

170. Jonah is an RN caring for a palliative client. At 0800 hrs, he pre-pours his client's medications for the day shift and signs the medication assessment record (MAR) sheet for the entire shift. At 1200 hrs, the client passes away and is transferred to the morgue at 1300 hrs. Upon audit of the client's chart, what would Jonah be accused of?
A. Efficiency and proficiency in time management.
B. Embarrassment because of the nature of the event.
C. Inappropriate charting of care provided.
D. Being a role model for junior staff.

171. The nurse leader of the risk management program in a hospital is providing orientation to new staff. She explains that the primary aim of a risk management program is which of the following?
A. Risk management provides the minimal health care required by law.
B. Risk management protects the family in cases of early discharge.
C. Risk management ensures that all staff nurses have the continuing education required for their job.
D. Risk management protects clients with regard to quality health care and safety.

172. A new graduate RN working on a mental health unit observes a senior nurse administer a parenteral dose of Haldol to a client against his wishes. What should the new nurse do in response to this observation?
A. Advise the nurse that he or she can be accused of battery.
B. Advise the nurse that he or she can be accused of negligence.
C. Ask the nurse if this is acceptable for this unit.
D. Notify the licensing body of the situation.

173. Molly is working at a community influenza immunization clinic. A client completes a consent form, and Molly reviews its contents. Molly asks the client how much her annual

income is. Which of the following would the nurse be liable for?
A. Collecting subjective data.
B. Collecting objective data.
C. Invasion of privacy.
D. Requesting appropriate data.

174. Kathleen is a new graduate RN who has begun working on a mental health unit. She receives report from the night nurse, who tells her that the newly admitted client is "a frequent flyer who is a chronic complainer and only seeking a rent-free stay." The new graduate nurse knows that the senior nurse could be accused of which of the following?
A. Slander.
B. Libel.
C. Battery.
D. Assault.

175. A client with asthma refuses treatment during an asthmatic episode, and the nurse respects the client's right to choose. What would be the nurse's priority action after this asthmatic episode?
A. Tell the client he should be thankful that he has free health care and should use it when needed.
B. Instruct the client that the next time he has an episode, no treatment will be offered.
C. Tell the client that he is being irresponsible and punishing his family by making this decision.
D. Provide an educational session regarding the importance of complying with treatment.

176. A client is in active labour and discloses to the nurse that she is HIV positive. She asks the nurse not to tell anyone. Which of the following would be the nurse's priority action?
A. Honour the client's request not to tell anyone that she is HIV positive.
B. Tell the physician that the client has disclosed her HIV status.
C. Advise the other nurses to ensure they wear gloves during the delivery.
D. Tell the client that she must not tell anyone she has HIV.

177. A nurse decides that she must "go public" with the knowledge of inappropriate allocation of public funds in a community health clinic. She approaches a director on the board of the organization with her information. She is doing which of the following?
A. Breaching confidentiality.
B. External whistleblowing.

C. Internal whistleblowing.
D. Reactive insignificance.

178. Michael has decided he can no longer work at a facility because of understaffing and lack of basic care provided to residents. After he has terminated his employment, he "goes public" with his observations and informs the local newspaper of the conditions in the facility. Which of the following describes Michael's actions?

A. Employee revenge.
B. External whistleblowing.
C. Internal whistleblowing.
D. Professional misconduct.

179. Jane and Mary have been living together as common law partners for 2 years. Mary is still legally married to Bill, but they have lived apart for 3 years and share joint custody of their two children. Paul, one of Mary and Bill's children, requires surgery after breaking his arm tobogganing. Jane and Mary are with Paul at the hospital. What is the nurse's responsibility when Bill telephones for information regarding Paul?

A. Give Bill the information regarding Paul.
B. Tell Bill he is not entitled to the information.
C. Ask Bill to come to the hospital and see for himself.
D. Refuse to speak to Bill and only speak to Jane and Mary.

180. Ethically and legally, informed consent requires all of the following *except*:

A. Discussion of pertinent information.
B. The client's agreement to the plan of care.
C. Freedom from coercion.
D. Caregiver preference and opinion.

181. Margaret, a nurse caring for a preoperative client, knows that clients don't always understand information concerning their treatment plan if the information contains medical jargon and terminology. Margaret wants to ensure that her client understands a scheduled procedure. Which of the following statements will best help Margaret evaluate her client's understanding of the treatment plan?

A. "In your own words, describe for me what you are having done."
B. "What is the name of the procedure you are having done today?"
C. "Do you understand what you are going to have done in the operating room?"
D. "Do you have any questions about the procedure you are having done?"

182. Patrick has been diagnosed with HIV at a sexual health clinic. He insists that his confidentiality be maintained and demands that his wife not be notified. Patrick discloses to the nurse that the clinic physician has informed him that he will notify the wife if Patrick does not. What would be the appropriate response by the clinic nurse?

A. Suggest that Patrick retain a lawyer to sue the doctor.
B. Encourage Patrick to disclose his diagnosis with his wife.
C. Suggest he contact the Human Rights Commission for advice.
D. Notify the provincial or territorial governing body for physicians.

183. Michelle, a nurse in a physician's office, observes a client driving a car. Michelle is aware that the client has a seizure disorder and her driver's license has been suspended. What would be the next best step for Michelle in this situation?

A. Follow the client home and call the police.
B. Notify the police department of the observation.
C. Call the client and ask whether he or she has been driving a car.
D. Discuss the observation with the physician.

184. Alison, an RN, is caring for a client with dysphagia. While she is feeding the client, the client begins to cough and becomes distressed. Alison tells the client to "get a grip and slow down." The nurse manager approaches Alison to discuss which of the following?

A. How to involve the family in feeding the client.
B. Alison's verbal abuse of the client during the meal.
C. How to better staff the unit so Alison has help at meal time.
D. The choice of menu items offered to a client affected with dysphagia.

185. Helene is an RN working on a postsurgical rehabilitation unit. To ensure that clients use their canes correctly, Helene would instruct clients to hold the cane in which manner?

A. On the unaffected side.
B. On the affected side.
C. In the dominant hand.
D. In either hand, depending on the activity.

***Case Study:*** *Leslie is concerned about the increased infection rate in postoperative clients on her unit. As a nurse educator, Leslie provides a refresher course* *on aseptic and sterile technique for the nursing staff. Questions 186 and 187 relate to this scenario.*

186. While demonstrating a sterile dressing change, Leslie begins to open a sterile dressing tray. While preparing to open the outer wrapper, she reminds the staff that they must do which of the following?
    A. Open the first flap of the wrapper toward them.
    B. Open the first flap of the wrapper away from them.
    C. Open the outer wrapper with sterile forceps only.
    D. Open the outer wrapper after donning sterile gloves.

187. The surgeon has asked that a culture swab be taken of a surgical wound. Leslie would demonstrate to the staff that the swab is taken at which point of the dressing change?
    A. After the removal of the old dressing before opening the dressing tray.
    B. After the dressing tray is open but before cleansing the wound.
    C. After cleansing the wound but before redressing the wound.
    D. At any point in the dressing change after the old dressing is removed.

188. A staff nurse mentions to Leslie that during a dressing change, her client reached into the sterile field and touched the wound. What would be the appropriate steps for the nurse to take in this situation?
    A. Tell the client not to do that again and continue to change the dressing because it was almost completed.
    B. Remind the client to avoid touching the wound and to recleanse the area and continue with the dressing change.
    C. Tell the client that he or she has caused an infection and take a culture swab immediately.
    D. Restrain the client's hands and continue with the dressing change after taking a culture swab.

189. The surgeon has not specifically ordered the solution to be used to cleanse the operative wound during a dressing change. In this instance, the nurse would know which of the following solutions should be used?
    A. Sterile water.
    B. Sterile Savlon solution.
    C. Sterile Saf-Clens solution.
    D. Sterile 0.9% sodium chloride.

190. Don, an infection control nurse, is preparing a presentation on various infectious control standards. Which of the following diseases requires droplet precautions?
    A. Avian flu.
    B. Dengue fever.
    C. SARS.
    D. Malaria.

191. When caring for a client with MRSA, which type of infection control precautions should the nurse implement?
    A. Contact precautions.
    B. Reverse isolation.
    C. Droplet precautions.
    D. Hand hygiene only.

192. A client develops a surgical site infection. The infection control nurse knows that the most common cause of this type of infection is which of the following?
    A. Contaminated surgical instruments.
    B. Lack of hand hygiene by the operating room staff.
    C. Contaminants in the air in the operating room.
    D. The client's skin flora entering the wound.

193. A nursing student asks her preceptor about digitally disimpacting her client. The preceptor tells the student that it would be unsafe to perform this intervention because of the client's history of which of the following conditions?
    A. Fecal impaction.
    B. Difficulty breathing.
    C. Cardiac problems.
    D. Constipation.

194. An unregulated health care worker (UHCW) in a long-term care facility asks the RN what the term "DNR" stands for. The nurse would correctly answer with which of the following?
    A. Do not resuscitate.
    B. Do not reuse.
    C. Do not recycle.
    D. Do not return.

195. Faye, an RN, is caring for a client who recently had abdominal surgery. The client refuses to turn in bed. What would be Faye's best action?
    A. Educate the client of the importance of turning in bed.

B. Not worry about it because the client will turn as he starts to feel better.

C. Call the surgeon and notify her of the client's refusal to turn in bed.

D. Roll him over and place him in restraints so he will stay positioned.

196. A 16-year-old client with a closed head injury has been intubated for 15 days. Although the neurologic surgeon has repeatedly discussed the risks and benefits of inserting a tracheotomy with the family, the client's family has repeatedly refused consent for this procedure. What is the best statement that the RN can make to the family?

A. "Do you know your son will die without the trach?"

B. "It is very unusual for someone to die during a tracheostomy insertion."

C. "We cannot transfer your son to another facility without the trach."

D. "I understand you have concerns regarding the tracheostomy."

197. An RN understands that the ultimate goal of improving clinical practice through research is to do which of the following?

A. Decrease the cost of patient care.

B. Improve health outcomes.

C. Promote standardized care.

D. Standardize health outcomes.

198. An RN working in the public health setting understands that primary prevention activities include which of the following?

A. Nutrition counseling for diabetics.

B. Cholesterol screenings.

C. Genetic counseling.

D. Routine blood testing to detect syphilis.

199. A nurse manager must make a decision and decides to base the decision on the advice of staff nurses who have experience and knowledge of the issue at hand. The nurse manager is using which decision-making style?

A. Authoritative.

B. Bureaucratic.

C. Consultative.

D. Facilitative.

200. After 6 weeks of negotiation between management and the union regarding a collective agreement for nurses in the hospital setting, the contract is going for ratification. Ratification occurs when which of the following takes place?

A. A majority of nurses on duty agree to the contract.

B. Both negotiating teams come to an agreement.

C. The Minister of Health signs the contract agreement.

D. Union members votes in favour of the agreement.

## ▶ Short Answer Questions

201. Anne has had a myocardial infarction and is on life support. Carol, her common law partner, wants to sign the organ donation consent to donate Anne's corneas if she is declared brain dead. Mark, Anne's estranged husband, shows up at the hospital and states that he will refuse to allow the donation to occur. In this situation, who has the legal right to make the decision? (1 point)

202. Agnes works for a visiting nursing service. At noon on Friday, Agnes decides to end her shift without visiting her afternoon clients but bills the agency for the visits. One week later, Agnes is terminated from her position. Identify three grounds the agency would have to terminate Agnes. (3 points)

203. A nurse is working on a medical unit. Three hours into her shift, she needs to leave the workplace because of a family emergency. The nurse assuming care for the first nurse's patients reviews the medication assessment record (MAR) sheets and notes that the nurse has signed for the medications for the entire shift. Identify three priority actions the nurse should take. (3 points)

204. The nurse is completing his computerized charting when a physician asks to use the nurse's password to access another client's file because she forgets her own password. Why should the

nurse refuse to give the doctor his password?
(1 point)

**205.** A nurse enters the nursing station to look at her client's most recent blood work on the computer. The previous nurse has not logged off of the computer. Identify two actions the nurse should take. (2 points)

*Case Study: Jane is a nurse working during the evening shift when she develops a headache. Jane asks her coworker, Mary, for a Tylenol #1 (acetaminophen with codeine 15 mg), which is available in the stock supply on this unit. Questions 206 and 207 relate to this scenario.*

**206.** List two reasons why the nurses would be found guilty of professional misconduct if Mary complies with the request of her coworker. (2 points)

**207.** When the nurse refuses to give Jane the Tylenol #1, Jane asks another nurse. This nurse complies with Jane's request by giving her one Tylenol #1 now and one for later. The Tylenol # 1 is taken from the stock medication. List two steps the nurse manager should follow when he or she becomes aware of this situation. (2 points)

**208.** A patient arrives in the emergency department in police custody. He is handcuffed to the stretcher rail. A nurse examines the patient but is concerned that he is in restraints. The nurse asks the officer to remove the handcuffs, but the officer refuses. Explain the nurse's responsibility regarding the handcuffs as a restraint. (1 point)

**209.** Mrs. Black is an 88-year-old patient who is receiving care in her home by a visiting nurse. The nurse shares with Mrs. Black that she is experiencing financial difficulty and has to work two jobs. Mrs. Black gives the nurse an envelope with a significant amount of money in it, stating, "It is a tip for the good care you give me." Identify two actions the nurse should take in response to this offer. (2 points)

**210.** The nurse returns to the client's bedside to restart the primary IV solution after the administration of a secondary piggyback medication. She now realizes that she administered the wrong medication to her client. What two priority actions should she take immediately? (2 points)

**211.** Rachelle is having difficulty getting her patient to take her medication. Fran, a second nurse, suggests she crush the pills and "put them in the client's mashed potatoes. She will never notice they are there, and your problem will be solved." Identify what is wrong with this solution. (1 point)

**212.** A surgeon examines a patient after an examination of another patient. The surgeon does not wash his hands between examining the patients. List two actions the nurse should take after observing this behaviour. (2 points)

**213.** A nurse observes another nurse preparing to administer an antihypertensive medication to a patient without assessing the client's blood pressure. Identify one nursing intervention the nurse should implement to address this situation. (1 point)

**214.** An RN is enrolled in the nurse practitioner program. While assessing his client, he is overheard behind a curtain "prescribing" digoxin to a patient. What is wrong with this order? (1 point)

**215.** After the discharge of a client from the hospital, the nurse cannot find the patient's chart. List three actions the nurse should take after a search of the unit for the chart. (3 points)

**216.** The nurse caring for a postoperative client hangs an IV solution that contains potassium chloride ($K^+$) 40 mEq/L. The client has had a urinary output of 20 mL/hr for each of the past 3 hours. Why would hanging this infusion be an unsafe practice? (1 point)

**217.** A physician orders doxycycline (Vibramycin) to be given every 6 hours via an intramuscular (IM) route. Product literature states that if doxycycline is given parenterally, it should only be administered intravenously. The nurse gives the medication as an IM injection, resulting in the patient's experiencing pain and swelling at the injection site. The damage is severe and has lead to a permanent disability. If the nurse is named in a lawsuit, on what grounds would she be liable for the outcome of the injection? (1 point)

**218.** A nurse administers meperidine (Demerol) as ordered for pain. The client experiences nausea and vomiting and a decrease in respiratory rate. Identify three priority areas the nurse should chart on regarding the client's adverse reaction to the medication. (3 points)

**219.** A nurse making rounds in a long-term care facility finds a client sitting on the floor beside his bed stating that he had fallen. Identify four significant pieces of information that the nurse should document when reporting the fall to ensure an accurate account of the incident is recorded. (4 points)

**220.** A 50-year-old man is admitted to the emergency department with a suspected forearm fracture. He has multiple tattoos and scars on his forearms, indicating that he could be an IV drug user. The physician orders a HIV test as part of the routine admission blood work. Provide three reasons why taking an HIV test based on these observations would be inappropriate. (3 points)

**221.** A client returns to the nursing unit at 1330 hrs after a total thyroidectomy. Eleanor, an RN, is caring for the client for the remainder of the shift and checks the patient's vital signs, dressing site, and ability to swallow. At 1900 hrs when the oncoming nurse assesses the client, she notes that the client has a positive Trousseau's sign and Chvostek sign. These tests had not been recorded in the nurse's notes or in the shift report. Why is Eleanor negligent in this case? (1 point)

**222.** A physician orders furosemide (Lasix) 40 mg PO to be given at 0800 hrs. The nurse has furosemide 20-mg tablets available. What would be the appropriate number of tablets for the nurse to administer? (1 point)

**223.** A nurse is to administer digoxin 0.25 mg PO at 1200 hrs. The nurse has digoxin 0.125-mg tablets in stock. How many tablets would the nurse administer? (1 point)

**224.** A 58-year-old man is admitted to the emergency department after a motorcycle accident in which the motorcycle landed on his left leg. The RN performs a vascular assessment before the emergency physician discharges the client. The RN notes that the client's left pedal pulse is neither palpable nor audible. She reports this finding to the physician, who still chooses to discharge the client. Twelve hours later, the client returns to the hospital in excruciating pain, and his foot is cyanotic. When the physician chose not to respond to the nurse's assessment of the client, what should have been the nurse's priority actions? (1 point)

**225.** Simon is applying for a position of RN on the pediatric unit of a hospital. During the interview, he states that he is competent to work with this age group of clients when he has actually not worked in this area before. Why is this an ethical nursing issue? (1 point)

**226.** Phil is an RN caring for a client who is confused and continually gets out of bed and walks in the halls, stating she is "going outside to meet my boyfriend in the park." Phil tells the client that the next time she gets out of bed, he is going to take her clothes away. Twenty minutes later, she is observed walking in the hallway naked, looking for her sweater. Why was Phil's behaviour inappropriate and unethical? (2 points)

**227.** Rodger, a nurse in the operating room, has been diagnosed with chronic fatigue syndrome. List two accommodations the nurse manager can offer Rodger to support him as he copes with his disability (2 points).

**228.** Sandra, a nurse in a long-term care facility, has developed minimal bilateral hearing loss. List three assistive devices the employer can provide for Sandra to accommodate her disability. (3 points)

---

*Case Study:* Michael is caring for a client who has had cancer treatment over the past 3 years. Michael is aware of the client's strong belief in not receiving a blood transfusion. Questions 229 to 231 relate to this scenario.

**229.** The client has low hemoglobin, and the physician orders a unit of packed blood cells to be infused. Michael brings it to the physician's attention that the client does not want blood or blood products. The physician's reply is, "Just do your job and hang the blood. Leave the thinking to me." What would be the consequences, if any, if Michael administers the blood? (1 point)

**230.** What would be the next appropriate action for Michael to take? (1 point)

**231.** Six months later, the cancer patient is admitted alone in a semi-comatose state to a hospital in another city. The emergency room physician orders a unit of blood because of the client's low hemoglobin. The emergency nurse administers the blood. What are the consequences, if any, for the nurse hanging the blood? (1 point)

**232.** During orientation for a student nurse, a clinic nurse points out the medication room that houses a fridge for storage of vaccines. The refrigerator has a thermometer attached to it, and the student asks why the nurse is looking at the thermometer and recording the temperature on a chart. What would be the most appropriate explanation by the nurse? (1 point)

**233.** Bonnie, an RN, is carrying out her morning assessment rounds. One of Bonnie's clients has a dressing on her left leg to cover a venous ulcer. Bonnie asks an unregulated health care worker (UHCW) to "turn the client." List two additional pieces of information Bonnie should provide to the UHCW. (2 points)

**234.** A client is in circulatory overload. Identify the impact this will have on a client's hemoglobin. (1 point)

**235.** Tony, a new graduate RN, observes another nurse administering the wrong dose of medication to a 2-year-old client. The nurse states to Tony that "a little extra antibiotic won't hurt" and proceeds to provide morning care. List two priority actions Tony should take in this situation. (2 points)

**236.** A new RN on a unit asks another nurse to provide feedback on his clinical competency. List three effective qualities for providing feedback when giving feedback to a nurse regarding his or her performance. (1 point)

### ▶ Answers and Rationales

**1. C.** Trust.

*Rationale*
When the nurse repeatedly follows through on a commitment made to a client, it fosters trust within the therapeutic relationship. Trust is a foundational quality within the therapeutic nurse–client relationship.

*Classification*
Competency Category: Nurse–Person Relationship
Taxonomic Level: Application

**2. C.** "I can offer you some information outlining a variety of ways to stop smoking."

*Rationale*
Every nurse has a responsibility to practice in a manner that promotes the patient's right to choose.

*Classification*
Competency Category: Professional Practice
Taxonomy Level: Application

**3. B.** Refuse and remind the manager that he or she is bound by confidentiality.

*Rationale*
It is the responsibility of the nurse to ensure that patient's confidentiality is held in utmost regard. In this scenario, the human resources manager has no authority or right to access confidential medical information. The nurse can summarize for the manager the types of injuries or illnesses cared for in the clinic to identify trends and for risk management purposes, but personal information is treated as confidential.

*Classification*
Competency Category: Professional Practice
Taxonomic Level: Critical Thinking

**4. D.** Appropriate because the focus of a therapeutic relationship is on the client.

*Rationale*
Every nurse has a responsibility to practice in a manner that is consistent with providing safe, competent, and ethical care. If John had shared personal information with Jessica, he would have crossed the boundary of a therapeutic relationship and changed the focus of the discussion from a client focus to a social focus. It is very important in all areas of care, particularly in the mental health setting, that the relationship between the nurse and the patient has very clear boundaries and a client focus.

*Classification*
Competency Category: Nurse–Person Relationship
Taxonomic Level: Application

**5. B.** "I must stay with you until we are sure you are not going to hurt yourself."

*Rationale*
Jessica is depressed and has expressed suicidal thoughts. She has been placed on constant supervision as required by the unit policy. Staying with Jessica, even when she is in the bathroom, demonstrates an understanding of constant observation. Staying with the patient also demonstrates exercising professional judgment regarding the policy and the situation.

*Classification*
Competency Category: Professional Practice
Taxonomic Level: Critical Thinking

**6. B.** "Before you leave the hospital, I will make sure you have the information about the crisis centre."

*Rationale*
The nurse realizes that in addition to crossing boundaries within the therapeutic relationship if they meet for coffee, it would not be consistent with promoting health and wellness. Providing the number for the crisis worker at the crisis centre is an example of promoting a healthy strategy if Jessica believes she is becoming depressed again.

*Classification*
Competency Category: Professional Practice
Taxonomic Level: Application

**7. A.** The worker has the appropriate knowledge and skills.

*Rationale*
The RN is accountable for her actions and for the delegation of tasks to UHCWs. The RN delegates tasks to UHCWs consistent with their level of expertise, education, job description, agency policy, legislation, and personal need. If the RN is confident that the UHCW has the appropriate knowledge regarding the task, the task can be delegated.

*Classification*
Competency Category: Professional Practice
Taxonomic Level: Critical Thinking

**8. D.** Discuss the overheard conversation directly with Carol.

*Rationale*
Planning to meet a client for a social event while he is still a patient could blur the boundaries of the therapeutic relationship, which may result in an unhealthy outcome for the client. Angela should take the second nurse aside and point out that her behaviour is inappropriate and not in the client's best interest.

*Classification*
Competency Category: Professional Practice
Taxonomic Level: Application

**9. C.** To protect the safety of the public.

*Rationale*
Provincial and territorial governing bodies, professional regulations, and laws are in place to protect the public by ensuring that nurses are accountable for safe, competent, and ethical nursing practice.

*Classification*
Competency Category: Professional Practice
Taxonomic Level: Knowledge/Comprehension

**10. B.** After the family has had time with the body.

*Rationale*
Every nurse has a responsibility to practice in a manner that promotes the patient's and family's right to dignity. Waiting until the family has had an opportunity to spend some time with the deceased demonstrates respect and dignity.

*Classification*
Competency Category: Professional Practice
Taxonomic Level: Application

**11. A.** "I will make sure this is noted on your chart to alert the evening staff."

*Rationale*
Every nurse has a responsibility to practice in a manner that promotes the patient's right to choose. There is no reason why the patient could not have a shower in the evening if he or she preferred it over a basin bath in the morning. Allowing choice promotes independence and self-efficacy and contributes to a self-care model adopted in many settings. Placing the information on the chart allows for communication of this client request among staff on all shifts.

*Classification*
Competency Category: Nurse–Person Relationship
Taxonomic Level: Application

**12. D.** Draw a line through the incorrect entry, date and initial it, and follow it with the correct data.

*Rationale*
Patient records are legal documents, so entries must not be erased, obliterated, or distorted in anyway. Incorrect entries should have a single line placed through them and then be dated, timed, and initialled. The correct entry should be placed in the next available space. By following these steps, the nurse maintains clear, concise, accurate, and timely documentation.

*Classification*
Competency Category: Professional Practice
Taxonomic Level: Application

**13. A.** The client has a right to make this choice about his or her treatment.

*Rationale*
Every nurse has a responsibility to practice in a manner that promotes the patient's right to choose. If the patient is competent and capable of making his or her own decisions, he or she should be allowed to do so.

*Classification*
Competency Category: Professional Practice
Taxonomic Level: Application

**14. C.** Consult the Compendium of Pharmaceuticals and Specialties (CPS) or another credible pharmacology resource.

*Rationale*
Nurses have a responsibility to recognize the limitations of their own competence and must seek assistance when necessary. It would be unsafe to administer a medication that is unfamiliar to the nurse. The CPS or a pharmacist would be appropriate resources.

*Classification*
Competency Category: Professional Practice
Taxonomic Level: Critical Thinking

**15. B.** Contact the nurse educator for an inservice and support.

*Rationale*
Nurses have the responsibility to recognize their limitations and to seek assistance when necessary. In this case, the nurse had not practiced this skill before even though it is a skill within the scope of practice of an RN. The nurse should contact the nurse educator for an inservice and support so the client can receive the medication on time and safely.

*Classification*
Competency Category: Professional Practice
Taxonomic Level: Critical Thinking

**16. A.** Develop a poster and pamphlet to be used at the sinks on each unit to promote hand washing.

*Rationale*
Abby has read and critiqued the evidence-based literature and can now use the research results to initiate changes in practice. Using posters and pamphlets is a good method to promote awareness regarding the importance of hand washing between client contacts.

*Classification*
Competency Category: Professional Practice
Taxonomic Level: Critical Thinking

**17. B.** Call a break in the meeting and talk to the nurse privately.

*Rationale*
When an individual is verbally acting out and others are present, it is advisable to isolate the acting-out individual by either removing him or her from the audience or removing the audience. By doing this, it gives the acting-out individual an opportunity to regain control of rational thinking without embarrassment in front of peers. It also avoids the audience from encouraging or coaching the individual and escalating the situation further.

*Classification*
Competency Category: Professional Practice
Taxonomic Level: Critical Thinking

**18. D.** "Please lower your voice or you will not be able to return to the meeting."

*Rationale*
When setting limits on behaviour, it is important to be clear about which behaviour you are addressing. It is important to tell the acting-out person what the consequences of not changing the behaviour will be. The consequences need to be reasonable, enforceable, and consistent.

*Classification*
Competency Category: Professional Practice
Taxonomic Level: Application

**19. A.** Consistent.

*Rationale*
To be effective, limits that are set on unacceptable behaviour should be consistent and should be all of the qualities mentioned in the stem of the question.

*Classification*
Competency Category: Professional Practice
Taxonomic Level: Knowledge/Comprehension

**20. C.** Discuss the situation with Emily, including the safety implications of her sleeping.

*Rationale*
Irene has a responsibility to immediately discuss this behaviour and its safety implications with Emily. Emily's behaviour can be interpreted both as abandoning her patients and as incompetence. If Emily did not change her behaviour, then Irene would be obligated to tell Emily that she must report her to the supervisor. The supervisor will keep a record of this incident for further reference. Reporting the incident to the supervisor will ensure that Irene is excluded from liability if complaints are made.

*Classification*
Competency Category: Professional Practice
Taxonomic Level: Knowledge/Comprehension

**21. A.** Inappropriate because it would be considered neglect of duty.

*Rationale*
Andrew was scheduled to visit the client, and the client expected the visit, as did the agency that Andrew works for. Not attending to the client would be inappropriate and would constitute neglect.

*Classification*
Competency Category: Professional Practice
Taxonomic Level: Knowledge/Comprehension

**22. A.** Report the situation to the immediate supervisor.

*Rationale*
Sylvia has a responsibility to report to the supervisor her suspicion that Ralph is not administering the medication to the client. The supervisor should discuss the concerns with Ralph and determine if Ralph needs assistance with his drug addiction. Ralph's clients need their pain medications, and this issue needs to be addressed as well.

*Classification*
Competency Category: Professional Practice
Taxonomic Level: Knowledge/Comprehension

**23. C.** He should wear a name tag to correct the misperception.

*Rationale*
All nurses must identify and present themselves as nurses, regardless of whether they are Registered Nurses, Registered Practical Nurses, or Nursing Attendants. Allowing clients to believe he is a doctor means Ralph is misrepresenting his scope of practice and professional designation.

*Classification*
Competency Category: Professional Practice
Taxonomic Level: Knowledge/Comprehension

**24. A.** Nonmaleficence.

*Rationale*
Nonmaleficence is the principle of creating no harm. It refers to preventing or minimizing harm to an individual.

*Classification*
Competency Category: Professional Practice
Taxonomic Level: Knowledge/Comprehension

**25. B.** Gross incompetence.

*Rationale*
Speaking about a client in a public setting outside of the professional environment is considered a breach of confidentiality. A breach of confidentiality is considered professional misconduct and behaviour unbecoming of the profession.

*Classification*
Competency Category: Professional Practice
Taxonomic Level: Knowledge/Comprehension

**26. C.** The nurse must treat each client equally without prejudice.

*Rationale*
The nurse must make a decision based on the needs of each client, not on personal values or on an opinion that is based on personal judgment of the client or client's actions.

*Classification*
Competency Category: Professional Practice
Taxonomic Level: Critical Thinking

**27. B.** Discuss the matter with the other nurse, reminding him or her not to leave client information in view of visitors.

*Rationale*
Leaving personal information in view of another person is a breach of confidentiality. The nurse should approach the nurse at the computer and inform him or her of the incident.

*Classification*
Competency Category: Professional Practice
Taxonomic Level: Critical Thinking

**28. B.** "Did you realize that accessing her chart is a breach of confidentiality?"

*Rationale*
Accessing medical records of clients that are not assigned to the nurse or for which the nurse has no professional reason to access is considered a breach of confidentiality.

*Classification*
Competency Category: Professional Practice
Taxonomic Level: Critical Thinking

**29. A.** Obtain consent from Cameron's next of kin.

*Rationale*
Before applying restraints, the nurse must obtain consent from the next of kin until the client is able to give consent himself.

*Classification*
Competency Category: Professional Practice
Taxonomic Level: Critical Thinking

**30. D.** Raising all side rails while Mrs. Brown is in bed.

*Rationale*
Raising all side rails on the bed would be considered a restraint and may contribute to greater risk of a fall if the patient climbs out of bed.

*Classification*
Competency Category: Professional Practice
Taxonomic Level: Critical Thinking

**31. A.** Ensure that the UHCW has the knowledge to care for the client.

*Rationale*
When delegating tasks to a UHCW, the RN must be sure that the individual has the knowledge to perform the task or provide the care to the client.

*Classification*
Competency Category: Professional Practice
Taxonomic Level: Critical Thinking

**32. A.** Discuss the observations with the other nurse.

*Rationale*
The first action one would take would be to discuss what was witnessed with the other nurse, expressing concern that this behaviour is unethical, unprofessional, and illegal. The nurse manager should be notified so he or she can follow up with the nurse. Documenting on a legal document vital

signs that were not actually taken is illegal and would result in professional misconduct. Additionally, the clients' health status and safety are concerns if their vital signs have not been assessed during the shift.

*Classification*
Competency Category: Professional Practice
Taxonomic Level: Critical Thinking

**33. B.** The patient should be treated with antibiotics for his pneumonia.

*Rationale*
The patient has signed a document indicating his wish not to be resuscitated. Treating the patient's pneumonia with antibiotics would not be considered a resuscitation measure.

*Classification*
Competency Category: Professional Practice
Taxonomic Level: Critical Thinking

**34. A.** Notify the physician that the patient has no vital signs.

*Rationale*
The patient has signed a document indicating his wish not to be resuscitated. The nurse should be aware of the resident's do not resuscitate (DNR) status and should not need to go to the desk to confirm this. This would delay the initiation of CPR if it were to be carried out. The nurse should notify the physician so he or she can pronounce the death and notify the family.

*Classification*
Competency Category: Professional Practice
Taxonomic Level: Critical Thinking

**35. C.** Assess the patient and notify the doctor.

*Rationale*
This is a medication error. The priority is to assess the patient and then call the physician to advise him or her of the error and seek further direction from the physician.

*Classification*
Competency Category: Professional Practice
Taxonomic Level: Critical Thinking

**36. A.** Slow the D5W to KVO (keep vein open) and call the physician.

*Rationale*
This could be a medication error if the wrong IV is running. If the IV order has been changed but not transcribed appropriately, the nurse needs to clarify

what the patient should be receiving. Slowing the IV to KVO will allow the nurse time to clarify the order without losing the site or giving a large amount of solution.

*Classification*
Competency Category: Professional Practice
Taxonomic Level: Critical Thinking

**37. D.** Document his choice and reassess his pain in 1 hour.

*Rationale*
Mr. Ralph has the right to choose whether he wants the medication. The nurse should assess the patient's pain on a regular basis and educate Mr. Ralph that taking the medication before the pain gets out of control will be a better pain management plan. Also, the nurse should try to determine Mr. Ralph's reason for not wanting the medication (e.g., side effects, fear of falling asleep and not waking) other than choice.

*Classification*
Competency Category: Professional Practice
Taxonomic Level: Critical Thinking

**38. B.** "Thank you. I will take them to the lounge to share with all the staff."

*Rationale*
A box of chocolates would be considered an appropriate gift for the care given, and refusing the gift might have a negative effect on the client. Sharing the gift with all the staff involved with the patient's care would also be appropriate because others may have also been involved in the care provided to Mr. Green during his hospitalization.

*Classification*
Competency Category: Professional Practice
Taxonomic Level: Critical Thinking

**39. B.** Discuss with the nurse that she needs to observe her patients taking their medications.

*Rationale*
The nurse administering the medication is responsible for signing that he or she observed the client actually take the medication. Having the nursing student administer the medication would be inappropriate. The patient should be aware that he or she is being given medication, so hiding the pills in food would be inappropriate because the patient would not know they are there.

*Classification*
Competency Category: Professional Practice
Taxonomic Level: Critical Thinking

**40. A.** Take the client to the operating room for surgery without informed consent.

*Rationale*
All attempts should be made to contact the family, but delaying life-saving surgery is not an option. The surgeon can perform surgery without consent if there is a risk of loss of life or limb if the surgery is not performed. The nurse should take the client to the operating room.

*Classification*
Competency Category: Professional Practice
Taxonomic Level: Critical Thinking

**41. A.** Notify the nursing supervisor of the situation.

*Rationale*
The nurse should notify the supervisor of the situation. The patient should not be disadvantaged by the fact that he or she is not receiving medication that is needed. The physician has not returned the nurse's telephone call, and the supervisor needs to assist and support the nurse. Failing to give the medication or giving a medication to which the patient is allergic would be a medication error. By notifying the supervisor, the nurse will be supported in the decision not to administer the medication.

*Classification*
Competency Category: Professional Practice
Taxonomic Level: Application

**42. C.** Approach the nurses individually before going to the manager.

*Rationale*
The team leader should approach the nurses individually to tell them that they must not administer medication to each other because there was neither a physician order nor documentation of the medication administration. The nursing manager should also be aware of the situation and document the incident.

*Classification*
Competency Category: Professional Practice
Taxonomic Level: Critical Thinking

**43. A.** Have a meeting with staff to see how they can improve on methods to decrease needlestick injuries.

*Rationale*
Based on research and occupational health and safety standards, employers must provide safety equipment for employees. When an accident is investigated and a plan is developed to prevent further accidents from occurring, the solution should be based on preventing

the accident at the source. Therefore, meeting with staff to determine the best way to prevent needlestick injuries for staff on the unit would be appropriate.

*Classification*
Competency Category: Professional Practice
Taxonomic Level: Critical Thinking

**44. B.** Relevance.

*Rationale*
Clients are more receptive and ready to learn if they see that the information is real and relevant to them.

*Classification*
Competency Category: Professional Practice
Taxonomic Level: Knowledge/Comprehension

**45. D.** Using repetition.

*Rationale*
Repetition is an effective means of reinforcing critical information and enhancing content retention.

*Classification*
Competency Category: Professional Practice
Taxonomic Level: Knowledge/Comprehension

**46. A.** Handouts.

*Rationale*
Visual learners retain a greater amount of information for a longer period if the presenter of the information reinforces the content by providing handouts. Visual learners prefer information that is presented and supported in a handout format.

*Classification*
Competency Category: Professional Practice
Taxonomic Level: Application

**47. A.** Obtaining information, developing trust, and showing caring.

*Rationale*
Therapeutic communication is client focused; goal directed; and includes an appropriate use of self, which includes empathy versus sympathy. Therapeutic communication conveys caring without crossing the boundaries of communication techniques unique to social and personal relationships.

*Classification*
Competency Category: Professional Practice
Taxonomic Level: Critical Thinking

**48. A.** Speak to Gilles directly, pointing out that he is harassing Stephen and that it will not be tolerated.

*Rationale*
It is the nursing manager's responsibility to intervene and advise Gilles that his comments are harassing and inappropriate and will not be tolerated in the work environment. This discussion should be clearly documented and the situation closely monitored in case Gilles makes similar comments in the future.

*Classification*
Competency Category: Professional Practice
Taxonomic Level: Critical Thinking

**49. D.** "As a nurse, you have a professional obligation to share your knowledge with students."

*Rationale*
Of the choices provided, D is the most appropriate. All nurses have a responsibility to provide teaching and learning opportunities to students. The nurse manager should further explore with the nurse the reasons why she does not want to work with a student. Strategies should be designed to support both the nurses and the students on this unit without resulting in any negative outcomes for clients.

*Classification*
Competency Category: Professional Practice
Taxonomic Level: Application

**50. A.** Notify the nurse manager and document the situation.

*Rationale*
The nurse has a responsibility to notify the manager of any behaviour that puts clients at risk or that is against hospital, legal, or professional standards. Linda may want to confront the nurse at some point, but this was not one of the options provided.

*Classification*
Competency Category: Professional Practice
Taxonomic Level: Critical Thinking

**51. C.** Battery.

*Rationale*
Assault is defined as "conduct that makes a person fearful and produces a reasonable apprehension of harm." Battery is defined as "an intentional and wrongful physical contact with a person that entails an injury or offensive touching." Performing a treatment without patient permission or without receiving informed consent might constitute both assault and battery. Battery suits have been won based on the use of restraints when dealing with confused clients.

*Classification*
Competency Category: Professional Practice
Taxonomic Level: Knowledge/Comprehension

**52. B.** Negligence.

*Rationale*
Negligence refers to careless acts on the part of an individual who is not exercising reasonable or prudent judgment. Negligence refers to the omission to do something that a reasonable person guided by the considerations that ordinarily regulate as situation would do or not doing something that a prudent and reasonable person (another nurse) would do.

*Classification*
Competency Category: Professional Practice
Taxonomic Level: Knowledge/Comprehension

**53. A.** Malpractice.

*Rationale*
Malpractice is the failure to act in a reasonable and prudent manner. Five elements must be in place for the nurse to be held liable for malpractice: the presence of a nurse–client relationship, a breach of duty, any foreseen ability of harm, failure to meet a standard of care with potential to injure the patient, and actual harm to the patient.

*Classification*
Competency Category: Professional Practice
Taxonomic Level: Critical Thinking

**54. B.** Slander.

*Rationale*
Slander is considered to be words that are communicated verbally to a third party and that harm or injure the personal or professional reputation of another person.

*Classification*
Competency Category: Professional Practice
Taxonomic Level: Knowledge/Comprehension

**55. D.** Libel.

*Rationale*
Libel is considered to be written words that harm or injure a person or the professional reputation of another person.

*Classification*
Competency Category: Professional Practice
Taxonomic Level: Knowledge/Comprehension

**56. D.** Malpractice.

*Rationale*
Malpractice is a negligent act on the part of a professional; it relates to the conduct of a person who is acting in a professional capacity. Five elements must be in place for the nurse to be held liable for malpractice: the presence of a nurse–client relationship, a breach of duty, any foreseen ability of harm, a failure to meet a standard of care with potential to injure the patient, and actual harm to the patient. The nurse is aware that a spike in temperature of 1°C or a headache is a significant symptom in a client receiving blood and should take further initiative to advocate for the client. The nurse must be aware that harm could come to the client as a result of not advocating for the patient.

*Classification*
Competency Category: Professional Practice
Taxonomic Level: Critical Thinking

**57. D.** The feedback is provided in front of the client.

*Rationale*
Feedback should be provided in a private setting, both for the benefit of the person receiving the feedback and to prevent the patient from becoming involved.

*Classification*
Competency Category: Professional Practice
Taxonomic Level: Knowledge/Comprehension

**58. A.** Assault.

*Rationale*
Assault is defined as "conduct that makes a person fearful and produces a reasonable apprehension of harm." Battery is defined as "an intentional and wrongful physical contact with person that entails an injury or offensive touching." Performing a treatment without patient permission or without receiving informed consent might constitute both assault and battery. Battery suits have been won based on the use of restraints when dealing with confused clients.

*Classification*
Competency Category: Professional Practice
Taxonomic Level: Critical Thinking

**59. B.** Battery.

*Rationale*
Assault is defined as "conduct that makes a person fearful and produces a reasonable apprehension of harm." Battery is defined as "an intentional and

wrongful physical contact with person that entails an injury or offensive touching." Performing a treatment without patient permission or without receiving informed consent might constitute both assault and battery. Battery suits have been won based on the use of restraints when dealing with confused clients.

*Classification*
Competency Category: Professional Practice
Taxonomic Level: Critical Thinking

**60. A.** Culture is a shared system of beliefs, values, and behaviours.

*Rationale*
Culture is defined as a shared system of beliefs, values, and behavioural expectations that provide social structure for daily living.

*Classification*
Competency Category: Professional Practice
Taxonomic Level: Knowledge/Comprehension

**61. A.** Abigail is a role model for healthy lifestyle choices.

*Rationale*
A role model is defined as someone worthy of imitation. Abigail's healthy lifestyle fits into the Health Canada guidelines for a healthy lifestyle, so she is role modeling healthy lifestyle choices regarding smoking, alcohol use, and exercise.

*Classification*
Competency Category: Professional Practice
Taxonomic Level: Critical Thinking

**62. B.** "After each client visit."

*Rationale*
A nurse must document in timely fashion after each client interaction. The documentation should be concise, timely, and sequential, reflecting the nursing care given and the response of the client to the care.

*Classification*
Competency Category: Professional Practice
Taxonomic Level: Application

**63. C.** Providing paternalistic care.

*Rationale*
Paternalism violates self-determination and advocacy by acting for another. Paternalistic acts and attitudes can limit the rights of a patient or client by providing care that is not wanted, requested, or consented for.

*Classification*
Competency Category: Professional Practice
Taxonomic Level: Critical Thinking

**64. A.** Find another nurse to cover this unit and send the nurse back to the surgery unit.

*Rationale*
Nurses are accountable for their practice and must recognize the limitations of their own competency. To the extent possible, the nurse manager must ensure nurses working on their units have the required knowledge, skills, and competencies.

*Classification*
Competency Category: Professional Practice
Taxonomic Level: Critical Thinking

**65. C.** "No, but thanks for asking. I don't like being a preceptor."

*Rationale*
Nurses should share their knowledge and provide mentorship and guidance for the professional development of nursing students and other colleagues and health care members.

*Classification*
Competency Category: Professional Practice
Taxonomic Level: Critical Thinking

**66. C.** Act as an advocate for James and request that the physician thoroughly explain the benefits and consequences of treatment.

*Rationale*
The nurse has a responsibility to James and should advocate for him. This may include notifying the physician of James' decision and ensuring that James understands the information he has been given by the doctor to make an informed decision.

*Classification*
Competency Category: Professional Practice
Taxonomic Level: Application

**67. A.** "I would take the unit of blood if I were you. It will help you feel better."

*Rationale*
The nurse's role is to provide information and clarification and to act as an advocate. Statement A is not focused on the client's needs but on the nurse's own personal view. The other three answers explore the client's understanding of the procedure and readiness to provide informed consent.

*Classification*
Competency Category: Professional Practice
Taxonomic Level: Critical Thinking

**68. D.** Remain in the operating room suite until another nurse arrives to relieve her.

*Rationale*
If nursing care is requested that is contrary to the nurse's personal values, the nurse must provide appropriate care until alternative care arrangements are in place to meet the client's needs.

*Classification*
Competency Category: Professional Practice
Taxonomic Level: Application

**69. A.** "Just as I will protect your privacy, I must protect the privacy of the other people involved."

*Rationale*
The nurse must maintain client confidentiality at all times. If people thought that their names were going to be shared with people they have identified as sexual partners, they would likely not disclose the names and would not want their names revealed. The nurse must assure all parties that no identifying information will be revealed.

*Classification*
Competency Category: Professional Practice
Taxonomic Level: Critical Thinking

**70. D.** "Do you have a physical disability?"

*Rationale*
The Canadian Human Rights Commission (http://www.chrc-ccdp.ca/discrimination/barrier_free-en.asp#duty) states: "During a formal job interview, conduct the same interview with someone with a disability as you would with anyone else. Unless the individual raises it him/herself, the job interview is not the appropriate time to discuss his/her disability. After a person has been given a conditional offer of employment, you can inquire about the accommodation necessary to achieve the expected outcomes of the job."

*Classification*
Competency Category: Professional Practice
Taxonomic Level: Critical Thinking

**71. D.** She does not have the credentials required of the position.

*Rationale*
If the individual does not have the required credentials advertised in the job posting, he or she may not be considered for the position.

*Classification*
Competency Category: Professional Practice
Taxonomic Level: Application

**72. C.** Abuse.

*Rationale*
The nurse should be client focused and act as an advocate for the client. An effective nurse is often a leader, but in this case, she has put her own biases before the needs of the client and may influence the client's decisions. This is considered abuse.

*Classification*
Competency Category: Professional Practice
Taxonomic Level: Critical Thinking

**73. A.** Verbal abuse.

*Rationale*
Reprimanding a resident for something that is beyond his control, especially in front of others, is considered abusive. It is also considered a breach of confidentiality.

*Classification*
Competency Category: Professional Practice
Taxonomic Level: Critical Thinking

**74. B.** Physical abuse.

*Rationale*
The nurse is guilty of physical abuse because she was forcing the client to do something he did not give consent for, and he expressed that he did not want to do it. Restraining the client's arms and undressing him against his will is considered physical abuse, and the nurse could be charged with battery.

*Classification*
Competency Category: Professional Practice
Taxonomic Level: Critical Thinking

**75. B.** The student may have been sexually abused.

*Rationale*
When a child appears to be preoccupied with sexual comments and is knowledgeable regarding sexual activities, the nurse should suspect that the child may have been sexually abused and should explore the situation.

*Classification*
Competency Category: Professional Practice
Taxonomic Level: Critical Thinking

**76. A.** Notify local Child Protective Services.

*Rationale*
If a nurse suspects abuse of any nature, it must be reported to the appropriate authorities such as the Children's Aid Society or Child Protective Services.

*Classification*
Competency Category: Professional Practice
Taxonomic Level: Critical Thinking

**77. B.** Ask the patient why he doesn't want to take the medication.

*Rationale*
All clients, including those on a mental health unit, have the right to refuse medication. It is important to find out why a patient is refusing to take a medication to understand if the cause can be eliminated or modified.

*Classification*
Competency Category: Professional Practice
Taxonomic Level: Critical Thinking

**78. A.** Complete an incident form and notify the doctor.

*Rationale*
This is a medication error. The nurse must document the error so the cause of the error can be identified and a plan put in place so it does not happen again. The nurse should notify the doctor so he or she can determine whether the patient needs to be contacted with follow-up instructions.

*Classification*
Competency Category: Professional Practice
Taxonomic Level: Critical Thinking

**79. C.** That Maureen has a conflict of interest.

*Rationale*
Maureen has offered advice outside of the scope of practice for an RN. She could be accused of diagnosing and prescribing. Maureen is also working outside of the therapeutic relationship. The client may feel pressured to purchase the supplements to get nursing care or assistance from Maureen. This puts Maureen in a "power" position over the client.

*Classification*
Competency Category: Professional Practice
Taxonomic Level: Critical Thinking

**80. A.** "I cannot do this, but I can help you get in contact with a lawyer."

*Rationale*
Becoming the client's power of attorney would not fall within the nurse–client relationship and would be considered financial abuse. The nurse could assist the client by contacting the client's lawyer for legal advice concerning her power of attorney.

*Classification*
Competency Category: Professional Practice
Taxonomic Level: Application

**81. A.** Tell the doctor to wash his hands.

*Rationale*
The nurse's priority is the safety of the patient. Therefore, she should tell the doctor to wash his hands. The nurse has an obligation to intervene and to take action to protect the client.

*Classification*
Competency Category: Professional Practice
Taxonomic Level: Critical Thinking

**82. A.** Contact the surgeon for clarification because this is not a complete order.

*Rationale*
When a patient goes to the operating room, all orders become null and void. After surgery, all orders must be renewed as full orders, which requires complete orders, including the drug name, route, dose, and frequency. The nurse should not transcribe and follow this order as written.

*Classification*
Competency Category: Professional Practice
Taxonomic Level: Critical Thinking

**83. B.** Advise the doctor that this is not a complete order and ask for a specific laxative to be ordered.

*Rationale*
This order leaves the nurse in the position of prescribing a medication. To be a complete order, the physician must write the drug, dose, frequency, route, and purpose for the drug. The nurse needs to clarify the order with the ordering physician.

*Classification*
Competency Category: Professional Practice
Taxonomic Level: Critical Thinking

**84. D.** Notify the supervisor and call the police.

*Rationale*
The supervisor should be made aware of the situation and should call the police to investigate the potential theft.

*Classification*
Competency Category: Professional Practice
Taxonomic Level: Application

**85. B.** Call the police and report the incident.

*Rationale*
The nurse should call the police because the individual has threatened the staff, and this is a chargeable offence under the Criminal Code of Canada. The individual's behaviour is unpredictable, and he could be a risk to himself and others.

*Classification*
Competency Category: Professional Practice
Taxonomic Level: Critical Thinking

**86. C.** Provide medication for pain relief as ordered by the physician.

*Rationale*
The client is alert and oriented and is in a position to make an informed choice. The nurse should advocate for the client to have adequate analgesia and monitor the client's condition.

*Classification*
Competency Category: Professional Practice
Taxonomic Level: Application

**87. A.** Inform the nurse that he or she is practicing outside of a nurse's legal scope of practice.

*Rationale*
Inserting an arterial line does not fall within the scope of practice of an RN, regardless of whether it is under the supervision of a physician.

*Classification*
Competency Category: Professional Practice
Taxonomic Level: Application

**88. D.** No. It is not within my scope of practice."

*Rationale*
Intubating a patient is not within the scope of practice for nurses, even with the anesthetist directing the procedure. This is not an emergency situation, and the nurse should refuse to place the tube into the patient. If the client were injured during the procedure, the nurse could be charged with malpractice.

*Classification*
Competency Category: Professional Practice
Taxonomic Level: Knowledge/Comprehension

**89. B.** Insist that the officers stay in the inmate's room at all times.

*Rationale*
A correctional officer should be with the inmate/client at all times. To protect the safety of the nurse and the clients being cared for, the nurse should refuse to administer care without the officer(s) present.

*Classification*
Competency Category: Professional Practice
Taxonomic Level: Critical Thinking

**90. A.** Practicing outside of the scope of nursing practice.

*Rationale*
The nurse acted outside of the scope of nursing practice by changing the route of the medication without a physician's order. This is also considered prescribing a medication.

*Classification*
Competency Category: Professional Practice
Taxonomic Level: Application

**91. A.** Unsafe because of the nature of the surgery.

*Rationale*
Because of the nature of the surgery, the nurse would know that replacing the NG tube could create bleeding or open the internal sutures, leading to possible injury to the client. The nurse should contact the surgeon to replace the tube. Replacing the tube would be an unsafe act by the RN.

*Classification*
Competency Category: Professional Practice
Taxonomic Level: Critical Thinking

**92. D.** Seek input and direction on time management and priority setting.

*Rationale*
The nurse should recognize the limitations of her own competence and seek assistance when necessary. She should also organize her workload effectively, which includes time management and delegation.

*Classification*
Competency Category: Professional Practice
Taxonomic Level: Critical Thinking

**93. B.** Appropriate; the nurse has 1 hour before and 1 hour after the established time to give a routine medication.

*Rationale*
Giving a routinely ordered medication within 1 hour before or after the established time on the

medication assessment record indicates that the nurse is practicing in a manner consistent with the acts governing nursing practice and the regulatory body's standards for nursing. This mechanism is in place to allow the nurse to administer medications to more than one client. Lasix (furosemide) is a diuretic and should be given in the morning not the evening so the client is not needing to urinate when he or she should be sleeping.

*Classification*
Competency Category: Professional Practice
Taxonomic Level: Knowledge/Comprehension

**94. A.** Not presenting a positive or professional image of nursing.

*Rationale*
The nurse has not demonstrated a positive or professional image of nursing in this situation.

*Classification*
Competency Category: Professional Practice
Taxonomic Level: Application

**95. D.** The nurse.

*Rationale*
It was the responsibility of the nurse to clarify the order when he or she initially could not read the doctor's handwriting.

*Classification*
Competency Category: Professional Practice
Taxonomic Level: Knowledge/Comprehension

**96. C.** "Client demonstrated, by repeating back to the nurse, steps to follow if wound becomes red and warm."

*Rationale*
By having the client repeat the instructions back to the nurse, the nurse can better assess the client's understanding of the health teaching provided. Documenting the statement as written substantiates the nurse's claim to not only provide health information but to also verify that the client understands the instructions.

*Classification*
Competency Category: Nursing Practice: Alterations in Health
Taxonomic Level: Critical Thinking

**97. A.** The nurses are responsible because hospital procedure was not followed.

*Rationale*
Agency and hospital policies and procedures establish standards of care. If a nurse deviates from the standard, liability could result if an injury is sustained. In this case, the baby suffered brain damage because the nurses failed to follow the procedure for restocking the crash cart immediately after a code.

*Classification*
Competency Category: Professional Practice
Taxonomic Level: Critical Thinking

**98. B.** Contact the physician's office to notify them of the error and shred the document as appropriate.

*Rationale*
The nurse should notify the doctor's office that mistakenly sent the fax in error because they are likely assuming that the document went to the appropriate recipient. After the notification, the fax should be shredded to prevent a further breach in confidentiality.

*Classification*
Competency Category: Professional Practice
Taxonomic Level: Application

**99. B.** "Now is not a good time to talk. I will telephone you later."

*Rationale*
Choices A, C, and D indicate to the neighbor that the nurse is working, which would identify the other person as a client. This would be considered a breach of confidentiality. Option B is clear but does not identify in the client in any way.

*Classification*
Competency Category: Professional Practice
Taxonomic Level: Application

**100. B.** The nurse was diligent in assessing the client before ambulating and is not negligent.

*Rationale*
Clients should ambulate after surgery to reduce the risk of developing deep vein thrombosis, pulmonary embolus, and respiratory complications. The nurse assessed the client before getting her out of bed by checking her vital signs and determining the presence of dizziness and nausea, which could all indicate reduced blood pressure and an increased risk for falls. The nurse was not negligent because she assessed the patient and recognized the importance of ambulation.

*Classification*
Competency Category: Professional Practice
Taxonomic Level: Critical Thinking

**101. B.** Refuse to administer the medication.

*Rationale*
The nurse should refuse to give the medication because the hospital policy would not support a nurse's giving it. Giving a medication and having someone else sign for it would be unethical and illegal. Asking another nurse would not be appropriate because the first nurse is aware that the drug should be given by a physician.

*Classification*
Competency Category: Professional Practice
Taxonomic Level: Critical Thinking

**102. A.** "Hoop earrings are not allowed because they present a safety issue for you and your clients."

*Rationale*
This statement is objective and based on fact and policy. By stating a fact, such as "It is a health and safety risk," it is the behaviour that is addressed, not the individual. This statement also does not include the manager's personal likes, dislikes, or biases, which the other answers do include.

*Classification*
Competency Category: Professional Practice
Taxonomic Level: Critical Thinking

**103. B.** "I understand your concern. Let me call the physician so she can review the results with you."

*Rationale*
It is not within the nurse's scope of practice to provide clients with diagnoses based on laboratory results. The nurse should advocate for the client to receive the results from the physician and facilitate that discussion.

*Classification*
Competency Category: Professional Practice
Taxonomic Level: Application

**104. A.** The spray should only be given in one nostril per day.

*Rationale*
Calcitonin salmon nasal spray is prescribed to postmenopausal women for the treatment of osteoporosis. Calcitonin salmon nasal spray should only be administered in one nostril per day. Many preprinted order sheets automatically print "adminis-ter in both nostrils" when a nasal spray is ordered. Nurses must be familiar with the directions for each medication they give before administering medications.

*Classification*
Competency Category: Professional Practice
Taxonomic Level: Knowledge/Comprehension

**105. B.** Gail acted appropriately.

*Rationale*
Gail, the nurse, acted appropriately because she assessed that her safety was at risk when the patient was becoming agitated and aggressive toward her. She needed to leave and obtain help in the form of a crisis response team.

*Classification*
Competency Category: Professional Practice
Taxonomic Level: Critical Thinking

**106. D.** "Making changes can be difficult. Would you like to make a shopping list?"

*Rationale*
Every nurse has a responsibility to practice in a manner that promotes the patient's right to make a choice. It is important for the nurse to understand what constitutes a therapeutic relationship and the process of making behaviour and lifestyle changes. Acknowledging that change is difficult, followed by offering a positive suggestion, promotes change versus the other options offered. Telling someone that they "must" do something can be perceived as a negative and paternalistic. The therapeutic relationship is focused on the client, not on the nurse.

*Classification*
Competency Category: Nurse–Person Relationship
Taxonomic Level: Critical Thinking

**107. C.** "I understand your concern. Have you asked the patient if she knows?"

*Rationale*
The nurse must maintain confidentiality. The clergy person may be well meaning but is trying to gather information that he or she is not privy to. The nurse should acknowledge the clergy person's concern and then suggest that he find out from the client if she understands why she is in the hospital. This allows the client to share with the clergy person whatever information she wants to disclose.

*Classification*
Competency Category: Professional Practice
Taxonomic Level: Critical Thinking

**108. C.** Refuse to administer the placebo to the client.

*Rationale*
The nurse should refuse to give the placebo and should also refuse to misinform the client. The nurse has a responsibility to explain to the client the medication that he or she is prescribed. The client can then make an informed decision about accepting or refusing the medication. If the nurse misinforms the client of the type of medication that is being administered, the client cannot provide informed consent.

*Classification*
Competency Category: Professional Practice
Taxonomic Level: Critical Thinking

**109. B.** "That information can only be released with a warrant."

*Rationale*
Information can only be released with a warrant. Disclosing or providing the information would put the nurse in a position of breaching confidentiality.

*Classification*
Competency Category: Professional Practice
Taxonomic Level: Critical Thinking

**110. B.** Hand washing or "hand hygiene."

*Rationale*
Hand washing, or "hand hygiene," is the single most important infection prevention and control practice. The College of Nurses of Ontario states: "Hand hygiene is the current evidence-based term used to describe all hand related practices that prevent infection. Hand hygiene refers to techniques such as hand washing, antiseptic hand wash and antiseptic hand rub, such as alcohol-based hand rinse or surgical hand antiseptic."

*Classification*
Competency Category: Nursing Practice: Health and Wellness
Taxonomic Level: Knowledge/Comprehension

**111. A.** "Personal protective equipment should be used when the potential exists for blood or other bodily fluids to come in contact with skin or mucous membranes."

*Rationale*
Personal protective equipment or a barrier should be used when a risk exists that blood or other bodily fluids may come in contact with the nurse's skin or mucous membranes. This is a decision that can be independently made by the nurse and can be used when the nurse deems it appropriate. It is not necessary to use personal protective equipment or a barrier in every client contact.

*Classification*
Competency Category: Nursing Practice: Health and Wellness
Taxonomic Level: Knowledge/Comprehension

**112. B.** Prepare labeled containers with medication taken from the patient's existing medication container.

*Rationale*
Taking a medication from an existing medication container that has already been dispensed to the patient by a pharmacist is referred to as "repackaging" and falls within the scope of practice of RNs. The container should be clearly labeled with the patient's name, the name of the drug, and instructions for taking the medication.

*Classification*
Competency Category: Professional Practice
Taxonomic Level: Critical Thinking

**113. A.** Cultural background.

*Rationale*
Pain is a complex experience influenced by a person's cultural background, the anticipation of pain, previous experience with pain, and the context in which pain occurs. It is also influenced by emotional and cognitive responses.

*Classification*
Competency Category: Nursing Practice: Health and Wellness
Taxonomic Level: Critical Thinking

**114. C.** Faces pain intensity rating scale.

*Rationale*
In this age group, it would be appropriate to use a nonverbal manner of pain assessment. The faces pain intensity rating scale consists of six faces with expressions ranging from happy and smiling to sad and tearful.

*Classification*
Competency Category: Nursing Practice: Health and Wellness
Taxonomic Level: Application

**115. B.** "Every 24 hours."

*Rationale*
To avoid microbial growth, IV solution should not be allowed to hang for longer than 24 hours. Allen has a responsibility to pass on or provide knowledge to the new nurse and to provide that information in a positive, supportive, and collegial fashion.

*Classification*
Competency Category: Professional Practice
Taxonomic Level: Knowledge/Comprehension

**116. D.** The arm where an arteriovenous shunt has been inserted.

*Rationale*
It would be unsafe to use the affected side of a client who has had a mastectomy, so the unaffected side would be appropriate. The nurse should avoid the arm with an arteriovenous shunt so the shunt is not jeopardized if the IV goes interstitial, if the area becomes infected or inflamed, or if a thrombosis develops.

*Classification*
Competency Category: Professional Practice
Taxonomic Level: Knowledge/Comprehension

**117. A.** Raise suspicion as to why the documentation was not completed.

*Rationale*
Nurses' notes should be completed at the time the care is provided. The documentation should be chronological, and if a late entry is made, it should indicate that it is a late entry. The appropriate date and time of the entry must be clear.

*Classification*
Competency Category: Professional Practice
Taxonomic Level: Critical Thinking

**118. B.** Questioning an incorrect order.

*Rationale*
Questioning an order that the nurse believes to be incorrect is not a medication error. The nurse has a responsibility to question orders when needed and to document the conversation and follow up. The other three examples would be considered medication errors if the nurse followed through on them.

*Classification*
Competency Category: Nursing Practice: Health and Wellness
Taxonomic Level: Knowledge/Comprehension

**119. B.** The nurse is reassuring the client by using a cliché.

*Rationale*
The nurse has given the client a false sense of hope. The nurse should explore with the patient how she feels about the pregnancy and then explore the feelings of anxiety associated with the news. The nurse has used a more social response that is not therapeutic.

*Classification*
Competency Category: Nurse–Person Relationship
Taxonomic Level: Application

**120. B.** "I would like to help. Why are you angry?"

*Rationale*
Statement B reflects a therapeutic response by offering intent to help while identifying the anger. Answer A is argumentative with the patient, answer C is inappropriate, and answer D is confrontational and value laden.

*Classification*
Competency Category: Nurse–Person Relationship
Taxonomic Level: Application

**121. D.** "You are right, you do have rights. Let's sit down and discuss them."

*Rationale*
Option D is the correct answer because it acknowledges Aiden's concern that he has rights. It also demonstrates that the nurse cares enough to sit down and discuss those rights and to establish some boundaries and limits. The other responses may be perceived as inappropriate and confrontational.

*Classification*
Competency Category: Nurse–Person Relationship
Taxonomic Level: Application

**122. A.** Behaviour that is within the definition of assault.

*Rationale*
The nurse's response is threatening and could be legally interpreted as assault. The manager must intervene in the best interest of the patient and take the opportunity to educate the nurse regarding his or her comments and potential actions.

*Classification*
Competency Category: Professional Practice
Taxonomic Level: Critical Thinking

**123. D.** "You are here for treatment of your injuries, not to be judged."

*Rationale*
Option D is the best answer because it shows respect and acknowledgment of the client's concern but also reassures him that the purpose of being in the hospital is for treatment, not judgment. This is an example of a nurse establishing a therapeutic relationship.

*Classification*
Competency Category: Nurse–Person Relationship
Taxonomic Level: Application

**124. A.** Discard the gauze and use another sterile piece.

*Rationale*
Option A is correct because it demonstrates that the nurse is aware that he or she contaminated the gauze and that it should not be used. This demonstrates that the nurse is providing safe, competent, and ethical care. Using the contaminated gauze, especially when the nurse is aware of the risk of transferring bacteria to the client's wound, would not be demonstrating safe and competent care.

*Classification*
Competency Category: Professional Practice
Taxonomic Level: Knowledge/Comprehension

**125. B.** "It is your opinion that is important. How do you feel about the transfusion?"

*Rationale*
Option B is the best response because it allows the nurse to recognize his own values and opinions but also leaves the focus of the therapeutic relationship on the client. This response also recognizes that the feelings and values of the client are important. In this case, Roger recognized that the client wants to discuss the transfusion, so he should explore it further.

*Classification*
Competency Category: Nurse–Person Relationship
Taxonomic Level: Critical Thinking

**126. C.** Request a different client assignment and arrange with the nurse educator a session on the care of a PICC line.

*Rationale*
Marilyn recognized that she does not have the knowledge, skill, and competency to flush the PICC line and needs further education. Gaining the appropriate knowledge, skill, and competency to complete this skill will require further education practice, not just a bedside session. The other options are neither appropriate nor safe.

*Classification*
Competency Category: Professional Practice
Taxonomic Level: Critical Thinking

**127. A.** Vary the layout of the medications on the shelves so that medications are not always in alphabetical order.

*Rationale*
Option A would be an appropriate action. Sometimes medication errors increase with drugs that are similar in name (SALAD names, that is, **s**ound-**a**like, **l**ook-**a**like **d**rugs). Not placing them together on the shelf or in alphabetical order will encourage the nurses to take the time to perform the three checks rather than automatically reaching in the same place without really looking. The other options are not appropriate.

*Classification*
Competency Category: Professional Practice
Taxonomic Level: Critical Thinking

**128. B.** Assess both of the clients and then call the clients' physicians to notify them of the error.

*Rationale*
Stephanie must admit to her mistake and take all the necessary actions to prevent or minimize harm arising from the adverse incident. After performing these steps, Stephanie should document her response. The other options are either incomplete or do not demonstrate that Stephanie has admitted to her mistake.

*Classification*
Competency Category: Professional Practice
Taxonomic Level: Application

**129. A.** Both nurses must admit to making the medication error.

*Rationale*
The correct answer is that both nurses are responsible for this error. Andrew transcribed the order incorrectly and did not recognize that the dose was too high when he administered the medication. Sylvia should have known the dose was too high. Both nurses must admit to the error. Options B and C do not reflect nurses' responsibility to admit error and prevent injury to clients.

*Classification*
Competency Category: Professional Practice
Taxonomic Level: Application

**130. C.** Contact the surgeon and inform him or her that the patient needs further clarification regarding her surgery.

*Rationale*
Monica should call the surgeon and have him or her clarify the extent of the surgery with the client and what is to be expected after surgery. The nurse acts as an advocate for the client. It is not the nurse's responsibility to explain the surgery to the client. Placing a note on the front of the chart is not acting in the best interest of the client because the note may get lost.

*Classification*
Competency Category: Nursing Practice: Health and Wellness
Taxonomic Level: Application

**131. A.** Mr. Brown will be reluctant to trust the nurse.

*Rationale*
Mr. Brown will likely have a change of attitude toward the relationship he has developed with his nurse based on what he has heard. He will lose any trust that has been established with the nurse. The nurse must be committed to building trusting relations as the foundation of meaningful communication.

*Classification*
Competency Category: Nurse–Person Relationship
Taxonomic Level: Application

**132. B.** "Talking about your son is important. When would be a good time?"

*Rationale*
Option B is correct because it reflects that the nurse respects the mother's right to choose and is sensitive to the timing of the information given. The other options do not demonstrate this understanding.

*Classification*
Competency Category: Nurse–Person Relationship
Taxonomic Level: Application

**133. A.** Dignity.

*Rationale*
Dignity includes the provision of privacy. Nurses must respect the physical privacy of persons when care is given. Nurses must also provide care in a discreet manner and limit the number of interruptions and intrusions during care.

*Classification*
Competency Category: Professional Practice
Taxonomic Level: Application

**134. C.** "The student was absent from her exam because of medical reasons."

*Rationale*
The nurse must protect the student's right to confidentiality. Stating that the student was absent because of medical reasons validates the absence but does not disclose the medical condition. The nurse should only address the absence and not make a recommendation regarding whether the student should be allowed to write the exam.

*Classification*
Competency Category: Professional Practice
Taxonomic Level: Application

**135. B.** Notify the wife that she may be in danger.

*Rationale*
The client is making statements that Arnold believes he may act upon. Arnold is obliged to notify the wife that she might be in danger. If he believes the statements reflect a new symptom, such as delusions, he should contact the attending psychiatrist for further direction.

*Classification*
Competency Category: Professional Practice
Taxonomic Level: Critical Thinking

**136. C.** Lower the bag of fluid.

*Rationale*
The nurse would be practicing safe and competent care as well as demonstrating knowledge regarding the procedure if she lowered the solution bag when the client complains of discomfort. The nurse would know that raising the bag would increase the rate of flow and may cause further discomfort. The client should not be asked to tolerate the discomfort because lowering the bag will likely relieve the discomfort. If the discomfort is not relieved, the nurse may then need to remove the tube from the rectum.

*Classification*
Competency Category: Professional Practice
Taxonomic Level: Application

**137. D.** Assessment of the bowel sounds.

*Rationale*
The nurse should assess bowel sounds on all clients, especially those who have had a lengthy anesthesia

or are vulnerable to complications of immobility. Prolonged immobility may lead to a paralytic ileus or a bowel obstruction. In response to a bowel obstruction, peristalsis may actually reverse and lead to fecal-smelling emesis.

*Classification*
Competency Category: Nursing Practice: Alterations in Health
Taxonomic Level: Application

**138. D.** Negligence.

*Rationale*
The nurse should have performed the abdominal assessment and listened for bowel sounds as part of the assessment of this client. By not performing the standard assessment expected of a nurse, he or she would be considered negligent.

*Classification*
Competency Category: Professional Practice
Taxonomic Level: Application

**139. A.** Paralytic ileus.

*Rationale*
Of the options provided, the nurse educator would include paralytic ileus as another risk factor to discuss in the education session with the nurse. Immobile clients do not usually have an increase in caloric intake, so they would have a decreased preload. Hirsutism is an endocrine disorder rather than a risk factor of immobility.

*Classification*
Competency Category: Professional Practice: Health and Wellness
Taxonomic Level: Application

**140. B.** Schedule Madeline on day shift until her blood glucose level has stabilized.

*Rationale*
The nurse manager and employer are responsible for accommodating disabilities in the workplace and should collaborate with the nurse to come to an arrangement that accommodates the nurse without causing "undue hardship" for the employer. The nurse manager would be providing appropriate accommodation for Madeline if she only scheduled her for day shifts until her blood glucose level becomes stable. The cost of this accommodation would be minimal. Working the evening and night shifts makes regulating blood glucose levels difficult. Asking Madeline to take time off as sick time is not an accommodation, and having her reassigned is not

an appropriate accommodation. **The employee assistance program will not provide Madeline with the means to stabilize her glucose level.**

*Classification*
Competency Category: Professional Practice
Taxonomic Level: Critical Thinking

**141. B.** Put her in a role in which she is not dispensing narcotics until the restriction is lifted.

*Rationale*
Option B is appropriate because it accommodates Shelly's disability and protects the public. Also, it does not cause undue hardship on the employer and allows a valuable employee to return to work. Options A and B are inappropriate because they violate confidentiality and do not address the restriction. Option D does not follow the restriction placed on Shelly's license to practice.

*Classification*
Competency Category: Professional Practice
Taxonomic Level: Critical Thinking

**142. B.** "A positive Mantoux test result is not definitive for a diagnosis of TB."

*Rationale*
Stella is aware that a positive Mantoux test result indicates that the individual has been exposed to tuberculosis (TB) and a follow-up assessment is required to rule out active TB. Option A is a breach of confidentiality. Option C is incorrect because the public health unit would only be notified of a confirmed active case of TB. Option D is incorrect and would be a breach of confidentiality.

*Classification*
Competency Category: Professional Practice
Taxonomic Level: Knowledge/Comprehension

**143. A.** "A positive test result indicates exposure to tuberculosis. Now we will rule out active TB and treat you if needed."

*Rationale*
Option A is correct because it provides accurate information regarding the test and the expected next steps. At this point, it is not reasonable to expect the nurse to predict the outcome of the follow-up assessment. The other options are incorrect, and option D is a cliché answer that is not based on fact.

*Classification*
Competency Category: Nurse–Person Relationship
Taxonomic Level: Application

**144. A.** "I understand that you want to put your lunch in the fridge, but it must not go in the drug fridge because of cross-contamination reasons."

*Rationale*
The clinic nurse is aware that food should not be placed in the refrigerator that houses medication. Option A is correct because it acknowledges the student's legitimate need to refrigerate her lunch but explains why she can't use the medication refrigerator. Options B and D do not address the reason why it is inappropriate, and option C is incorrect information.

*Classification*
Competency Category: Nursing Practice: Health and Wellness
Taxonomic Level: Critical Thinking

**145. C.** Offering false reassurance.

*Rationale*
Roseanne's response represents offering false reassurance. This is an ineffective communication technique in the therapeutic setting.

*Classification*
Competency Category: Nurse–Person Relationship
Taxonomic Level: Knowledge/Comprehension

**146. D.** Empathy and observation.

*Rationale*
Reg is demonstrating empathy by stating that this is difficult for the client. He is also acknowledging the client's frustration. The other options are therapeutic techniques but are not reflected in Reg's statement.

*Classification*
Competency Category: Nurse–Person Relationship
Taxonomic Level: Knowledge/Comprehension

**147. C.** Self-disclosure.

*Rationale*
Maintaining the therapeutic relationship is important, and some self-disclosure followed by refocusing on the client is therapeutic and may encourage engagement in the conversation. The other options are therapeutic communication techniques but are not reflected in Mary's statement.

*Classification*
Competency Category: Nurse–Person Relationship
Taxonomic Level: Knowledge/Comprehension

**148. B.** Summarizing.

*Rationale*
Karen is summarizing what she has heard to ensure that she understands the cause of the conflict among the staff. The other options are effective communication techniques but are not reflected in Karen's statement.

*Classification*
Competency Category: Nurse–Person Relationship
Taxonomic Level: Knowledge/Comprehension

**149. B.** "Your report was subjective and not reflective of the cause of the behaviour."

*Rationale*
The nurse's report was subjective regarding her observed behaviour of the client. It was value laden and did not establish the cause of the behaviour, which could have been anything from anxiety to uncontrolled pain. The other options are incorrect.

*Classification*
Competency Category: Professional Practice
Taxonomic Level: Application

**150. A.** Volume per hour divided by infusion time in minutes multiplied by the drip factor of the tubing.

*Rationale*
Option A reflects the accurate formula used to calculate drip rate of the IV.

*Classification*
Competency Category: Nursing Practice: Health and Wellness
Taxonomic Level: Knowledge/Comprehension

**151. B.** "A two-step test involves an injection given on day one, and if the test result is negative, a second test given 1 to 4 weeks later."

*Rationale*
A two-step Mantoux skin test consists of an intradermal injection given on day one and if the test result is interpreted as negative 48 to 72 hours later, a second test is given 1 to 4 weeks later. This test is also interpreted 48 to 72 hours later.

*Classification*
Competency Category: Nursing Practice: Health and Wellness
Taxonomic Level: Knowledge/Comprehension

**152. D.** A positive test result consists of greater than 10 mm of induration.

*Rationale*
According to the guidelines of the Canadian Lung Association, a positive Mantoux test result is defined as induration of greater than 10 mm. In the United States, the guidelines may differ.

*Classification*
Competency Category: Professional Practice
Taxonomic Level: Knowledge/Comprehension

**153. A.** "It is your responsibility to obtain informed consent from the client."

*Rationale*
It is the surgeon's responsibility to obtain the informed consent after he or she has explained to the client the procedure, including the risks, benefits, and alternatives.

*Classification*
Competency Category: Professional Practice
Taxonomic Level: Application

**154. C.** Inform the surgeon that the consent is not signed and the client has received morphine.

*Rationale*
A client can only provide informed consent when he or she is competent to do so. A client who has been given morphine may not be considered competent to give consent.

*Classification*
Competency Category: Professional Practice
Taxonomic Level: Application

**155. A.** Suggest that the physician have a hospital interpreter explain the procedure to the client before the client signs the consent form.

*Rationale*
The nurse must intervene as an advocate on behalf of the client if he or she believes that the client does not understand the information provided because of a language barrier. The nurse should suggest the services of a hospital interpreter to ensure that the client is providing informed consent based on understanding the risks and benefits of the surgery. Option B would not allow the nurse to ensure that the client understands the full risks of the procedure. Option C would not ensure that the information was being translated accurately. A hospital interpreter should be accessed.

*Classification*
Competency Category: Professional Practice
Taxonomic Level: Critical Thinking

**156. A.** "Signing the appraisal indicates that the meeting took place and you received the information."

*Rationale*
The nurse manager should give an accurate and honest answer to the staff member regarding the reason he or she is asked to sign the appraisal document. By signing the document, the staff member is acknowledging that he or she has received the information but is not necessarily agreeing to the information in the appraisal. Options B, C, and D do not provide the staff person with an honest or accurate answer.

*Classification*
Competency Category: Professional Practice
Taxonomic Level: Critical Thinking

**157. D.** A strict lecture format.

*Rationale*
Options A, B, and C follow the principle of adult learning outlined in literature pioneered by Malcolm Knowles. Option D does not fit into the model of effective adult education principles because it is self-limiting and not always effective.

*Classification*
Competency Category: Nursing Practice: Health and Wellness
Taxonomic Level: Knowledge/Comprehension

**158. A.** Canadian Blood Services except in the province of Quebec (Hema-Quebec collects it there).

*Rationale*
Canadian Blood Services collects blood in all provinces and territories except Quebec. In Quebec, Hema-Quebec is responsible for collecting blood. Nurses should be aware of this so they can access appropriate services and information.

*Classification*
Competency Category: Professional Practice
Taxonomic Level: Knowledge/Comprehension

**159. D.** Failure to verify the client's identification before transfusion.

*Rationale*
Not verifying the client's identify before initiating a transfusion is the major cause of acute hemolytic

transfusion reaction. This is the last opportunity to verify that the client is receiving the correct unit of blood.

*Classification*
Competency Category: Professional Practice
Taxonomic Level: Critical Thinking

**160. A.** Both units should be given at the same time in two separate sites.

*Rationale*
In a non-emergency setting, each unit of blood should be given separately so that the client does not become fluid overloaded. If an adverse reaction occurs, it will be easier to identify the unit of blood that is causing the reaction and the transfusion can be stopped or slowed. Options B, C, and D reflect safe blood administration practices.

*Classification*
Competency Category: Nursing Practice: Health and Wellness
Taxonomic Level: Knowledge/Comprehension

**161. D.** After meals.

*Rationale*
The term "p.c." is the acceptable abbreviation for "after meals."

*Classification*
Competency Category: Professional Practice
Taxonomic Level: Knowledge/Comprehension

**162. B.** Hang the piggyback infusion higher than the primary infusion.

*Rationale*
For the piggyback or secondary infusion to infuse, the piggyback infusion must hang higher than the solution in the primary infusion. If the piggyback infusion is lower than the primary infusion, the fluid in the piggyback infusion will travel into the primary solution bag. If the bags are at the same height, the solutions will not infuse.

*Classification*
Competency Category: Professional Practice
Taxonomic Level: Knowledge/Comprehension

**163. C.** A crushed enteric-coated tablet.

*Rationale*
Option C should not be administered through the nasogastric tube. Crushing the enteric-coated tablet alters the properties of the tablet and the benefit of the enteric coating. The other options are acceptable forms of medication to be administered by this route.

*Classification*
Competency Category: Professional Practice
Taxonomic Level: Knowledge/Comprehension

**164. D.** Allergy serum.

*Rationale*
Options A and B do not require that the nurse aspirate before administering. Option C is given intradermally and does not require aspiration. Option D and any other subcutaneous injection should be aspirated before administration.

*Classification*
Competency Category: Nursing Practice: Health and Wellness
Taxonomic Level: Critical Thinking

**165. A.** Protamine sulfate.

*Rationale*
The nurse should ensure that adequate quantities of protamine sulfate are on the unit to be used in an emergency heparin overdose situation.

*Classification*
Competency Category: Professional Practice
Taxonomic Level: Knowledge/Comprehension

**166. B.** Vitamin K.

*Rationale*
Nurses should be aware that an INR of 12 would be because of an overdose of warfarin, and the reversal agent for this medication is vitamin K, which is injectable and should be kept in the refrigerator.

*Classification*
Competency Category: Professional Practice
Taxonomic Level: Critical Thinking

**167. B.** 24 hours.

*Rationale*
IV solution should not hang for longer than 24 hours. It should be replaced every 24 hours to prevent the growth of bacteria in the solution.

*Classification*
Competency Category: Professional Practice
Taxonomic Level: Critical Thinking

**168. D.** When spiking a new IV bag.

*Rationale*
The nurse would not be required to wear protective gloves while spiking or hanging a new bag of solution. However, the nurse should wear protective gloves for all the other procedures mentioned because of the risk of exposure to blood and bodily fluids.

*Classification*
Competency Category: Professional Practice
Taxonomic Level: Knowledge/Comprehension

**169. B.** Discuss her concerns with the nursing manager and ask for advice.

*Rationale*
Abby should take her concern to the nurse manager for direction and to bring her concerns of unsafe care to his or her attention. Ignoring the situation is not condoned in the standards of nursing practice. Compromising her practice and following these "short cuts" would put her in a position of negligence. Just because something has become the norm on a unit does not supersede the established standards of practice for nursing.

*Classification*
Competency Category: Professional Practice
Taxonomic Level: Application

**170. C.** Inappropriate charting of care provided.

*Rationale*
Jonah charted care before it was given, which goes against the standards of nursing practice. Nursing records are legal documents of care given. Signing the MAR indicates that the medication was given to the client. If Jonah had poured and signed for a narcotic, he could put himself in a position where he could be accused of taking the medication himself.

*Classification*
Competency Category: Professional Practice
Taxonomic Level: Critical Thinking

**171. D.** Risk management protects clients regarding quality health care and safety.

*Rationale*
Elements of a risk management program are client safety, product safety, and quality assurance.

*Classification*
Competency Category: Professional Practice
Taxonomic Level: Knowledge/Application

**172. A.** Advise the nurse that he or she can be accused of battery.

*Rationale*
Battery is defined as an intentional and wrongful physical contact with person that entails an injury or offensive touching.

*Classification*
Competency Category: Professional Practice
Taxonomic Level: Critical Thinking

**173. C.** Invasion of privacy.

*Rationale*
The nurse should request only the necessary information to provide safe care. In this case, information regarding annual income is not required and would constitute an invasion of the client's privacy.

*Classification*
Competency Category: Professional Practice
Taxonomic Level: Knowledge/Comprehension

**174. A.** Slander.

*Rationale*
The statement by the senior nurse would fall into the definition of slander and defamation of character.

*Classification*
Competency Category: Professional Practice
Taxonomic Level: Application

**175. D.** Provide an educational session regarding the importance of complying with treatment.

*Rationale*
The nurse would continue to respect the client's right to choose but would ensure that the choice is based on accurate and complete information.

*Classification*
Competency Category: Nursing Practice: Health and Wellness
Taxonomic Level: Critical Thinking

**176. B.** Tell the physician that the client has disclosed her HIV status.

*Rationale*
The nurse has a responsibility to tell the physician of the mother's HIV status so that steps can be taken to ensure the safety of the unborn child. When the nurse is aware of information that could impact on the health and safety of another person, the nurse must disclose the information and cannot hold the information confidential.

*Classification*
Competency Category: Professional Practice
Taxonomic Level: Critical Thinking

**177. C.** Internal whistleblowing.

*Rationale*
Whistleblowing is the disclosure of illegal, immoral, or illegitimate practices that are under an employer's control. Whistleblowing is the public disclosure of organizational wrongdoing. In this case, the whistleblowing is internal because the information was disclosed to a member of the board of directors.

*Classification*
Competency Category: Professional Practice
Taxonomic Level: Application

**178. B.** External whistleblowing.

*Rationale*
Whistleblowing is the disclosure of illegal, immoral, or illegitimate practices that are under an employer's control. Whistleblowing includes the exposure of serious wrongdoing, such as negligence or maltreatment, that exists in the workplace. By going to the media, it is considered external whistleblowing.

*Classification*
Competency Category: Professional Practice
Taxonomic Level: Application

**179. A.** Give Bill the information regarding Paul.

*Rationale*
Bill has joint custody with Mary of Paul, a child who is a minor. Bill is entitled to knowing Paul's medical information.

*Classification*
Competency Category: Professional Practice
Taxonomic Level: Critical Thinking

**180. D.** Caregiver preference and opinion.

*Rationale*
Informed consent does not include coercion and caregiver preference. Caregiver opinion could be perceived as coercion.

*Classification*
Competency Category: Professional Practice
Taxonomic Level: Knowledge/Comprehension

**181. A.** "In your own words, describe for me what you are having done."

*Rationale*
Margaret's goal is to assess her client's understanding of the treatment plan. Option A provides an opportunity for the client to describe the plan in his or her own words, allowing the client to use lay terms to describe his or her understanding of the procedure. Option B may be answered correctly by the client but does not demonstrate an understanding of the procedure. Options C and D are closed-ended questions and do not allow for evaluation of understanding. Clients may answer "yes" out of embarrassment of not wanting to admit they do not understand what they have been told.

*Classification*
Competency Category: Nurse–Person Relationship
Taxonomic Level: Critical Thinking

**182. B.** Encourage Patrick to disclose his diagnosis with his wife.

*Rationale*
Exceptions to confidentiality are warranted when certain conditions are present. One of these conditions includes serious potential harm to a third party. Disclosure should be limited to information essential for the intended purpose, and only persons with a need to know should receive the information. Voluntary disclosure with the support of the physician would be the ideal approach to this situation.

*Classification*
Competency Category: Professional Practice
Taxonomic Level: Critical Thinking

**183. D.** Discuss the observation with the physician.

*Rationale*
The physician has a responsibility to report to the Ministry of Transportation any client who has a condition that impairs his or her ability to drive safely. The Ministry of Transportation (Department of Motor Vehicles) will determine the consequences regarding the person's driver's license. The nurse cannot breach confidentiality by reporting the client to the authorities.

*Classification*
Competency Category: Professional Practice
Taxonomic Level: Application

**184. B.** Alison's verbal abuse of the client during the meal.

*Rationale*
Alison was verbally abusive toward the client when the client became distressed during the meal. The

nurse manager has an obligation to address the behaviour and offer Alison feedback and consequences if the behaviour continues.

*Classification*
Competency Category: Professional Practice
Taxonomic Level: Critical Thinking

**185. A.** On the unaffected side.

*Rationale*
It is appropriate for the client to hold the cane on the unaffected side to avoid further injury and to promote ambulation.

*Classification*
Competency Category: Nursing Practice: Health and Wellness
Taxonomic Level: Knowledge/Comprehension

**186. B.** Open the first flap of the wrapper away from them.

*Rationale*
To maintain sterility of the field, the first flap of the outer wrapper of a sterile dressing tray is opened away from oneself. Opening the flap toward oneself would result in leaning across the sterile field to open the other flap. The outer wrapper is considered nonsterile on the outside and is opened before donning sterile gloves. This step can be performed with clean hands.

*Classification*
Competency Category: Nursing Practice: Health and Wellness
Taxonomic Level: Knowledge/Comprehension

**187. C.** After cleansing the wound but before redressing the wound.

*Rationale*
The wound culture is collected after the wound has been cleansed. This allows for exudate consisting of dead white blood cells and debris to be removed and colonized tissue cultured.

*Classification*
Competency Category: Nursing Practice: Health and Wellness
Taxonomic Level: Application

**188. B.** Remind the client to avoid touching the wound and to recleanse the area and continue with the dressing change.

*Rationale*
The nurse should remind the client not to reach over and touch the wound. The wound should be recleansed

to remove any organisms that may have been introduced, and the dressing change should then continue. It would be prudent of the nurse to include this in her documentation. Culturing the wound immediately is not likely to provide an accurate response. Restraining the client's hands would not be appropriate.

*Classification*
Competency Category: Nursing Practice: Health and Wellness
Taxonomic Level: Application

**189. D.** Sterile 0.9% sodium chloride.

*Rationale*
A nurse should know that the solution must be sterile and would choose 0.9% sodium chloride because it is an isotonic solution that will not affect cellular homeostasis. Sterile water is hypertonic and would be absorbed by cells and possibly cause cells to burst. A solution such as Saf-Clens is not a cleansing solution. Any other solution must be ordered by the surgeon.

*Classification*
Competency Category: Professional Practice
Taxonomic Level: Critical Thinking

**190. C.** SARS.

*Rationale*
Severe acute respiratory syndrome (SARS) is passed on from person to person by exposure to respiratory droplets within 3 feet. Droplet precautions, including appropriate personal protective equipment, reduces the transmission of the infection.

*Classification*
Competency Category: Nursing Practice: Health and Wellness
Taxonomic Level: Knowledge/Comprehension

**191. A.** Contact precautions.

*Rationale*
A client with MRSA should be cared for with contact precautions. Contact precautions include placing the client in a private room, gowning, gloving, and limiting the movement of the client outside of the room.

*Classification*
Competency Category: Nursing Practice: Alterations in Health
Taxonomic Level: Knowledge/Comprehension

**192. D.** The client's skin flora entering the wound.

*Rationale*
The client's own flora entering the wound during surgery is the main cause of surgical site infections.

*Classification*
Competency Category: Nursing Practice: Alterations in Health
Taxonomic Level: Knowledge/Comprehension

**193. C.** Cardiac problems.

*Rationale*
Because digital disimpaction can result in the stimulation of the vagus nerve, disimpaction is contraindicated in clients with cardiac conditions. Stimulation of the vagus nerve can result in bradycardia or dysrhythmia.

*Classification*
Competency Category: Nursing Practice: Alterations in Health
Taxonomic Level: Knowledge/Comprehension

**194. A.** Do not resuscitate.

*Rationale*
"DNR" stands for "do not resuscitate." The nurse should ensure that the UHCW understands exactly what this means in relation to the care he or she is providing to residents.

*Classification*
Competency Category: Nursing Practice: Health and Wellness
Taxonomic Level: Knowledge/Comprehension

**195. A.** Educate the client of the importance of turning in bed.

*Rationale*
Option A represents the best option for this patient. The nurse needs to inform the client of the importance of turning in bed to prevent postoperative complications. If the client still refuses to turn, the nurse may need to inform the physician, especially if the client needs his or her pain management adjusted or if physiotherapy is required. Option B does not help the client. Option D would be inappropriate and would put the patient at risk of being charged with battery.

*Classification*
Competency Category: Nursing Practice: Health and Wellness
Taxonomic Level: Application

**196. D.** "I understand you have concerns regarding the tracheostomy."

*Rationale*
Option D is the appropriate statement because it allows for the family to discuss their concerns, fears, and questions with the nurse.

*Classification*
Competency Category: Professional Practice
Taxonomic Level: Application

**197. B.** Improve health outcomes.

*Rationale*
Improving health outcomes is the ultimate goal of improving clinical practice through research.

*Classification*
Competency Category: Professional Practice
Taxonomic Level: Knowledge/Comprehension

**198. C.** Genetic counselling.

*Rationale*
Genetic counselling is an example of primary prevention.

*Classification*
Competency Category: Nursing Practice: Health and Wellness
Taxonomic Level: Knowledge/Comprehension

**199. C.** Consultative.

*Rationale*
Asking for input and basing a decision on the expertise and knowledge of those with previous and direct experience with the issue at hand is considered a consultative style of decision making.

*Classification*
Competency Category: Professional Practice
Taxonomic Level: Knowledge/Comprehension

**200. D.** Union members votes in favour of the agreement.

*Rationale*
Ratification occurs when union members have an opportunity to vote. When they vote in favor of the contract, it is considered ratified.

*Classification*
Competency Category: Professional Practice
Taxonomic Level: Knowledge/Comprehension

**201. Answer:** Mark, the estranged husband, has the legal right to make the decision because Anne and Mark are still legally married.

*Rationale*
In this situation, Mark would be considered next of kin and would have to provide consent for the donation.

*Classification*
Competency Category: Professional Practice
Taxonomic Level: Critical Thinking

## 202. Answers:

- Misappropriating funds from the company
- Fraud
- Abandonment of patient care
- Falsifying documents

*Rationale*
All of these answers could be applied to this situation.

*Classification*
Competency Category: Professional Practice
Taxonomic Level: Knowledge/Comprehension

## 203. Answers:

- Notify the supervisor.
- Call the previous nurse to establish which medications were actually given and when and notify him or her that this is an inappropriate action.
- Complete an incident report.
- Ensure that the patients receive the medications that they should receive on time.

*Rationale*
The nursing supervisor needs to be notified and an incident report completed to track this behaviour. Doing this also allow the manager to follow up on previous occurrences. If this is behaviour occurs routinely on this unit, it needs to be addressed in an educational session. The previous nurse should be aware of the inappropriate behaviour and should clarify with the oncoming nurses which medications have been given. The patients still require medication as prescribed.

*Classification*
Competency Category: Professional Practice
Taxonomic Level: Critical Thinking

## 204. Answer: Computer passwords should be kept private and not shared because they are used to ensure patient confidentiality and to track access to records.

*Rationale*
Most agencies require staff members to sign a contract indicating that they will not share their passwords. Doing so could lead to a reprimand.

*Classification*
Competency Category: Professional Practice
Taxonomic Level: Critical Thinking

## 205. Answers:

- Log off the previous nurse.
- Log on using her own password.
- Speak to the previous nurse about leaving the computer while still being logged on.

*Rationale*
Take steps to protect patient confidentiality by logging off the previous nurse. The system should only be accessed by using your own password. This situation should be addressed with the nurse who did not log off previously to ensure that he or she understands appropriate computer access protocol.

*Classification*
Competency Category: Professional Practice
Taxonomic Level: Knowledge/Comprehension

## 206. Answers:

- There has been no doctor order for a prescription medication.
- There is no medical chart to document the medication.
- There is likely an agency policy that states that this should not be done.
- The nurse would be considered to be prescribing and dispensing.

*Rationale*
All answers are based on the legality and scope of practice of nursing. Nurses are answerable for their practice, and they must act in a manner consistent with their professional responsibilities and standards of practice.

*Classification*
Competency Category: Professional Practice
Taxonomic Level: Critical Thinking

## 207. Answers:

- Notify Jane and the other nurse involved that they should not dispense medication without an order.
- Notify the nurse manager (supervisor) of the situation.

*Rationale*
There is no order for these medications nor is there a mechanism for documentation. Jane would be considered to be dispensing medication, which falls within the scope of practice of a pharmacist and is outside the scope of practice of nurses. Nurses must practice in a manner consistent with the acts governing nursing practice and the regulatory body's standards of practice. The nurses must practice within the scope of practice of nursing.

*Classification*
Competency Category: Professional Practice
Taxonomic Level: Application

**208. Answer:** The police, not the nurse, have put the client in restraint, so the nurse was not responsible for the application of the restraint.

*Rationale*
The nurse would be responsible if he or she applied any form of restraint. The police and correctional officers have their own policies regarding restraints and take responsibility for this action. However, the nurse should assess the skin around and underneath the handcuffs to ensure there is no damage as a result.

*Classification*
Competency Category: Professional Practice
Taxonomic Level: Critical Thinking

**209. Answer:**

- Refuse to take the money.
- Advise the nursing supervisor.
- Document the conversation and her actions.

*Rationale*
The nurse should not accept the gift from the client. The nursing supervisor should be notified and the conversation documented to ensure it is clear that the nurse did not accept the gift. Gifts appropriate in value for the care given, such as chocolates or a donation that is made to a nursing unit for all the staff to access, would be appropriate. Accepting a significant amount of money from a client would be considered abuse and crosses the boundaries of the nurse–client relationship.

*Classification*
Competency Category: Professional Practice
Taxonomic Level: Critical Thinking

**210. Answer:** Assess the client and call the doctor.

*Rationale*
The primary responsibly of the nurse is to assess that no harm has come to the client and to notify the physician for further direction.

*Classification*
Competency Category: Professional Practice
Taxonomic Level: Application

**211. Answer:** Patients have the right to refuse medication. Hiding medications in food is unethical and unprofessional and is considered abuse.

*Rationale*
Patients have the right to refuse medication. The nurse should find out why the patient does not want the medication. Hiding medications in food is unethical and unprofessional and is considered abuse.

*Classification*
Competency Category: Professional Practice
Taxonomic Level: Critical Thinking

**212. Answers:**

- Tell the surgeon that he must wash his hands between patients.
- Complete an incident report.
- Notify the nursing manager or infection control department.

*Rationale*
The surgeon needs to be made aware of his infection control risk, and the manager needs to be made aware of the situation. An incident report should be completed to track trends because patients' risk of infection is of utmost importance.

*Classification*
Competency Category: Professional Practice
Taxonomic Level: Application

**213. Answer:** The nurse should intervene on the client's behalf and tell the other nurse that he or she should assess the blood pressure before administering the antihypertensive medication. The nurse should notify the nursing manager so he or she can offer training to the other nurse to prevent repeat incidents.

*Rationale*
The nurse must intervene on behalf of the client before the medication is administered. Assessing blood pressure before administering an antihypertensive is appropriate. Nurses should notify the appropriate person if they observe unsafe practices by a nursing colleague.

*Classification*
Competency Category: Professional Practice
Taxonomic Level: Application

**214. Answer:** He would be practicing outside of his scope of practice because he is not yet registered as a nurse practitioner.

*Rationale*
Although registered nurse practitioners are allowed to prescribe certain medications, they are not allowed to do so independently outside of the delegated list of medications. Digoxin is not a drug that could be ordered by the RN in the extended class category (nurse practitioner).

*Classification*
Competency Category: Professional Practice
Taxonomic Level: Application

### 215. Answers:

- Notify the physician.
- Notify security.
- Notify the supervisor.
- Notify the patient.
- Complete an incident report.

*Rationale*
All of these steps should be taken to recover the chart and to ensure that the appropriate individuals are notified. The nurse and the nursing unit are responsible for the chart, and if it is "lost," they need to take action regarding the confidentiality of the record and the recovery of the information.

*Classification*
Competency Category: Professional Practice
Taxonomic Level: Application

### 216. Answer: The client does not have enough urinary output to demonstrate adequate kidney function to eliminate excess $K^+$. The client is predisposed to becoming hyperkalemic.

*Rationale*
The nurse who hangs the IV with $K^+$ while knowing that the patient's urinary output is less than sufficient (30 mL/hr) does not recognize that the client has decreased urinary function and, as a result, $K^+$ is not being diuresed at an appropriate rate. This would lead to hyperkalemia, which would be a negative outcome for the client. If the $K^+$ is hung, the nurse would be acting in an unsafe and negligent manner.

*Classification*
Competency Category: Professional Practice
Taxonomic Level: Critical Thinking

### 217. Answer: The nurse would be liable because nurses are responsible for knowing the accepted routes for administration for medications they are giving and must question orders that are incorrect, inconsistent, or inappropriate.

*Rationale*
Knowing the appropriate route to administer a medication is a fundamental part of medication administration and is the responsibility of nurses. Giving the medication by a route not approved or recommended would make the nurse liable for negative outcomes to the client.

*Classification*
Competency Category: Professional Practice
Taxonomic Level: Critical Thinking

### 218. Answers:

- Document the event and assessment in the nurse's notes.
- Document the notification of the event to the physician.
- Document the nursing interventions.
- Document the client's response to the nursing interventions.

*Rationale*
Documenting each of these actions will establish a record of events and will demonstrate that the nurse met the standards of patient care during and after administration of the medication.

*Classification*
Competency Category: Professional Practice
Taxonomic Level: Application

### 219. Answers:

- The condition and position of the client when he was found
- Fall prevention measures that were in place
- Statements made by the client regarding pain
- The time of and response to the call placed to the physician
- The time of the physician's arrival, if applicable
- The time of the call and time of response by EMS, if applicable
- The time of contact to client's family or next of kin
- Diagnostic and assessment measures used and their results

*Rationale*
Documenting these observations and steps will provide background information and support the safety measures taken to prevent falls and further injury. Documenting timelines and response times will support the nurse's claims of providing competent care.

*Classification*
Competency Category: Professional Practice
Taxonomy Level: Application

### 220. Answers:

- This test is being ordered based on a subjective observation of the client (i.e., tattoos and needle scars).

- The client's HIV status would not affect the cause or outcome of the injury for which he was admitted.
- The client did not give informed consent for the test to be done.
- Universal precautions should be taken with all clients.

*Rationale*
The client's HIV status will not affect the cause or treatment of his forearm fracture. If the client had been admitted with a condition that could warrant investigation of HIV as a cause, then the physician should discuss the test with the client. Informed consent is necessary before testing is done.

*Classification*
Competency Category: Professional Practice
Taxonomic Level: Critical Thinking

**221. Answer:** Eleanor did not carry out the appropriate postoperative assessment for a client who has had a total thyroidectomy.

*Rationale*
Trousseau's sign and Chvostek' s sign are required and routine postoperative assessments for patients who have undergone a thyroidectomy. When a client has had thyroid surgery or any surgery or injury that might injure the parathyroid glands, assessment of calcium deficit is required. A calcium deficit will lead to a positive T and C test result. The nurse caring for the client should have included this assessment technique as part of the routine postoperative assessment. By missing the signs of a low calcium level, the nurse is negligent.

*Classification*
Competency Category: Professional Practice
Taxonomic Level: Application

**222. Answer:** Two tablets.

*Rationale*
The nurse is responsible for administering the appropriate dose of medication.

*Classification*
Competency Category: Professional Practice
Taxonomic Level: Knowledge/Comprehension

**223. Answer:** Two tablets.

*Rationale*
The nurse is responsible for administering the correct dose of medication.

*Classification*
Competency Category: Professional Practice
Taxonomic Level: Knowledge/Comprehension

**224. Answers:**

- Report her concerns to the supervisor.
- Thoroughly document the assessment findings.
- Document the conversation with the physician.

*Rationale*
The nurse has a responsibility to advocate for the patient and ensure that he receives appropriate care. The nurse should have taken her assessment finding and concerns to her supervisor before the client left the hospital.

*Classification*
Competency Category: Professional Practice
Taxonomic Level: Critical Thinking

**225. Answer:** Simon has a responsibility to practice within his level of competence. When seeking employment, he must accurately state his area of competence. In this situation, Simon has not done this and is breaching an ethical standard that could lead to unsafe patient care.

*Rationale*
Simon has a professional responsibility to present himself accurately when applying for a job.

*Classification*
Competency Category: Professional Practice
Taxonomic Level: Application

**226. Answer:** Nurses must avoid any punishment, unusual treatment, or action that is inhumane or degrading. Taking the client's clothes away, which resulted in her walking in the hall naked, is unethical, degrading, and unprofessional. This is not an appropriate means to change patient behaviour.

*Rationale*
The Code of Ethics for Canadian Nurses clearly states that nurses must recognize and respect the inherent worth of each person and advocate for respectful treatment of all persons. This behaviour does not reflect this kind of ethical behaviour.

*Classification*
Competency Category: Professional Practice
Taxonomic Level: Application

**227. Answers:**

- Have him work the day shift only.
- Ensure that he gets his regular breaks.

- Reduce his work load.
- Ensure that he does not work more than four shifts in a row.

*Rationale*
All of these options would accommodate the nurse's disability without causing undue hardship to the employer.

*Classification*
Competency Category: Professional Practice
Taxonomic Level: Application

**228. Answers:**

- Amplification on the telephone
- Amplified stethoscopes
- Automated blood pressure cuffs with digital readout displays
- Pulse oximetry with digital readout displays
- Vibrating pager
- Taped reports that can be replayed as needed
- Smoke alarms and other alarms that have lights as well as sound

*Rationale*
All of these assistive devices assist nurses experiencing hearing loss and assist employers to meet their obligations to accommodate workers' disabilities.

*Classification*
Competency Category: Professional Practice
Taxonomic Level: Knowledge/Comprehension

**229. Answer:** Michael should not hang the blood because he is aware of the client's wishes. He could be found liable for battery if he proceeds.

*Rationale*
Michael is aware of the client's right to refuse treatment and believes the client made this decision as a competent person. He understands that he is an advocate for the client and should not provide a treatment he knows that the client has refused.

*Classification*
Competency Category: Professional Practice
Taxonomic Level: Critical Thinking

**230. Answer:** He should call his manager to report the situation and ask for support.

*Rationale*
Clients have the right to refuse treatment. Consent for or against treatment must be made by competent individuals. Nurses must contact their supervisors when they believe the client has refused treatment.

*Classification*
Competency Category: Professional Practice
Taxonomic Level: Application

**231. Answer:** The client was not able to give or refuse consent because of her cognitive state. The underlying assumption is that the client has come to the hospital for care and the unit of blood is an appropriate treatment for her low hemoglobin.

*Rationale*
There was no one with the client to give consent. The nurse would not be liable for battery in this case.

*Classification*
Competency Category: Professional Practice
Taxonomic Level: Critical Thinking

**232. Answer:** Immunizations must be stored at a temperature of 4° to 8°C. It is important to document the temperature of the refrigerator to record and maintain the "cold chain" and integrity of vaccines.

*Rationale*
The nurse is aware of the safety measures and safe storage of vaccines. Documentation will protect the nurse, the facility, and the public by ensuring a record of the temperature the refrigerator is kept at and the appropriate steps taken if the temperature moves outside the acceptable range.

*Classification*
Competency Category: Professional Practice
Taxonomic Level: Knowledge/Comprehension

**233. Answers:**

- Instructions regarding the dressing on the venous ulcer
- Safety precautions regarding protecting the venous ulcer and other skin areas
- Bonnie's expectations regarding the UHCW's reporting back to her after turning the patient

*Rationale*
Bonnie is within her rights to delegate the turning of the client to an UHCW as long as she gives specific instructions regarding special circumstances such as how to ensure safe turning when the client has a dressing and a venous ulcer. Bonnie should also ensure that the UHCW has the knowledge, skill, and ability to perform the task and knows what information Bonnie requires after completing the task.

*Classification*
Competency Category: Professional Practice
Taxonomic Level: Knowledge/Comprehension

**234. Answer:** The client's hemoglobin may be falsely low.

*Rationale*
The nurse should be aware of the impact of overhydration on hemoglobin so that he or she can advocate for the client for appropriate treatment.

*Classification*
Competency Category: Professional Practice
Taxonomic Level: Knowledge/Comprehension

**235. Answers:**

- This is a medication error and must be reported.
- Ensure that the nursing manager is notified.
- Ensure that the physician is notified.
- Ensure that an incident report is completed.
- Ensure that the child is assessed for adverse effects.

*Rationale*
Tony has witnessed a medication error. He is responsible for following up on what he has observed. He must ensure that the child has not been injured and then must report the error. Ideally, the nurse who made the mistake should report the incident and should demonstrate that he or she is responsible for his or her own acts.

*Classification*
Competency Category: Professional Practice
Taxonomic Level: Critical Thinking

**236. Answers:** The feedback is:

- Immediate
- Frequent
- Specific
- Objective
- Based on observable behaviour
- Communicated appropriately
- Communicated in private
- Accompanied by suggestions for change

*Rationale*
All of these qualities are essential when giving effective feedback regarding performance to adults. These qualities will avoid defensiveness on the part of the receiver. This type of feedback leads to a greater chance of positive behaviour changes or modification.

*Classification*
Competency Category: Professional Practice
Taxonomic Level: Critical Thinking

## ▶ Self-Analysis for Chapter 3

200 Multiple choice questions × 1 point each = /200 points
+
36 Short answer questions for a total of 61 points = /61 points

*Total Professional Practice review questions =/261 points*

## PROFESSIONAL PRACTICE BIBLIOGRAPHY

Alfaro-LeFevre, R. (2006) *Applying nursing process: A tool for critical thinking*. Philadelphia: Lippincott Williams & Wilkins.

Bandman, E., & Bertram B. (2002). *Nursing ethics through the life span* (4th ed.). Upper Saddler River, NJ: Pearson Education.

Canadian Nurses Association (2002). *Code of ethics for registered nurses*. Ottawa, ON: Author.

Fortinash, K.M., & Holoday-Warret, P.A. (2007). *Psychiatric nursing care plans* (5th ed.). St. Louis: Mosby Elsevier.

Huston, C.J. (2006). *Professional issues in nursing: Challenges & opportunities*. Philadelphia: Lippincott Williams & Wilkins.

Ignatavicius, D., & Workman, M.L. (2006). *Medical surgical nursing: Critical thinking for collaborative care*. Philadelphia: WB Saunders.

Lo, B. (2005). *Resolving ethical dilemmas: A guide for clinicians*. Philadelphia: Lippincott Williams & Wilkins.

Marquis, B.L., & Huston, C.J. (2006). *Leadership roles and management functions in nursing theory and applications* (5th ed.). Philadelphia: Lippincott Williams & Wilkins.

Morris, D.G. (2006). *Calculate with confidence*. St. Louis: Mosby Elsevier.

Tappen, R. (2001). *Nursing leadership and management: Concepts and practice* (4th ed.). Philadelphia: F.A. Davis Company.

Taylor C., Lillis, C., & LeMone, P. *Fundamentals of nursing* (5th ed.). Philadelphia: Lippincott Williams & Wilkins.

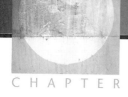

# 4 Care of Adults and Older Adults

**Directions:** Below are 354 multiple-choice questions and short answer questions totalling 448 points. These questions will test your knowledge of nursing with the care of adults and older adults. These questions offer a wide array of case-based and stand-alone questions representing the taxonomies of critical thinking, application, and knowledge/comprehension. Also reflected in these questions are the nursing competencies of health and wellness, alterations in health, professional practice, and nurse–person relationship. After completing these multiple-choice and short answer questions, compare your work with the Answers and Rationales provided at the end of the chapter. Please make note of the questions you found difficult and develop a plan to help increase your knowledge of these areas.

## ▶ Multiple-Choice Questions

1. The nursing unit manager on a medical teaching unit says that she would like a nurse to present a case study at interdisciplinary rounds on a patient who has compartment syndrome from a leg injury. This is the first patient you have cared for with this complication, and you have difficulty presenting your ideas in front of a group. What would you do?

   A. Ask to attend the rounds to increase your understanding of the condition.
   B. Research the condition and present what you have learned as well as your assessment findings and care measures.
   C. Suggest that a more experienced nurse be selected to present this case study.
   D. Approach the unit manager, explain your difficulty presenting in front of interdisciplinary team members, and ask to be excused from presenting.

2. Which of the following situations would indicate a professional boundary violation?

   A. To empathize with a patient's situation, sharing a personal experience with a patient that is very similar to the situation the patient is experiencing.
   B. Reminding a patient who has dementia that certain sexual touch behaviours are not acceptable.
   C. Being concerned about a patient's welfare and seeking ways to protect the client's best interests.
   D. Having well-intentioned behaviours that detract from achievable health outcomes for patients.

3. An important component of professional practice is self-awareness. Why is self-awareness an important basis for nursing practice?

   A. It may prevent biases and assumptions from affecting relationships.
   B. It may allow the nurse to examine how biases and assumptions could interfere with therapeutic effectiveness.
   C. It may enable the nurse to treat people from different cultural backgrounds according to the dominant beliefs of their culture.
   D. It allows for more objectivity in facilitating the healing process.

4. Which of the following is a theoretical perspective that underlies group process and effectiveness?

   A. The personality style theory acknowledges that the nature of individuals in a group helps us understand group dynamics and sources of conflict in the group.
   B. When groups are formed to complete a task, the task functions need to be assigned to individuals to ensure effective group functioning.

C. Considering the roles and functions of groups would explain the developmental theory of groups.

D. For group effectiveness, a group needs to have homogeneity and common views and interests.

5. Which of the following group principles interferes with the effectiveness of a group?

A. Groups get to know each other while focusing on accomplishing tasks.

B. Groups set norms, cooperate, and monitor progress.

C. Groups encourage similarity of viewpoints and minimize differing opinions.

D. Groups deal with conflicts and allow members to express their differences.

6. Janna, age 27 years, a single mother, appreciates the help you have given her through the birth of her first child. When you conclude your last follow-up community visit, she expresses gratitude and suggests that you come back and visit her and the baby for regular outings. How would you respond?

A. Acknowledge your appreciation of this experience, explain that her nursing needs have been met, and tell her you have to leave to care for other new mothers.

B. Thank her for the offer and tell her that you will have to give her a call to see whether you will be able to work in outings in your personal schedule.

C. Tell her this would be unprofessional.

D. State that you would really like to do this but you are too busy with your other commitments.

_____

**Case Study:** *The night before heart surgery involving a quadruple bypass, Mr. Carlson has signed his consent. The morning of the surgery, he states that he has changed his mind and wants to cancel the surgery. Questions 7 and 8 relate to this scenario.*

7. How would you respond to Mr. Carlson?

A. Remind him that he has signed the consent and that the surgery has been scheduled.

B. Discuss his fears regarding the surgery and reassure him that many patients want to change their minds as the surgery draws near.

C. Explore reasons why he wishes to cancel the surgery, clarify his concerns, and reinforce that he can change his mind if he chooses.

D. Tell him not to make up his mind until the doctor comes to talk to him again.

8. Mr. Carlson makes the decision to sign himself out of the hospital. What actions would you take?

A. Ensure that he signs the release form and contact the doctor and the operating room staff.

B. Convince him to stay because heart surgery is very important.

C. Contact the nursing unit manager and document it in the chart.

D. Realistically explain the wait list for surgery and what could happen to him.

9. You are admitting Darlene, age 40 years, who has come in for regulation of her insulin-dependent diabetes. When she is unpacking, you note that she has a bag with some of her used syringes with needles, which she places in the top drawer of her bedside table. What would you do?

A. Reinforce that she should keep the syringes in her suitcase so there are no injuries to staff members.

B. Ask her why she is keeping the used syringes and ensure they are disposed of safely.

C. Ask her to glove and dispose of the contaminated syringes in the needle receptacle.

D. Report the incident to the diabetic care team so effective teaching can be done.

10. You are supervising a nursing student during a dressing change. When the student is removing the dressing from a leg ulcer, the patient begins to yell and swear at both of you. He threatens to throw the water pitcher if both of you don't leave his room immediately. What should you do?

A. Leave the leg ulcer undressed and exit the room immediately.

B. Report the incident to the doctor and have him or her explain that this behaviour will not be tolerated.

C. Temporarily dress the wound, explain that verbal abuse is not tolerated, leave the room, and return later to discuss alternate wound dressing strategies.

D. Firmly explain that that behaviour will not be tolerated, remove the water pitcher, and continue applying the dressing.

11. You have completed your initial assessment and charting on a patient with chronic obstructive pulmonary disease. When you go back into the room 1 hour later, you note that his status has changed: He has become confused and does not know where he is; is taking short, rapid breaths

at 34 breaths/min; has to sit up to breathe; and has a bluish tinge around his lips. His oxygen saturation levels have gone from 94% to 84%. What would you document for the assessment?

A. Confused and disoriented X3. Dyspneic. Pallor of lips. Oxygen saturation dropped from 94% to 84%.

B. Confused. Cheyne Stokes breathing at rate of 34/min. Positioned in Fowler's position. Blue lips.

C. Disoriented. Tachypneic breathing at 34/min. Short of breath. Oxygen saturation at 84%.

D. Disoriented to place, tachypneic, shallow breathing at 34/min, orthopneic with circumoral cyanosis. Oxygen saturation at 84%.

12. Laurana, age 24 years, is being discharged today after the birth of her first baby. She is concerned about how she will manage at home and wonders how she can get her questions answered. What sources of information would you suggest?

A. Parents and friends.

B. A retired nurse in her neighbourhood and web sites.

C. Community health clinics, telehealth, and hospital-based web site.

D. Pamphlets, library books, husband, parents, and in-laws.

13. What is the most important responsibility when inserting a nasogastric (NG) tube?

A. Accurate measurement and lubrication of the NG tube.

B. Asking the patient to breathe deeply when the tube is inserted past the nasopharynx.

C. Encouraging the patient to swallow sips of water to facilitate the insertion.

D. Checking the placement of the tube by aspiration and testing the pH of the contents.

---

*Case Study:* Mrs. April Hume, age 86 years, has been admitted with advanced liver metastasis after a mastectomy. She is very weak and is experiencing abdominal pain, has ascites, and is having difficulty breathing. She has requested that only supportive measures be given. Questions 14 and 15 relate to this scenario.

14. Which would be priority nursing interventions?

A. Addressing concerns she might have regarding death and dying, encouraging family support, and promoting her independence in meeting her needs.

B. Initiating oxygen therapy, Fowler's positioning, pain control, and addressing her questions and concerns.

C. Encouraging her to eat, mobilizing her every 2 hours, and having her perform deep breathing and coughing exercises every half hour.

D. Ensuring that she understands that she is on a palliative care unit and explaining that only comfort measures she requests will be followed.

15. Mrs. Hume is anxious and concerned about her breathing difficulties. She states that she feels that breathing is taking so much energy that she is hardly able to eat. She is having difficulty mobilizing because of the pain and spends most of her time in bed. She says that her family is concerned about her lack of progress. What would you do?

A. Explore other ways to more effectively control her symptoms and advocate for her when approaching her family.

B. Reinforce the meaning of supportive care to her family and restrict their visits so Mrs. Hume has more rest time.

C. Provide support for the family and encourage Mrs. Hume to become more actively involved in her care.

D. Determine where the patient is regarding the stages of dying and discuss the findings with her family.

16. If a mass casualty occurs near your acute care unit, what would be included in a disaster preparedness plan?

A. An informal fanout to contact and inform all registered nurses about the disaster and elicit their help in assisting with the casualties.

B. A formal written plan of action for coordinating the response of the hospital staff and to designate how different areas will be used.

C. A designation of levels of casualty care and having nurses volunteer services at different levels.

D. A formal plan to ensure that medical supplies and medications are available for the great number of casualties.

17. Mrs. Jones recently had a cystectomy for bladder cancer. She has an ileal conduit (urostomy). What teaching would you include?

A. How to protect the skin, how to apply a dressing over the ostomy site, and the importance of reporting shreds of mucus in the urine as evidence of a urinary tract infection.

B. Stoma care and application of an ostomy pouch and drainage bag, increasing intake of fluids, observing amount and the colour of the urine.

C. Odour control, skin cleansing, and irrigation of the ostomy.

D. Signs of infection or skin breakdown, intermittent application of the appliance, and the importance of dietary restrictions.

18. Which of the following patients require increased sensory stimulation to prevent sensory deprivation?

   A. A 24-year-old patient who has been admitted with an anxiety disorder and appears very agitated.

   B. A 60-year-old patient who is blind, reads books through use of Braille, listens to the radio, and regularly takes walks around the unit.

   C. A 65-year-old patient who has employment-induced presbycusis and advanced glaucoma.

   D. An 84-year-old patient who has hemiparesis and ambulates with a walker.

19. Mrs. Starface, age 62 years, a First Nations patient, has been admitted with a chronic cough and progressive weight loss. She has a positive Mantoux test result, and is placed in isolation for suspected tuberculosis. What isolation precautions should the nurse take?

   A. Have her wear a disposable mask when she is transported to the radiography department.

   B. Wear a gown and gloves while in her isolation room.

   C. Wear a disposable mask, gown, and gloves while giving care.

   D. Discourage visitors from spending time with the patient to reduce transmission.

20. Mrs. Mames, age 27 years, gravida 1, para 0, is admitted in active labour. She states that her contractions are very intense and that she needs pain medication. What is the most important factor to assess before analgesic administration?

   A. Her respiratory rate and fetal heart rate during contractions.

   B. The frequency, duration, and intensity of her contractions.

   C. The effectiveness of the coaching from her husband.

D. How well she manages through the next five contractions.

21. Mrs. Davies, gravida 2, para 1, is admitted at 8 weeks gestation for a moderate amount of bleeding and abdominal cramps. A day later, the bleeding stops, and she is being discharged. What would you include in discharge teaching?

   A. Ask her how badly she wants this baby and what she would be willing to do to ensure carrying the baby to term.

   B. Ask her if she understands the reason for the cramping and bleeding and explain what precautions she could take to retain the pregnancy.

   C. Explain that nature aborts the fetus if it is abnormal and that bleeding and cramps may indicate an abnormality.

   D. Ask her if she has been eating nutritious meals and restricting her activity during pregnancy.

22. Mr. Jones, age 64 years, had a transurethral resection of the prostate yesterday. How could you detect hypovolemic shock in this client?

   A. Slow, irregular heart rate and pulse deficit.

   B. Bounding pulse and hypotension.

   C. Pallor, cold extremities, and tachycardia.

   D. Dark red–tinged urine, shivering, and confusion.

23. Jennifer, age 16 years, is admitted to the postanesthesia recovery room after wiring of a fractured jaw. She is conscious. Her breathing has become noisy and shallow. Her oxygen saturation levels were at 98 and now are at 90. What actions would you take?

   A. Position her in Sims position with her head to the side, give oxygen as ordered, and suction if needed.

   B. Position her in Fowler's position to assist her in breathing and give oxygen as ordered.

   C. Insert an airway, suction her, and position her in the supine position.

   D. Encourage her to breathe deeply, position her in the prone position, and give oxygen as ordered.

24. Daniel, age 16 years, had a cast applied after a fracture of the tibia. When teaching him before discharge about detecting signs of impaired circulation and nervous system functioning, which signs would indicate problems?

   A. Pallor, coolness, and numbness of the toes.

   B. Pain at the fracture site and a small amount of bleeding through the cast.

C. Inability to move the leg at the fracture site.

D. Slight edema of the foot and presence of pedal pulse.

25. Mr. Blair had a bowel resection 2 days ago and has had a nasogastric (NG) tube inserted. He is complaining of increased abdominal pain and nausea. What assessments or actions would be most appropriate?

A. Check the patency and amount of drainage from the NG tube.

B. Give him an analgesic and antiemetic as ordered.

C. Irrigate the NG tube with water and give an analgesic as ordered.

D. Explain that nausea is common because the NG tube irritates the gag reflex.

26. Mr. Evans has ascites secondary to cirrhosis of the liver. He is jaundiced and malnourished. Which of the following problems is not associated with cirrhosis of the liver?

A. Eupnea related to esophageal varices.

B. Potential for pressure ulcers related to malnourishment.

C. Concentrated, dark urine related to kidney excretion of bile byproducts.

D. Confusion and disorientation related to increase in circulating toxins.

27. Mrs. Chu had a cholecystectomy 2 days ago. Which signs would indicate a wound infection?

A. Serosanguineous drainage, temperature of 38°C, and abdominal pain.

B. Purulent drainage, pain in the mid incision, and temperature of 38.5°C.

C. Serous drainage, temperature of 38°C, and redness of the incision line.

D. Sanguinous drainage, temperature of 37.5°C, and bradycardia.

28. Dillon is 7 years old and weighs 30 kg. He has acute streptococcal pharyngitis. He is prescribed Keflex (cephalexin) 26.67 mg/kg q6h. How much would he receive in each dose?

A. 150 mg.

B. 200 mg.

C. 400 mg.

D. None of the above.

29. Jane, age 18 years, has an asthma attack when in the hospital. She is in respiratory distress. What initial action would you take?

A. Position her in the supine position and administer oxygen and bronchodilators as ordered.

B. Position her in the Sims position and give bronchodilators as ordered.

C. Position her in Fowler's position, initiate oxygen, and give bronchodilators as ordered.

D. Give bronchodilators and steroid medication as ordered.

30. Mrs. Jones, age 34 years, returns from the recovery room after bowel surgery. She is receiving morphine sulfate through a patient-controlled analgesia (PCA) pump. When you assess her pain levels, her pain intensity is 8 of 10. When you ask her if she has been using the button to relieve her pain, she states, "I'm afraid that I'll become addicted if I use too much morphine." Which would be the best response to her concern?

A. "Morphine is not addicting in these circumstances."

B. "You need to take the morphine to help you rest and recuperate from the surgery; you can deal with the addiction later."

C. "When morphine is used to alleviate severe pain for 2 to 3 days, there is little likelihood of becoming addicted."

D. "Have you had problems with drug addiction before?"

31. Mr. Keaton, age 65 years, has aplastic anemia and is going to receive a transfusion of packed blood cells. In addition to taking vital signs and verifying that packed blood cells are matched to the patient, what other assessments would you make?

A. Assess pain at the transfusion site and transfuse the packed blood cells over 5 hours to lessen reactions.

B. Check the patient regarding chills, low back pain, dyspnea, and skin itching during the transfusion.

C. Ask the patient about headaches, maintaining bed rest during the transfusion, and reducing intake of fluids to reduce the likelihood of fluid overload.

D. Transfuse the blood quickly for the first 15 minutes and then check for abnormal breath sounds and other symptoms.

32. Mrs. Kilts, age 84 years, has hypostatic pneumonia. When you complete your assessment, which of the following would indicate hypoxia?

A. Tachypnea, orthopnea, tachycardia, and circumoral cyanosis.

B. Hypotension, bradycardia, bradypnea, and use of accessory muscles in the neck.

C. Eupnea, hypertension, bradycardia, and cyanosis of the nail beds.

D. Occasional productive cough, pursed-lip breathing, and nasal flaring.

33. When you enter the recreation room, you observe Sara Jones, age 20 years, pacing, speaking in a threatening manner, and appearing to defend herself. She has been diagnosed with paranoid schizophrenia. What approach would you take?

A. Approach her directly and tell her you are going to get her some medication to help her calm down.

B. Ignore her until she calms down and then approach her gently and ask what is wrong.

C. Ask her if she is hallucinating and whether she has taken her medication today.

D. Approach her calmly and find out what is causing her to be upset.

34. Mr. Pritchard, age 55 years, has been informed by his doctor that his pancreatic cancer is inoperable and that it has spread to his liver. When you enter the room, he states, "The doctor feels that things are hopeless. I hate this place. You're all so useless. Just leave me alone." What would be a therapeutic response?

A. "This is devastating news for you. I'll let you have some time and will come back later."

B. "You are much too young to have inoperable cancer. How does your family feel about this?"

C. "You'll need to get over this. Your family needs you to get your affairs in order."

D. "Why are you upset with us? You need some time to calm down."

35. Mr. Corwin, age 74 years, has had an open reduction and internal fixation (ORIF) after a right hip fracture. What are important priorities on the first postoperative day?

A. Supporting the leg to maintain adduction, ensuring adequate pain control, and maintaining bed rest.

B. Assessing the neurovascular status in the right leg; providing pain control; and encouraging deep breathing and coughing exercises, position changes, and early ambulation.

C. Assessing for skin integrity, enhancing his nutritional status, and restricting his movement and activity in bed.

D. Preventing confusion and disorientation, restricting analgesics, and encouraging pursed-lip breathing.

36. Mr. Balm, age 70 years, comes into the emergency department with acute onset of severe chest pain, dyspnea, and anxiety. His respirations are 28 breaths/min, and he has circumoral cyanosis with an oxygen saturation of 84%. What would your immediate actions be?

A. Gather information regarding the nature and intensity of the chest pain.

B. Place him in Fowler's position, initiate oxygen therapy, and get an analgesic ordered.

C. Keep him in the supine position, encourage deep breathing, and request an ECG.

D. Get an order for an analgesic, position him in the side-lying position, and encourage pursed-lip breathing.

37. During a gymnastics practice, 18-year-old Tracey falls and fractures her right tibia. The doctor asks to be notified if anterior compartment syndrome presents in the right extremity. What signs and symptoms would indicate this syndrome?

A. Edema of the right foot, loss of sensation in the right leg, and hypotension.

B. Edema of the right foot, redness on the skin surface of the calf, and poor capillary refill in the toenails.

C. Severe pain aggravated by plantarflexion, tense and tender muscles in the lateral right calf, and paresthesia.

D. Painful contracture of the calf muscles, inability to extend the leg, and redness and warmth in the calf region.

38. Mr. Harris, age 65 years, had an abdominal perineal resection for cancer of the rectum. He is receiving morphine via a patient-control analgesia (PCA) pump. What would your priority assessment be regarding the analgesia?

A. The rate and depth of respiration.

B. The pulse rate and blood pressure.

C. The effectiveness of pain control.

D. The accuracy of the programming on the pump.

39. You are caring for Shauna, an 18-year-old gymnast who has been admitted for investigation of seizures. She weighs 50 kg. For two meals, you observe that she eats a very small amount of salad and skim milk. What approach would you take?

A. Tell her you will have a dietician come to assess her eating habits.

B. Ask her about her usual eating patterns and reason for her low intake.

C. Inform the doctor regarding her poor intake and suggest an appetite stimulant.

D. Inform her that if she isn't eating foods, a nasogastric feeding tube will have to be inserted.

40. When you complete the initial postoperative assessment for Mr. Violini, age 55 years, you note that his IV is infusing at 200 cc/hr. You check the order, which reads: "IV of 1000 cc D5S to infuse over 8 hours." What actions would you take?

    A. Continue infusing the IV at 200 cc/hr and observe his hydration status.
    B. Change the rate to 125 cc/hr and observe for fluid overload.
    C. Reduce the rate to 150 cc/hr and observe for fluid overload.
    D. Tell him that he should not adjust the flow clamp on the IV.

41. Dana Evans, age 19 years, has been admitted after an asthma attack. When you complete your assessment, you observe that she is anxious, has audible wheezing, and is using her neck muscles when breathing. What would you do?

    A. Position her in orthopneic position, encourage coughing exercises, and ask her to calm down.
    B. Position her in Fowler's position, administer oxygen, and give her the ordered prn lorazepam (Ativan) 2 mg.
    C. Encourage her to lie in a semi-prone position, perform diaphragmatic breathing, and give her the ordered prn beclomethasone dipropionate (Beclovent) inhaler.
    D. Position her in Fowler's position, administer oxygen as ordered, and give her the ordered prn med salbutamol (Ventolin) by inhaler.

42. Mr. Lexus, age 33 years, comes into the emergency department with severe back pain radiating to the left lower groin region. The doctor suspects renal calculi and orders meperidine HCl (Demerol) 100 mg IM q3–4h prn. One hour after Mr. Lexus receives the medication, he states that the pain is still at 8 of 10. What actions would you take?

    A. Explain that the medication takes longer than 1 hour to exert its effects.
    B. Tell him he will have to wait for 2 more hours before he can get his next injection.
    C. Contact the doctor, explain that the pain is still at 8 of 10, and request a higher dosage.
    D. Ask Mr. Lexus if he has routinely taken painkillers or street drugs.

43. Which of the following indicates that the nurse is using critical thinking skills?

    A. The nurse follows the routine of the unit and encourages others to do the same.
    B. The nurse asks another nurse to outline the steps in performing a wound packing.
    C. The nurse does not know the answer and checks to find the answer on the unit or in the library.
    D. The nurse asks the patient about the symptoms she is experiencing and lists them on the care plan.

44. Which is the most important step in the nursing process?

    A. The assessment step because it involves collecting, organizing, and validating information that is used for the remaining steps.
    B. The nursing diagnosis step because it involves identifying the problems.
    C. The planning step because it identifies ways to reduce, prevent, and resolve problems.
    D. The implementation step because it ensures that interventions are effective.

45. When identifying the nursing diagnosis or patient problems, which statement is most accurate?

    A. The nursing diagnosis helps to clarify the medical diagnosis and the problems that result from this diagnosis.
    B. Critical thinking skills are used to interpret, analyze, and cluster the assessment data to determine the problems.
    C. The nursing diagnosis focuses on ways to prevent, reduce, or resolve the identified problems.
    D. The identification of patient problems provides the means of measuring the degree to which the goals are met.

46. When performing a psychosocial assessment, which areas should be assessed?

    A. Breathing patterns, circulation patterns, and metabolic needs.
    B. Health habits, family, and social and sexual patterns.
    C. General survey, movement, eating habits, and activities of daily living.
    D. Rest and sleep patterns, activity and exercise patterns, and coping and stress tolerance.

47. What is the primary purpose of conducting a health history?

    A. Identify the risk factors and how to promote health for the client.

B. Obtain information to identify the level of health of the client and his or her past illnesses.

C. Examine the chief complaint of the client and related factors.

D. Provide for health teaching opportunities.

48. When completing the physical assessment of the abdomen, which is the first skill used in the assessment?

A. Palpation.

B. Auscultation.

C. Percussion.

D. Inspection.

49. Which of the following statements heard during shift report identifies an important priority for action?

A. A patient is reluctant to ambulate on the evening of surgery.

B. A postoperative patient's pulse has been increasing, and his blood pressure is decreasing.

C. A postoperative patient is drowsy and slow to respond when the analgesic is at its maximal effect.

D. A postoperative patient has not voided for 5 hours after surgery.

50. Upon completion of teaching related to Lanoxin (digoxin), a client is able to explain the effects of the medication and when not take it and can also identify the radial pulse site. What would this indicate?

A. An accurate assessment of her teaching needs.

B. An evaluation of psychomotor and cognitive learning.

C. A high degree of motivation.

D. An independent learner.

51. When teaching a group of middle-aged women, what would you include when discussing primary prevention?

A. Prevention of anemia and type 1 diabetes.

B. Prevention of ulcers and inflammatory bowel disease.

C. Fall prevention and maintaining joint mobility.

D. Prevention of osteoporosis and the importance of regular breast self-examinations and regular Pap smears.

52. A community health nurse is planning to address the needs of elderly adults living in their homes. What primary areas should be included in this discussion?

A. Importance of exercise, balanced nutrition and hydration, and safety and fall prevention.

B. Prevention of joint deterioration and mobility problems.

C. Prevention of hearing and visual deficits.

D. Importance of frequent doctor visits and access to health care resources.

53. Which of the following legal definitions is true?

A. Good Samaritan laws are designed to protect victims in emergency situations.

B. Negligence is intentional failure to act responsibly or deliberate omission of a professional act.

C. Malpractice is failure to perform professional duties that result in patient injury.

D. Scope of practice involves general guidelines that define nursing.

54. A nurse has delegated the taking of vital signs for an unregulated health care provider. When a client's blood pressure is reported as high, the registered nurse rechecks the blood pressure and other vital signs for the patient. What would these actions be called?

A. Obligation to the patient.

B. Reversing of delegation.

C. Empowerment of the patient.

D. Accountability for care.

55. When suctioning a tracheotomy, which actions are correct?

A. Insert the suction catheter as far as patient can tolerate and suction for 25 seconds.

B. Oxygenate the patient and then suction for 10 to 15 seconds while withdrawing the catheter.

C. Suction every 15 minutes to prevent secretions from accumulating.

D. Commence suctioning upon insertion of the catheter and continue for 5 seconds while withdrawing the catheter.

56. A patient has been admitted to the emergency department after a car accident. He is sent to the hospital unit after emergency chest tube insertion. What would constitute an emergency situation with the chest tube?

A. Bubbling of air in the underwater seal chamber.

B. Improper suction setting on the wall suction.

C. Disconnection of the connecting tubing from the chest tube.

D. Drainage of bloody material into the drainage chamber.

57. A postoperative patient after bowel surgery has orders for DAT (diet as tolerated). What assessments would indicate return of peristalsis?

A. Distended abdomen and tympany on percussion.

   B. Soft abdomen and absence of bowel sounds
      on auscultation.
   C. Intermittent cramping, abdominal pain, and
      bowel sounds in all four quadrants.
   D. Nausea, vomiting, and pain on palpation.

58. A patient has a patient-controlled analgesia
    (PCA) pump with morphine after a bowel
    resection. What are the nursing responsibilities
    after the client has self-administered a bolus of
    medication?

    A. Have the client mobilize to reduce the
       harmful effects of morphine.
    B. Ensure that the client understands that a
       bolus may take up to 15 minute to alleviate
       the pain.
    C. Encourage deep breathing and coughing
       exercises to lessen respiratory depression.
    D. Reduce the amount of IV pain medication
       being administered on a regular basis.

59. Your assigned patient has been requesting a
    stronger pain medication. In response, the doctor
    has ordered morphine combined with a
    nonsteroidal antiinflammatory drug (NSAID) for
    pain relief. How would you explain the effective-
    ness of these two medications?

    A. Combining these two drugs will increase pain
       relief without the increased side effects of
       increasing the morphine dose.
    B. The two drugs are antagonistic, so they will
       relieve the pain but will counteract the side
       effects.
    C. Combining the two drugs will lessen the
       incidence of addiction.
    D. The NSAID will relieve muscle pain; the
       morphine will act centrally on the central
       nervous system to relieve pain.

60. In addition to the pain medication, what other
    measures help promote comfort and alleviate
    pain?

    A. Encouraging ambulation and vigorous
       rubbing of the inflamed tissues.
    B. Gentle massage of the area, warm and cold
       applications, guided imagery, and TENS.
    C. Prolonged heat applications followed by
       prolonged cold application to the area.
    D. Encouraging tensing of muscles and
       performing distraction exercises.

61. Which of the following would be indicators of
    severe hypoxia?

    A. Generalized pallor and eupnea.
    B. Circumoral cyanosis and $PaO_2$ of 70 mm Hg.
    C. Low oxygen saturation levels of 95%.
    D. Increased anxiety and drowsiness.

62. What nursing measures are important when a
    Foley retention catheter has been inserted?

    A. The Foley catheter should be left unsecured
       to prevent urethral irritation.
    B. Urine samples should be obtained by discon-
       necting the catheter from the drainage bag.
    C. The patient should limit fluid intake to keep
       the catheter patent.
    D. Reflux of urine from the tubing to the bladder
       should be prevented.

63. You read through your assigned patient's chart.
    The history states: "Paroxysmal nocturnal dyspnea;
    reduced CSWM in left leg." What do these medical
    history terms and abbreviations indicate?

    A. The patient is experiencing intermittent
       shortness of breath, is unable to breathe
       unless in a supine position, and has impaired
       venous return in the left leg.
    B. The patient is experiencing painful breathing
       and shortness of breath with exertion and has
       impaired arterial flow to the left leg.
    C. The patient is experiencing periods of severe
       shortness of breath at night and impaired cir-
       culation and sensory and motor functioning
       in the left leg.
    D. The patient has reduced breathing capacity,
       loss of breathing reserve, and impaired motor
       movement of the left leg.

64. Which sexuality alterations might emerge after a
    myocardial infarction (MI)?

    A. The patient may be concerned that a heart
       attack may occur during orgasm.
    B. Emotional concerns may interfere with the
       phase of resolution.
    C. The arousal phase may be affected by
       personal concerns.
    D. Sexual dysfunction may present because of
       reduced ventricular contractions.

65. Which of the following signs and symptoms
    would indicate impaired arterial circulation in
    the lower extremities?

    A. Capillary refill in the toenails within 2 seconds.
    B. Absence of dorsalis pedis pulse; coolness and
       decreased sensation in the feet.
    C. Edema and coolness in the ankles and feet.
    D. Redness, inflammation, and sharp pain with
       calf muscle contraction.

66. Which of the following isolation precautions
    would be relevant for the communicable illness
    identified?

    A. Airborne precautions are indicated for
       varicella (chickenpox) and involve wearing a
       mask when in the room.

B. Gloves, a mask, and a gown are worn when changing a wound dressing infected with *Staphylococcus* spp.

C. If a patient is infected with VRE (vancomycin-resistant *Enterococcus*), vital signs equipment is brought into the room every time it is needed.

D. Specimens obtained from a contaminated wound would be transferred directly to the laboratory without special precautions.

67. You are developing a care plan for a patient with tuberculosis. What isolation precautions would you take?

A. Use a special mask to prevent inhaling infected airborne droplets.

B. Wear a mask, gown, and gloves when providing care.

C. Wear a gown and gloves when in contact with the patient.

D. Prevent visitors from visiting to reduce the possibility of transmission.

68. You are assessing a patient who has been in a car accident. He complains about sore ribs and painful breathing on the left side of his chest cage. What assessment findings would alert you to a pneumothorax?

A. Pain on exhalation; fatigue.

B. Dyspnea; decreased breath sounds on the affected side.

C. Bradycardia and hypertension.

D. Tachypnea and hyperventilation.

69. A patient has been diagnosed with deep vein thrombosis (DVT). Suddenly, the patient develops chest pain and severe dyspnea. He looks anxious and is very apprehensive. What actions would you take?

A. Position him in Fowler's position, initiate oxygen, and call the physician.

B. Auscultate for abnormal breath sounds and encourage deep breathing.

C. Encourage pursed-lip breathing and coughing exercises.

D. Ambulate the patient, encourage deep breaths, and take the apical pulse.

70. Your patient has a cerebrovascular accident (CVA). Which of the following neurologic deficits may present after a CVA?

A. Visual field deficits such as homonymous hemianopsia.

B. Emotional changes such as lack of emotional response and enhanced coping.

C. Motor deficits such as paresthesia with numbness and tingling.

D. Verbal deficits such as dysphagia and memory loss.

71. Which of the following assessment findings are associated with cholelithiasis?

A. Associated risk factors include being male and athletic.

B. Jaundice is seen if the calculus lodges in the common bile duct.

C. Biliary colic attacks occur when there is stone formation in the gallbladder.

D. Symptoms of pain include steady LUQ pain radiating to the left scapula.

72. Which of the following assessment findings are seen in patients with cancer of the head of the pancreas?

A. Early onset of pain.

B. Anorexia, nausea, and vomiting.

C. Early onset of jaundice and pruritus.

D. Presence of steatorrhea, melena stools, and dilute urine.

73. A client presents with cirrhosis of the liver secondary to alcohol abuse. What assessment findings would indicate portal hypertension?

A. Ascites and hematemesis.

B. Pulmonary edema.

C. Absence of jugular vein distension.

D. Cramps and watery diarrhea.

74. After a total hip arthroplasty, what are the most important precautions to prevent dislocation?

A. Limit movements resulting in internal rotation and adduction of the affected hip.

B. Use a pillow under the knees to prevent hip flexion.

C. Reduce extension and hyperextension of the affected hip.

D. Use toilet seats to prevent circumduction of the hip joint.

75. Without hand washing between activities, a nurse makes an occupied bed and then assists another patient with meal preparation. Considering the chain of infection, which statement is true?

A. The new portal of entry of microorganisms could be through the mouth.

B. The mode of transmission is through direct contact.

C. Microorganisms from the bed making would be spread by direct contact.

D. An epidemic infection would occur if pathogens from the health care agency caused an illness.

76. What are characteristics of effective decision-making strategies in a nurse?

A. Reviewing the chart and duplicating the actions of previous nurses.

B. Gathering assessment data and analyzing and identifying priority problems.

C. Independently developing a plan of care based on the nurse's workload.

D. Willingness to follow the doctor's orders and directions without questioning his or her rationale.

77. What are important considerations when assessing and caring for a patient with pyrexia?

A. The patient usually experiences a decrease in vital signs.

B. The patient usually exhibits flushing of the skin and jaundice.

C. The patient may experience dehydration and convulsions from a high temperature.

D. The patient may experience increased urine output and dilute urine.

78. Which of the following statements is true regarding wound healing when an infection is present?

A. The infected portion of the wound will likely heal by primary intention.

B. The inflammatory phase of healing will be shortened.

C. The proliferative or regeneration phase will be delayed and prolonged.

D. There will be less formation of granulation tissue because of the infection.

79. Which of the following assessment factors would indicate a need for oral pharyngeal suctioning?

A. Thin sputum and a weak cough.

B. Breathing rate of 36 breaths/min; noisy, gurgling respirations.

C. Auscultation of fluid (rales and rhonchi) in the lower lobes of the lungs.

D. Oxygen saturation levels of 95%; use of diaphragmatic breathing.

80. Which of the following is an important consideration when performing oral–pharyngeal suctioning?

A. Oxygen provided before suctioning limits the effectiveness of the suction.

B. The nurse should only suction when the patient agrees to the procedure.

C. Fluid intake should be limited to reduce the secretions produced.

D. The duration of each suctioning episode should be 10 to 15 seconds.

81. What important postoperative care measures related to care of chest tubes should be done the day after a lobectomy?

A. Disconnect the tubing to empty and measure drainage at the end of each shift.

B. Frequently check the dressing and chest tube for drainage.

C. Ensure that all connections are securely taped.

D. Position the patient in the prone or supine position to permit optimal drainage.

82. Nutrients are important for wound healing. Which of the following is true regarding the role of specific nutrients in healing?

A. Vitamin C is needed for building capillaries and fibroblasts in the inflammatory phase.

B. Essential amino acids are needed to ensure building blocks are present for building or proliferative phase.

C. Nonessential fatty acids to provide a good supply of glucose for energy.

D. Vitamin K is needed for the convalescent phase to help restore energy and nutrient needs.

83. Mr. John G. has a history of cramps and has been experiencing diarrhea for the past 2 days. His urine is concentrated. You would assess for:

A. Dehydration by checking tissue turgor and checking mucous membranes.

B. Impaction as a result of the surgery.

C. Signs of kidney suppression because of the concentrated urine.

D. Absence of bowel sounds in the abdomen.

84. What assessment findings would indicate circulatory overload from too rapid an IV infusion?

A. Decreased pulse, decreased blood pressure, and jugular vein distension.

B. Increased pulse, increased respirations, and jugular vein distension.

C. Headache, paleness, and hypertension.

D. Increased temperature, peripheral edema, and decreased pulse rate.

85. Which is the priority system to assess when a patient has severe hypothyroidism?

A. Respiratory system.

B. Heart and circulation.

C. Neurologic system.

D. Integumentary system.

**86.** A patient with diabetes is being tested for glycosylated hemoglobin. How would you explain the reason for this diagnostic test?

A. It determines the fasting blood glucose level.

B. It determines the average blood glucose level in the previous 4 months.

C. It determines the ratio of glucose to hemoglobin.

D. It is used to identify a reduction in hemoglobin because of high glucose levels.

---

***Case Study:*** *Mr. Evan Jenkins, age 65 years, has had type 2 diabetes for 20 years and has been admitted to the hospital with chronic renal failure. Questions 87 to 90 relate to this scenario.*

**87.** When completing the initial assessment, which signs would indicate circulatory overload?

A. Increased blood pressure, apprehension, and shock.

B. Weight gain, coughing of frothy sputum, and jugular vein distension.

C. Cool, dry skin; gastric distension; and pleural edema.

D. Apprehension, poor tissue turgor, and bradycardia.

**88.** Which of the following statements is true regarding end-stage renal failure?

A. A common cause of renal failure is pyelonephritis.

B. It results in an increase in erythropoietin, leading to chronic fatigue.

C. It results in a decrease in creatinine and blood urea nitrogen.

D. It is characterized by fluid volume excess, hypernatremia, and hyperkalemia.

**89.** What are important nursing care measures for a patient with chronic renal failure?

A. Prepare the client for temporary peritoneal dialysis or hemodialysis.

B. Restrict sodium and potassium; restrict fluids as ordered.

C. Provide a diet high in protein; restrict fluids as ordered.

D. Monitor for hypotension and maintain accurate intake and output records.

**90.** Mr. Jenkins makes this comment just before his hemodialysis treatment: "What have I got to live for? I'd just like this to be over." How would you interpret these comments?

A. This indicates feelings of depression associated with a long-term, incurable disease.

B. This response will be temporary, and he will feel much better after his hemodialysis is initiated.

C. His family is not providing the support he needs at this time.

D. This is an unusual response and indicates that his cognitive abilities have become impaired by the disease.

**91.** A client has just been transferred to the postanesthesia recovery room. What are the most important initial assessments that need to be completed?

A. Skin color, warmth of extremities, and mental status assessment.

B. Temperature, metabolic rate, and presence of reflexes.

C. Vital signs, level of consciousness, pain level, and wound dressing.

D. Emotional status, response to anaesthesia, and social support.

**92.** Which factors increase the risk of postoperative complications?

A. Hypotension and athletic bradycardia.

B. Hypertension and obesity, chronic lung condition.

C. Poor gag reflex and optimal nutritional status.

D. High hemoglobin and negative midstream urine analysis.

---

***Case Study:*** *Mrs. Jane Everly, age 65 years, had a left cerebrovascular accident (CVA) with right-sided hemiplegia. She is confused and disoriented and has a nasogastric (NG) feeding tube inserted. Questions 93 to 98 relate to this scenario.*

**93.** Which is the most important consideration before administering tube feedings through an NG tube?

A. Ensure that the anchoring tape is intact.

B. Determine placement of the tube by aspiration of gastric contents.

C. Position the patient in the supine position to prevent aspiration.

D. Flush out the tube with 50 cc of water before the feeding to prevent obstruction of the tube.

**94.** Mrs. Everly's family is upset that this CVA has happened to her at such a young age. They ask you what she should be doing differently and what they should do to prevent having a CVA. What risk factors are associated with the incidence of CVA?

A. Genetics plays the most important role in its incidence.

B. Lack of exercise and effective stress management.
C. Smoking, high cholesterol levels, and hypertension.
D. Low weight, dehydration, and aerobic exercise.

95. Mrs. Everly is prescribed warfarin sodium (Coumadin) 8.5 mg after her prothrombin time and INR (International Normalized Ratio) laboratory report were reviewed. She has warfarin tablets of the following strengths: 5 mg/tab, 3 mg/tab, and 2 mg/tab. Which of the following would you give?
    A. 1 tablet of 5 mg, 1 tablet of 3 mg, and ½ tablet of 2 mg.
    B. ½ tablet of 5 mg, 1 tablet of 3 mg, and 1 tablet of 2 mg.
    C. 1 tablet of 5 mg and ½ tablet of 5 mg.
    D. 1 tablet of 5 mg, 1 tablet of 2 mg, and ½ tablet of 3 mg.

96. Mrs. Everly undergoes intense rehabilitation and is discharged with residual hemiparesis. As the home care coordinator, what would be important for you to do before Mrs. Everly's return home?
    A. Reduce risk factors and implement measures to prevent a subsequent CVA.
    B. Identify complications of immobility and reinforce measures to prevent them.
    C. Reduce nutritional intake and fluid intake to promote weight loss.
    D. Assess the home and demonstrate effective use of assistive devices.

97. What are important factors to consider in helping her integrate back into the community?
    A. Financial resources, ability to afford home care nursing.
    B. Independence, adjustment to moving back home, sleeping patterns.
    C. Coping abilities, emotional lability, physical deficits, family supports.
    D. Redefining her community involvement, daily checks of blood pressure.

98. What community resources could help her and her family learn more about stroke and rehabilitation?
    A. Heart and Stroke Foundation and Canadian Stroke Network.
    B. Internet resources and products to help stroke patients.
    C. Community drop-in center for retired persons and community health center.
    D. Hospital outpatient department and mediclinic.

***Case Study:*** *Jeffrey Brim, age 18 years, has been admitted unconscious to the neurosurgical unit after a car accident that resulted in a head injury. He was not wearing a seatbelt. Questions 99 to 103 relate to this scenario.*

99. When caring for an unconscious patient, which is the most important nursing measure?
    A. Maintaining a patent airway.
    B. Maintaining integrity of the skin and mucous membranes.
    C. Maintaining fluid and nutritional balance.
    D. Preventing urinary incontinence.

100. You are asked to complete a neurologic assessment. Which of the following would indicate an abnormal neurologic finding?
    A. The client is conscious and responds to verbal commands.
    B. Temperature, 37, pulse, 86 bpm; and blood pressure, 120/80 mm Hg.
    C. The pupils are equal and sluggish in reaction to light.
    D. The patient has equal strength in hand grasps and foot pushes.

101. What change in vital signs would indicate increased intracranial pressure?
    A. Hypotension and tachycardia.
    B. Increase in temperature and tachypnea.
    C. Increasing systolic blood pressure.
    D. Widening pulse pressure and bradycardia.

102. The doctor has indicated a poor prognosis for recovery, and the client's family is very concerned. How would you support the family?
    A. Listen to them, explain what is happening, and encourage them to be involved in their family member's care.
    B. Encourage them to have realistic expectations of recovery and reinforce the poor prognosis.
    C. Identify the strongest family member and communicate with that person.
    D. Explain the parents never get over the horrors of such massive injuries.

103. Jeffrey's teachers have asked for a nurse to speak regarding prevention of injuries caused by car accidents. Considering the age group and injury risks, what would you address?
    A. Allow open discussion of what went wrong with this accident.
    B. Discuss the downfalls of inexperienced drivers and the omnipotence that young drivers feel.

C.  Discuss the purpose of seatbelts, the effects of drinking and driving, and the effects of speed.

D.  Explain how accidents can be prevented and discuss the high cost of injuries in this age group.

104. Mrs. Ava J., age 58 years, has had a bone density test indicating osteoporosis. What risk factors would predispose a person to osteoporosis?

A.  Excessive sunlight exposure and increased calcium intake.

B.  Increased weight-bearing activities.

C.  Heavy smoking, sedentary lifestyle, and diet low in calcium.

D.  Diet deficient in vegetables and fruits; increased alcohol intake.

105. Persons in a retirement residence are asking for assistance in preventing falls and reducing injuries. What would you *omit* from the discussion?

A.  Explanation of the importance of a health professional evaluating gait and assessing for motor deficits.

B.  Discussion of instability and effective use of ambulatory aids.

C.  Teaching about stabilizing by sitting for a few minutes before standing to lessen dizziness.

D.  Talk about decreasing activity and the regular use of restraints to prevent falls.

106. Which statement is true regarding informed consent before a surgical procedure?

A.  Consent must be signed after explanations of the benefits and risks of the procedure.

B.  The nurse is responsible for giving the explanations and providing information regarding the risks.

C.  The patient cannot decide not to have the surgery after the consent has been signed.

D.  Informed consents are documents of understanding, not legal documents.

107. A patient comes into the preoperative clinic and states that she has decreased her nutritional intake and has lost 15 kg in the past 2 months. Which of the following statements is true regarding wound healing when poor nutritional status is present?

A.  The wound is likely to become infected and will then heal by primary intention.

B.  The inflammatory phase of healing will be shortened.

C.  The proliferative or regeneration phase will be prolonged.

D.  There will be less formation of scar tissue because of the client's nutritional state.

108. John Smith has been diagnosed with lung cancer. He approaches you about his diagnosis and states, "I can hardly face my family. They have been after me to quit smoking for so long, but I never really believed this would happen to me." What elements of family-centered care would be important?

A.  Assessing his guilt and identifying how each member is affected by his diagnosis.

B.  Assuring family members that this is not the time to be judging but to be supporting him in his recovery.

C.  Encouraging him to stop smoking and apologize to his family.

D.  Developing a sense of trust, discussing feelings, and identifying the family's strengths and coping strategies.

109. Mary Lane, age 72, is admitted to the hospital with a GI disorder. Which disorder would contraindicate abdominal palpation?

A.  Aortic aneurysm

B.  Bowel obstruction

C.  Cirrhosis

D.  Umbilical hernia

---

**Case Study:** *As a nurse, you are taking care of Mr. Jackson, age 56 years, who has been admitted with a myocardial infarction. Questions 110 to 113 relate to this scenario.*

110. You observe that Mr. Jackson is very sad and dejected. He states, "Life will never be the same." How would you respond to him?

A.  "This makes you really sad."

B.  "Why do you think life will never be the same?"

C.  "Could you be a little more hopeful of your recovery from this heart attack?"

D.  "You're concerned when you think about how this will change your life?"

111. What questions would you ask to determine his coping abilities?

A.  "What could you have done to prevent this illness?

B.  "How is this illness impacting you and your family?"

C. "How can we take away your worries while you are in hospital?"

D. "What are the worst challenges that you have faced?"

112. Mr. Jackson has been taking a diuretic, furosemide (Lasix). His serum potassium level is 3.2 mmol/L. Which assessment findings would confirm hypokalemia?

A. Muscle weakness and a weak, irregular pulse.

B. Diarrhea and cramps.

C. Tetany and tremors.

D. Headaches and poor tissue turgor.

113. When Mr. Jackson goes home, he enters a community heart rehabilitation program. What lifestyle changes will be reviewed?

A. Reduced intake of unsaturated fats, anaerobic activity, increase fluids.

B. Reduced intake of calcium, increased intake of sodium, rest periods.

C. Reduced cholesterol levels, progressive activity levels, coping strategies.

D. Increasing homocysteine levels, reducing weight, sedentary lifestyle.

114. Upon inspecting a client's abdomen, the nurse notes a distinct rhythmic pulsation in the midline. Although this pulsation may be normal in a thin client, the nurse should:

A. Call the physician immediately, as this finding usually indicates abdominal aneurysm.

B. Palpate the area to determine the extent of the pulsation, then call the physician with this information.

C. Auscultate the area to determine whether a bruit is present.

D. Percuss the area to determine whether the bowel is displaced.

115. When practicing according to ethical principles, what is the principle of beneficence?

A. It consists of the patient's having freedom to make decisions and take appropriate actions.

B. It uses the principle of loyalty to ethical beliefs as a guideline for behaviour.

C. It means ensuring that nursing virtues serve as the basis of practice.

D. It is to act in the best interests of others; to become a client advocate.

*Case Study:* Mr. Jules Hilt, age 22 years, has been injured in a snowmobile accident. He suffered a neck injury when he was thrown from the snowmobile. Questions 116 to 118 relate to this scenario.

116. When completing your assessment, what findings would indicate an incomplete spinal cord injury (SCI)?

A. Immediate flaccid paralysis that persists for months.

B. Evidence of voluntary motor and sensory function below the level of injury.

C. Presence of spinal shock response with hypertension and tachycardia.

D. Presence of paralytic ileus and urinary retention.

117. What emergency interventions would need to be implemented if the injury is at C4 level?

A. Measures to reverse hypertension.

B. Mechanical ventilation.

C. Measures to control hyperthermia.

D. Use of a catheter to intervene in urinary retention.

118. Corticosteroids (methylprednisolone) are given IV within 8 hours of the injury. Why would methylprednisolone be administered?

A. To reverse spinal shock.

B. To reduce damage and improve functional recovery.

C. To assist the body in maintaining the stress response.

D. To reduce spinal cord edema.

119. Which of the following are important considerations when providing culturally competent care in a community clinic?

A. Knowing about different cultural practices and generalizing when caring for clients from that culture.

B. Asking about cultural beliefs related to health, illness, treatments, and dietary practices.

C. Making decisions for the client and informing him or her about appropriate health interventions.

D. Explaining that multiculturalism in Canada means all cultures melting to join the dominant culture.

120. When you enter a female client's room, you find her passionately kissing and embracing another woman. What action would you take?

A. Quietly leave the room, come back later, and state that this behaviour is unacceptable in the hospital.

B. Announce your presence by excusing yourself and proceed to conduct the health history.

C. Do not disturb the couple, leave the room, and allow them privacy.

D. Explain that intimate encounters are better facilitated in the privacy of their home.

___

**Case Study:** *You are a health nurse in an elderly seniors' residence. Your role is to individualize health teaching and assessment and focus on risk identification and injury prevention. Questions 121 to 125 relate to this scenario.*

121. What methods would you use to identify the clients' educational needs?

A. Have the families meet together as a group to identify primary needs of each senior.

B. Conduct focus group interviews and have the clients fill out a survey.

C. Develop a list of the seniors' common interests and have them select their preferred choices.

D. Discuss with attendants what the primary interests of the clients are.

122. Safe medication administration is an issue. What factors influence medication effectiveness for elderly adults?

A. There is a lower risk of drug interactions.

B. There is usually less need for medications.

C. There is an increase in lipid solubility and distribution throughout the body.

D. There is less efficient absorption, detoxification, and elimination.

123. Several clients are concerned that they are taking too many medications and are unsure of the reasons for taking some of the medications. What would you do?

A. Review all the medications and their actions and side effects with each client.

B. Have a pharmacist discuss the medications and interactions and initiate physician referrals as needed.

C. Give a general presentation on common groupings of medications and indications.

D. Ask each client to research the medications prescribed and identify the reasons they were prescribed.

124. A health assessment of visual alterations is scheduled. Which of the following is true regarding visual alterations or deficits in seniors?

A. Cataracts are seen individuals older than age 65 years and occur when the cornea becomes opaque and impairs the visual field.

B. Glaucoma is a painless blockage in the circulation of the vitreous humour in the eye, leading to increased intraocular pressure.

C. Diabetic retinopathy is the leading cause of blindness and occurs because of ischemic retinal blood vessel changes.

D. Macular degeneration occurs when there is blurring and distortion of visual images caused by destruction of peripheral visual fields.

125. Some of the clients are not participating in activities and appear to be becoming more reserved and isolated, as reported by their families and other residents. What would be your approach?

A. Respect each client's choice of not participating in activities and leave the clients alone.

B. Encourage family members to visit as often as they are able to provide socialization.

C. Assess for depression and signs of sensory deprivation; take action as needed.

D. Explain to the clients that participation is mandatory and that it is for their health and benefit.

126. Nurse Hanes has completed discharge teaching of a dressing change to a patient. The next day, Nurse Pane observes that the client seems confused about the dressing and reminds Nurse Hanes about a video on dressing technique. In demonstrating that she is open to feedback about her own practice, what would Nurse Hanes' response be?

A. "He really didn't seem motivated to learn, so I'm not sure that would help."

B. "I actually don't think that videos are very useful for patient teaching."

C. "My client did seem to have difficulty; maybe the video would help."

D. "I wonder if you would reteach him; you have so much more experience."

127. Two registered nurses are working nights with a senior student nurse and an unregulated health care worker (UHCW). While one RN is on break, a client requests his pain medication. The nurse knows he will have to waste 0.5 mL of Demerol to administer the ordered dosage. Which of the following actions would be indicated?

A. Draw up the medication and discard the wastage. The amount of wastage is too small to need to be recorded.

B. Draw up the medication; lock up the wastage in the medication cabinet until the other RN returns and can witness and cosign the wastage.

C. Call the student nurse to witness the wastage and cosign for its proper disposal.

D. Ask the UHCW to witness the wastage and confirm to the other RN that the medication was disposed of appropriately.

128. Sanchea Jones notices the smell of marijuana on a colleague upon return from lunch break. Shortly after, Sanchea notices that the colleague is having difficulty drawing up a dose of insulin; she appears uncoordinated and is unaware that she has contaminated the needle several times. What is the best action for Sanchea to take?

A. Take the syringe and insulin vials from her and draw up the insulin for her. Instruct her to be very careful when she is giving the injection.

B. Take the insulin vials and needle from her; draw up the insulin and administer it for her. Ask a colleague to help keep an eye on her for the rest of the shift.

C. Reassign her responsibilities and inform her she will have to report her if it happens again.

D. Stop her from drawing up the insulin. Call a supervisor, inform him or her about the incident, and document the observations.

***Case Study:*** *Tara Fisher, age 43 years, has had symptoms of systemic lupus erythematosus (SLE) for years, but she was just recently diagnosed with the condition. She has been taking corticosteroids for the past 1.5 years. Questions 129 to 133 relate to this scenario.*

129. What are some of the effects of corticosteroids when they have been administered for a long period of time?

A. Hypoglycemia and cognitive changes.
B. Skeletal muscle atrophy and osteoporosis.
C. Hyponatremia and hypokalemia.
D. Edema and hyperpigmentation of the skin.

130. When teaching Tara regarding the long-term effects of corticosteroids, how would you explain the importance of not suddenly discontinuing this medication?

A. Long-term use of these hormones has resulted in depression of your body's own production, and a crisis could occur if you suddenly stop taking them.

B. Corticosteroids assist in the responding to stress by stimulating your stress hormones, epinephrine and norepinephrine.

C. Corticosteroid administration causes Cushing's syndrome, and sudden stoppage results in more serious aggravation of this syndrome.

D. The feedback mechanism results in extra stimulation of the pituitary gland to increase production of the corticosteroids.

131. Tara is very dejected that she needs to continue taking the corticosteroids to control her symptoms of SLE. When you come in to administer her medication, she refuses to take it, stating, "This is turning me into an old woman before my time." How would you respond?

A. Explain that the symptoms of the disease are chronic and progressive and are much worse than the side effects from the drugs.

B. Ask her about the medication side effects and explain why suddenly stopping the drug can cause problems.

C. Encourage her to take the medication until she is able to consult with her doctor regarding the side effects.

D. Document her refusal to take the medication and notify the doctor.

132. Tara states that she is not sure how she can handle the long-term effects of this disease and that her multiple hospitalizations are really affecting the family and her role in the family. How would you respond to her?

A. "Have you discussed with your family ways they could take the burden off you at this time?"

B. "Who in your family is the strongest and could manage to take over your role in addition to theirs?"

C. "This illness has really taken its toll on you and your family. Which effects are most difficult to handle?"

D. "Which roles are you not able to handle? Maybe we could consult with a social worker regarding these."

133. Tara tells you she feels "so alone with this illness" and asks you what resources may be available to assist her. What community resources might you suggest?

A. Chronic illness support group or SLE support group.
B. Internet resources and chat lines.
C. Medical library to find out more about the illness.
D. Nursing texts to help her better understand this condition.

***Case Study:*** *Jeremy Brook, a 29-year-old bisexual male, comes to the sexual health clinic. He has symptoms of night sweats, fatigue, and weight loss. His* *temperature is 39°C. He has a history of syphilis and hepatitis B and is being investigated for HIV infection. He has a chronic lung infection and is being investigated for digestive problems. Questions 134 to 138 relate to this scenario.*

**134.** Which of the following groups have an increased risk of contracting HIV?

A. Having a recent blood transfusion; being a heterosexual monogamous woman or man.

B. Participating in unprotected sex with multiple sexual partners; sharing IV needles.

C. Health care workers working in emergency settings, bisexuals, and hemophiliacs.

D. Individuals from developing countries, oral drug abusers, and alcoholics with nutritional deficiencies.

**135.** What is the primary risk factor for health care workers contracting HIV when providing patient care for Jeremy?

A. Needlestick injuries or contact with the client's blood.

B. Contact with saliva or urine drainage.

C. Droplet transmission from coughing and sneezing.

D. Accidental injury.

**136.** When the results of the tests come back confirming Jeremy is HIV positive, he asks about the significance of this diagnosis. What opportunistic infections or cancers tend to develop with AIDS?

A. Hepatitis B, chicken pox, measles, and leukemia.

B. *Pneumocystis carinii* pneumonia, Kaposi's sarcoma, and herpes simplex.

C. Uterine sarcoma, melanoma, and *E. coli* infection.

D. Prostate cancer, lung cancer, urinary tract infections, and prostatitis.

**137.** Jeremy is started on antiviral medications. In addition to teaching regarding medications, what should the nurse include to reinforce health and prevent illness for Jeremy?

A. Prevention of transmission, isolation precautions, and avoidance of infection.

B. Medications and side effects; nutritional supplementation.

C. Prevention of transmission, optimal nutrition, and exercise.

D. Safe sex practices, choices of medications, and hospice care.

**138.** Jeremy states: "Why did this ever have to happen to me? I can't even bring myself to tell my family." What would this indicate?

A. Denial of the disease.

B. Guilt and remorse regarding the disease.

C. Realization of the seriousness of the disease.

D. Anger over contracting the disease.

**139.** When students in a health class are discussing birth control and safer sex, which would indicate that teaching was effective?

A. A student indicates that safe sex means preventing pregnancy through use of birth control.

B. A student states that the rhythm method means not having sex just before menstruation.

C. A student indicates that responsible sex involves using condoms for protection and birth control.

D. A student states that the intrauterine device is the most effective way to prevent pregnancy.

**140.** Three college students in the class have indicated that they have never gone to the doctor to have a Pap test done even though they have been sexually active for several years. You have read a research article regarding factors that increase cancer of the cervix. What would be important information to reinforce?

A. Teens can be vulnerable to developing cancer of the cervix if they are exposed to certain strains of human papilloma virus (HPV).

B. Uterine cancer is more common in sexually active teens.

C. Breast cancer is more common in sexually active teens.

D. Teens having unprotected sex are more vulnerable to ectopic pregnancies, which can be identified with a Pap test.

**141.** Some female college students discuss that they have encountered situations that almost culminated in date rape. When considering preventive precautions, which statement is *false*?

A. Alcohol is usually involved in date rape.

B. Date rape drugs, such as ketamine, are not detectable in a drink.

C. If rape occurs, the victim should not douche or wash and should go to the police station.

D. Date rape is usually a misinterpretation of responsive cues.

142. In another college health class, the topic of risk-taking behaviours, or "living dangerously," is being discussed. What topic would *not* be included?

    A. Effects of cigarette smoking.
    B. Responsible drinking patterns.
    C. Motor vehicle accidents.
    D. Aerobic exercise.

*Case Study:* *James Edwards, age 42 years, is admitted with steam burns to his face, neck, and chest region. Questions 143 to 148 relate to this scenario.*

143. During the initial assessment, it is important to include the rule of nines to estimate the extent of the burn and to assess its depth. In addition, what would be the most important assessment priority?

    A. Assessing tolerance of the pain.
    B. Checking for airway patency.
    C. Observing for facial swelling and disfiguration.
    D. Determining oxygen saturation levels.

144. James is assessed and has fluid replacement ordered. What important assessment data will help ensure accurate replacement?

    A. Vital signs and presence of edema.
    B. Age, weight, vital signs, and tissue turgor.
    C. Urine output, mucous membrane hydration, and orientation.
    D. Capillary refill, specific gravity of urine, and blood pressure readings.

145. Which replacement fluid is most likely to be used during the initial 24 hours after a burn?

    A. Ringer's lactate is used as long as the urine output is maintained at an adequate level.
    B. Packed blood cells are used to replace the red blood cells that have been lost.
    C. Dextrose with water are used to rehydrate the patient.
    D. Albumin is used to restore plasma proteins.

146. Fluid therapy has been ordered at 1500 cc/8 hr. The drip administration set is 10 gtt/mL. How fast will the IV run (drops/minute)?

    A. 19 gtt/min.
    B. 31 gtt/min.
    C. 26 gtt/min.
    D. 36 gtt/min.

147. When you assess the IV at the beginning of the shift, it is 0.5 hour behind. Your assessment indicates that it is safe to catch up the IV to the ordered rate, and you decide to do this in the next 2 hours. What is the adjusted rate per hour for the next 2 hours?

    A. 150 cc/hr.
    B. 234 cc/hr.
    C. 281 cc/hr.
    D. 225 cc/hr.

148. The nurse notices that in the recuperation phase, James has become very quiet and withdrawn. What concerns should the nurse explore?

    A. Concerns regarding dependence and unwillingness to be discharged.
    B. Body image and self-esteem concerns.
    C. Concerns regarding coping abilities and family response.
    D. Financial concerns.

*Case Study:* *Dawn Mar, age 36 years, has been diagnosed with myasthenia gravis. Her history indicates progressive myopathy, dysphagia, diplopia, and dysarthria. Questions 149 to 154 relate to this scenario.*

149. Assessments confirming Dawn's history would include:

    A. Atrophy of the muscles, difficulty chewing, strabismus, and difficulty moving.
    B. Muscle inflammation, choking when eating, nearsightedness, and painful joints.
    C. Muscle weakness, difficulty swallowing, double vision, and difficulty speaking.
    D. Muscle pain, difficulty speaking, headaches, and arthritic changes.

150. Dawn asks you, "What is this disease? I have never even heard about it before." How would you respond?

    A. "It is a debilitating disease in which patches of nerves lose their myelin sheath, which interferes with nerve transmission to the muscles."
    B. "It is a chronic disease in which there is a disturbance in nerve transmission to the muscle, resulting in fatigue and muscle weakness."
    C. "It is an inherited disorder in which there is progressive destruction of the basal ganglia in the cerebral cortex."
    D. "It is a progressive degenerative process involving spinal and lower motor neurons with spastic changes in cranial and spinal nerves."

151. Diagnosis of myasthenia gravis is confirmed by evaluating the patient's response to an IV injection of the cholinesterase inhibitor edrophonium (Tensilon). If the patient responds positively, what would the nurse expect?

    A. Exaggeration of the symptoms.
    B. A rapid and dramatic increase in muscle strength.
    C. A slight increase in muscle strength followed by exaggerated muscle fatigue.
    D. Partial relief of muscle weakness.

152. What assessment findings would indicate an emergency myasthenic crisis?

    A. Airway obstruction, profound muscle weakness, and inability to move.
    B. Paralysis of the muscles and hyperventilation.
    C. Severe dyspnea, intensification of dysphagia, and dysarthria.
    D. Impairment of functioning of the autonomic and skeletal muscles.

153. What emergency procedures may be implemented during a myasthenic gravis crisis?

    A. Tracheotomy with mechanical ventilation.
    B. Insertion of a nasogastric tube.
    C. Insertion of an endotracheal tube.
    D. Insertion of an oral airway.

154. Dawn is very concerned about the impact of her illness on her family, particularly her two daughters. What question would help in family assessment of her concerns?

    A. "Do your daughters know that they will have to fulfill your role until your disease is under control?"
    B. "Why is your condition having such a disruptive effect on your family?"
    C. "How is your condition affecting your family members and their usual roles?"
    D. "How can we help your family adjust to this illness and give you the support you need to recover?"

155. What question would you ask to assess coping abilities of a family?

    A. "How has your family handled difficult situations before? What strengths emerged from these situations?"
    B. "Has your family been able to handle chronic illness management before?"
    C. "What is the best way your family resolves crisis situations?"

    D. "Does your family have the strength to deal with the changes and still support you through this difficult time?"

156. Which therapeutic interventions may be implemented for individuals with myasthenia gravis?

    A. Cholinergic medications, muscle relaxants, and nervous system antagonists.
    B. Anticholinergic medications, muscle stimulants, and nervous system stimulants.
    C. Cholinesterase inhibitors, thymectomy, and corticosteroids.
    D. Cholinergic inhibitors, immunosuppressants, and antibodies.

157. A patient who is overweight asks for information regarding diet counselling. What action should the nurse take?

    A. Suggest a diet with a very limited number of calories from fat and carbohydrates so that she will have reinforcement from quick initial weight loss.
    B. Assess the patient's eating and exercise patterns and together develop a weight control program that allows for gradual weight loss.
    C. Examine emotional eating issues and identify the foods that are most harmful and are contributing to the weight gain.
    D. Identify which diet would be most suited to her needs and body type and then have her follow through with the diet principles.

158. A client is receiving IV therapy with 5% dextrose in water (D5W). When assessing the IV site, you note that there is a red line and pain and edema at the insertion site. What actions would you take?

    A. Slow the infusion rate and apply warm compresses to the site.
    B. Discontinue the infusion and apply a warm compress to the IV site.
    C. Reposition the IV access device to lessen the vein irritation.
    D. Apply antibacterial ointment to the IV site and slow the IV infusion.

159. A physician in a clinic asks you to perform an IV insertion. You have not done an IV start for many years. What would you do?

    A. Quickly review the procedure and perform the IV insertion.
    B. Explain that you are unable to perform the IV start until you have completed an inservice and practice session on IV insertions.

C. State that it is not within your scope of practice as a nurse working in a clinic.

D. Explain that you do not have malpractice insurance to cover this skill.

160. You are working with a licensed practical nurse (LPN) and have delegated the taking of vital signs for a preoperative patient. When you are reviewing the chart as the patient is leaving for the operating room, you note that his temperature is 38.4°C and pulse is 110 bpm. What should you do?

A. Have the LPN take the vital signs again, phone the operating room, and cancel the surgery.

B. Take the vital signs yourself and do not delegate this preoperative responsibility in the future.

C. Notify the surgeon and await his or her decision; reinforce with the LPN the importance of reporting abnormal preoperative vital signs.

D. Sign off the chart but flag that the vital signs are abnormal; allow the patient to go to the operating room.

161. You are on a surgical unit and have been assigned four patients. When you receive your report, you find out that you have a patient who had a transurethral resection of the prostate (TURP) today. A postoperative patient from yesterday is requesting pain medication. A patient with a postoperative infection needs to have an IV antibiotic given in ½ an hour. Another patient is to be discharged shortly when his family arrives. Which patient would be your first priority to complete an initial assessment?

A. The patient who had the TURP.

B. The patient requesting pain medication.

C. The patient with the postoperative infection to get IV medication ready.

D. The patient being discharged.

162. A 62-year-old male client had drainage of a pelvic abscess secondary to diverticulitis 6 days ago. While drinking water, he begins to cough violently. His daughter runs to the nurse's station, screaming that her father has "exploded." Upon entering the room, the nurse observes that the client has experienced dehiscence, and a small segment of bowel is protruding. What should be the nurse's priority action?

A. Ask the client what has occurred, call the physician, have the daughter stay with her father, and cover the area with the bed sheet soaking in water.

B. Have a nursing assistant hold the incision together while you obtain the vital signs, call the physician, and flex the client's knees.

C. Obtain vital signs, call the physician, obtain emergency orders, and explain to the daughter exactly what has occurred.

D. Have the nursing assistant call the physician while you remain with the client, flex the client's knees, and cover the incision with sterile gauze.

163. A patient is receiving external-beam radiation therapy to her thoracic and lumbar spine because of metastatic breast cancer. Which of the following people should be permitted to visit?

A. Her pregnant granddaughter.

B. Her husband, who is recovering from the flu.

C. Her grandson and his family, including his wife and four children, who are between the ages of 4 and 8 years.

D. Her elderly sister, who has a history of chronic obstructive pulmonary disease and frequent respiratory infections.

164. When monitoring a patient who is at risk for hemorrhage, which assessment data would be significant?

A. Warm, dry skin; hypotension; and bounding pulse.

B. Hypertension; bounding pulse; and cold, clammy skin.

C. Weak, thready pulse; hypertension; and warm, dry skin.

D. Hypotension; cold, clammy skin; and weak, thready pulse.

165. A patient who has had multiple hospital admissions for congestive heart failure is returned to the hospital by her daughter. The patient is admitted to the coronary care unit for observation. She states, "I know I'm sick, but I understand what is needed to take care of myself at home." The nurse recognizes that the patient is attempting to:

A. Deny her illness.

B. Suppress her fears.

C. Reassure her daughter.

D. Maintain her independence.

166. When teaching a patient newly diagnosed with inflammatory bowel disease, the nurse must first consider the influence of the:

A. Patient's personal resources.

B. Type of onset of the disease.

C. Total stress of the situation.

D. Patient's past experiences.

**167.** A nurse is caring for a patient admitted to the hospital for treatment of infection secondary to AIDS. The patient is experiencing night fevers and as a result is perspiring profusely. Which of the following is the least helpful in managing this symptom?

   A.  Keep a change of bed linen nearby and change as required.
   B.  Administer an antipyretic agent after the patient spikes a fever.
   C.  Ensure that the patient's pillow has a plastic pillowcase.
   D.  Keep liquids for hydration available at the bedside.

**168.** An elderly client is apprehensive about being hospitalized. The nurse realizes that one of the stresses of hospitalization is the strangeness of the environment and activity. This stress can be reduced by:

   A.  Listening to what the client has to say.
   B.  Using the client's first name.
   C.  Visiting the client frequently.
   D.  Explaining procedures and unit routines to the client.

**169.** A client who has recently had a fractured hip repaired must be transferred from his bed to a wheelchair. While assisting with this, the nurse should remember that:

   A.  During a weight-bearing transfer, the client's knees should be slightly bent.
   B.  Transfers to and from a wheelchair will be easier if the bed is higher than the wheelchair.
   C.  The transfer can be accomplished by instructing the patient to pivot while placing his weight on both upper extremities rather than on his legs.
   D.  The appropriate proximity and visual relationship of the wheelchair to the bed must be maintained.

**170.** When teaching a client about diabetes and self-administration of insulin, what should the nurse's first action be?

   A.  Begin the teaching program at the client's level of understanding.
   B.  Determine what the client knows about the health problem.
   C.  Set specific short and long-term goals.
   D.  Collect equipment needed to demonstrate giving an injection.

**171.** An elderly client with primary degenerative dementia has difficulty following simple directions and selecting clothes to be worn for the day. The nurse recognizes that these problems are the result of:

   A.  Clouding of consciousness.
   B.  Impaired judgment.
   C.  Loss of abstract thinking ability.
   D.  Decreased attention span.

**172.** During the day, a nurse puts one side rail up on the bed of a 73-year-old client admitted to the unit after a hip fracture. What is the reason for putting up the side rail?

   A.  Because all clients over 65 years of age should use side rails.
   B.  Because elderly people are often disoriented for several days after anaesthesia.
   C.  To be used as handholds and to facilitate the client's mobility in bed.
   D.  As a safety measure because of the client's age.

**173.** Mr. Unter's family physician uses an electronic medical record. The primary objective of an electronic medical record is to support health care providers with:

   A.  Reminders, alerts, support systems, and links to medical knowledge.
   B.  Referrals, clinical decision support systems, and hospital records.
   C.  Laboratory results, alerts, and medical knowledge.
   D.  All of the above.

**174.** Nursing informatics includes:

   A.  Use of decision-making systems to support the use of the nursing process.
   B.  Research related to the information nurses use when making patient care decisions.
   C.  Nursing use of a hospital information system.
   D.  All of the above.

---

***Case Study:*** *Mrs. Kennedy, age 78 years, is admitted to a rehabilitation unit after a cerebrovascular accident (CVA). She is bedridden and aphasic. The next morning, the physician orders an indwelling catheter because Mrs. Kennedy has been incontinent during the night. Questions 175 to 178 relate to this scenario.*

**175.** Mrs. Kennedy's niece expresses that her aunt had not been incontinent while at home. She insists that the nurse failed to communicate the need for catheterization with her aunt or get consent. This is an example of:

A. Treatment without consent of the patient, which is an invasion of rights.
B. Treatment for the patient's benefit.
C. Inability to obtain consent for treatment because the patient was aphasic.
D. Treatment that does not need special consent.

176. Mrs. Kennedy's emotional responses to her illness would be most influenced by:

A. Her past experiences and coping abilities.
B. The fact that she is incontinent.
C. Her relationship with the health care staff.
D. Her ability to understand her illness.

177. In aiding Mrs. Kennedy to develop independence, her nurse should:

A. Demonstrate ways she can regain independence in activities.
B. Reinforce success in tasks accomplished.
C. Establish long-term goals for the patient.
D. Point out her errors in performance.

178. Because of symptoms experienced after her CVA, the nurse discovers that Mrs. Kennedy needs assistance using utensils while eating. What would the nurse do to support this?

A. Encourage Mrs. Kennedy to participate in the feeding process to the best of her abilities.
B. Feed another patient and wait in the dining room until Mrs. Kennedy feeds herself.
C. Request that Mrs. Kennedy's food be pureed by dietary staff working at the facility.
D. Have Mrs. Kennedy's niece feed her at every meal to reduce staffing limitations.

179. As a nurse, you are facilitating a cancer screening inservice for colorectal cancer. Which of the following clients presents the fewest risk factors for colon cancer?

A. A 45-year-old woman with a 25-year history of ulcerative colitis.
B. A 50-year-old man whose father died of colon cancer.
C. A 60-year-old man who follows a diet low in fat and high in fibre.
D. A 72-year-old woman with a history of breast cancer.

180. A 52-year-old woman has a blood pressure of 146/96 mm Hg. Upon hearing the reading, she exclaims, "Wow! My pressure seems high. Will I need to take medication?" Which of the following is the best response by the nurse?

A. "Yes. Hypertension is now more prevalent among women. It's fortunate we caught this during your routine examination."
B. "We will need to reevaluate your blood pressure because your age places you at a high risk for hypertension."
C. "A single elevated blood pressure does not confirm hypertension. You will need to have your blood pressure reassessed several times before a diagnosis can be made."
D. "You have no need to worry. Your blood pressure is probably elevated because you're in the doctor's office."

181. A client with a positive Mantoux test result is taking isoniazid as prescribed. Which of the following should the nurse assess for during the client's next clinic visit?

A. Yellowing of the skin or eyes.
B. Peripheral edema.
C. Shortness of breath.
D. Pruritus.

182. A client comes to the clinic because of low-grade afternoon fevers, night sweats, and a productive cough. The physician suspects pulmonary tuberculosis, especially after the client remarks that his wife was recently diagnosed with the disease. A positive acid-fast bacillus sputum culture confirms the diagnosis of tuberculosis. During the initial nursing history, you observe that the client refers to his diagnosis by using the impersonal pronoun "it." What would your best response be?

A. "Let's not talk about it. How long have you been having night sweats?"
B. "Tell me how you feel about the diagnosis of tuberculosis."
C. "'It will not kill you if you take your medications."
D. "You should not be embarrassed that you have tuberculosis."

183. To promote early and efficient ambulation after an above-the-knee amputation, the client should be encouraged to keep the hip:

A. In a flexed position.
B. Extended and abducted.
C. In functional alignment.
D. Slightly raised when moving the stump.

184. The nurse should be aware that a client with rheumatoid arthritis would most often have pain and limited movement of the joints:

A. When the latex fixation test result is positive.
B. When the room is cool.

C. In the morning upon awakening.

D. After assistive exercise.

185. To prepare a client with a long leg cast for walking with crutches, the nurse should encourage the client to:

A. Sit up straight in a chair to develop the back muscles.

B. Keep the affected limb in extension and abduction.

C. Do exercises in bed to strengthen the upper extremities.

D. Use a trapeze to strengthen the biceps muscles.

186. Which of the following nursing measures would be inappropriate to include when planning care for a client receiving chemotherapy via an IV access device?

A. Clean the insertion site and change the dressing within 24 to 72 hours.

B. Periodically flush the catheter with heparin.

C. Monitor for redness, drainage, and swelling at the insertion site.

D. Rotate the insertion site every 72 hours.

187. A client taking lithium carbonate is going home for a 3-day pass. The nurse should advise the client to:

A. Adjust the lithium dosage if mood changes are noted.

B. Have a snack with milk before going to bed.

C. Avoid participation in controversial discussions.

D. Continue to maintain normal sodium intake while at home.

188. A female client with a diagnosis of alcohol abuse appears untidy and disorganized. The plan that would best gain the client's involvement in personal care would include:

A. Giving her a schedule and requiring her to bathe and dress herself every morning.

B. Drawing up a schedule with her and making certain that she adheres to it.

C. Bathing and dressing her each morning until she is willing to perform self-care independently.

D. Assisting her in bathing and dressing by giving her clear, simple directions.

**Case Study:** *A nurse is developing a plan of care for Betty, who is experiencing anxiety after the recent loss of her job. Betty is verbalizing her concerns regarding her ability to meet her role expectations and financial obligations. Questions 189 and 190 relate to this scenario.*

189. Which nursing diagnosis would Betty be most at risk for?

A. Altered family process.

B. Altered thought process.

C. Potential for anxiety.

D. Ineffective individual coping.

190. Betty is now in a crisis state. When developing a care plan for Betty, what should the nurse consider?

A. Presenting symptoms in a crisis situation are similar for all individuals experiencing a crisis.

B. A crisis state indicates that the individual has an emotional illness.

C. A crisis state indicates that the individual has a mental illness.

D. Presenting symptoms of a crisis are unique and vary from one person to another.

191. Pressure ulcers most often occur in clients who:

A. Are immobilized.

B. Have psychiatric diagnoses.

C. Experience respiratory distress.

D. Need close supervision for safety.

**Case Study:** *Brian, a 60-year-old retired plumber, falls and is unable to get up. His wife calls an ambulance, and he is brought to the emergency room, where it is found that he has a fracture of the neck of the left femur. Brian is admitted to the orthopaedic unit, put in Buck's traction, and prepared for surgery the next day. Questions 192 and 193 relate to this scenario.*

192. On examination of Brian, what would the nurse expect?

A. Lengthening of the affected extremity with internal rotation.

B. Shortening of the affected extremity with external rotation.

C. Abduction with external rotation.

D. Abduction with internal rotation.

193. Part of the nursing care for Brian is assessment of the peripheral pulses. What characteristics are important to note when assessing the peripheral pulses?

A. Contractility and rate.

B. Color of the skin and rhythm.

C. Amplitude and symmetry.

D. Local temperature and visible pulsations.

194. To prevent pulmonary complications after surgery, patients should be instructed to perform:

A. Incisional splinting.

B. Progressive ambulation.

C. Diaphragmatic breathing.

D. Range of motion exercises.

---

**Case Study:** *Mrs. Doreen, age 69 years, was involved in a serious fall at her home. She has a fractured right hip and left tibia. She is scheduled for a right hip replacement and cast application to the left leg. She is currently in Buck's traction on the right side. She lives alone, and her daughter lives in the same community. Questions 195 to 201 relate to this scenario.*

**195.** Mrs. Doreen fears surgery. This fear may depend on past experiences with surgery or preconceptions of surgery. To alleviate Mrs. Doreen's fears and misconceptions about surgery, what should the nurse do first?

A. Provide an explanation about procedures involved in the planned surgery.

B. Explain all nursing care and possible discomfort that may result.

C. Tell her that preoperative fear is normal.

D. Ask her to discuss her understanding of the planned surgery.

**196.** Identifying a patient upon admittance to the surgical suite is one of the circulating nurse's responsibilities. Which of the following would be the most appropriate verification of Mrs. Doreen's identification upon admittance to the surgical suite?

A. Call the client by name before administering the anaesthetic.

B. Check her name on the surgical list and suite assignment.

C. Compare her arm bracelet with the information in the chart.

D. Question the orderly who brought down the client and ask him to identify her.

**197.** Mrs. Doreen has just returned from the operating room with a Foley catheter, an IV line, and an oral airway and is unresponsive. Which of the following is the priority nursing assessment?

A. Check the surgical dressing to ensure that it is intact.

B. Confirm the placement of the oral airway.

C. Examine the IV site for infiltration.

D. Observe the Foley catheter for drainage.

**198.** Mrs. Doreen is on prolonged bed rest. The nurse caring for her should plan nursing care to avoid

which common hazard associated with immobility?

A. Increased heart rate.

B. Shearing forces.

C. Increased bone density.

D. Hypertension.

**199.** The nurse encourages Mrs. Doreen to turn frequently in bed to prevent everything except:

A. Pneumonia.

B. Urinary stasis.

C. Abdominal pain.

D. Deep vein thrombosis.

**200.** When turning Mrs. Doreen, the nurse notices a reddened area on the coccyx. Which of the following is a priority nursing action?

A. Test for blanching.

B. Rub the reddened area.

C. Check for perspiration.

D. Use powder to minimize shear forces.

**201.** Mrs. Doreen is being discharged from the hospital. Which of the following is the most appropriate intervention for fall prevention?

A. Eliminating home safety hazards.

B. Encouraging an exercise regimen.

C. Maintaining medication administration.

D. Ensuring adequate nutrition.

---

**Case Study:** *Donna, age 20 years, is scheduled for a cholecystectomy. Questions 202 and 203 relate to this scenario.*

**202.** After the nurse completes the preoperative teaching, Donna states, "If I lie still and avoid turning, I will avoid pain. Do you think this is a good idea?" What is the nurse's best response?

A. "It is always a good idea to rest quietly after surgery."

B. "You need to turn from side to side every 2 hours."

C. "The doctor will probably order you to lie flat for 24 hours."

D. "Why don't you decide about activity after you return from the recovery room?"

**203.** Donna has returned from the operating room. When assessing her respiratory status as she recovers from general anaesthesia, it is of primary importance for the nurse to evaluate the patient's ability to:

A. Inhale voluntarily.

B. Breathe deeply.

C. Swallow.

D. Speak.

204. Through the prevention of postoperative complications, the nurse promotes rapid convalescence. Which of the following would be most indicative of a potential postoperative complication requiring further observation?

   A. Urinary output of 20 mL/hr.
   B. Temperature of 37.6°C.
   C. Serous drainage on the surgical dressing.
   D. Blood pressure of 100/70 mm Hg.

205. After a resection of a lower lobe of the lung, a client has a large amount of respiratory secretions. Nursing care should include:

   A. Turning and positioning.
   B. Administration of an expectorant.
   C. Intermittent positive-pressure breathing.
   D. Postural drainage.

206. When determining the method of oxygen administration to be used for a specific client, the major concern is:

   A. Facial anatomy.
   B. Pathologic condition.
   C. Age and mental capacity.
   D. Level of activity.

207. What preventive measure should be taken by the nurse regarding the untoward effects of oxygen therapy?

   A. Padding elastic bands of the face mask.
   B. Humidifying the gas before delivery.
   C. Taking the apical pulse before starting therapy.
   D. Placing the client in the orthopneic position.

208. Clients are encouraged to perform deep breathing exercise after surgery. Deep breathing exercises help to:

   A. Counteract respiratory acidosis.
   B. Expand the residual volume.
   C. Increase the blood volume.
   D. Decrease the partial pressure of oxygen.

209. When oxygen therapy via nasal cannula is ordered for a patient, what is the priority nursing action?

   A. Post an "Oxygen in use" sign.
   B. Adjust the oxygen level before applying the cannula.
   C. Explain fire safety and oxygen use.
   D. Lubricate the nares with water-soluble gel.

210. What is the most therapeutic position for a patient diagnosed with cardiopulmonary disease?

   A. Supine position.
   B. Prone position.
   C. High Fowler's position.
   D. 45-degree semi-Fowler's position.

211. A patient is diagnosed with thrombophlebitis. What is the appropriate level of activity for this patient?

   A. Bed rest with the affected extremity in the dependent position.
   B. Bed rest with bathroom privileges.
   C. Bed rest, keeping the affected extremity flat.
   D. Bed rest with elevation of the affected extremity.

212. Which patient assessment made by the nurse would require immediate intervention?

   A. Ten respirations per minute by a sleeping patient.
   B. Rattling sound in the pharynx of an unconscious patient.
   C. Coughing and expectorating large amounts of thick mucus.
   D. Slight shortness of breath after returning from the bathroom.

---

***Case Study:*** *Mr. Kenn, age 39 years, arrives at the hospital to undergo a total laryngectomy and radical neck dissection. Questions 213 to 218 relate to this scenario.*

213. Mr. Kenn enters the operating room and appears relaxed. Then he begins talking rapidly, commenting, "I'm really nervous and scared about the operation." What is the client experiencing, and what action should the nurse take next?

   A. The client is experiencing anxiety; the nurse should listen attentively and provide realistic verbal reassurance.
   B. The client is experiencing an adverse effect of meperidine; the nurse should report it to the physician.
   C. The client is typically anxious; the nurse should proceed with the assessment and preparation for surgery.
   D. The client needs additional sedation; the nurse should request an order from the anaesthesiologist.

214. It is Mr. Kenn's first postoperative day. What is a priority goal?

   A. Communicate by use of esophageal speech.
   B. Improve body image and self-esteem.
   C. Prevent aspiration.
   D. Maintain a patent airway.

**215.** When preparing to suction Mr. Kenn's tracheostomy, the nurse should be aware that the maximum recommended time frame for intermittent suction is:

   A. 1 to 5 seconds.
   B. 5 to 10 seconds.
   C. 10 to 15 seconds.
   D. 16 to 20 seconds.

**216.** Which of the following must you consider regarding positioning Mr. Kenn for suctioning?

   A. When performing suctioning on Mr. Kenn, who has a gag reflex, position him in the semi-Fowler's position.
   B. When performing oral and oropharyngeal suctioning on Mr. Kenn, ensure that his head is turned to one side.
   C. When performing nasal and nasopharyngeal suctioning on Mr. Kenn, ensure that his neck is hyperextended.
   D. All of the above.

**217.** Mr. Kenn is receiving mechanical ventilation. What nursing action is appropriate in relation to cuff care for his tracheostomy?

   A. Inflate the cuff during suctioning.
   B. Allow the cuff to be deflated for 10 minutes every hour.
   C. Assess cuff pressure for a minimal air leak.
   D. Ensure the cuff pressure allows for a gradual decrease in tidal volume.

**218.** When performing deep tracheal suctioning for Mr. Kenn, the nurse should:

   A. Be sure the cuff of the tracheotomy is inflated during suctioning.
   B. Instil acetylcysteine (Mucomyst) into the tracheotomy before suctioning.
   C. Apply negative pressure as the catheter is being inserted.
   D. Hyperoxygenate the client before suctioning.

*Case Study:* Mr. Ray, age 83 years, presents at the emergency department after falling on the ice outside his senior citizens' housing facility. The admitting diagnosis is right hip fracture, and surgical repair is planned. Questions 219 to 221 relate to this scenario.

**219.** What is the most important initial assessment finding by the nurse?

   A. Leg shortening on the affected side.
   B. Complaints of pain.
   C. Neurovascular compromise.
   D. Internal or external rotation of the hip.

**220.** A progressive ambulation schedule is to be instituted for Mr. Ray after surgery. Mr. Ray has been receiving antihypertensive medication as well as morphine sulfate for pain. When getting the client out of bed, the nurse should first have him sit on the edge of the bed with his feet dangling. This action is taken because the nurse is anticipating:

   A. Postural or orthostatic hypotension.
   B. Respiratory distress.
   C. Initial hypertension.
   D. Hip pain.

**221.** When assisting Mr. Ray to ambulate after repair of his fractured right hip, where should the nurse stand?

   A. In front of the client.
   B. Behind the client.
   C. On the client's left side.
   D. On the client's right side.

*Case Study:* Mr. Schultz is skiing. During his last ski run, he falls awkwardly and breaks his left leg. Questions 222 and 223 relate this scenario.

**222.** Mr. Shultz's leg is set in a long leg cast. The nurse should observe for signs indicative of compromised circulation, such as:

   A. Foul odour of the affected leg.
   B. Increased swelling of the toes.
   C. Increased body temperature.
   D. Purulent drainage on the cast.

**223.** During afternoon rounds, the nurse finds Mr. Schultz using a pencil to scratch inside his cast. Mr. Schultz is complaining of severe itching in the ankle area. Which action should the nurse take?

   A. Encourage him to scratch more gently with a pencil.
   B. Give him a sterile metal object to use for scratching.
   C. Administer diphenhydramine as ordered for the relief of severe itching.
   D. Obtain an order for a sedative, such as diazepam (Valium), to prevent him from scratching.

*Case Study:* Mr. Chorn is a patient with kidney failure. Questions 224 and 225 relate to this scenario.

**224.** Mr. Chorn is placed on fluid restriction of 1000 mL of fluid over a 24-hour period. The nurse should:

A. Eliminate the liquids between meal times.
B. Divide the fluids equally among the three nursing shifts.
C. Indicate just clear liquids in the restriction plan.
D. Proportion more fluids in the day than during the night.

**225.** Mr. Chorn has an IV started. At what rate should the IV be set to infuse 3000 mL of D5W in a 24-hour period (drop factor, 10)?

A. 125 mL/hr; 21 gtt/min.
B. 100 mL/hr; 17 gtt/min.
C. 150 mL/hr; 23 gtt/min.
D. 200 mL/hr; 34 gtt/min.

**226.** In relation to extracellular body fluids, normal saline is:

A. Hypertonic.
B. Hypotonic.
C. Isotonic.
D. Acidotic.

---

***Case Study:*** *Hannah York has Addison's disease. She is admitted to the hospital because of complications. Questions 227 and 228 relate to this scenario.*

**227.** Which assessment finding would most probably warrant a nursing diagnosis of fluid volume deficit?

A. Leathery, pliable skin.
B. Pretibial pitting edema.
C. Pedal pulses of 4+.
D. Dry skin with poor turgor.

**228.** Hannah is drinking 3000 mL of fluid a day. When assessing her urine, the nurse can expect the urine to be:

A. Dark and straw coloured.
B. Straw coloured.
C. Light amber.
D. Dark amber.

**229.** Mrs. Anderson is receiving furosemide (Lasix) and digoxin. Nursing care should include observation for symptoms of electrolyte depletion caused by:

A. Sodium restriction.
B. Inadequate oral intake.
C. Continuous dyspnea.
D. Diuretic therapy.

**230.** Martin Fechner enters the hospital with diarrhea, anorexia, weight loss, and abdominal cramps. A tentative diagnosis of colitis has been made. He is scheduled for a sigmoidoscopy and barium enema. Symptoms of fluid and electrolyte imbalance the nurse should report immediately are:

A. Extreme muscle weakness and tachycardia.
B. Development of tetany with muscle spasms.
C. Nausea, vomiting, and leg and stomach cramps.
D. Skin rash, diarrhea, and diplopia.

**231.** Total parental nutrition (TPN) solution contains all of the following nutrients except:

A. Dextrose.
B. Amino acids.
C. Electrolytes.
D. Fat emulsions.

**232.** What is an appropriate nursing action to detect early signs of metabolic complications of total parental nutrition (TPN)?

A. Assess lung sounds.
B. Weigh the patient daily.
C. Monitor urine output.
D. Monitor vital signs.

**233.** The nurse should be aware that the patient's serum blood glucose should be maintained below which level when receiving TPN?

A. 3 mmol/L.
B. 4.2 mmol/L.
C. 5.5 mmol/L.
D. 8.3 mmol/L.

**234.** If symptoms of an air embolism occur, the patient should be placed in which of the following positions?

A. On the back in semi-Fowler's position.
B. On the left side in the deep Trendelenburg position.
C. On the right side in the deep Trendelenburg position.
D. On the left in semi-Fowler's position.

**235.** Symptoms of hyperglycemic hyperosmolar non-ketotic (HHNK) coma include all of the following except:

A. Glycosuria.
B. Seizures.
C. Coma.
D. Anuria.

**236.** After a laminectomy, a male client has a palpable bladder and complains of lower abdominal discomfort. He is voiding 60 to 80 mL of urine every 4 hours. What is the best nursing intervention?

A. Observe for worsening discomfort.

B. Administer the prescribed analgesic.

C. Obtain an order for urinary catheterization.

D. Reassure the client that this is a normal voiding pattern.

**237.** Which complication is a client who is receiving hemodialysis for chronic renal failure at risk of developing?

A. Peritonitis.

B. Renal calculi.

C. Bladder infection.

D. Serum hepatitis.

**238.** What is a major disadvantage of an ileal conduit?

A. Stool continuously oozes from it.

B. Absorption of nutrients is diminished.

C. Peristalsis is greatly decreased.

D. Urine drains from it continuously.

*Case Study: Mrs. Jules is a 77-year-old woman who has had problems with urinary urgency for the past 3 years. She is trying to deal with the problem herself by using an absorbent pad, but she is self-conscious and believes that "everyone notices it." She states that the bulkiness and odour are embarrassing and now she does not like to go out. Questions 239 and 240 relate to this scenario.*

**239.** When caring for Mrs. Jules, who is now on a bladder-retraining program, the nurse should recognize that an intervention always implemented during a bladder-retraining program is toileting:

A. Every 2 hours when awake.

B. At 8 a.m., 2 p.m., 8 p.m., and 2 a.m.

C. Every 4 hours and through the night.

D. When the patient goes to bed at night.

**240.** What would be the most common reason why Mrs. Jules became incontinent of urine?

A. Older adults tend to drink less fluid than younger patients.

B. Older adults' slow metabolism increases pressure from their intestines onto their bladder.

C. Older adults use incontinence to manipulate and control others.

D. The muscles that control urination have weakened.

**241.** A physician orders daily stool examinations for a client with chronic bowel inflammation. These stool examinations are ordered to determine:

A. Culture and sensitivity.

B. Occult blood and organisms.

C. Ova and parasites.

D. Fat and undigested food.

**242.** A physician orders a low-residue diet for a client with an acute exacerbation of colitis. The nurse would know that the dietary teaching is understood when the client states, "I can eat:"

A. "Cream soup and crackers, omelettes, mashed potatoes, peas, orange juice, and coffee."

B. "Stewed chicken, baked potatoes with butter, strained peas, white bread, plain cake, and milk."

C. "Baked fish, macaroni with cheese, strained carrots, fruit gelatine, and milk."

D. "Lean roast beef, buttered white rice with egg slices, white bread with butter and jelly, and tea with sugar."

*Case Study: Mrs. Hillster has a diagnosis of a bowel obstruction. She complains of nausea; is vomiting dark bile material; and has severe cramping, intermittent abdominal pain. This condition is caused by intussusceptions, and surgery is scheduled. Questions 243 to 245 relate to this scenario.*

**243.** Four days after surgery, Mrs. Hillster has not passed any flatus, and bowel sounds are not present. Even though her abdomen has become more distended, she feels little discomfort. Paralytic ileus is suspected. What causes this condition?

A. Impaired blood supply to the bowel.

B. Impaired neural functioning.

C. Perforation of the bowel wall.

D. Obstruction of the bowel wall.

**244.** Mrs. Hillster requires additional surgery, and an ileostomy is performed. What knowledge should guide the nurse when caring for Mrs. Hillster's ostomy?

A. Expect the stoma to start draining 72 hours after surgery.

B. Explain that the drainage can be controlled with daily irrigations.

C. Anticipate that emotional stress can increase intestinal peristalsis.

D. Be aware that bleeding from the stoma is a medical emergency.

**245.** Why is Mrs. Hillster at risk for the development of anemia?

A. The hemopoietic factor is absorbed only in the terminal ileum.

B. Folic acid is absorbed only in the terminal ileum.

C. Iron absorption depends on simultaneous bile salt absorption in the terminal ileum.

D. The trace elements required for hemoglobin synthesis occur only in the ileum.

*Case Study:* Mr. Kerry is admitted to the hospital with extensive carcinoma of the descending portion of the colon with metastasis to the lymph nodes. He has undergone surgery and now has a colostomy. Questions 246 to 248 relate to this scenario.

246. Which product should the nurse use to protect the skin surrounding the colostomy opening?

A. Tincture of benzoin.
B. Mineral oil.
C. Stomahesive.
D. Petroleum jelly.

247. What action should the nurse take if Mr. Kerry complains of abdominal cramps during his colostomy irrigation?

A. Raise the irrigating container to quickly complete the irrigation.
B. Reassure him and continue the irrigation.
C. Pinch the tubing so that less fluid enters the colon.
D. Clamp the tubing and allow the client to rest.

248. What should the nurse emphasize when discussing the regaining of bowel control with Mr. Kerry?

A. An irrigation routine.
B. A soft, low-residue diet.
C. Managing fluid intake.
D. A high-protein diet.

249. Mrs. Lyste is an immobile client. When a nurse repositions her, redness over a bony prominence is noticed. When this area is assessed, the red spot blanches with fingertip touch indicating:

A. A local skin infection requiring antibiotics.
B. Abnormal reactive hyperemia.
C. Deep tissue damage.
D. The reactive hyperemia is likely transient.

*Case Study:* Sue Kang is a 38-year-old woman. She had a panniculectomy (tummy tuck) and experienced wound dehiscence 3 days after surgery. Questions 250 to 252 relate to this scenario.

250. Sue has yellowish discharge on her dressing every time the dressing is changed. The nurse notices that the amount of discharge is increasing. The nurse recognizes that the yellow drainage is from serum. Serous drainage from a wound is defined as:

A. Fresh, red bleeding.
B. Clear, watery plasma.
C. Thick and yellow.
D. Beige to brown and foul smelling.

251. Sue has a binder placed around her surgical incision. What is the purpose of applying a binder after panniculectomy surgery?

A. Collection of wound drainage from the incision.
B. Keeping her abdominal pain under control.
C. Reducing stress on the abdominal incision.
D. Stimulation of peristalsis from direct pressure.

252. Sue is receiving hydrocolloid dressings for her abdomen. What is the purpose of this dressing?

A. A dressing that is highly absorptive and prevents dehiscence of the wound.
B. A dressing that is premoistened and promotes granulation of the wound.
C. A dressing that contains a debriding enzyme that is used to remove necrotic tissue.
D. A dressing that forms a paste that interacts with the surface of the wound.

253. Parenteral preparations of potassium must be administered slowly and cautiously to prevent:

A. Acidosis.
B. Cardiac arrest.
C. Hypertension.
D. Hyperglycemia.

254. When caring for a client within the first 24 hours after a cardiac catheterization, the nurse should:

A. Keep the patient NPO for 2 to 4 hours after catheterization.
B. Check the pulse distal to the catheter insertion site.
C. Ensure that the patient is kept flat in bed for 8 hours after the procedure.
D. Ensure that the doctor has order antiarrhythmic medications for the patient.

*Case Study:* Mr. McKay, age 44 years, comes into the emergency department as he is passing a kidney stone. Mr. McKay requires increased volume, and a physician orders normal saline 125 mL/hr. You are the nurse, and you need to start his IV line. Questions 255 to 257 relate to this scenario.

**255.** An air embolism may be avoided by:

    A. PICC insertion.

    B. Valsalva manoeuvre.

    C. Pneumocentesis.

    D. Fluoroscopy.

**256.** Mr. McKay's catheter has become occluded. What is the most common cause of catheter occlusion?

    A. Improper dressing.

    B. Catheter defects.

    C. Infection.

    D. Thrombosis.

**257.** Mr. McKay now complains of pain. Pain with infusion is a sign of which of the following?

    A. Catheter malposition.

    B. Pinch-off syndrome.

    C. Fibrin sheath occlusion.

    D. External compression.

---

***Case Study:*** *As a result of an all-terrain vehicle mishap, Mr. Jool, age 60 years, has a punctured right lung. He is admitted to the hospital, and a chest tube is inserted. Questions 258 to 261 relate to this scenario.*

**258.** While turning Mr. Jool, his chest tube accidentally becomes disconnected. As a nurse, you should:

    A. Immediately tell him to breathe shallowly while you cover the wound.

    B. Immediately tell him to cough or exhale forcibly while you cover the wound.

    C. Calling for assistance and then cover the wound with a sterile dressing.

    D. Call for assistance and cover the insertion site with clean gauze.

**259.** To prevent Mr. Jool's chest tube from disconnecting again, the tubing should be:

    A. Coiled flat on the bed and positioned loosely beside him.

    B. Coiled flat on the bed and secured without putting tension on the tube.

    C. Coiled flat and secured to his bedrail.

    D. Coiled flat and secured in dependent loops along the side of the bed.

**260.** Mr. Jool has his chest tube attached to a Pleur-evac system. When caring for Mr. Jool, the nurse should:

    A. Change the dressing daily using aseptic technique.

    B. Palpate the surrounding area for crepitus.

    C. Empty the drainage chamber at the end of the shift.

    D. Clamp the chest tubes when suctioning the client.

**261.** When scheduling postural drainage treatments for Mr. Jool, when would be the most appropriate time of day for him to receive this treatment?

    A. Immediately upon awakening.

    B. One hour before a meal.

    C. Before bedtime.

    D. One hour after a meal.

**262.** The purpose of the water in the closed chest drainage chamber is to:

    A. Facilitate emptying bloody drainage from the chest.

    B. Foster removal of chest secretions by capillarity.

    C. Prevent entrance of air into the pleural cavity.

    D. Decrease the danger of sudden change in pressure in the tube.

**263.** A doctor orders a nurse to monitor the amount of chest tube drainage. The normal amount of drainage in 24 hours is approximately:

    A. 300 mL.

    B. 750 mL.

    C. 1200 mL.

    D. 1500 mL.

**264.** While delivering a tube feeding by gravity, the observation that indicates that the client is unable to tolerate a continuation of the feeding is:

    A. A passage of flatus.

    B. Rapid flow of the feeding.

    C. Epigastric tenderness.

    D. A rise of formula in the tube.

**265.** After a modified radical mastectomy, a client has two Jackson-Pratt portable wound drainage systems in place. When caring for these drains, the nurse should:

    A. Leave them open to the air to ensure maximum drainage.

    B. Ensure that the drainage receptacles are kept compressed to maintain suction.

    C. Attach the tubes to straight drainage to monitor the output.

    D. Irrigate the drains with normal saline to ensure patency.

**266.** A semi-Fowler's position is used to:

    A. Minimize flexion contractures of the hip.

    B. Relieve pressure on the ischial tuberosities.

C. Prevent aspiration during nasogastric tube feeding.

D. Reduce the development of pressure (decubitus) ulcers.

---

**Case Study:** *A physician has ordered insertion of a nasogastric (NG) tube for Mr. Brucks. Questions 267 and 268 relate to this scenario.*

267. During the insertion of the NG tube, the nurse would report that Mr. Brucks was experiencing difficulty if he demonstrates:

A. Choking.

B. Cyanosis.

C. Flushing.

D. Gagging.

268. To ensure that Mr. Brucks' NG tube is positioned correctly, the nurse should insert the tube a distance:

A. That is equal to the distance from the patient's ear lobe to his nose plus the distance from his nose to the tip of his xiphoid process.

B. That is equal to the distance from the tip of his nose to the tip of the ear lobe down to the xiphoid process of the sternum.

C. To the second or third black marking on the NG tube.

D. From the tip of his ear to the tip of his xiphoid process.

269. Which of the following is true concerning the height of the IV solution bag?

A. It should be placed 90 cm above the injection site.

B. It should be placed 30 cm above the injection site.

C. The greater the height, the lower the force.

D. The lower the height, the greater the force.

270. The term "vasovagal reaction" refers to an autonomic nervous system response to:

A. Stress.

B. Fluid resuscitation.

C. Sudden hydration.

D. Circulatory overload.

---

**Case Study:** *Mrs. Bezler is a 59-year-old widow who was diagnosed 25 years ago with type 2 diabetes mellitus. She has recently been diagnosed with thyroid cancer. Mrs. Bezler is currently receiving total parenteral nutrition (TPN) therapy. Questions 271 and 272 relate to this scenario.*

271. The doctor has ordered a central venous pressure (CVP) catheter for Mrs. Bezler. In assessing Mrs. Belzer's CVP reading, a nurse should place the client:

A. In a horizontal position.

B. In a low Fowler's position.

C. Side-lying on the affected side.

D. Side-lying opposite to the manometer.

272. Which of the following statements concerning Mrs. Bezler's CVP catheter patency is correct?

A. Patency includes the ability to infuse through and aspirate blood from the catheter.

B. The risk for occlusion increases with dehydration and atrial fibrillation.

C. Occlusions can lead to superior vena cava syndrome.

D. All of the above.

273. Which of the following veins has the least risk for catheter-related bloodstream infections?

A. Brachycephalic.

B. Femoral.

C. Internal jugular.

D. Subclavian.

274. The most important aspect of hand washing is:

A. Water.

B. Soap.

C. Friction.

D. Time.

275. When performing tracheotomy care, the nurse must:

A. Monitor the client's temperature after the procedure.

B. Use sterile gloves during the procedure.

C. Use Betadine to clean the inner cannula when it is removed.

D. Place the client in the semi-Fowler's position.

276. When transferring an immobilized client, the nurse should remember to use which principle of body mechanics?

A. Bending at the waist to provide the power for lifting.

B. Keeping the body straight when lifting to reduce pressure on the abdomen.

C. Placing the feet apart to increase the stability of the body.

D. Relaxing the abdominal muscles and using the extremities to prevent strain.

**277.** The most important aspect in reducing the risk of bloodborne infections for nurses working in the operating room is:

A. The avoidance of percutaneous injury.
B. The awareness of emerging infectious diseases.
C. The avoidance of doing invasive procedures.
D. The awareness of potential risks.

**278.** Mr. Lee comes to the hospital for open heart surgery. After 3 days, he is diagnosed with an antibiotic-resistant organism. Which precautions should be used with Mr. Lee?

A. Droplet.
B. Airborne.
C. Contact.
D. Isolation.

**279.** Mr. James, age 55 years, has a history of hypertension and has just been prescribed a new antihypertension medication. He complains of feeling dizzy at times. Which of the following is the best way to assess his blood pressure related to his complaints?

A. Assess his blood pressure in the supine, sitting, and standing positions.
B. Have him walk around the room and then assess his blood pressure.
C. Assess his blood pressure at the beginning and the end of the examination.
D. Take his blood pressure on the left arm and again in 5 minutes on the right arm.

---

***Case Study:*** *Mr. Metivier, age 46 years, has presented to the emergency department for treatment of chest pain. After the pain subsides, he is admitted to a medical-surgical unit with telemetry because no cardiac unit beds are available. Questions 280 to 284 relate to this scenario.*

**280.** Mr. Metivier is scheduled for an EEG. Which of the following is the client permitted to ingest 24 hours before the test?

A. Solid foods.
B. Stimulants.
C. Coffee and tea.
D. Tranquilizers.

**281.** While in the hospital, Mr. Metivier has a myocardial infarction. The medical team is concerned about reducing the workload of his heart. Mr. Kerry's orders include strict bed rest and a clear liquid diet. The nurse should

explain that the primary reason for this diet is to reduce:

A. Gastric acidity of the stomach.
B. The metabolic workload of digestion.
C. Mr. Metivier's current weight.
D. The amount of fecal elimination.

**282.** Two days after the myocardial infarction, Mr. Metivier's temperature is elevated. From his cardiac episode, which of the following would be most likely related to his infarction?

A. Possible infection.
B. Tissue necrosis.
C. Pulmonary infarction.
D. Pneumonia.

**283.** When creating a therapeutic environment for Mr. Metivier, the nurse should encourage:

A. Daily papers in the morning.
B. Telephone communication.
C. Short family visits.
D. Television for short periods.

**284.** Mr. Metivier, who is receiving multiple medications for a myocardial infarction, complains of severe nausea. Assessments reveal that his heartbeat is irregular and slow. The nurse should recognize these symptoms as toxic effects of which medication?

A. Lanoxin (Digoxin).
B. Aminosalicylic acid.
C. Morphine sulfate (morphine).
D. Meperidine hydrochloride (Demerol).

**285.** A 92-year-old patient has suffered a cerebrovascular accident (CVA). The right side of his face has visible ptosis. Knowing this, you may also suspect which of the following?

A. Agenesis.
B. Epistaxis.
C. Dysphagia.
D. Xerostomia.

**286.** An 18-year-old young man has suffered a C5 spinal cord contusion that has resulted in quadriplegia. His mother is crying in the waiting room 2 days after the surgery has occurred. The mother asks you whether her son will ever play football again. Which of the following would be the most therapeutic approach when working with this mother?

A. Reassure her that given time and motivation, he will return to his functional ability before the injury.

B. Advise her that it is not in his best interest for her to be so upset and explain the importance of moral support.

C. Reflect on how she is feeling and encourage her to express other fears that she has about his injury.

D. Leave the waiting room, call the son's physician, and ask that the physician speak to his mother right away.

287. A 72-year-old client has been admitted to the medical-surgery unit from the emergency department with a diagnosis of left-sided vascular accident. In transferring him from the stretcher to his bed, the nurse notices that the client's respirations have a snoring quality. Which of the following is the priority nursing action?

A. Place the client in a Fowler's position with the head of the bed at a 45-degree angle.

B. Assess the client's ability to communicate his needs to the health care team.

C. Position the client on his side with the head of the bed slightly elevated.

D. Place all items that the client may need to the left side of the bed.

288. A client has been admitted and has been diagnosed with having a cerebrovascular accident. Twenty-four hours after admission, the client has right-sided hemiplegia. Which of the following neurologic deficits is closely associated with this type of hemiplegia?

A. Difficulty speaking and understanding.

B. Loss of consciousness.

C. Inability to see to the left.

D. Poor judgement and impulsive behaviour.

289. An 18-year-old young man has fractured his spine in a diving accident. Upon initial admission to hospital, what is the best position for the client?

A. Prone with his head to the side.

B. Side-lying with his head midline.

C. High Fowler's position with his head to the side.

D. Supine position with his head midline.

290. A patient has an impairment of cranial nerve II. Knowing the function of this nerve, a nurse must do which of the following to ensure the patient's safety?

A. Clear any obstacles in a path for walking.

B. Test the water temperature of the shower.

C. Speak loudly to the patient.

D. Check the temperature of hot tea the client is going to drink.

291. A nurse assesses a client who is in cardiogenic shock. The nurse understands that this type of shock is:

A. A failure of peripheral circulation.

B. An irreversible phenomenon.

C. Generally caused by decreased blood volume.

D. Usually a fleeting reaction to tissue injury.

292. A client has sustained a head injury and is to receive mannitol (Osmitrol) by IV push. In evaluating the effectiveness of the drug, the nurse should expect to find which of the following?

A. Increased lung expansion.

B. Decreased cerebral edema.

C. Decreased cardiac workload.

D. Increased cerebral circulation

293. A 64-year-old woman is found on the floor of her apartment. She had apparently fallen and hit her head on the bathtub. On admission to the neurology unit, she has a decreased level of consciousness. The physician's orders for positioning are as follows: "Elevate the head of the bed; keep the head in neutral alignment with no neck flexion or head rotation; avoid sharp hip flexion." Which of the following is the best rationale for this positioning?

A. To decrease cerebral arterial pressure.

B. To avoid impeding venous outflow.

C. To prevent flexion contractures.

D. To prevent aspiration of stomach contents.

294. The first-line treatment of cardiogenic shock involves all the following except:

A. Supplying supplemental oxygen

B. Controlling chest pain.

C. Hemodynamic monitoring.

D. Enhancing safety and comfort.

295. A traumatic tension pneumothorax can be caused by:

A. A penetrating injury resulting in air moving into the thoracic cavity without being able to exit.

B. A blunt or penetrating injury resulting in air moving into the pleural space without being able to exit.

C. A blunt injury in which air enters and exits the pleural cavity through the pressure deficit created by injury.

D. A penetrating injury that causes air to be sucked into the lungs during both inhalation and exhalation.

**296.** Which of the following are considered normal respiratory parameters?

A. Respiratory rate of 10 to 20 breaths/min, $SpO_2$ of 98%, and retraction and bulging of the interspaces on inspiration.

B. Respiratory rate of 10 to 20 breaths/min, $SpO_2$ of 97% to 98%, and even breathing with occasional sighs.

C. Accessory muscles are used to enhance respiration, restlessness, and pale lips and nail beds.

D. None of the above.

**297.** A client with heart failure develops pink frothy sputum, coarse crackles, and restlessness. Of the following, which is the priority nursing action?

A. Check the client's blood pressure.

B. Place the client in high Fowler's position.

C. Calculate the client's fluid balance.

D. Notify the physician.

**298.** What position would be contraindicated for a client who has dyspnea?

A. Supine.

B. Contour.

C. Fowler's position.

D. Orthopneic.

**299.** From the following, which assessment findings would most likely indicate that a client is having difficulty breathing?

A. 16 breaths/min and deep in character.

B. 18 breaths/min and inhaled through the mouth.

C. 20 breaths/min and shallow in character.

D. 28 breaths/min and noisy.

**300.** A 57-year-old client is admitted to the hospital for exacerbation of chronic obstructive pulmonary disease (COPD). Which of the following would the nurse expect to find during a nursing assessment?

A. Dyspnea, cough, and bradycardia.

B. Wheezing, tachycardia, and restlessness.

C. Barrel chest, tachycardia, and hypertension.

D. Hypotension, confusion, and weight gain.

**301.** A client's arterial blood gas analysis reveals an excess of carbon dioxide. The nurse should recognize that this is consistent with which of the following?

A. Metabolic acidosis.

B. Metabolic alkalosis.

C. Respiratory acidosis.

D. Respiratory alkalosis.

**302.** Mrs. Schneidar, age 82 years, is admitted with congestive heart failure and pulmonary edema. To help alleviate Mrs. Schneidar's distress, the nurse should:

A. Elevate her lower extremities.

B. Place her in an orthopneic position.

C. Encourage frequent coughing.

D. Prepare for modified postural drainage.

**303.** A 65-year-old man comes to the emergency department with severe chest pain and shortness of breath. He is diaphoretic, pale, and weak. Suddenly, he collapses and becomes unresponsive. What should the nurse do first when assessing this client?

A. Check for a carotid pulse.

B. Check for spontaneous respirations.

C. Maintain an open airway.

D. Gently shake him and shout, "Are you OK?"

**304.** A 48-year-old foreman at a local electric company comes to the emergency department complaining of severe substernal chest pain that radiates down his left arm. He is admitted to the coronary care unit with a diagnosis of myocardial infarction (MI). Which of the following should the nurse do first when the patient is admitted to the coronary care unit?

A. Begin EGG monitoring.

B. Obtain a family health history.

C. Auscultate the lung fields bilaterally.

D. Determine the quality of the client's pain.

**305.** When performing external cardiac compression, the nurse should exert downward vertical pressure on the lower sternum by placing:

A. The heels of each hand side by side, extending the fingers over the chest.

B. The heel of one hand on the sternum and the heel of the other on top of it with the fingers interlocking.

C. The fingers of one hand on the sternum and the fingers of the other hand on top of them.

D. The heel of one hand on the sternum and the fleshy part of a clenched fist on the lower sternum.

**306.** A client's cardiac monitor is indicative of ventricular fibrillation. The nurse from the coronary care unit should prepare for:
   A. An IM injection of digoxin (Lanoxin).
   B. An IV line for emergency medications.
   C. Immediate defibrillation.
   D. Elective cardioversion.

***Case Study:*** *Mr. and Mrs. Donald Reitz have been married almost 7 years when a physical examination confirms that Mrs. Reitz is 8 to 10 weeks pregnant. Mr. and Mrs. Reitz are overjoyed. About 10 days after her visit to the physician, at the time of her normal menstrual period, Mrs. Reitz starts to spot but denies pain. Her physician tells her to remain on complete bed rest for at least 72 hours. Questions 307 to 309 refer to this scenario.*

**307.** What is the most appropriate diagnosis for Mrs. Reitz?
   A. Threatened abortion.
   B. Inevitable abortion.
   C. Ectopic pregnancy.
   D. Missed abortion.

**308.** After a few hours, Mrs. Reitz begins to experience bearing-down sensations and suddenly expels tissue. A priority nursing action at this time would be to:
   A. Take her immediately to the delivery room.
   B. Check the fundus for firmness.
   C. Give her the sedation ordered.
   D. Immediately notify the physician.

**309.** When the nurse returns to the room, she notices that both Mrs. Reitz and her husband are visibly upset. Mr. Reitz has tears in his eyes, and Mrs. Reitz has her face turned to the wall, sobbing quietly. The best approach for the nurse to take is to go over to Mrs. Reitz and say:
   A. "I know how you feel, but you should not be so upset now. It will make it more difficult for you to get better."
   B. "I can understand that you are upset, but be glad it happened early in your pregnancy and not after you carried the baby to full term."
   C. "I know that you are upset now, but hopefully you will become pregnant again very soon."
   D. "I see that both of you are very upset. I will be here if you want to talk."

**310.** Diabetic coma results from an excess accumulation of which substance in the blood?
   A. Ketones from rapid fat breakdown, causing acidosis.
   B. Glucose from rapid carbohydrate metabolism, causing drowsiness.
   C. Sodium bicarbonate, causing alkalosis.
   D. Nitrogen from protein catabolism, causing ammonia intoxication.

**311.** A client with diabetes mellitus has had declining renal function over the past several years. He is placed on hemodialysis because of persistently elevated creatinine levels. Which diet regimen would be best for the client on days between dialysis?
   A. High-protein with a prescribed amount of water.
   B. Low-protein diet with a prescribed amount of water.
   C. Low-protein diet with an unlimited amount of water.
   D. No protein in the diet and use of a salt substitute.

**312.** A 28-year-old woman has had type I diabetes for 10 years. She is doing home blood glucose monitoring and urinary dipsticks for acetone. She asks the nurse why she has to dipstick her urine, too. Upon which of the following rationales would the nurse base her answer?
   A. A positive test reaction indicates too much glucose.
   B. A positive test reaction indicates too much insulin.
   C. A positive test reaction indicates ketoacidosis
   D. The test measures protein in the urine.

**313.** When working with a diabetic patient, the nurse must know that the difference between diabetic coma and hyperglycemic hyperosmolar nonketotic coma is that clients in diabetic coma experience:
   A. Fluid loss.
   B. Glycosuria.
   C. Increased blood glucose.
   D. Kussmaul respirations.

***Case Study:*** *Mr. Hanif Mulji, age 28 years, is found in a coma in his hospital room. There was a strong odour of acetone on his breath. He is married, climbs mountains, and is a triathlete. Previous health records do not reveal that Mr. Mulji had diabetes mellitus. Emergency measures are instituted immediately. Questions 314 and 315 refer to this scenario.*

314. A nursing intervention that should be included in the plan of care for Mr. Mulji is:
    A. Withholding glucose in any from until the ketoacidosis is corrected.
    B. Observing for signs of hypoglycemia as a result of treatment.
    C. Giving fruit juices, broth, and milk as soon as he is able to take fluids orally.
    D. Regulating insulin dosage according to the amount of ketones found in the urine.

315. Important to both Mr. Mulji and his wife, Salima, is an understanding that a diabetic diet:
    A. Is based on nutritional requirements that are the same for all clients.
    B. Can be planned around a wide variety of commonly available foods.
    C. Should be rigidly controlled to avoid similar diabetic emergencies.
    D. Must not include processed foods because they have too many variable seasonings.

---

*Case Study:* Melanie, a 28-year-old college student, is admitted to the hospital for diabetic acidosis. Questions 316 to 318 relate to this scenario.

316. After blood work and observation of urinary volume, the physician orders 20 mEq of potassium chloride to be added to the IV solution. The primary purpose for administering this drug to Melanie is:
    A. Replacement of potassium deficit.
    B. Treatment of hypercapnia.
    C. Prevention of flaccid paralysis.
    D. Treatment of cardiac dysrhythmias.

317. The nurse should recognize that Melanie needs further teaching when, after reviewing the dietary exchange system, Melanie she states that:
    A. 1 scoop ice milk = 1 slice bread.
    B. 1 oz cheese = 1 cup milk.
    C. 1 egg = 1 oz meat.
    D. 1 slice bacon = 2 Tbsp cream.

318. Melanie's nursing care plan indicates that before discharge, she will know how to self-administer insulin, adjust the dosage, understand her diet, and perform glucose monitoring. She progresses well and is discharged 10 days after admission. Legally:
    A. The physician was responsible, and the nurse should have cleared the care with him or her.
    B. The nurse was properly functioning as a health teacher.

C. The visiting nurse should do health teaching in the home.
    D. A family member should have also been taught to administer the insulin.

319. Early indications of lithium toxicity include:
    A. Torticollis.
    B. Tinnitus.
    C. Akathisia.
    D. Diarrhea.

320. Why is important for nurses to assess blood pressure in patients receiving antipsychotic drugs?
    A. Orthostatic hypotension is a common side effect.
    B. Most antipsychotic drugs cause elevated blood pressure.
    C. This provides additional support for the patient.
    D. It will indicate the need to institute anti-parkinsonian drugs.

321. Alcohol withdrawal delirium is a medical emergency. Which of the following symptoms would alert the nurse to the potential for delirium tremors?
    A. Fever, hypertension, changes in level of consciousness, and hallucinations.
    B. Hypertension, stupor, agitation, headache, and auditory hallucinations.
    C. Vomiting, ataxia, muscular rigidity, and tactile hallucinations.
    D. Coarse hand tremor, agitation, hallucinations, and hypertension.

---

*Case Study:* Jane Bryant, age 29 years, is involved in an automobile accident. She is brought to the emergency department with head trauma, but she is awake and able to speak. Questions 322 and 323 relate to this scenario.

322. Which of the following questions would best assess her cerebral function?
    A. Can you tell me your address?
    B. How would you describe your eyesight?
    C. Have you noticed a change in your coordination?
    D. Have you noticed a change in your muscle strength?

323. As the nurse, you assess the following change in Jane's status: Initially her pupils were equal; now the right pupil is fully dilated and nonreactive, and the left pupil is 4 mm and reacts to light. What would this suggest?

A. Increased intracranial pressure.
B. Decreased intracranial pressure.
C. The test was not performed accurately.
D. Normal response after a head injury.

**324.** The parents of a critically ill infant are practicing Roman Catholics. The nurse is aware that baptism is an important religious ritual. Which of the following is the best action for the nurse to take?

A. Ask the hospital chaplain to baptize the baby.
B. Ask the doctor to baptize the baby.
C. Ask the parents what their wishes are regarding baptism.
D. Do nothing because discussing baptism will make the parents more anxious.

**325.** A patient recovering from surgery in the hospital requests spiritual support from a parish nurse. A parish nurse is:

A. A registered nurse who works in a community with religious organizations.
B. Only concerned with how spirituality interacts with physical health.
C. Someone who is called to the ministry to promote health.
D. A nurse who believes faith and health are separate.

**326.** A 78-year-old woman has been discharged recently from the hospital after experiencing heart failure relating to long-standing hypertension and coronary artery disease. A community health nurse is evaluating her compliance with medication therapy. Which of the following factors best indicates that the client is complying with digoxin (Lanoxin) therapy?

A. Her ability to correctly count her radial pulse.
B. Her weight gain of 2 lb in less than a week.
C. An apical heart rate of 101 bpm.
D. Absence of a pericardial friction rub.

**327.** The nurse is teaching a female client with osteoporosis about her prescribed diet. Which of the following foods is the best source of calcium?

A. 1 cup of low-fat yogurt.
B. 1 cup of skim milk.
C. 1 oz of cheddar cheese.
D. 1 cup of ice cream.

**328.** A client is being discharged after successful same-day cataract surgery. The nurse instructs the client about permitted activities and those to avoid. Which of the following activities is permitted?

A. Cooking.
B. Driving.
C. Vacuuming.
D. Showering.

**329.** A client with chronic obstructive pulmonary disease (COPD) is being discharged after treatment for an acute exacerbation. Which statement by the client indicates proper understanding of the discharge instructions?

A. "I should take my bronchodilator at bedtime to prevent insomnia."
B. "I should do my most difficult activities when I first get up in the morning."
C. "I should try to eat several small meals during the day."
D. "I should plan to do my exercises after I eat."

**330.** Which aging characteristic increases the risk of falls in elderly individuals?

A. Forward-flexed posture.
B. Decreased ability to adapt.
C. Inability to take responsibility.
D. Increased reaction time.

**331.** Many falls in older adults are related to:

A. Tripping.
B. Wearing slippers.
C. The urge to urinate.
D. Barriers between the bed and bathroom.

**332.** A 63-year-old female client has a 10-year history of rheumatoid arthritis. Her 40-year-old daughter has recently noticed that she herself wakes up with stiff joints. The client shares her concerns regarding her daughter with you. What would be the most appropriate response?

A. Explain that rheumatoid arthritis does not have a genetic basis, so there is nothing for her to be concerned about.
B. Tell her that there is some evidence that a genetic basis for the disease may exist and suggest that the daughter be evaluated.
C. Have her suggest that her daughter take aspirin for a few days to see if the stiffness is relieved.
D. Reassure her that it is normal for a 40-year-old woman to have aches and pains and that her concern is probably unwarranted.

**333.** A plan of care for a client with osteoporosis includes active and passive exercises, calcium supplements, and daily vitamins. The desired effect of therapy would be noted by the nurse if the client:

A. Had fewer bruises than on admission.
B. Developed an increase in her mobility.
C. Developed fewer cardiac irregularities.
D. Developed fewer muscular spasms.

334. A community health nurse visits an older adult client whose husband has recently passed away. The client says, "No one cares about me anymore. All the people I loved are dead." Which of the following responses by the nurse conveys therapeutic communication?

    A. "That seems rather unlikely to me."
    B. "You must be feeling lonely at this time."
    C. "I don't believe that, and neither do you."
    D. "That's true. Why don't you just give up?"

335. Mrs. McDonald, an 84-year-old widow, has been diagnosed with metastatic melanoma and is admitted for hospice care. The nurse caring for Mrs. MacDonald knows that clients in the initial stage of accepting the diagnosis of terminal illness often:

    A. Ask for other medical opinions.
    B. Cry uncontrollably over the diagnosis.
    C. Criticize medical care received.
    D. Isolate themselves and refuse visitors.

336. A male client, age 78 years, has recently been diagnosed with hypothyroidism. He lives in his own apartment in a community facility designed for elderly people. He asks the nurse assigned to the complex for advice about his condition. What would be the best advice the nurse could give this client?

    A. "Stop taking your prescribed daily aspirin."
    B. "Stop attending your group activities."
    C. "Increase your daily caloric consumption."
    D. "Increase fibre and fluids in your diet."

337. Which clinical signs would indicate to a nurse caring for a terminally ill patient that death may be imminent?

    A. Cold, clammy skin and irregular, noisy breathing.
    B. Apnea and a body temperature of 37°C.
    C. Swallowing reflex and bowel sounds present.
    D. Respirations regular at 18 breaths/min and pedal pulse present.

338. When a disaster occurs, the nurse may have to treat mass hysteria first. The person or persons to be cared for immediately would be those in which of the following states?

    A. Depressive.
    B. Euphoric.

    C. Panic.
    D. Comatose.

339. In any disaster concerning a number of people, the function that contributes most to saving lives is triage. When determining the priority of needs, the people who need immediate care are those with:

    A. A second-degree burn covering 10% of the body.
    B. Severe lacerations involving open fractures of major bones.
    C. Closed fractures of major bones.
    D. Pain from whiplash and soft tissue injuries.

340. There has just been a 25-vehicle collision in your community. You are the first on the scene. From the options below, who would require immediate care?

    A. Those with severe head injuries.
    B. Those with multiple fractures.
    C. Those with minor bleeding.
    D. Those with controlled severe bleeding.

341. A client is placed on home oxygen therapy using a nasal cannula at 2 L/min and an oxygen concentrator. The client expresses a fear of using oxygen at home, stating, "I just know it will blow up." What is the nurse's best response?

    A. "You have nothing to worry about. That never happens anymore."
    B. "I would like to further discuss your concerns about this. What have you heard about using oxygen at home?"
    C. "I've brought information that I want you to read. After you go through it, you'll see that you don't have anything to worry about."
    D. "Thousands of people use oxygen therapy safely in their homes every day."

342. A female client is discharged from the hospital after having an exacerbation of congestive heart failure. She is prescribed a daily oral doses furosemide (Lasix). Two days later, she tells her community health nurse that she feels weak and frequently feels her heart "flutter." What would be the nurse's priority action?

    A. Call the physician and tell the client to rest more often to decrease her symptoms.
    B. Tell the client to stop taking the digoxin, call the physician, and have the client stop all physical activity.
    C. Call the physician; report the symptoms; and upon the physician's order, send a blood

sample to the laboratory to determine the client's potassium level.

D. Give firm and clear instructions about avoiding foods that contain caffeine.

343. A nurse is teaching a client about the use of a respiratory inhaler. Which of the following would not be a component of the teaching plan?

A. Remove the cap and shake the inhaler well before use.

B. Press the canister down with your finger as you breathe in.

C. Inhale the mist and quickly exhale.

D. Wait 1 minute between puffs if more than 1 puff has been prescribed.

344. Mr. Tse has been recently diagnosed with kidney failure. A fluid restriction order of 1000 mL q24h is in effect. Knowing this, the nurse caring for Mr. Tse should:

A. Eliminate all liquids between meal times.

B. Divide fluids equally over three nursing shifts.

C. Indicate just clear liquids in the restriction plan.

D. Proportion more fluids during the day than during the night.

345. The nurse should provide a confused client with an environment that is:

A. Challenging.

B. Nonstimulating.

C. Variable.

D. Familiar.

346. Mr. Jones, age 78 years, has Parkinson's disease. He slept very poorly last night, was nauseated when he got up this morning, and feels weak and tired. He ate a small portion of his breakfast. He is scheduled to go down to physiotherapy in 1 hour. What action should the nurse take?

A. Give him an antiemetic to reduce the nausea and get him up and dressed to go to physiotherapy.

B. Assess his nausea and sleep interferences; call physiotherapy to cancel or reschedule his appointment.

C. Notify the dietician to change his diet to clear fluids; cancel physiotherapy until his strength resumes.

D. Ask the dietician to visit with him regarding food preferences and recommend that the doctor order sleeping pills for him.

**Case Study:** *Jennifer Hall, age 43 years, has been admitted for a left mastectomy after confirmation of cancer from the biopsy report. She has a daughter who is 12 years old. Questions 347 to 351 relate to this scenario.*

347. Communication is very important when preparing Jennifer for the mastectomy. What are important issues to discuss with her?

A. How body image changes will affect her sexual relationship.

B. Concerns regarding the cancer and how the surgery will affect her.

C. Impact of surgery on the family's coping abilities.

D. History of breast cancer in the family.

348. Jennifer states that her husband has been very supportive but says, "I've been a basket case just thinking of what implications this has for us as a family." How would you respond?

A. "Sounds like you are still in denial about the diagnosis."

B. "This is a very difficult adjustment period for you and your family."

C. "You need to talk to someone who has gone through this same experience."

D. "Let's discuss this problem with your husband and daughter."

349. What would you include in Jennifer's preoperative teaching before a mastectomy?

A. Informing her regarding a Hemovac, pressure dressing, and deep breathing exercises.

B. Explaining that a catheter will be inserted and removed on the first postoperative day.

C. Informing her that she will not be allowed food or fluids for the first 2 days.

D. Explaining that she will have minimal effects from the anaesthetic because the surgery is superficial and quick.

350. Jennifer's husband has arrived to be with her before her surgery. When she leaves for the operating room, what would you tell her husband?

A. Encourage him to go to work and come back later in the evening when the anaesthetic effects are gone.

B. Inform him that he can see her as soon as she comes out of the operating room.

C. Inform him that she will be going to the recovery room after the operation; they will notify the unit when she is ready to come back.

D. Take this opportunity to discuss the concerns she expressed regarding the implications this has for her family.

351. When Jennifer returns from the recovery room, which of the following is *not* included in the initial postoperative assessment?

    A. Assessing the vital signs and oxygen saturation levels.
    B. Checking the dressing, drain, and amount of drainage.
    C. Checking the neurologic responses and level of pain.
    D. Checking for urinary retention and the need to void.

352. Mr. Gupta, age 44 years, is admitted to the hospital. His religious beliefs require that he meditate and pray several times every day. He tells the nurse he is uncomfortable praying in his semi-private room. How would the nurse respond?

    A. "It's unfortunate you feel uncomfortable. Could you pull the drapes around your bed for privacy?"
    B. "I'm sure this is difficult for you; I'll see when a private room may become available."
    C. "I can see you're concerned about this. I could arrange a private place for you to pray."
    D. "I'm sorry for your discomfort. Could I call the hospital chaplain to assist you?"

353. Mrs. Li is receiving chemotherapy through a central venous catheter into her right subclavian vein. The nurse observes that she is dyspneic and cyanotic; her blood pressure has dropped to 86/48 mm Hg and she has a weak, rapid pulse. Mrs. Li is complaining of pain in her chest and shoulder. What complication would the nurse suspect?

    A. Circulatory overload.
    B. Air embolism.
    C. Infection.
    D. Infiltration.

354. You are caring for a patient who has returned from the operating room after an exploratory laparotomy. He has an IV infusion at 150 cc/hr. He has not voided for 8 hours. Postoperative orders read: "Catheterize prn. Conservative measures to stimulate voiding have not been successful." What assessments and actions would you take?

    A. Palpate all four abdominal quadrants and assess his intake and output record.
    B. Inspect and palpate the lower abdomen; if it is distended and uncomfortable, insert a straight catheter.

    C. Give him pain medication and catheterize him as soon as possible to lessen the possibility of a bladder and kidney infection.
    D. Wait until the patient experiences considerable discomfort in the bladder region and then catheterize.

## Short Answer Questions

355. Identify four criteria for evaluating nursing research information on the Internet. (4 points)

356. Define nursing informatics. (1 point)

357. Describe how a nurse could implement informatics into the work setting. (1 point)

358. Identify two objectives for standardized interdisciplinary electronic documentation. (2 points)

359. As the nurse, you are conducting therapeutic range of motion exercises on your client. Identify the purposes of passive, active, and resistive range of motion exercises. (3 points)

360. A nurse is planning care for a client who is depressed and may be suicidal. Identify two signs that would indicate that a client is suicidal (2 points).

**361.** A home care nurse visits a client. The client tells the nurse that the physician told him to take ibuprofen 0.4 g for mild pain. The medication bottle states ibuprofen is available in 200-mg tablets. In planning the pain medications for the client, how many tablets should the nurse tell the client to take? (1 point)

**362.** Identify and briefly describe three outcomes you would observe in a patient who has adapted to having an ostomy. (3 points)

**363.** If the patient's postoperative pain is not controlled, the risk for pressure ulcer development increases because pain will limit the patient's ability to change position frequently. What actions should the nurse take to reduce the risk for pressure ulcer development? (1 point)

**364.** A physician orders an IV solution of 1000 mL of D5W to be administered at 100 mL/hr. The drop factor of the IV administration set is 15 drops/hr. How many drops per minute should the patient receive? (1point)

**365.** Identify three criteria for consent for surgery to be valid. (3 points)

**366.** Identify and briefly describe two reasons why repositioning a patient every 2 hours increases both circulation and respiration. (2 points)

**367.** Identify two reasons why body fluid losses may exceed fluid intake. (2 points)

**368.** Describe one characteristic of a healthy stoma. (1 point)

---

**Case Study:** *Mrs. Marge Evenrude, age 88 years, is admitted to the unit from the emergency department after having a cerebrovascular accident (CVA) affecting the right side of her body. She is aphasic and chokes when taking fluids. Her daughter was at her home and witnessed the CVA 2 hours ago. The doctor has ordered IV tissue plasminogen activator (TPA) to be given. Questions 369 to 370 relate to this scenario.*

**369.** Describe two measures you would take to enhance communication with Mrs. Evenrude. (2 points)

**370.** Identify two health team members and their role in the rehabilitation of Mrs. Evenrude. (2 points)

**371.** Describe one characteristic of a necrotic stoma. (1 point)

**372.** Identify three complications of endotracheal suctioning. (3 points)

**373.** Describe the purpose of antiembolism stockings. (1 point)

**374.** Joint mobility is limited by ligaments, muscles, and the nature of the joint. Describe three joint movements used in range of motion exercises. (3 points)

**375.** Identify two precautions taken to prevent dislodgement or disconnection of a central line. (2 points)

**376.** Describe the purpose of postural drainage. (1 point)

**377.** A stage II pressure ulcer is partial-thickness skin loss involving the epidermis or dermis. Describe two observations of a stage II pressure ulcer and identify the treatment objectives. (2 points)

**378.** Explain the three phases of wound healing. (3 points)

**379.** A tornado has just hit your community. Reports indicate that many people are dead and approximately 500 people are injured. As an RN, you are helping to provide round-the-clock first aid services. What is your plan of action? (1 point)

**380.** Describe the difference between multi-trauma and multiple casualties. (2 points)

**381.** Provide two suggestions that can help a client regain control of urinary incontinence. (2 points)

**382.** Identify three vascular structures (veins) used for central venous access. (3 points)

**383.** Some medical conditions may create complications when inserting a venous device. Identify two such conditions. (2 points)

**384.** Describe two purposes of closed chest drainage. (2 points)

**385.** Describe three considerations a nurse must make before administering a nasogastric (NG) tube feeding. (3 points)

**386.** Identify three reasons a physician may order insertion of a tube. (3 points)

**387.** Identify two priority nursing actions that must be taken before infusing blood products. (2 points)

**Case Study:** *Mr. Ramsay, a 43-year-old patient, is admitted with a gastrointestinal (GI) hemorrhage. His physician has ordered a blood transfusion. Mr. Ramsay has an IV infusion of 100 mL 5% dextrose/lactated Ringer's solution infusing in his left arm. Question 388 relates to this scenario.*

**388.** What type of blood transfusion is Mr. Ramsay most likely to receive? (1 point)

**389.** Describe the causes, signs and symptoms, prevention, and treatment of hyperglycemia. (3 points)

**390.** Describe the causes, symptoms, and prevention, and treatment of hypoglycemia. (3 points)

**391.** Identify when central line catheters are more effective in the delivery of medications and solutions than peripherally placed catheters. (1 point)

**392.** Identify one bacterial respiratory infection spread by droplet and one viral infection spread by droplet transmission. (2 points)

**Case Study:** *Mr. Lechelt comes to the hospital for open heart surgery. After 3 days, he is diagnosed with an antibiotic-resistant organism. Questions 393 and 394 relate to this scenario.*

**393.** When caring for Mr. Lechelt, the nurse should adhere to good hand washing techniques. Hand washing is one example of universal standard precautions. Describe two other examples. (2 points)

**394.** Even though the nurse caring for Mr. Lechelt is wearing gloves, she washes her hands after removing the gloves. What is the reason she adheres to this routine? (1 point)

**395.** A nurse notices that a patient's creatinine kinase (CK) levels are markedly elevated. What is a normal range for CK? (1 point)

**396.** How many hours after a cardiac infarction occurs might creatinine kinase levels increase? (1 point)

**397.** Identify two contraindications for administration of thrombolytic therapy. (2 points)

**398.** Describe two key causes of hyponatremia. (2 points)

**399.** Identify two vasoactive medications used to treat patients in shock. (2 points)

**400.** Which two laboratory results would indicate respiratory acidosis? (2 point)

**401.** Identify and briefly describe three health promotion strategies nurses could implement to assist clients diagnosed with chronic illnesses. (3 points)

**402.** Describe one way a patient may exhibit that he or she is working through the grieving process. (1 point)

> **Answers and Rationales**

**1. B.** Research the condition and present what you have learned as well as your assessment findings and care measures.

*Rationale*
This is an opportunity for new learning about a complication that pertains to your patient and an important safety consideration when assessing and performing care measures. Presenting this case would also provide a professional growth opportunity.

*Classification*
Competency Category: Professional Practice
Taxonomic Level: Critical Thinking

**2. D.** Having well-intentioned behaviours that detract from achievable health outcomes for patients.

*Rationale*
Professional boundaries focus on provision of professional care that assists clients in achieving health outcomes.

*Classification*
Competency Category: Nurse–Person Relationship
Taxonomic Level: Knowledge/Comprehension

**3. B.** It may allow the nurse to examine how biases and assumptions could interfere with therapeutic effectiveness.

*Rationale*
Self-awareness in nurses allows openness and a willingness to enhance therapeutic relationships. Answer B is an example of ways nurses can examine their biases and examine how they interfere with rapport building.

*Classification*
Competency Category: Nurse–Person Relationship
Taxonomic Level: Application

**4. A.** The personality style theory acknowledges that the nature of individuals in a group helps us understand group dynamics and sources of conflict in the group.

*Rationale*
Effective principles of group process emphasize getting to know individuals and understanding the diverse nature of participants.

*Classification*
Competency Category: Nurse–Person Relationship
Taxonomic Level: Knowledge/Comprehension

**5. C.** Groups encourage similarity of viewpoints and minimize differing opinions.

*Rationale*
When groups are forced to conform and when there is little acknowledgement of differing opinions, group effectiveness is limited.

*Classification*
Competency Category: Nurse–Person Relationship
Taxonomic Level: Knowledge/Comprehension

**6. A.** Acknowledge your appreciation of this experience, explain that her nursing needs have been met, and tell her you have to leave to care for other new mothers.

*Rationale*
Clarification of the professional role is important so the patient understands the boundaries of the professional relationship and that it differs from a social relationship.

*Classification*
Competency Category: Nurse–Person Relationship
Taxonomic Level: Critical Thinking

**7. C.** Explore reasons why he wishes to cancel the surgery, clarify his concerns, and reinforce that he can change his mind if he chooses.

*Rationale*
Although he has signed the consent, he still has the choice of whether to follow through and have the surgery. The reason for the change in decision also needs to be explored to see if he is lacking important information.

*Classification*
Competency Category: Nurse–Person Relationship
Taxonomic Level: Application

**8. A.** Ensure that he signs the release form and contact the doctor and the operating room staff.

*Rationale*
The nurse needs to respect the patient's decision and ensure that team members are appropriately notified regarding his choice and the cancellation of surgery.

*Classification*
Competency Category: Professional Practice
Taxonomic Level: Application

**9. B.** Ask her why she is keeping the used syringes and ensure they are disposed of safely.

*Rationale*
It is important to find out the reason underlying her retention of the syringes and to ensure that she is not reusing contaminated syringes. Safe disposal is also important so needlestick injuries do not occur.

*Classification*
Competency Category: Nursing Practice: Health and Wellness
Taxonomic Level: Application

**10. C.** Temporarily dress the wound, explain that verbal abuse is not tolerated, leave the room, and return later to discuss alternate wound dressing strategies.

*Rationale*
The wound needs to be left protected, but the verbal abuse should also be addressed. Other strategies need to be explored (e.g., analgesics before the dressing change) so the patient can better tolerate the dressing change.

*Classification*
Competency Category: Nursing Practice: Health and Wellness
Taxonomic Level: Critical Thinking

**11. D.** Disoriented to place, tachypneic, shallow breathing at 34/min, orthopneic with circumoral cyanosis. Oxygen saturations of 84%.

*Rationale*
This documentation most accurately describes the findings of the assessment using appropriate medical terminology.

*Classification*
Competency Category: Professional Practice
Taxonomic Level: Critical Thinking

**12. C.** Community health clinics, telehealth, and hospital-based web site.

*Rationale*
Outlining credible resources is important for nurses to do for new mothers. This choice contains the most reliable resources.

*Classification*
Competency Category: Nursing Practice: Alterations in Health
Taxonomic Level: Application

**13. D.** Checking the placement of the tube by aspiration and testing the pH of the contents.

*Rationale*
Checking to ensure the proper placement of the NG tube is most important. The presence of acidic stomach contents is the most reliable of the tests outlined.

*Classification*
Competency Category: Nursing Practice: Alterations in Health
Taxonomic Level: Knowledge

**14. B.** Initiating oxygen therapy, Fowler's positioning, pain control, and addressing her questions and concerns.

*Rationale*
Addressing the patient's priority physical needs and promoting comfort are very important. Psychosocial concerns can be addressed next.

*Classification*
Competency Category: Nursing Practice: Alterations in Health
Taxonomic Level: Application

**15. A.** Explore other ways to more effectively control her symptoms and advocate for her when approaching her family.

*Rationale*
Trying other nursing measures may more effectively alleviate her symptoms, and the nurse's role as advocate is very important to explain what is happening to the family and support her.

*Classification*
Competency Category: Nursing Practice: Alterations in Health
Taxonomic Level: Critical Thinking

**16. B.** A formal written plan of action for coordinating the response of the hospital staff and to designate how different areas will be used.

*Rationale*
These are important components of a disaster preparedness plan.

*Classification*
Competency Category: Nursing Practice: Alterations in Health
Taxonomic Level: Knowledge/Comprehension

**17. B.** Stoma care and application of an ostomy pouch and drainage bag, increasing intake of fluids, observing amount and the colour of the urine.

*Rationale*
Teaching regarding care of the ostomy, the importance of fluids, and observing urine output are the most important teaching components for care of a urostomy.

*Classification*
Competency Category: Nursing Practice: Alterations in Health
Taxonomic Level: Application

**18. C.** A 65-year-old patient who has employment-induced presbycusis and advanced glaucoma.

*Rationale*
This patient is most at risk for sensory deprivation because of two sensory deficits.

*Classification*
Competency Category: Nursing Practice: Alterations in Health
Taxonomic Level: Application

**19. A.** Have her wear a disposable mask when she is transported to the radiography department.

*Rationale*
Because tuberculosis is airborne and spread by droplet infection, having her wear a mask is necessary to prevent transmission.

*Classification*
Competency Category: Nursing Practice: Health and Wellness
Taxonomic Level: Knowledge/Comprehension

**20. B.** The frequency, duration, and intensity of her contractions.

*Rationale*
Assessment of the contractions and the frequency between contractions is important before analgesic administration.

*Classification*
Competency Category: Nursing Practice: Alterations in Health
Taxonomic Level: Application

**21. B.** Ask her if she understands the reason for the cramping and bleeding and explain what precautions she could take to retain the pregnancy.

*Rationale*
The patient needs to be able to identify when cramps and bleeding could indicate a threat to the fetus and herself and to monitor this carefully, consult with the doctor, and restrict her activity.

*Classification*
Competency Category: Nursing Practice: Health and Wellness
Taxonomic Level: Knowledge/Comprehension

**22. C.** Pallor, cold extremities, and tachycardia.

*Rationale*
These three signs indicate hypovolemic shock and the body's compensation for the blood loss.

*Classification*
Competency Category: Nursing Practice: Alterations in Health
Taxonomic Level: Knowledge/Comprehension

**23. A.** Position her in Sims position with her head to the side, give oxygen as ordered, and suction if needed.

*Rationale*
Sims position is indicated for patients regaining consciousness and to ensure patency of the airway by allowing secretions and blood to pool in the cheek and drain out the side of the mouth. If secretions are accumulating too quickly, suctioning may be required.

*Classification*
Competency Category: Nursing Practice: Alterations in Health
Taxonomic Level: Application

**24. A.** Pallor, coolness, and numbness of the toes.

*Rationale*
Teaching should include recognition of these important signs and symptoms that would indicate that circulation or nervous system functioning is impaired.

*Classification*
Competency Category: Nursing Practice: Alterations in Health
Taxonomic Level: Understanding

**25. A.** Check the patency and amount of drainage from the NG tube.

*Rationale*
Subjective assessment data indicate that the NG tube may not be functioning, so assessment of its patency and the amount of drainage would be the first step. Then appropriate action can be taken if the tube is not patent.

*Classification*
Competency Category: Nursing Practice: Alterations in Health
Taxonomic Level: Application

**26. A.** Eupnea related to esophageal varices.

*Rationale*
Eupnea is normal respirations and does not represent a problem. It is not related to esophageal varices, which can present with cirrhosis of the liver.

*Classification*
Competency Category: Nursing Practice: Alterations in Health
Taxonomic Level: Knowledge/Comprehension

**27. B.** Purulent drainage, pain in the mid incision, and temperature of 38.5°C.

*Rationale*
Signs of systemic temperature elevation, increased inflammation, and drainage of purulent exudate all indicate wound infection.

*Classification*
Competency Category: Nursing Practice: Alterations in Health
Taxonomic Level: Knowledge/Comprehension

**28. B.** 200 mg.

*Rationale*
Math calculations are as follows:
$30 \times 26.67 = 800.1$
800.1/4 doses = 200 mg/dose

*Classification*
Competency Category: Nursing Practice: Alterations in Health
Taxonomic Level: Application

**29. C.** Position her in Fowler's position, initiate oxygen, and give bronchodilators as ordered.

*Rationale*
Correct positioning, oxygenating, and relieving the bronchospasm are critical for patients during asthma attacks.

*Classification*
Competency Category: Nursing Practice: Alterations in Health
Taxonomic Level: Application

**30. C.** "When morphine is used to alleviate severe pain for 2 to 3 days, there is little likelihood of becoming addicted."

*Rationale*
Patients need to understand that when pain is present, morphine is used therapeutically to alleviate the pain and there is less likelihood of addiction.

*Classification*
Competency Category: Nursing Practice: Alterations in Health
Taxonomic Level: Knowledge/Comprehension

**31. B.** Check the patient regarding chills, low back pain, dyspnea, and skin itching during the transfusion.

*Rationale*
Checking for the possibility of transfusion reactions is an important responsibility. Answer B outlines some of the signs associated with transfusion reactions.

*Classification*
Competency Category: Nursing Practice: Alterations in Health
Taxonomic Level: Application

**32. A.** Tachypnea, orthopnea, tachycardia, and circumoral cyanosis.

*Rationale*
When the body is hypoxic, the person will increase the heart rate and breathing to alleviate the problem; reduced hemoglobin results in cyanosis.

*Classification*
Competency Category: Nursing Practice: Alterations in Health
Taxonomic Level: Knowledge/Comprehension

**33. D.** Approach her calmly and find out what is causing her to be upset.

*Rationale*
Using a calm approach and asking a clarifying question will help address the patient's concerns and help the nurse build a trusting rapport.

*Classification*
Competency Category: Nurse–Person Relationship
Taxonomic Level: Application

**34. A.** "This is devastating news for you. I'll let you have some time and will come back later."

*Rationale*
Acknowledging to the patient the magnitude of the diagnosis and responding to his cues to be alone are the most appropriate responses.

*Classification*
Competency Category: Nurse–Person Relationship
Taxonomic Level: Application

**35. B.** Assessing the neurovascular status in the right leg; providing pain control; and encouraging deep breathing and coughing exercises, position changes, and early ambulation.

*Rationale*
These assessments and measures are most important priorities after an ORIF.

*Classification*
Competency Category: Nursing Practice: Alterations in Health
Taxonomic Level: Application

**36. B.** Place him in Fowler's position, initiate oxygen therapy, and get an analgesic ordered.

*Rationale*
Initiating measures to increase oxygenation and control pain are most important.

*Classification*
Competency Category: Nursing Practice: Alterations in Health
Taxonomic Level: Application

**37. C.** Severe pain aggravated by plantarflexion, tense and tender muscles in the lateral right calf, and paresthesia.

*Rationale*
Compartment syndrome is an emergency situation that can present in a trauma situation. Answer C outlines the characteristics of this syndrome.

*Classification*
Competency Category: Nursing Practice: Alterations in Health
Taxonomic Level: Knowledge/Comprehension

**38. A.** The rate and depth of respiration.

*Rationale*
Morphine depresses respiration, so the nurse should assess the patient's respiratory rate.

*Classification*
Competency Category: Nursing Practice: Alterations in Health
Taxonomic Level: Application

**39. B.** Ask her about her usual eating patterns and reason for her low intake.

*Rationale*
You would ask her about her eating and identify the observations you have made regarding low intake; anorexia nervosa may be presenting.

*Classification*
Competency Category: Nursing Practice: Alterations in Health
Taxonomic Level: Application

**40. B.** Change the rate to 125 cc/hr and observe for fluid overload.

*Rationale*
The rate of infusion is too rapid; it should be 125 cc/hr. The nurse should observe for signs indicating too rapid an infusion.

*Classification*
Competency Category: Nursing Practice: Alterations in Health
Taxonomic Level: Critical Thinking

**41. D.** Position her in Fowler's position, administer oxygen as ordered, and give her the ordered prn med salbutamol (Ventolin) by inhaler.

*Rationale*
These are appropriate actions during an asthma attack to ensure that breathing is optimized and bronchospasm is counteracted.

*Classification*
Competency Category: Nursing Practice: Alterations in Health
Taxonomic Level: Application

**42. C.** Contact the doctor, explain that the pain is still at 8 of 10, and request a higher dosage.

*Rationale*
Renal colic can be one of the most severe pain experiences. The medication has not provided relief, so additional intervention is appropriate.

*Classification*
Competency Category: Nursing Practice: Alterations in Health
Taxonomic Level: Critical Thinking

**43. C.** The nurse does not know the answer and checks to find the answer on the unit or in the library.

*Rationale*
This activity indicates that the nurse recognizes his or her own learning need and then seeks to find the answer. This process includes elements of critical thinking.

*Classification*
Competency Category: Professional Practice
Taxonomic Level: Application

**44. A.** The assessment step because it involves collecting, organizing, and validating information that is used for the remaining steps.

*Rationale*
The assessment step is most important because if data collection is inaccurate or incomplete, it will influence the effectiveness of each of the subsequent steps.

*Classification*
Competency Category: Professional Practice
Taxonomic Level: Knowledge/Comprehension

**45. B.** Critical thinking skills are used to interpret, analyze, and cluster the assessment data to determine the problems.

*Rationale*
Critical thinking skills are used to interpret and analyze the assessment data to determine the patient's problems.

*Classification*
Competency Category: Nursing Practice: Alterations in Health
Taxonomic Level: Knowledge/Comprehension

**46. B.** Health habits, family, and social and sexual patterns.

*Rationale*
This answer represents the most complete answer pertaining to aspects of psychosocial assessment.

*Classification*
Competency Category: Nursing Practice: Alterations in Health
Taxonomic Level: Knowledge/Comprehension

**47. B.** Obtain information to identify the level of health of the client and his or her past illnesses.

*Rationale*
Subjective information is collected with the health history to determine the current level of health and past illnesses that could impact the current situation.

*Classification*
Competency Category: Nursing Practice: Health and Wellness
Taxonomic Level: Knowledge/Comprehension

**48. D.** Inspection.

*Rationale*
Inspection is usually completed followed by auscultation. If percussion or palpation is done before auscultation, the findings may change.

*Classification*
Competency Category: Nursing Practice: Alterations in Health
Taxonomic Level: Knowledge/Comprehension

**49. B.** A postoperative patient's pulse has been increasing, and his blood pressure is decreasing.

*Rationale*
This indicates that the status of the patient is rapidly changing and may indicate that the body was initially compensating but is now decompensating, as evidenced by the decrease in blood pressure.

*Classification*
Competency Category: Nursing Practice: Alterations in Health
Taxonomic Level: Critical Thinking

**50. B.** An evaluation of psychomotor and cognitive learning.

*Rationale*
The client has learned new skills as well as new information related to medications.

*Classification*
Competency Category: Nursing Practice: Alterations in Health
Taxonomic Level: Application

**51. D.** Prevention of osteoporosis and the importance of regular breast self-examinations and regular Pap smears.

*Rationale*
Primary prevention teaching should focus on risk factors for the population and include teaching to prevent these problems. Answer D is the most complete of the choices.

*Classification*
Competency Category: Nursing Practice: Health and Wellness
Taxonomic Level: Critical Thinking

**52. A.** Importance of exercise, balanced nutrition and hydration, and safety and fall prevention.

*Rationale*
This choice provides teaching regarding health promotion and illness and injury prevention for elderly clients living in their homes.

*Classification*
Competency Category: Nursing Practice: Health and Wellness
Taxonomic Level: Critical Thinking

**53. C.** Malpractice is failure to perform professional duties that result in patient injury.

*Rationale*
The only legal definition that is accurate is the malpractice one, which is failure to perform duties that result in injury.

*Classification*
Competency Category: Professional Practice
Taxonomic Level: Application

**54. D.** Accountability for care.

*Rationale*
Abnormalities need to be checked so current assessments can be completed and vital sign abnormalities can be verified.

*Classification*
Competency Category: Professional Practice
Taxonomic Level: Application

**55. B.** Oxygenate the patient and then suction for 10 to 15 seconds while withdrawing the catheter.

*Rationale*
Safe suctioning should be preceded by oxygenation, and suctioning should last a maximum of 15 seconds.

*Classification*
Competency Category: Nursing Practice: Alterations in Health
Taxonomic Level: Application

**56. C.** Disconnection of the connecting tubing from the chest tube.

*Rationale*
All of the other situations can happen with chest tubes, but the one that requires emergency intervention is disconnection of the tubing from the chest tube.

*Classification*
Competency Category: Nursing Practice: Alterations in Health
Taxonomic Level: Critical Thinking

**57. C.** Intermittent cramping, abdominal pain, and bowel sounds in all four quadrants.

*Rationale*
Return of peristalsis will be evident by cramping pain and active sounds in all four quadrants.

*Classification*
Competency Category: Nursing Practice: Alterations in Health
Taxonomic Level: Application

**58. B.** Ensure that the client understands that a bolus may take up to 15 minute to alleviate the pain.

*Rationale*
Patients need to be informed regarding self-administration of pain medication and anticipation of effects.

*Classification*
Competency Category: Nursing Practice: Alterations in Health
Taxonomic Level: Application

**59. A.** Combining these two drugs will increase pain relief without the increased side effects of increasing the morphine dose.

*Rationale*
Providing explanations regarding potentiation effects of medications is the most important point, and evaluating effectiveness of the combination is the second most important point.

*Classification*
Competency Category: Nursing Practice: Alterations in Health
Taxonomic Level: Application

**60. B.** Gentle massage of the area, warm and cold applications, guided imagery, and TENS.

*Rationale*
The alternative measures to reduce pain and enhance comfort are most completely identified in this choice.

*Classification*
Competency Category: Nursing Practice: Alterations in Health
Taxonomic Level: Application

**61. B.** Circumoral cyanosis and $PaO_2$ of 70 mm Hg.

*Rationale*
Severe hypoxia would be indicated by low oxygen saturation levels and reduced haemoglobin, resulting in cyanosis.

*Classification*
Competency Category: Nursing Practice: Alterations in Health
Taxonomic Level: Critical Thinking

**62. D.** Reflux of urine from the tubing to the bladder should be prevented.

*Rationale*
Urinary reflux should be prevented to lessen the possibility of cystitis.

*Classification*
Competency Category: Nursing Practice: Alterations in Health
Taxonomic Level: Knowledge/Comprehension

**63. C.** The patient is experiencing periods of severe shortness of breath at night and impaired circulation and sensory and motor functioning in the left leg.

*Rationale*
The terms and abbreviations are best described by this choice.

*Classification*
Competency Category: Professional Practice
Taxonomic Level: Application

**64. A.** The patient may be concerned that a heart attack may occur during orgasm.

*Rationale*
One of the most common concerns after MI is fear of having another MI during orgasm.

*Classification*
Competency Category: Nursing Practice: Health and Wellness
Taxonomic Level: Application

**65. B.** Absence of dorsalis pedis pulse; coolness and decreased sensation in the feet.

*Rationale*
This choice is the most accurate description of an interference with arterial circulation.

*Classification*
Competency Category: Nursing Practice: Alterations in Health
Taxonomic Level: Application

**66. A.** Airborne precautions are indicated for varicella (chickenpox) and involve wearing a mask when in the room.

*Rationale*
This represents the correct isolation precautions to be taken. The other choices are incorrect.

*Classification*
Competency Category: Nursing Practice: Health and Wellness
Taxonomic Level: Knowledge/Comprehension

**67. A.** Use a special mask to prevent inhaling infected airborne droplets.

*Rationale*
This choice represents the use of transmission-based precautions to prevent the spread of tuberculosis.

*Classification*
Competency Category: Nursing Practice: Health and Wellness
Taxonomic Level: Knowledge/Comprehension

**68. B.** Dyspnea; decreased breath sounds on the affected side.

*Rationale*
Shortness of breath and decreased breath sounds present if there is collapse of the lung because of loss of integrity of the pleural space.

*Classification*
Competency Category: Nursing Practice: Alterations in Health
Taxonomic Level: Knowledge/Comprehension

**69. A.** Position him in Fowler's position, initiate oxygen, and call the physician.

*Rationale*
A pulmonary embolism may be presenting; this would account for the chest pain and severe dyspnea. The physician needs to be notified.

*Classification*
Competency Category: Nursing Practice: Alterations in Health
Taxonomic Level: Critical Thinking

**70. A.** Visual field deficits such as homonymous hemianopsia.

*Rationale*
Visual field deficits can occur after a CVA.

*Classification*
Competency Category: Nursing Practice: Alterations in Health
Taxonomic Level: Knowledge/Comprehension

**71. B.** Jaundice is seen if the calculus lodges in the common bile duct.

*Rationale*
When calculus obstructs the common bile duct, a backup of bile occurs and causes pressure in the hepatic ducts and congestion in the liver. Liver functioning is affected, resulting in jaundice.

*Classification*
Competency Category: Nursing Practice: Alterations in Health
Taxonomic Level: Knowledge/Comprehension

**72. B.** Anorexia, nausea, and vomiting.

*Rationale*
Interference with digestive enzymes can result in loss of appetite, nausea, and vomiting.

*Classification*
Competency Category: Nursing Practice: Alterations in Health
Taxonomic Level: Critical Thinking

**73. A.** Ascites and hematemesis.

*Rationale*
Patients who have an accumulation of fluid in the peritoneal cavity and hematemesis from esophageal varices can present with portal hypertension.

*Classification*
Competency Category: Nursing Practice: Alterations in Health
Taxonomic Level: Knowledge/Comprehension

**74. A.** Limit movements resulting in internal rotation and adduction of the affected hip.

*Rationale*
Dislocation after hip replacement is minimized when the patient avoids movements resulting in internal rotation and adduction of the affected hip.

*Classification*
Competency Category: Nursing Practice: Alterations in Health
Taxonomic Level: Application

**75. A.** The new portal of entry of microorganisms could be through the mouth.

*Rationale*
According to the chain of infection, the nurse would transmit the microorganisms by indirect contact through the new portal of entry, the mouth.

*Classification*
Competency Category: Nursing Practice: Health and Wellness
Taxonomic Level: Application

**76. B.** Gathering assessment data and analyzing and identifying priority problems.

*Rationale*
Effective decision making starts with gathering assessment data and analyzing and then identifying patient problems.

*Classification*
Competency Category: Professional Practice
Taxonomic Level: Application

**77. C.** The patient may experience dehydration and convulsions from a high temperature.

*Rationale*
The worst consequence of an untreated temperature would be dehydration and convulsions.

*Classification*
Competency Category: Nursing Practice: Alterations in Health
Taxonomic Level: Application

**78. C.** The proliferative or regeneration phase will be delayed and prolonged.

*Rationale*
The physiologic sequence of healing and is impaired by a wound infection. The regeneration phase is delayed by a longer inflammatory phase, and healing is prolonged as the body focuses on removing the infectious matter.

*Classification*
Competency Category: Nursing Practice: Alterations in Health
Taxonomic Level: Knowledge/Comprehension

**79. B.** Breathing rate of 36 breaths/min; noisy, gurgling respirations.

*Rationale*
These signs indicate an airway interference.

*Classification*
Competency Category: Nursing Practice: Alterations in Health
Taxonomic Level: Application

**80. D.** The duration of the suctioning episode should be 10 to 15 seconds each time.

*Rationale*
The correct answer limits the suctioning episode to a short time so that breathing is not compromised.

*Classification*
Competency Category: Nursing Practice: Alterations in Health
Taxonomic Level: Knowledge/Comprehension

**81. B.** Frequently check the dressing and chest tube for drainage.

*Rationale*
Important postoperative considerations include checking the dressing and chest tube and ensuring that connections are securely taped.

*Classification*
Competency Category: Nursing Practice: Alterations in Health
Taxonomic Level: Critical Thinking

**82. B.** Essential amino acids are needed to ensure building blocks are present for building or proliferative phase.

*Rationale*
This statement is true regarding the role of essential amino acids in the healing process.

*Classification*
Competency Category: Nursing Practice: Alterations in Health
Taxonomic Level: Application

**83. A.** Dehydration by checking tissue turgor and checking mucous membranes.

*Rationale*
When a patient has diarrhea, the nurse should assess for a fluid volume deficit.

*Classification*
Competency Category: Nursing Practice: Alterations in Health
Taxonomic Level: Critical Thinking

**84. B.** Increased pulse, increased respirations, and jugular vein distension.

*Rationale*
These signs indicate complications from too rapid an IV perfusion.

*Classification*
Competency Category: Nursing Practice: Alterations in Health
Taxonomic Level: Application

**85. B.** Heart and circulation.

*Rationale*
Assessment of the effects of severe hypothyroidism on the circulatory system is important. Serum cholesterol levels are also elevated in clients with hypothyroidism.

*Classification*
Competency Category: Nursing Practice: Alterations in Health
Taxonomic Level: Knowledge/Comprehension

**86. B.** It determines the average blood glucose level in the previous 4 months.

*Rationale*
Glycosylated hemoglobin gives a measure of blood glucose controls over the previous 4 months and gives an indication of diabetes control.

*Classification*
Competency Category: Nursing Practice: Alterations in Health
Taxonomic Level: Knowledge/Comprehension

**87. B.** Weight gain, coughing of frothy sputum, and jugular vein distension.

*Rationale*
Signs of fluid overload from renal insufficiency are indicated by weight gain, jugular vein distension, and pulmonary edema.

*Classification*
Competency Category: Nursing Practice: Alterations in Health
Taxonomic Level: Application

**88. D.** It is characterized by fluid volume excess, hypernatremia, and hyperkalemia.

*Rationale*
When chronic renal failure occurs, the body is unable to process and eliminate the body fluids resulting in fluid volume overload, hypernatremia and hyperkalemia.

*Classification*
Competency Category: Nursing Practice: Alterations in Health
Taxonomic Level: Application

**89. B.** Restrict sodium and potassium; restrict fluids as ordered.

*Rationale*
Important care measures include diet and fluid restrictions.

*Classification*
Competency Category: Nursing Practice: Alterations in Health
Taxonomic Level: Application

**90. A.** This indicates feelings of depression associated with a long-term, incurable disease.

*Rationale*
The client's psychosocial adaptation is impaired. Depression associated with chronic illness is a likely result.

*Classification*
Competency Category: Nursing Practice: Alterations in Health
Taxonomic Level: Application

**91. C.** Vital signs, level of consciousness, pain level, and wound dressing.

*Rationale*
Important postoperative considerations are captured in this response.

*Classification*
Competency Category: Nursing Practice: Alterations in Health
Taxonomic Level: Knowledge/Comprehension

**92. B.** Hypertension, obesity, and chronic lung condition.

*Rationale*
The client has an increased risk of complications if these three factors are present.

*Classification*
Competency Category: Nursing Practice: Health and Wellness
Taxonomic Level: Knowledge/Comprehension

**93. B.** Determine placement of the tube by aspiration of gastric contents.

*Rationale*
Ensuring correct placement in the stomach is the most important consideration before tube feeds.

*Classification*
Competency Category: Nursing Practice: Alterations in Health
Taxonomic Level: Knowledge/Comprehension

**94. C.** Smoking, high cholesterol levels, and hypertension.

*Rationale*
These are modifiable factors associated with increased risk of CVA.

*Classification*
Competency Category: Nursing Practice: Health and Wellness
Taxonomic Level: Knowledge/Comprehension

**95. D.** 1 tablet of 5 mg, 1 tablet of 2 mg, and 1/2 tablet of 3 mg.

*Rationale*
This is the most accurate combination to give 8.5 mg of warfarin.

*Classification*
Competency Category: Nursing Practice: Alterations in Health
Taxonomic Level: Critical Thinking

**96. D.** Assess the home and demonstrate effective use of assistive devices.

*Rationale*
Her situation has changed, and her safety at home is critical because of the residual effects from the hemiparesis.

*Classification*
Competency Category: Nursing Practice: Alterations in Health
Taxonomic Level: Application

**97. C.** Coping abilities, emotional lability, physical deficits, family supports.

*Rationale*
Her reintegration will be most influenced by her coping abilities, emotional response, physical deficits, and family support.

*Classification*
Competency Category: Nursing Practice: Health and Wellness
Taxonomic Level: Application

**98. A.** Heart and Stroke Foundation and Canadian Stroke Network.

*Rationale*
These two resources provide current research-based information to prevent strokes and help in rehabilitation after stroke.

*Classification*
Competency Category: Nursing Practice: Health and Wellness
Taxonomic Level: Knowledge/Comprehension

**99. A.** Maintaining a patent airway.

*Rationale*
Maintenance of a patent airway is most important priority because of increased probability of relaxation of the tongue and jaw and resultant obstruction.

*Classification*
Competency Category: Nursing Practice: Alterations in Health
Taxonomic Level: Knowledge/Comprehension

**100. C.** The pupils are equal and sluggish in reaction to light.

*Rationale*
This choice is the only one in which the patient has abnormal neurologic response.

*Classification*
Competency Category: Nursing Practice: Alterations in Health
Taxonomic Level: Critical Thinking

**101. D.** Widening pulse pressure and bradycardia.

*Rationale*
Widening pulse pressure and bradycardia both indicate compromised neurologic functioning.

*Classification*
Competency Category: Nursing Practice: Alterations in Health
Taxonomic Level: Critical Thinking

**102. A.** Listen to them, explain what is happening, and encourage them to be involved in their family member's care.

*Rationale*
The family is grieving the loss of the dreams they had for their loved one. They need to be listened to, encouraged, and supported.

*Classification*
Competency Category: Nursing Practice: Alterations in Health
Taxonomic Level: Critical Thinking

**103. C.** Discuss the purpose of seatbelts, the effects of drinking and driving, and the effects of speed.

*Rationale*
This is a very important time to address the risks and implications associated with car accidents. The students' motivation is increased because of the consequences to a classmate.

*Classification*
Competency Category: Nursing Practice: Health and Wellness
Taxonomic Level: Knowledge/Comprehension

**104. C.** Heavy smoking, sedentary lifestyle, and diet low in calcium.

*Rationale*
These three factors increase the risk of osteoporosis.

*Classification*
Competency Category: Nursing Practice: Health and Wellness
Taxonomic Level: Knowledge/Comprehension

**105. D.** Talk about decreasing activity and the regular use of restraints to prevent falls.

*Rationale*
Decreasing activity will cause limitations in mobility. Restraints are not ethically indicated.

*Classification*
Competency Category: Nursing Practice: Health and Wellness
Taxonomic Level: Application

**106. A.** Consent must be signed after explanations of the benefits and risks of the procedure.

*Rationale*
The nurse needs to ensure that the patient understood what the surgeon has explained, including the risks of the procedure. If the patient does not understand, the nurse is professionally obligated to contact the surgeon and ensure that he or she explains these benefits and risks.

*Classification*
Competency Category: Nurse–Person Relationship
Taxonomic Level: Knowledge/Comprehension

**107. C.** The proliferative or regeneration phase will be prolonged.

*Rationale*
The physiologic sequence of healing and is impaired by a wound infection. The regeneration phase is delayed by a longer inflammatory phase, and healing is prolonged as the body focuses on removing the infectious matter.

*Classification*
Competency Category: Nursing Practice: Alterations in Health
Taxonomic Level: Knowledge/Comprehension

**108. D.** Developing a sense of trust, discussing feelings, and identifying the family's strengths and coping strategies.

*Rationale*
It is important that the family is the focus of care and that a trusting relationship is developed. This will

facilitate them discussing their concerns with the nurse allowing for identification of strengths, resources and coping strategies to assist the family to manage the health situation.

*Classification*
Competency Category: Nursing Practice: Alterations in Health
Taxonomic Level: Application

**109. A.** Aortic aneurysm.

*Rationale*
Palpation over an aortic aneurysm may result in perforation of the aneurysm which could be a life-threatening situation.

*Classification*
Competency Category: Nursing Practice: Alterations in Health
Taxonomic Level: Application

**110. D.** "You're concerned when you think about how this will change your life?"

*Rationale*
The response should be attune to the feelings of sadness and dejection as well as the content of the patient's statement.

*Classification*
Competency Category: Nurse–Person Relationship
Taxonomic Level: Critical Thinking

**111. B.** "How is this illness impacting you and your family?"

*Rationale*
This question helps to assess the impact of the stressor and his coping abilities.

*Classification*
Competency Category: Nursing Practice: Health and Wellness
Taxonomic Level: Application

**112. A.** Muscle weakness and a weak, irregular pulse.

*Rationale*
Muscle weakness and heart irregularities would be evident with hypokalemia.

*Classification*
Competency Category: Nursing Practice: Alterations in Health
Taxonomic Level: Knowledge/Comprehension

**113. C.** Reduced cholesterol levels, progressive activity levels, coping strategies.

*Rationale*
Dietary changes, a progressive increase in activity, and effective coping strategies for stress reduction should all be included to assist in rehabilitation and reduce the risk of recurrence.

*Classification*
Competency Category: Nursing Practice: Health and Wellness
Taxonomic Level: Application


**114. C.** Auscultate the area to determine whether a bruit is present.

*Rationale*
The symptoms indicate an aortic aneurysm. The safest and most effective assessment of this is auscultation of the area to determine if a bruit is heard. If a bruit is heard, the patient likely has an aneurysm.

*Classification*
Competency Category: Nursing Practice: Alterations in Health
Taxonomic Level: Application


**115. D.** It is to act in the best interests of others; to become a client advocate.

*Rationale*
The ethical principle of beneficence involves advocating for the patient.

*Classification*
Competency Category: Professional Practice
Taxonomic Level: Knowledge/Comprehension


**116. B.** Evidence of voluntary motor and sensory function below the level of injury.

*Rationale*
Initial assessment that indicates some motor and sensory functioning below the level of injury indicates an incomplete SCI with a potential for recovery.

*Classification*
Competency Category: Nursing Practice: Alterations in Health
Taxonomic Level: Application


**117. B.** Mechanical ventilation.

*Rationale*
If the injury is at C3 or C4 level, paralysis of respiratory muscles is of concern, so emergency intervention with mechanical ventilation is critical.

*Classification*
Competency Category: Nursing Practice: Alterations in Health
Taxonomic Level: Knowledge/Comprehension


**118. B.** To reduce damage and improve functional recovery.

*Rationale*
Use of corticosteroids reduces the inflammation and damage after the injury and contributes to functional recovery by protecting the neuromembrane from further destruction.

*Classification*
Competency Category: Nursing Practice: Health and Wellness
Taxonomic Level: Application


**119. B.** Asking about cultural beliefs related to health, illness, treatments, and dietary practices.

*Rationale*
This answer elicits key information regarding the client's beliefs, values, and cultural practices.

*Classification*
Competency Category: Nurse–Person Relationship
Taxonomic Level: Application


**120. C.** Do not disturb the couple, leave the room, and allow them privacy.

*Rationale*
This statement reflects respect for diversity in choices and practices.

*Classification*
Competency Category: Nurse–Person Relationship
Taxonomic Level: Application


**121. B.** Conduct focus group interviews and have the clients fill out a survey.

*Rationale*
Gathering information from the clients by using survey and focus groups would help identify the clients' needs and interests. Focus groups will also help generate discussion of needs.

*Classification*
Competency Category: Nursing Practice: Health and Wellness
Taxonomic Level: Application

**122. D.** There is less efficient absorption, detoxification, and elimination.

*Rationale*
When giving medications to elderly individuals, consideration needs to be made for physiologic changes associated with aging.

*Classification*
Competency Category: Nursing Practice: Alterations in Health
Taxonomic Level: Knowledge/Comprehension

**123. B.** Have a pharmacist discuss the medications and interactions and initiate physician referrals as needed.

*Rationale*
Having the pharmacist review the importance of medications and possible interactions and initiate physician referrals if indicated uses the skills of this health team member.

*Classification*
Competency Category: Nursing Practice: Health and Wellness
Taxonomic Level: Critical Thinking

**124. C.** Diabetic retinopathy is the leading cause of blindness and occurs because of ischemic retinal blood vessel changes.

*Rationale*
Diabetic retinopathy causes blindness through destruction of retinal blood vessels.

*Classification*
Competency Category: Nursing Practice: Alterations in Health
Taxonomic Level: Application

**125. C.** Assess for depression and signs of sensory deprivation; take action as needed

*Rationale*
It is important for the nurse to assess the clients for depression and sensory deprivation to identify early signs of mental health problems and intervene appropriately. Finding out the reason for clients' nonparticipation is important. Family visits are important, but the remaining time could impact mental health.

*Classification*
Competency Category: Nursing Practice: Health and Wellness
Taxonomic Level: Critical Thinking

**126. C.** "My client did seem to have difficulty; maybe the video would help."

*Rationale*
This statement indicates that Nurse Hanes is open and willing to review her teaching approach based on the evaluative comments from her colleague and ensure that another approach helps to reinforce the concept for the patient.

*Classification*
Competency Category: Professional Practice
Taxonomic Level: Application

**127. C.** Call the student nurse to witness the wastage and cosign for its proper disposal.

*Rationale*
Calling the senior student nurse would be most appropriate to witness the wastage. Otherwise, the patient would have to wait for the pain medication until the return of the other registered nurse.

*Classification*
Competency Category: Professional Practice
Taxonomic Level: Critical Thinking

**128. D.** Stop her from drawing up the insulin. Call a supervisor, inform him or her about the incident, and document the observations.

*Rationale*
Protection of the patient is a professional responsibility. Calling the supervisor is important so the patient can be reassigned and the supervisor can deal with the problem.

*Classification*
Competency Category: Professional Practice
Taxonomic Level: Critical Thinking

**129. B.** Skeletal muscle atrophy and osteoporosis.

*Rationale*
Two long-term effects of corticosteroid administration are muscle atrophy and osteoporosis.

*Classification*
Competency Category: Alterations in Heath; Health and Wellness
Taxonomic Level: Critical Thinking

**130. A.** Long-term use of these hormones has resulted in depression of your body's own production, and a crisis could occur if you suddenly stop taking them.

*Rationale*
This description indicates that the body is no longer producing these hormones, so sudden withdrawal could cause a crisis.

*Classification*
Competency Category: Alterations in Heath; Health and Wellness
Taxonomic Level: Critical Thinking

**131. B.** Ask her about the medication side effects and explain why suddenly stopping the drug can cause problems

*Rationale*
It is important to explore the client's concerns regarding the side effects and reinforce the desired effect of the drug and the importance of not suddenly discontinuing its use.

*Classification*
Competency Category: Alterations in Heath; Health and Wellness
Taxonomic Level: Critical Thinking

**132. C.** "This illness has really taken its toll on you and your family. Which effects are most difficult to handle?

*Rationale*
Acknowledgement of her difficulty in adjusting as well as her family's concerns is very important. An important next step is to consider what she thinks the most difficult changes are.

*Classification*
Competency Category: Alterations in Heath; Health and Wellness
Taxonomic Level: Critical Thinking

**133. A.** Chronic illness support group or SLE support group.

*Rationale*
A chronic illness support group and one that provides support for persons dealing with the chronic challenges of SLE would be best so she can discuss the illness and its management and restore hope.

*Classification*
Competency Category: Alterations in Heath; Health and Wellness
Taxonomic Level: Critical Thinking

**134. B.** Participating in unprotected sex with multiple sexual partners; sharing IV needles.

*Rationale*
There is an increased risk of contracting HIV if a person participates in unprotected sex with several sexual partners or shares needles.

*Classification*
Competency Category: Nursing Practice: Health and Wellness
Taxonomic Level: Knowledge/Comprehension

**135. A.** Needlestick injuries or contact with the client's blood.

*Rationale*
The principal method of contracting HIV is through needlestick injuries or blood contamination from an infected patient.

*Classification*
Competency Category: Nursing Practice: Health and Wellness
Taxonomic Level: Application

**136. B.** *Pneumocystis carinii* pneumonia, Kaposi's sarcoma, and herpes simplex.

*Rationale*
With the immune system suppressed in individuals with AIDS, rare pneumonias, cancers, and viral eruptions are common.

*Classification*
Competency Category: Nursing Practice: Health and Wellness
Taxonomic Level: Knowledge/Comprehension

**137. C.** Prevention of transmission, optimal nutrition, and exercise.

*Rationale*
Prevention of transmission is an important legal prevention consideration, and support of the immune

system through proper exercise and nutrition is important.

*Classification*
Competency Category: Nursing Practice: Health and Wellness
Taxonomic Level: Application

**138. B.** Guilt and remorse regarding the disease.

*Rationale*
Sensitivity to his plight and his inability to share this diagnosis with the family indicate guilt and remorse.

*Classification*
Competency Category: Nursing Practice: Health and Wellness
Taxonomic Level: Critical Thinking

**139. C.** A student indicates that responsible sex involves using condoms for protection and birth control.

*Rationale*
This comment indicates an understanding of ways to lessen the incidence of sexually transmitted illnesses and to prevent unwanted pregnancies.

*Classification*
Competency Category: Nursing Practice: Health and Wellness
Taxonomic Level: Critical Thinking

**140. A.** Teens can be vulnerable to developing cancer of the cervix if they are exposed to certain strains of human papilloma virus (HPV).

*Rationale*
Many teens are unaware of the increased incidence of cancer of the cervix if they have been exposed to certain strains of HPV.

*Classification*
Competency Category: Nursing Practice: Health and Wellness
Taxonomic Level: Application

**141. D.** Date rape is usually a misinterpretation of responsive cues.

*Rationale*
Date rape occurs when sex is not consensual, even if the person is drugged or intoxicated.

*Classification*
Competency Category: Nursing Practice: Health and Wellness
Taxonomic Level: Application

**142. D.** Aerobic exercise.

*Rationale*
Aerobic exercise is not a risk-taking behaviour.

*Classification*
Competency Category: Nursing Practice: Health and Wellness
Taxonomic Level: Knowledge/Comprehension

**143. B.** Checking for airway patency.

*Rationale*
Because the client has received facial burns, he may have gasped for air during the steam burn, resulting in the possibility that the steam may have been inhaled and airway swelling may be present.

*Classification*
Competency Category: Nursing Practice: Alterations in Health
Taxonomic Level: Critical Thinking

**144. B.** Age, weight, vital signs, and tissue turgor.

*Rationale*
Considering the client's physiologic status by age and weight is important. Monitoring vital signs and tissue turgor levels will indicate how his body is compensating.

*Classification*
Competency Category: Nursing Practice: Alterations in Health
Taxonomic Level: Critical Thinking

**145. A.** Ringer's lactate is used as long as the urine output is maintained at an adequate level.

*Rationale*
Replacement fluid should be monitored to prevent signs of hypovolemic shock and restore circulating fluid volume. Kidney perfusion is important to assess to ensure that acute renal failure is not presenting.

*Classification*
Competency Category: Nursing Practice: Alterations in Health
Taxonomic Level: Application

**146. B.** 31 gtt/min.

*Rationale*
1500 × 10 gtt = 15,000 gtt/8 hr = 1875 gtt/60 min = 31.25 gtt/min.

*Classification*
Competency Category: Nursing Practice: Alterations in Health
Taxonomic Level: Application

**147. B.** 234 cc/hr.

*Rationale*
The adjusted rate takes into consideration gradual increase to catch the IV to the ordered amount of fluid intake. Rate/hr = 187 cc/hr. IV is behind 187/2 = 93.5 mL. Increase/each of 2 hrs = 46.88 Rate/hr = 187 + 47 = 234 cc/hr.

*Classification*
Competency Category: Nursing Practice: Alterations in Health
Taxonomic Level: Critical Thinking

**148. B.** Body image and self-esteem concerns.

*Rationale*
During the recuperation phase, the patient is likely to consider the body image implications of this injury. Sensitivity to body image and self-esteem issues are anticipated concerns.

*Classification*
Competency Category: Nursing Practice: Health and Wellness
Taxonomic Level: Application

**149. C.** Muscle weakness, difficulty swallowing, double vision, and difficulty speaking.

*Rationale*
Understanding the meaning of the terms and the assessment implications is important. The terms refer to the finding identified in answer C.

*Classification*
Competency Category: Nursing Practice: Alterations in Health
Taxonomic Level: Knowledge/Comprehension

**150. B.** "It is a chronic disease in which there is a disturbance in nerve transmission to the muscle, resulting in fatigue and muscle weakness."

*Rationale*
This is the most accurate description of the problems and effects of myasthenia gravis. Answer A describes multiple sclerosis, answer B describes Huntington's chorea, and answer D describes amyotrophic lateral sclerosis.

*Classification*
Competency Category: Nursing Practice: Alterations in Health
Taxonomic Level: Application

**151. B.** A rapid and dramatic increase in muscle strength.

*Rationale*
With IV administration of a cholinesterase inhibitor, edrophonium, the individual should have a rapid and dramatic increase in muscle strength, which helps confirm the diagnosis of myasthenia gravis.

*Classification*
Competency Category: Nursing Practice: Alterations in Health
Taxonomic Level: Application

**152. C.** Severe dyspnea, intensification of dysphagia, and dysarthria.

*Rationale*
Intensification of all of the symptoms would indicate a myasthenia crisis; these assessment findings call for emergency actions.

*Classification*
Competency Category: Nursing Practice: Alterations in Health
Taxonomic Level: Application

**153. A.** Tracheotomy with mechanical ventilation.

*Rationale*
Initiation and maintenance of mechanical ventilation is a priority emergency procedure.

*Classification*
Competency Category: Nursing Practice: Alterations in Health
Taxonomic Level: Application

**154. C.** "How is your condition affecting your family members and their usual roles?"

*Rationale*
Clarification of the concerns she has regarding the impact of her illness on the family is very important. This answer asks about how members are affected. This is an important step before examining ways that the nurse support the family in adjustment.

*Classification*
Competency Category: Nursing Practice: Alterations in Health
Taxonomic Level: Application

**155. A.** "How has your family handled difficult situations before? What strengths emerged from these situations?"

*Rationale*
Assessing how the family has handled difficult situations in the past and identifying some of the emergent strengths assists in identifying coping strategies and resilience within the family.

*Classification*
Competency Category: Nursing Practice: Health and Wellness
Taxonomic Level: Knowledge/Comprehension

**156. C.** Cholinesterase inhibitors, thymectomy, and corticosteroids.

*Rationale*
These therapeutic interventions are indicated to control the signs and symptoms of myasthenia gravis.

*Classification*
Competency Category: Nursing Practice: Alterations in Health
Taxonomic Level: Knowledge/Comprehension

**157. B.** Assess the patient's eating and exercise patterns and together develop a weight control program that allows for gradual weight loss.

*Rationale*
A safe way to lose weight includes assessment of eating patterns and exercise and getting involved in gradual weight loss program.

*Classification*
Competency Category: Nursing Practice: Health and Wellness
Taxonomic Level: Application

**158. B.** Discontinue the infusion and apply a warm compress to the IV site.

*Rationale*
The red line, pain, and edema all indicate phlebitis. The infusion needs to be discontinued and warm compresses applied to enhance the inflammatory response in the area.

*Classification*
Competency Category: Nursing Practice: Alterations in Health
Taxonomic Level: Application

**159. B.** Explain that you are unable to perform the IV start until you have completed an inservice and practice session on IV insertions.

*Rationale*
This is a skill that requires knowledge and supervised practice because of the invasive nature of the procedure. Honest acknowledgement of lack of competency in a skill is an important professional responsibility and should be followed by actions to ensure you acquire the skill.

*Classification*
Competency Category: Professional Practice
Taxonomic Level: Critical Thinking

**160. C.** Notify the surgeon and await his or her decision; reinforce with the LPN the importance of reporting abnormal preoperative vital signs.

*Rationale*
The purpose of a registered nurse's signing off the chart is to ensure that the safety of the patient has been assessed. Abnormal vital signs identify that priority systems indicate that a stressor or infection is present.

*Classification*
Competency Category: Professional Practice
Taxonomic Level: Critical Thinking

**161. A.** The patient who had the TURP.

*Rationale*
The priority is to assess the potential for bleeding after a TURP because this could quickly compromise the status of the patient. Hemorrhage in this patient could become an emergency situation.

*Classification*
Competency Category: Nursing Practice: Health and Wellness
Taxonomic Level: Critical Thinking

**162. D.** Have the nursing assistant call the physician while you remain with the client, flex the client's knees, and cover the incision with sterile gauze.

*Rationale*
This is an emergency situation: The physician must be notified, but further injury must be prevented immediately by flexing the client's knees and moistening the area with sterile towels and sterile saline. The moistening reduces the chance of infection and prevents dehydration of the intestines, which could result in necrosis.

*Classification*
Competency Category: Nursing Practice: Alterations in Health
Taxonomic Level: Critical Thinking

**163. A.** Her pregnant granddaughter

*Rationale*
The pregnant granddaughter is in no danger from external-beam radiation therapy, and the visitor would pose no health threat to the patient.

*Classification*
Competency Category: Nursing Practice: Health and Wellness
Taxonomic Level: Application

**164. D.** Hypotension; cold, clammy skin; and weak, thready pulse.

*Rationale*
The decreased blood pressure volume associated with hemorrhage will reduce the individual's blood pressure and create a weak, thready pulse. The skin becomes cold and clammy from the constriction of peripheral blood vessels caused by the compensatory activation of the sympathetic nervous system.

*Classification*
Competency Category: Nursing Practice: Alterations in Health
Taxonomic Level: Knowledge/Comprehension

**165. D.** Maintain her independence.

*Rationale*
The patient is really saying, "I can manage this myself. I am capable."

*Classification*
Competency Category: Nurse–Person Relationship
Taxonomic Level: Critical Thinking

**166. D.** Patient's past experiences.

*Rationale*
Past experiences have the most meaningful influence on present learning.

*Classification*
Competency Category: Nursing Practice: Health and Wellness
Taxonomic Level: Critical Thinking

**167. B.** Administer an antipyretic agent after the patient spikes a fever.

*Rationale*
Because fever and night sweats occur serially, it is most helpful to give the antipyretic agent before sleep as a prophylactic measure.

*Classification*
Competency Category: Nursing Practice: Alterations in Health
Taxonomic Level: Application

**168. D.** Explaining procedures and unit routines to the client.

*Rationale*
Explaining procedures and routines decreases the client's anxiety about the unknown.

*Classification*
Competency Category: Nurse–Person Relationship
Taxonomic Level: Application

**169. D.** The appropriate proximity and visual relationship of the wheelchair to the bed must be maintained.

*Rationale*
The wheelchair should be angled close to the bed so the client can pivot on his stronger leg. When the wheelchair is within the client's visual field, the client will be aware of the distance and direction his body must navigate to transfer safely and avoid falling.

*Classification*
Competency Category: Nursing Practice: Health and Wellness
Taxonomic Level: Knowledge/Comprehension

**170. B.** Determine what the client knows about the health problem.

*Rationale*
Before planning and implementing a teaching plan, the nurse must assess the client's attitudes, experience, knowledge, and understanding of the health problem.

*Classification*
Competency Category: Nursing Practice: Health and Wellness
Taxonomic Level: Knowledge/Comprehension

**171. C.** Loss of abstract thinking ability.

*Rationale*
Impairment of abstract thinking interferes with interpretation and defining of words. Skill in abstract thinking is required to follow directions and select clothes.

*Classification*
Competency Category: Nursing Practice: Health and Wellness
Taxonomic Level: Critical Thinking

**172. C.** To be used as handholds and to facilitate the client's mobility in bed.

*Rationale*
Devices such as side rails can help clients increase their mobility by facilitating movement in bed. Side rails are immovable objects that provide a handhold for leverage when changing positions.

*Classification*
Competency Category: Nursing Practice: Health and Wellness
Taxonomic Level: Critical Thinking

**173. D.** All of the above.

*Rationale*
The vision for electronic medical records is that all data documenting a person's contact with health care providers, interventions, knowledge, supports, and potential alerts should be included. Linking all information would make communication more efficient.

*Classification*
Competency Category: Nursing Practice: Health and Wellness
Taxonomic Level: Knowledge/Comprehension

**174. D.** All of the above.

*Rationale*
Nursing informatics refers to the use of information technologies in relation to that function within the purview of nursing, completed by nurses when performing their duties. Therefore, all of these items are part of nursing informatics.

*Classification*
Competency Category: Professional Practice
Taxonomic Level: Knowledge/Comprehension

**175. D.** Treatment that does not need special consent.

*Rationale*
This is considered a routine procedure to meet a basic physiologic need and is covered by the consent to treatment form signed at the time of admission.

*Classification*
Competency Category: Nursing Practice: Alterations in Health
Taxonomic Level: Application

**176. A.** Her past experiences and coping abilities.

*Rationale*
The major factors determining the reaction to illness are past experiences and coping mechanisms.

*Classification*
Competency Category: Nursing Practice: Health and Wellness
Taxonomic Level: Critical Thinking

**177. B.** Reinforce success in tasks accomplished.

*Rationale*
To aid motivation, the nurse should focus on the positive aspects of the patient's progress.

*Classification*
Competency Category: Nursing Practice: Health and Wellness
Taxonomic Level: Application

**178. A.** Encourage Mrs. Kennedy to participate in the feeding process to the best of her abilities.

*Rationale*
As a part of rehabilitative process after a CVA, clients must be encouraged to participate in their own care to the extent that they are able to extend their ability by establishing mutually agreed-upon short-term goals.

*Classification*
Competency Category: Nursing Practice: Health and Wellness
Taxonomic Level: Knowledge/Comprehension

**179. C.** A 60-year-old man who follows a diet low in fat and high in fibre.

*Rationale*
Although the man is older than age 40 years, he follows an appropriate diet for avoiding colorectal cancer and does not have other common risk factors.

*Classification*
Competency Category: Nursing Practice: Health and Wellness
Taxonomic Level: Knowledge/Comprehension

**180. C.** "A single elevated blood pressure does not confirm hypertension. You will need to have your blood pressure reassessed several times before a diagnosis can be made."

*Rationale*
Hypertension is confirmed by three readings with systolic pressure of at least 140 mm Hg and diastolic pressure of at least 90 mm Hg.

*Classification*
Competency Category: Nursing Practice: Health and Wellness
Taxonomic Level: Application

**181. A.** Yellowing of the skin or eyes.

*Rationale*
Clients taking isoniazid may show signs of hepatic stress. The nurse should assess for signs of liver dysfunction.

*Classification*
Competency Category: Nursing Practice: Health and Wellness
Taxonomic Level: Knowledge/Comprehension

**182. B.** "Tell me how you feel about the diagnosis of tuberculosis."

*Rationale*
This encourages the client to express his feelings about the diagnosis.

*Classification*
Competency Category: Nurse–Person Relationship
Taxonomic Level: Application

**183. C.** In functional alignment.

*Rationale*
Muscles that originate at the vertebrae or pelvic girdle and insert on the femur act to abduct, adduct, flex, extend, and rotate the femur. Normal body alignment should be maintained because it facilitates the safe and efficient use of muscle groups for balance and stability.

*Classification*
Competency Category: Nursing Practice: Alterations in Health
Taxonomic Level: Critical Thinking

**184. C.** In the morning on awakening.

*Rationale*
Symptoms of rheumatoid arthritis include localized pain, stiffness, and decreased joint mobility after a period of rest, such as after sleeping. This can be more localized, which causes symptoms such as pain or stiffness. Lack of mobility over a period of time can increase the symptoms.

*Classification*
Competency Category: Nursing Practice: Alterations in Health
Taxonomic Level: Knowledge/Comprehension

**185. C.** Do exercises in bed to strengthen the upper extremities.

*Rationale*
When walking with crutches, the client engages the triceps, trapezius, and latissimus muscles. A client who has been immobilized may need to implement an exercise program to strengthen these shoulder and upper arm muscles before initiating crutch walking.

*Classification*
Competency Category: Nursing Practice: Health and Wellness
Taxonomic Level: Critical Thinking

**186. D.** Rotate the insertion site every 72 hours.

*Rationale*
Venous access devices are commonly used for clients receiving long-term chemotherapy, total parenteral nutrition, or frequent medication or fluids. These devices may remain in place for several weeks to more than 1 year if no complications develop.

*Classification*
Competency Category: Nursing Practice: Health and Wellness
Taxonomic Level: Critical Thinking

**187. D.** Continue to maintain normal sodium intake while at home.

*Rationale*
Lithium decreases sodium reabsorption by the renal tubules. If sodium intake is decreased, sodium depletion can occur. In addition, lithium retention is increased when sodium intake is decreased. A reduced sodium intake can lead to lithium toxicity.

*Classification*
Competency Category: Nursing Practice: Health and Wellness
Taxonomic Level: Application

**188. D.** Assisting her in bathing and dressing by giving her clear, simple directions.

*Rationale*
This action would provide a disorganized client with the necessary structure to encourage participation and support of self-image.

*Classification*
Competency Category: Nursing Practice: Health and Wellness
Taxonomic Level: Critical Thinking

**189. D.** Ineffective individual coping.

*Rationale*
Ineffective individual coping may be evidenced because of the inability to meet her basic needs, inability to meet her role expectations, and altered social participation.

*Classification*
Competency Category: Nurse–Person Relationship
Taxonomic Level: Critical Thinking

**190. D.** Presenting symptoms of a crisis are unique and vary from one person to another.

*Rationale*
Crisis for an individual is unique to that individual. Being in a crisis does not mean the individual has an emotional illness.

*Classification*
Competency Category: Nursing Practice: Alterations in Health
Taxonomic Level: Application

**191. A.** Are immobilized.

*Rationale*
Clients who are immobilized and are in stationary positions without regular position changes are more likely to develop pressure ulcers because of pressure on the skin for extended periods.

*Classification*
Competency Category: Nursing Practice: Alterations in Health
Taxonomic Level: Knowledge/Comprehension

**192. B.** Shortening of the affected extremity with external rotation.

*Rationale*
As a result of the muscles contracting and pulling on the two portions of bone, there is a characteristic shortening of the femur with external rotation of the extremity.

*Classification*
Competency Category: Nursing Practice: Alterations in Health
Taxonomic Level: Critical Thinking

**193. C.** Amplitude and symmetry.

*Rationale*
Assessment of any peripheral pulse should include the characteristics of the pulse (e.g., amplitude, rhythm, rate). The presence or lack of symmetry in the peripheral pulses must also be assessed.

*Classification*
Competency Category: Nursing Practice: Alterations in Health
Taxonomic Level: Knowledge/Comprehension

**194. C.** Diaphragmatic breathing.

*Rationale*
Diaphragmatic breathing helps promote alveolar expansion and facilitates exchange of oxygen and carbon dioxide.

*Classification*
Competency Category: Nursing Practice: Health and Wellness
Taxonomic Level: Knowledge/Comprehension

**195. D.** Ask her to discuss her understanding of the planned surgery.

*Rationale*
Upon assessing Mrs. Doreen's knowledge base regarding her upcoming surgery, the nurse can clarify inaccurate information and provide further patient education as needed.

*Classification*
Competency Category: Nurse–Person Relationship
Taxonomic Level: Critical Thinking

**196. C.** Compare her arm bracelet with the information in the chart.

*Rationale*
Comparing the name and hospital number on the arm bracelet with the chart best verifies the client's identity.

*Classification*
Competency Category: Professional Practice
Taxonomic Level: Knowledge/Comprehension

**197. B.** Confirm the placement of the oral airway.

*Rationale*
Confirming the placement of the oral airway ensures a patent air passage. Oxygen is essential for life, so this action takes priority.

*Classification*
Competency Category: Nursing Practice: Alterations in Health
Taxonomic Level: Critical Thinking

**198. B.** Shearing forces.

*Rationale*
Prolonged bed rest increases the risk of skin shearing caused by a lack of mobility. Shearing forces are a

hazard when clients are frequently moved and repositioned.

*Classification*
Competency Category: Nursing Practice: Health and Wellness
Taxonomic Level: Critical Thinking

**199. C.** Abdominal pain.

*Rationale*
By frequently changing positions in bed, the patient can prevent the development of pneumonia, urinary stasis, and deep vein thrombosis. These movements promote blood, oxygen, and fluid circulation throughout the body systems and prevent stasis.

*Classification*
Competency Category: Nursing Practice: Health and Wellness
Taxonomic Level: Knowledge/Comprehension

**200. A.** Test for blanching.

*Rationale*
When a fingertip is pressed over the reddened area and the area does not blanch but remains consistently reddened, it is an indication of deep tissue injury.

*Classification*
Competency Category: Nursing Practice: Alterations in Health
Taxonomic Level: Critical Thinking

**201. A.** Eliminating home safety hazards.

*Rationale*
Falls in the home occur most frequently from hazards in the home, such as loose rugs, cluttered hallways, power chords, and so on.

*Classification*
Competency Category: Nursing Practice: Health and Wellness
Taxonomic Level: Critical Thinking

**202. B.** "You need to turn from side to side every 2 hours."

*Rationale*
To prevent venous stasis and improve muscle tone, circulation, and respiratory function, the client should be encouraged to move around after surgery. Pain medication will be administered to permit movement.

*Classification*
Competency Category: Nursing Practice: Health and Wellness
Taxonomic Level: Critical Thinking

**203. C.** Swallow.

*Rationale*
Anaesthesia interferes with the gag reflex. Until the gag reflex returns, the patient cannot swallow without a risk of aspiration.

*Classification*
Competency Category: Nursing Practice: Alterations in Health
Taxonomic Level: Knowledge/Comprehension

**204. A.** Urinary output of 20 mL/hr.

*Rationale*
Urine output is maintained at a minimum of at least 30 mL/hr in adults. Less than this for 2 consecutive hours should be reported to the physician.

*Classification*
Competency Category: Nursing Practice: Alterations in Health
Taxonomic Level: Critical Thinking

**205. A.** Turning and positioning.

*Rationale*
Turning and positioning prevent pooling of secretions in the lung and maximize lung expansion and can be implemented immediately after surgery without a physician's order.

*Classification*
Competency Category: Nursing Practice: Alterations in Health
Taxonomic Level: Application

**206. B.** Pathologic condition.

*Rationale*
Several modes may be used for the administration of oxygen. Selection is based on the disease and the client's adaptation. For example, oxygen-induced hypoventilation is a particular concern for clients with chronic obstructive pulmonary disease.

*Classification*
Competency Category: Nursing Practice: Alterations in Health
Taxonomic Level: Critical Thinking

**207. B.** Humidifying the gas before delivery.

*Rationale*
Oxygen can dry the mucous membranes of the respiratory tract, which predisposes the client to infection.

*Classification*
Competency Category: Nursing Practice: Alterations in Health
Taxonomic Level: Application

**208. A.** Counteract respiratory acidosis.

*Rationale*
Retention of carbon dioxide in the blood lowers the pH, causing respiratory acidosis. Deep breathing maximizes gaseous exchange, ridding the body of excess carbon dioxide.

*Classification*
Competency Category: Nursing Practice: Alterations in Health
Taxonomic Level: Knowledge/Comprehension

**209. C.** Explain fire safety and oxygen use.

*Rationale*
Patient and staff safety is a priority. Oxygen is a combustible gas, and patients must understand the guidelines related to oxygen use in the home, hospital, and community.

*Classification*
Competency Category: Nursing Practice: Alterations in Health
Taxonomic Level: Critical Thinking

**210. D.** 45-degree semi-Fowler's position.

*Rationale*
This position is most effective because gravity assists in lung expansion and reduces pressure from the abdomen on the diaphragm.

*Classification*
Competency Category: Nursing Practice: Alterations in Health
Taxonomic Level: Application

**211. D.** Bed rest with elevation of the affected extremity.

*Rationale*
Elevation of the affected leg facilitates blood flow by the force of gravity and also decreases venous pressure, which in turn relieves edema and pain.

*Classification*
Competency Category: Nursing Practice: Alterations in Health
Taxonomic Level: Knowledge/Comprehension

**212. B.** Rattling sound in the pharynx of an unconscious patient.

*Rationale*
Rattling would indicate that mucus is in the airway. Suctioning may be necessary to maintain a patent airway because an unconscious patient cannot voluntarily cough.

*Classification*
Competency Category: Nursing Practice: Alterations in Health
Taxonomic Level: Critical Thinking

**213. A.** The client is experiencing anxiety; the nurse should listen attentively and provide realistic verbal reassurance.

*Rationale*
Clients routinely experience preoperative anxiety. Nurses should use basic communication skills to reduce their apprehension.

*Classification*
Competency Category: Nurse–Person Relationship
Taxonomic Level: Application

**214. D.** Maintain a patent airway.

*Rationale*
Although all of the options are appropriate postoperative goals, maintaining a patent airway takes priority, especially on the first postoperative day. A laryngectomy tube is most likely to be in place, and suctioning is commonly needed to clear secretions. Edema and hematoma formation at the surgical site may increase the risk of a blocked airway.

*Classification*
Competency Category: Nursing Practice: Alterations in Health
Taxonomic Level: Application

**215. B.** 5 to 10 seconds.

*Rationale*
The total procedure from catheter insertion to removal should not take longer than 15 seconds. Intermittent suction removes pharyngeal secretions and minimizes stress to the patient. Suctioning that takes longer than 10 seconds can cause cardiopulmonary compromise as a result of hypoxemia or vagal overload.

*Classification*
Competency Category: Nursing Practice: Alterations in Health
Taxonomic Level: Application

**216. D.** All of the above.

*Rationale*
All of the positions are correct. Although these are the recommended suctioning positions, variations based on the patient's condition may warrant an alteration in these positions. For example, a patient with a newly fractured cervical spine must remain in the supine position.

*Classification*
Competency Category: Nursing Practice: Alterations in Health
Taxonomic Level: Application

**217. C.** Assess cuff pressure for a minimal air leak.

*Rationale*
Cuff underinflation may allow aspiration, and overinflation may cause ischemia or necrosis of tracheal tissue

*Classification*
Competency Category: Nursing Practice: Alterations in Health
Taxonomic Level: Application

**218. D.** Hyperoxygenate the client before suctioning.

*Rationale*
Preoxygenation and deep breathing assist in reducing suction-induced hypoxemia. Preoxygenation decreases the risk of atelectasis caused by negative pressure of suctioning.

*Classification*
Competency Category: Nursing Practice: Alterations in Health
Taxonomic Level: Application

**219. C.** Neurovascular compromise.

*Rationale*
Because impaired circulation can cause permanent damage, neurovascular assessment of the affected leg is always a priority assessment.

*Classification*
Competency Category: Nursing Practice: Alterations in Health
Taxonomic Level: Critical Thinking

**220. A.** Postural or orthostatic hypotension.

*Rationale*
After the administration of certain antihypertensive or narcotics, the client's neurocirculatory reflexes may have some difficulty adjusting to the force of gravity when he or she assumes an upright position. Postural or orthostatic hypotension may then occur, causing a temporarily decreased blood supply to the brain.

*Classification*
Competency Category: Nursing Practice: Alterations in Health
Taxonomic Level: Critical Thinking

**221. C.** On the client's left side.

*Rationale*
When ambulating a client, the nurse walks on the client's stronger or unaffected side. This provides a wide base of support and therefore increases stability during the phase of ambulation that calls for weight bearing on the affected side as the unaffected limb moves forward.

*Classification*
Competency Category: Nursing Practice: Alterations in Health
Taxonomic Level: Application

**222. B.** Increased swelling of the toes.

*Rationale*
Constriction of circulation decreases venous return and increases pressure within the vessels. Fluid then moves into the interstitial spaces, causing edema.

*Classification*
Competency Category: Nursing Practice: Alterations in Health
Taxonomic Level: Knowledge/Comprehension

**223. C.** Administer diphenhydramine as ordered for the relief of severe itching.

*Rationale*
Patients should be discouraged from scratching because of the risk of skin breakdown and potential damage to the cast if they scratch with a sharp object. Itching can be relieved by administering a mild antihistamine such as diphenhydramine.

*Classification*
Competency Category: Nursing Practice: Alterations in Health
Taxonomic Level: Knowledge/Comprehension

**224. D.** Proportion more fluids in the day than during the night.

*Rationale*

The patient and nurse should make a fluid schedule that takes into consideration factors such as periods of wakefulness, number of meals, oral medications, and personal preferences.

*Classification*

Competency Category: Nursing Practice: Alterations in Health

Taxonomic Level: Application

**225. A.** 125 mL/hr; 21 gtt/min.

*Rationale*

To arrive at the answer, you would have to perform the following calculation:

$$\frac{\text{Volume to be infused} \times \text{Drop factor}}{\text{Number of hours} \times 60 \text{ minutes}}$$

$$\frac{3000 \times 10}{24 \times 60}$$

$$= \frac{30,000}{1440} = 21 \text{ drops/min}$$

*Classification*

Competency Category: Nursing Practice: Alterations in Health

Taxonomic Level: Knowledge/Comprehension

**226. C.** Isotonic.

*Rationale*

Normal body fluids have a neutral pH, so any extremes of hypo- or hypertonic can be eliminated.

*Classification*

Competency Category: Nursing Practice: Alterations in Health

Taxonomic Level: Knowledge/Comprehension

**227. D.** Dry skin with poor turgor.

*Rationale*

Fluid volume deficit is characterized by dry skin and mucous membranes, decreased skin turgor, hypotension, tachycardia, increased body temperature, and weakness.

*Classification*

Competency Category: Nursing Practice: Alterations in Health

Taxonomic Level: Application

**228. B.** Straw coloured.

*Rationale*

The more fluid the person drinks, the lighter the color of the urine.

*Classification*

Competency Category: Nursing Practice: Alterations in Health

Taxonomic Level: Knowledge/Comprehension

**229. D.** Diuretic therapy.

*Rationale*

Diuretic therapy generally involves the use of drugs that directly or indirectly increase urinary sodium excretion.

*Classification*

Competency Category: Nursing Practice: Alterations in Health

Taxonomic Level: Application

**230. A.** Extreme muscle weakness and tachycardia.

*Rationale*

Potassium, the major intracellular cation, functions with sodium and calcium to regulate neuromuscular activity and contraction of muscle fibres, particularly the heart muscle. These symptoms develop in hypokalemia.

*Classification*

Competency Category: Nursing Practice: Alterations in Health

Taxonomic Level: Critical Thinking

**231. D.** Fat emulsions.

*Rationale*

TPN is a hypertonic solution that consists of dextrose, proteins, and electrolytes.

*Classification*

Competency Category: Nursing Practice: Alterations in Health

Taxonomic Level: Knowledge/Comprehension

**232. C.** Monitor urine output.

*Rationale*

Hyperosmolar hyperglycemia is a metabolic complication of TPN. Expansion of the blood volume combined with hyperglycemia may cause osmotic diuresis presenting as increased urine output. Intake and output should be recorded so that a fluid imbalance can be readily detected. Urine can also be tested for hyperosmolar diuresis.

*Classification*

Competency Category: Nursing Practice: Health and wellness

Taxonomic Level: Application

**233. D.** 8.3 mmol/L.

*Rationale*
Blood glucose should be maintained below 8.3 mmol/L because hyperglycemia has been shown to be associated with decreased immune function.

*Classification*
Competency Category: Nursing Practice: Alterations in Health
Taxonomic Level: Knowledge/Comprehension

**234. B.** On the left side in the deep Trendelenburg position.

*Rationale*
Positioning the patient on the left side in the deep Trendelenburg position keeps the air in the right atrium and out of pulmonary circulation, preventing obstruction of the right ventricle.

*Classification*
Competency Category: Nursing Practice: Alterations in Health
Taxonomic Level: Application

**235. D.** Anuria.

*Rationale*
Osmotic diuresis accompanied by dehydration, electrolyte imbalance, and decreased level of consciousness may result in glycosuria, seizures, and coma.

*Classification*
Competency Category: Nursing Practice: Alterations in Health
Taxonomic Level: Critical Thinking

**236. C.** Obtain an order for urinary catheterization.

*Rationale*
The client has "overflow retention." A catheter relieves the discomfort by draining urine from the bladder. Permitting further distension could injure the bladder. Although an analgesic may relieve the discomfort, it will not resolve the primary cause.

*Classification*
Competency Category: Nursing Practice: Alterations in Health
Taxonomic Level: Application

**237. D.** Serum hepatitis.

*Rationale*
Serum hepatitis (hepatitis B) is transmitted by blood or blood products. The hemodialysis and routine transfusions needed for a client in renal failure constitute a great risk of exposure.

*Classification*
Competency Category: Nursing Practice: Alterations in Health
Taxonomic Level: Knowledge/Comprehension

**238. D.** Urine drains from it continuously.

*Rationale*
The ureters are implanted in a segment of the ileum, and urine drains continually because there is no sphincter.

*Classification*
Competency Category: Nursing Practice: Alterations in Health
Taxonomic Level: Knowledge/Comprehension

**239. D.** When the patient goes to bed at night.

*Rationale*
All patients, regardless of the specifics of their own bladder-retraining program, will be toileted before going to bed at night and after awakening in the morning.

*Classification*
Competency Category: Nursing Practice: Alterations in Health
Taxonomic Level: Knowledge/Comprehension

**240. D.** The muscles that control urination have weakened.

*Rationale*
Muscles, particularly the perineal muscles, tend to lose strength as people age.

*Classification*
Competency Category: Nursing Practice: Alterations in Health
Taxonomic Level: Knowledge/Comprehension

**241. B.** Occult blood and organisms.

*Rationale*
Occult blood in the stool could indicate active bleeding; the stool should also be examined for microorganisms to detect early infections that could easily become systemic by spreading through the damaged mucosa.

*Classification*
Competency Category: Nursing Practice: Alterations in Health
Taxonomic Level: Knowledge/Comprehension

**242. D.** "Lean roast beef, buttered white rice with egg slices, white bread with butter and jelly, and tea with sugar."

*Rationale*
This is a low-residue diet and is necessary in the acute phase of ulcerative colitis to prevent irritation of the colon. Orange juice contains cellulose, which is not absorbed and irritates the colon; creamed soups and contain lactose, which is irritating to the colon and is contraindicated in people with colitis.

*Classification*
Competency Category: Nursing Practice: Health and Wellness
Taxonomic Level: Application

**243. B.** Impaired neural functioning.

*Rationale*
Paralytic ileus occurs when neurologic impulses are diminished, as from anaesthesia, infection, or surgery.

*Classification*
Competency Category: Nursing Practice: Alterations in Health
Taxonomic Level: Critical Thinking

**244. C.** Anticipate that emotional stress can increase intestinal peristalsis.

*Rationale*
Emotional stress of any kind can stimulate peristalsis and thereby increase the volume of drainage and continuous, so irrigations are not indicated.

*Classification*
Competency Category: Nursing Practice: Alterations in Health
Taxonomic Level: Application

**245. A.** The hemopoietic factor is absorbed only in the terminal ileum.

*Rationale*
Vitamin B12 (extrinsic factor) combines with intrinsic factor, a substance secreted by the parietal cells of the gastric mucosa, forming hemopoietic factor. Hemopoietic factor is only absorbed in the ileum, from which it travels to bone marrow and stimulates erythropoiesis.

*Classification*
Competency Category: Nursing Practice: Alterations in Health
Taxonomic Level: Knowledge/Comprehension

**246. C.** Stomahesive.

*Rationale*
Stomahesive provides a protective coating that provides a barrier to gastrointestinal enzymes and protects against allergic reactions to the tape on the appliance.

*Classification*
Competency Category: Nursing Practice: Alterations in Health
Taxonomic Level: Application

**247. D.** Clamp the tubing and allow the client to rest.

*Rationale*
Rapid instillations of fluid into the colon may cause abdominal cramps. By clamping off the tubing, the nurse allows the cramps to subside so the irrigation can be continued.

*Classification*
Competency Category: Nursing Practice: Alterations in Health
Taxonomic Level: Application

**248. A.** An irrigation routine.

*Rationale*
Colostomy irrigations done daily at the same time help establish normal patterns of bowel evacuation.

*Classification*
Competency Category: Nursing Practice: Health and Wellness
Taxonomic Level: Application

**249. D.** The reactive hyperemia is likely transient.

*Rationale*
If the area blanches white and the erythema returns when the finger is removed, the reactive hyperemia is likely transient.

*Classification*
Competency Category: Nursing Practice: Alterations in Health
Taxonomic Level: Knowledge/Comprehension

**250. B.** Clear, watery plasma.

*Rationale*
Serous drainage is clear, watery plasma; sanguineous drainage is fresh, red bleeding; purulent drainage is thick and yellow; and purulent drainage with

infection is beige to brown and foul smelling, which indicate infection.

*Classification*
Competency Category: Nursing Practice: Alterations in Health
Taxonomic Level: Knowledge/Comprehension

**251. C.** Reducing stress on the abdominal incision.

*Rationale*
Using a binder provides even support to a wound and immobilizes a body part. A binder is cloth and therefore would not be a good collection of drainage.

*Classification*
Competency Category: Nursing Practice: Alterations in Health
Taxonomic Level: Knowledge/Comprehension

**252. C.** A dressing that contains a debriding enzyme that is used to remove necrotic tissue.

*Rationale*
These dressing have complex formulations of colloids and elastomeric and adhesive components and are used for autolytic debridement of necrotic tissue.

*Classification*
Competency Category: Nursing Practice: Alterations in Health
Taxonomic Level: Knowledge/Comprehension

**253. B.** Cardiac arrest.

*Rationale*
Potassium is a drug that must be administered slowly and monitored closely and cautiously by the nurse. Failure to conduct rigorous potassium monitoring and thorough nursing assessments can result in cardiac arrest from potassium overload.

*Classification*
Competency Category: Nursing Practice: Alterations in Health
Taxonomic Level: Knowledge/Comprehension

**254. B.** Check the pulse distal to the catheter insertion site.

*Rationale*
The pulse should be assessed because a trauma at the insertion site may interfere with blood flow distal to the site. There is also danger of bleeding or occlusion.

*Classification*
Competency Category: Nursing Practice: Alterations in Health
Taxonomic Level: Application

**255. B.** Valsalva manoeuvre.

*Rationale*
Having the patient perform Valsalva manoeuvre while assuming a left lateral decubitus position may prevent air embolus. The increased venous pressure created by the manoeuvre prevents air from entering the blood stream during catheter insertion.

*Classification*
Competency Category: Nursing Practice: Alterations in Health
Taxonomic Level: Application

**256. D.** Thrombosis.

*Rationale*
The catheter occlusion may have been caused by inadequate flushing. It is usually a lipid build use, not particulate matter.

*Classification*
Competency Category: Nursing Practice: Alterations in Health
Taxonomic Level: Knowledge/Comprehension

**257. A.** Catheter malposition.

*Rationale*
The catheter pressing against the vein causes the pain.

*Classification*
Competency Category: Nursing Practice: Alterations in Health
Taxonomic Level: Knowledge/Comprehension

**258. B.** Immediately tell him to cough or exhale forcibly while you cover the wound.

*Rationale*
Telling Mr. Jool to exhale forces air out and allows the space to be covered before a sucking chest wound occurs.

*Classification*
Competency Category: Nursing Practice: Alterations in Health
Taxonomic Level: Application

**259. B.** Coiled flat on the bed and secured without putting tension on the tube.

*Rationale*
Tubing that is coiled flat on the bed and secured without putting tension of the tube maintains a patent, free draining system. This prevents fluid accumulation and decreases the risk of infection, atelectasis, and tension pneumothorax.

*Classification*
Competency Category: Nursing Practice: Alterations in Health
Taxonomic Level: Application

**260. B.** Palpate the surrounding area for crepitus.

*Rationale*
Leakage of air into the subcutaneous tissue is evidenced by a crackling sound when the area is gently palpated. This is referred to as crepitus.

*Classification*
Competency Category: Nursing Practice: Alterations in Health
Taxonomic Level: Knowledge/Comprehension

**261. B.** One hour before a meal.

*Rationale*
Productive coughing induced by postural drainage may cause nausea and vomiting. Upon awakening, mucus secretions are plentiful and tenacious, so postural drainage at this time would be most beneficial. Approximately 1 hour before meals is a preferred time for postural drainage; the resulting cough and mucus production will be less likely to affect the client's dietary intake.

*Classification*
Competency Category: Nursing Practice: Alterations in Health
Taxonomic Level: Application

**262. C.** Prevent entrance of air into the pleural cavity.

*Rationale*
Atmospheric pressure is greater than the pressure inside the pleural space. If a chest tube were not attached to underwater seal drainage, air would enter the pleural space and collapse the lung (pneumothorax). The water seal does not affect the amount of suction used.

*Classification*
Competency Category: Nursing Practice: Alterations in Health
Taxonomic Level: Knowledge/Comprehension

**263. B.** 750 mL.

*Rationale*
Between 100 and 300 mL of fluid may drain in the chest tube in an adult during the first 3 hours. This rate then decreases, and 500 to 1000 mL of drainage can be expected within the first 24 hours.

*Classification*
Competency Category: Nursing Practice: Alterations in Health
Taxonomic Level: Knowledge/Comprehension

**264. D.** A rise of formula in the tube.

*Rationale*
A rise in the level of formula within the tube indicates a full stomach. Passage of flatus reflects intestinal motility, which does not pose a potential problem.

*Classification*
Competency Category: Nursing Practice: Alterations in Health
Taxonomic Level: Critical Thinking

**265. B.** Ensure that the drainage receptacles are kept compressed to maintain suction.

*Rationale*
Portable wound drainage systems are self-contained and can be emptied and compressed to reestablish negative pressure, which promotes drainage.

*Classification*
Competency Category: Nursing Practice: Alterations in Health
Taxonomic Level: Application

**266. C.** Prevent aspiration during nasogastric tube feeding.

*Rationale*
Raising the head of the bed keeps the nasogastric tube feeding in the stomach via the principle of gravity.

*Classification*
Competency Category: Nursing Practice: Alterations in Health
Taxonomic Level: Knowledge/Comprehension

**267. B.** Cyanosis.

*Rationale*
Inability to pass air can indicate that the tube is through the client's vocal cords and into the lungs. The tube may also coil around itself in the back of the throat causing gagging and eventually obstruction.

*Classification*
Competency Category: Nursing Practice: Alterations in Health
Taxonomic Level: Knowledge/Comprehension

**268. B.** That is equal to the distance from the tip of his nose to the tip of the ear lobe down to the xiphoid process of the sternum.

*Rationale*
Measure distance form tip of nose to earlobe to xiphoid process, which approximates the distance from the nose to the stomach. The tube should extend from the nares to the stomach.

*Classification*
Competency Category: Nursing Practice: Alterations in Health
Taxonomic Level: Application

**269. A.** It should be placed 90 cm above the injection site.

*Rationale*
Container heights of approximately 90 cm (1 m) are usually sufficient to overcome venous pressure and other resistance from the tubing and the catheter.

*Classification*
Competency Category: Nursing Practice: Alterations in Health
Taxonomic Level: Knowledge/Comprehension

**270. A.** Stress.

*Rationale*
This is a transient vascular and neurogenic reaction. It is most often evoked by emotional stress associated with fear or pain.

*Classification*
Competency Category: Nursing Practice: Alterations in Health
Taxonomic Level: Knowledge/Comprehension

**271. A.** In a horizontal position.

*Rationale*
The CVP is to be recorded when the patient is horizontal and the zero point of the manometer is at the midaxillary line.

*Classification*
Competency Category: Nursing Practice: Alterations in Health
Taxonomic Level: Application

**272. D.** All of the above.

*Rationale*
All of the answers are correct because they can all lead to complications if the catheter is not patent.

*Classification*
Competency Category: Nursing Practice: Alterations in Health
Taxonomic Level: Knowledge/Comprehension

**273. D.** Subclavian.

*Rationale*
The subclavian vein is in an area for decreased potential of contamination. There are limited natural skin folds in this area, and its location has limited movement.

*Classification*
Competency Category: Nursing Practice: Alterations in Health
Taxonomic Level: Knowledge/Comprehension

**274. C.** Friction.

*Rationale*
Soap helps by reducing surface tension of water, but friction is necessary for the removal of microorganisms.

*Classification*
Competency Category: Nursing Practice: Health and Wellness
Taxonomic Level: Knowledge/Comprehension

**275. B.** Use sterile gloves during the procedure.

*Rationale*
The tracheostomy site is a portal of entry for microorganisms. Sterile technique must be used.

*Classification*
Competency Category: Nursing Practice: Alterations in Health
Taxonomic Level: Application

**276. C.** Placing the feet apart to increase the stability of the body.

*Rationale*
Placing the feet apart creates a wider base of support and brings the center of gravity closer to the ground. This improves stability.

*Classification*
Competency Category: Nursing Practice: Alterations in Health
Taxonomic Level: Application

**277. A.** The avoidance of percutaneous injury.

*Rationale*
Extreme care is essential in handling sharp objects, especially with needles, which should not be recapped.

*Classification*
Competency Category: Nursing Practice: Alterations
in Health
Taxonomic Level: Critical Thinking

**278. C.** Contact.

*Rationale*
Contact precautions are designed to emphasize
cautious technique for organisms that have serious epi-
demiologic consequences or those easily transmitted by
contact between health care workers and patients.

*Classification*
Competency Category: Nursing Practice: Alterations
in Health
Taxonomic Level: Application

**279. A.** Assess his blood pressure in the supine, sitting, and standing positions.

*Rationale*
By assessing his blood pressure in these positions, you
can calculate his postural pressure, understanding the
increase or decrease in blood pressure from a lying to
sitting or sitting to standing positions.

*Classification*
Competency Category: Nursing Practice: Health and
Wellness
Taxonomic Level: Application

**280. A.** Solid foods.

*Rationale*
Solid foods are permitted. Stimulants, including the
caffeine in coffee and tea, and tranquilizers can alter
EEG wave patterns or mask abnormal patterns.
Therefore, such substances must be avoided for
24 hours before the test.

*Classification*
Competency Category: Nursing Practice: Alterations
in Health
Taxonomic Level: Application

**281. B.** The metabolic workload of digestion.

*Rationale*
Acute care of the client with a myocardial infarction is
aimed at reducing the cardiac workload. Clear liquids
are easily digested to help reduce this workload. Sympathetic nervous system involvement causes decreased
peristalsis and gastric secretion, so limiting food intake
helps prevent gastric distension and cardiac workload.

*Classification*
Competency Category: Nursing Practice: Alterations
in Health
Taxonomic Level: Critical Thinking

**282. B.** Tissue necrosis.

*Rationale*
The body's general inflammatory response to
myocardial necrosis causes an elevation of
temperature as well as leukocytosis within 24
to 48 hours.

*Classification*
Competency Category: Nursing Practice: Alterations
in Health
Taxonomic Level: Critical Thinking

**283. C.** Short family visits.

*Rationale*
Visits by family members can alleviate anxiety and
consequently reduce emotional stress.

*Classification*
Competency Category: Nursing Practice: Alterations
in Health
Taxonomic Level: Application

**284. A.** Lanoxin (Digoxin).

*Rationale*
Signs of digitalis toxicity include cardiac
dysrhythmias, anorexia, nausea, vomiting, and visual
disturbances. Cardiac dysrhythmias result from the
inhibition, by digitalis, of myocardial $Na+$ and $K+$.
Extracardiac effects may be caused by central nervous
system or local disturbances.

*Classification*
Competency Category: Nursing Practice: Alterations
in Health
Taxonomic Level: Critical Thinking

**285. C.** Dysphagia.

*Rationale*
Dysphagia is difficulty in swallowing. The same
nerve that controls the drooping of the face can cause
dysphagia.

*Classification*
Competency Category: Nursing Practice: Alterations
in Health
Taxonomic Level: Critical Thinking

**286. C.** Reflect on how she is feeling, and encourage
her to express other fears that she has about his
injury.

*Rationale*
Listening and encouraging the client's mother to express her feelings will be most therapeutic and will allow the nurse to gather more data about understanding the injury.

*Classification*
Competency Category: Nurse–Person Relationship
Taxonomic Level: Application

**287. C.** Position the client on his side with the head of the bed slightly elevated.

*Rationale*
Stroke in evolution refers to neurologic changes that continue for 24 to 48 hours. The snoring respirations indicate airway obstruction caused by the tongue falling backward, so turning the client on his side will clear the obstruction.

*Classification*
Competency Category: Nursing Practice: Alterations in Health
Taxonomic Level: Critical Thinking

**288. A.** Difficulty speaking and understanding.

*Rationale*
Right-sided hemiplegia is caused by damage to the left hemisphere of the brain. Expressive and receptive dysphasias are associated with damage to the left hemisphere, where the dominant speech centers are located in most people.

*Classification*
Competency Category: Nursing Practice: Alterations in Health
Taxonomic Level: Knowledge/Comprehension

**289. D.** Supine with his head midline.

*Rationale*
The best initial position for a person with a cervical fracture is supine with the head immobilized and midline. This position prevents flexion, rotation, and extension of the neck.

*Classification*
Competency Category: Nursing Practice: Alterations in Health
Taxonomic Level: Application

**290. A.** Clear any obstacles in a path for walking.

*Rationale*
Cranial nerve II is the optic nerve, which guides vision. Clearing the path of obstacles will provide safety for this patient.

*Classification*
Competency Category: Nursing Practice: Alterations in Health
Taxonomic Level: Critical Thinking

**291. A.** A failure of peripheral circulation.

*Rationale*
Shock may have different causes (e.g., hypovolemic, cardiogenic, septic) but always involves a decrease in blood pressure and failure of the peripheral circulation because of sympathetic nervous system involvement.

*Classification*
Competency Category: Nursing Practice: Alterations in Health
Taxonomic Level: Knowledge/Comprehension

**292. B.** Decreased cerebral edema.

*Rationale*
Mannitol, an osmotic diuretic, is used to decrease cerebral edema in clients with head injuries.

*Classification*
Competency Category: Nursing Practice: Alterations in Health
Taxonomic Level: Critical Thinking

**293. B.** To avoid impeding venous outflow.

*Rationale*
Any activity or position that impedes venous outflow from the head may contribute to increased volume inside the skull and possibly increase intracranial pressure.

*Classification*
Competency Category: Nursing Practice: Alterations in Health
Taxonomic Level: Critical Thinking

**294. D.** Enhancing safety and comfort.

*Rationale*
Enhancing safety and comfort is important throughout any type of shock; however, this is not a priority action when initially treating a person experiencing shock.

*Classification*
Competency Category: Nursing Practice: Alterations in Health
Taxonomic Level: Application

**295. B.** A blunt or penetrating injury resulting in air moving into the pleural space without being able to exit.

*Rationale*
Blunt trauma such as a rib fracture or penetrating chest trauma can cause pneumothorax. This is considered a tension pneumothorax because air that enters the chest cavity is trapped and cannot be expelled out.

*Classification*
Competency Category: Nursing Practice: Alterations in Health
Taxonomic Level: Critical Thinking

**296. B.** Respiratory rate of 10 to 20 breaths/min, $SpO_2$ of 97% to 98%, and even breathing with occasional sighs.

*Rationale*
Normal respiratory parameters include easy breathing. Easy breathing would be considered even breaths that are not creating noticeable use of muscles.

*Classification*
Competency Category: Nursing Practice: Alterations in Health
Taxonomic Level: Knowledge/Comprehension

**297. B.** Place the client in high Fowler's position.

*Rationale*
Proper positioning can help reduce venous return to the heart. Placing the patient in the high Fowler's position also decreases lung congestion.

*Classification*
Competency Category: Nursing Practice: Alterations in Health
Taxonomic Level: Application

**298. A.** Supine.

*Rationale*
In the supine position, the abdominal contents press against the diaphragm, impeding expansion of the lungs.

*Classification*
Competency Category: Nursing Practice: Alterations in Health
Taxonomic Level: Application

**299. D.** 28 breaths/min and noisy.

*Rationale*
Twenty-eight breaths are outside the normal range of 14 to 20 breaths/min. Breathing should be without effort or adventitious sounds. Based on these abnormal assessment findings, this patient may be experiencing respiratory distress.

*Classification*
Competency Category: Nursing Practice: Alterations in Health
Taxonomic Level: Application

**300. B.** Wheezing, tachycardia, and restlessness.

*Rationale*
Wheezing results when air is expired against resistance, such as from a collapsed airway. Tachycardia results from hypoxia, and restlessness is a result of cerebral hypoxia.

*Classification*
Competency Category: Nursing Practice: Alterations in Health
Taxonomic Level: Knowledge/Comprehension

**301. C.** Respiratory acidosis.

*Rationale*
An increased level of dissolved carbon dioxide ($PaCO_2$) indicates respiratory acidosis.

*Classification*
Competency Category: Nursing Practice: Alterations in Health
Taxonomic Level: Critical Thinking

**302. B.** Place her in an orthopneic position.

*Rationale*
The orthopneic position allows maximum lung expansion because gravity reduces the pressure of the abdominal viscera on the diaphragm and lungs.

*Classification*
Competency Category: Nursing Practice: Alterations in Health
Taxonomic Level: Application

**303. D.** Gently shake him and shout, "Are you OK?"

*Rationale*
Assessing the client's level of consciousness is the first step in basic life support. Unconsciousness is assessed by shaking the client's shoulders and shouting, "Are you OK?"

*Classification*
Competency Category: Nursing Practice: Alterations in Health
Taxonomic Level: Application

**304. A.** Begin EGG monitoring.

*Rationale*
EGG monitoring should be started as soon as possible; life-threatening arrhythmias are the leading cause of death in the first hours after an MI.

*Classification*
Competency Category: Nursing Practice: Alterations in Health
Taxonomic Level: Application

**305. B.** The heel of one hand on the sternum and the heel of the other on top of it with the fingers interlocking.

*Rationale*
This provides the best leverage for depressing the sternum, adequately compressing the heart and forcing blood into the arteries. Grasping the fingers keeps them off the chest and concentrates the energy expended in the heel of the hand while minimizing the possibility of fracturing the client's ribs.

*Classification*
Competency Category: Nursing Practice: Alterations in Health
Taxonomic Level: Knowledge/Comprehension

**306. C.** Immediate defibrillation.

*Rationale*
When ventricular fibrillation is verified, the first intervention is defibrillation, which is the only intervention that will terminate this lethal dysrhythmia.

*Classification*
Competency Category: Nursing Practice: Alterations in Health
Taxonomic Level: Application

**307. A.** Threatened abortion.

*Rationale*
Spotting in the first trimester may indicate that the pregnancy is in jeopardy. Bed rest and avoidance of physical and emotional stress are recommended. Abortion is usually inevitable if the bleeding is accompanied by pain with dilation and effacement of the cervix.

*Classification*
Competency Category: Nursing Practice: Alterations in Health
Taxonomic Level: Application

**308. B.** Check the fundus for firmness.

*Rationale*
After a spontaneous abortion, the fundus should be checked for firmness, which would indicate

effective uterine tone. If the uterus is not firm, it is hypotonic, and hemorrhage may occur. A soft or boggy uterus may also indicate retained placental tissue.

*Classification*
Competency Category: Nursing Practice: Alterations in Health
Taxonomic Level: Application

**309. D.** "I see that both of you are very upset. I will be here if you want to talk."

*Rationale*
This allows the husband and wife to comfort each other while letting them know the nurse is available. It also allows them to recognize and accept their feelings of loss.

*Classification*
Competency Category: Nurse–Person relationship
Taxonomic Level: Critical Thinking

**310. A.** Ketones from rapid fat breakdown, causing acidosis.

*Rationale*
Ketones are released when fat is broken down for energy.

*Classification*
Competency Category: Nursing Practice: Alterations in Health
Taxonomic Level: Knowledge/Comprehension

**311. B.** Low-protein diet with a prescribed amount of water.

*Rationale*
Although dialysis removes water, creatinine, and urea from the blood, the client's diet must still be monitored.

*Classification*
Competency Category: Nursing Practice: Health and Wellness
Taxonomic Level: Critical Thinking

**312. C.** A positive test reaction indicates ketoacidosis.

*Rationale*
Urinary acetone indicates the development of ketoacidosis from the body's breakdown of fats.

*Classification*
Competency Category: Nursing Practice: Alterations in Health
Taxonomic Level: Critical Thinking

**313. D.** Kussmaul respirations.

*Rationale*
Kussmaul respirations occur in diabetic coma as the body attempts to correct a low pH caused by accumulation of ketones (ketoacidosis). It affects people with type II diabetes who still have some insulin production because insulin prevents the breakdown of fats into ketones.

*Classification*
Competency Category: Nursing Practice: Alterations in Health
Taxonomic Level: Knowledge/Comprehension

**314. B.** Observing for signs of hypoglycemia as a result of treatment.

*Rationale*
During treatment for acidosis, the client may develop hypoglycaemia. Careful observation for this complication should be made by the nurse.

*Classification*
Competency Category: Nursing Practice: Alterations in Health
Taxonomic Level: Application

**315. B.** Can be planned around a wide variety of commonly available foods.

*Rationale*
Each client should be given an individually devised diet selecting commonly used foods from the Canadian Diabetic Association exchange diet. Family members should be included in the diet teaching.

*Classification*
Competency Category: Nursing Practice: Alterations in Health
Taxonomic Level: Knowledge/Comprehension

**316. A.** Replacement of potassium deficit.

*Rationale*
After treatment with insulin for diabetic acidosis is begun, potassium ions reenter the cells, causing hypokalemia. Therefore, potassium, along with the replacement fluids, is generally supplied.

*Classification*
Competency Category: Nursing Practice: Alterations in Health
Taxonomic Level: Knowledge/Comprehension

**317. A.** 1 scoop ice milk = 1 slice bread.

*Rationale*
In the food groups, all the answers are grouped according to grains, dairy, proteins, and fats, except the ice milk and bread choice. This indicates that the patient does not know the food groups and requires further teaching.

*Classification*
Competency Category: Nursing Practice: Health and Wellness
Taxonomic Level: Application

**318. B.** The nurse was properly functioning as a health teacher.

*Rationale*
The Canadian Nurses Association identifies that the nurse will do health teaching and administer nursing care supportive to life and well-being.

*Classification*
Competency Category: Nursing Practice: Health and Wellness
Taxonomic Level: Knowledge/Comprehension

**319. D.** Diarrhea.

*Rationale*
Gastrointestinal symptoms are the initial symptoms of lithium toxicity.

*Classification*
Competency Category: Nursing Practice: Alterations in Health
Taxonomic Level: Knowledge/Comprehension

**320. A.** Orthostatic hypotension is a common side effect.

*Rationale*
Orthostatic hypotension is common during the first few weeks of treatment with antipsychotic drugs.

*Classification*
Competency Category: Nursing Practice: Alterations in Health
Taxonomic Level: Critical Thinking

**321. A.** Fever, hypertension, changes in level of consciousness, and hallucinations.

*Rationale*
The most common symptoms of alcohol withdrawal delirium are anxiety, insomnia, anorexia, hypertension, disorientation, hallucinations, changes in level of consciousness, agitation, fever, and delusions.

*Classification*
Competency Category: Nursing Practice: Alterations
in Health
Taxonomic Level: Application

**322. A.** Can you tell me your address?

*Rationale*
This question requires recall and no memory loss.
The other questions are based on opinion rather
than fact. There should be one clear answer for this
question.

*Classification*
Competency Category: Nursing Practice: Alterations
in Health
Taxonomic Level: Application

**323. A.** Increased intracranial pressure.

*Rationale*
Movement of the eyes should be a balanced and
coordinated function. Both pupils should be
equal, reactive, and responsive to light and
accommodation.

*Classification*
Competency Category: Nursing Practice: Alterations
in Health
Taxonomic Level: Critical Thinking

**324. C.** Ask the parents what their wishes are
regarding baptism.

*Rationale*
Although the nurse may have her own beliefs, she
should discuss with the parents their knowledge and
decisions regarding baptism.

*Classification*
Competency Category: Nurse–Person Relationship
Taxonomic Level: Application

**325. C.** Someone who is called to the ministry to
promote health.

*Rationale*
Although parish nursing can be defined in multiple
ways, it is usually a calling and related to promoting
health and well-being. This person may be a trusted
spiritual leader for the patient.

*Classification*
Competency Category: Nurse–Person Relationship
Taxonomic Level: Knowledge/Comprehension

**326. A.** Her ability to correctly count her radial
pulse.

*Rationale*
A client who complies with drug therapy is less likely
to have a recurrence of cardiac failure. Client knowledge of how to check a radial pulse and actions to
take if it is not within normal limits can prevent a
toxic digoxin reaction.

*Classification*
Competency Category: Nursing Practice: Alterations
in Health
Taxonomic Level: Critical Thinking

**327. A.** 1 cup of low-fat yogurt.

*Rationale*
One cup of low-fat yogurt contains 415 mg of
calcium.

*Classification*
Competency Category: Nursing Practice: Health and
Wellness
Taxonomic Level: Knowledge/Comprehension

**328. A.** Cooking.

*Rationale*
Cooking will not cause increased ocular pressure.

*Classification*
Competency Category: Nursing Practice: Health and
Wellness
Taxonomic Level: Critical Thinking

**329. C.** "I should try to eat several small meals
during the day."

*Rationale*
The respiratory workload is increased in individuals
with COPD. Because digestion also is energy
consuming, clients with COPD may feel full after
only a small meal. They may tolerate smaller, more
frequent, high-calorie meals better than larger
meals.

*Classification*
Competency Category: Health and Wellness
Taxonomic Level: Application

**330. A.** Forward-flexed posture.

*Rationale*
As people age, the spine tends to flex forward, causing
a shift in balance and an increased risk for falls.

*Classification*
Competency Category: Nursing Practice: Alterations
in Health
Taxonomic Level: Knowledge/Comprehension

**331. C.** The urge to urinate.

*Rationale*
The urgency to urinate may result in the need to increase ambulation speed and therefore may result in falls.

*Classification*
Competency Category: Nursing Practice: Alterations in Health
Taxonomic Level: Knowledge/Comprehension

**332. B.** Tell her that there is some evidence that a genetic basis for the disease may exist and suggest that the daughter be evaluated.

*Rationale*
Some research has indicated that a genetic link may be present. Unexplained joint stiffness at age 40 years should be evaluated by a physician before aspirin therapy is initiated on a regular basis.

*Classification*
Competency Category: Nurse–Person Relationship
Taxonomic Level: Application

**333. B.** Developed an increase in her mobility.

*Rationale*
This regimen limits bone demineralization. It also reduces osteoporotic pain, which promotes increased activity.

*Classification*
Competency Category: Nursing Practice: Alterations in Health
Taxonomic Level: Critical Thinking

**334. B.** "You must be feeling lonely at this time."

*Rationale*
The client is experiencing loss and is feeling hopeless. The most therapeutic response by the nurse is the one that attempts to translate feelings into words.

*Classification*
Competency Category: Nurse–Person Relationship
Taxonomic Level: Critical Thinking

**335. A.** Ask for other medical opinions.

*Rationale*
Seeking other opinions to disprove the inevitable is a form of denial used by individuals with illnesses that have a poor prognosis.

*Classification*
Competency Category: Nursing Practice: Health and Wellness
Taxonomic Level: Critical Thinking

**336. D.** "Increase fibre and fluids in your diet."

*Rationale*
Clients with hypothyroidism typically have constipation. A diet high in fibre and fluids can help prevent this.

*Classification*
Competency Category: Nurse–Person Relationship
Taxonomic Level: Application

**337. A.** Cold, clammy skin and irregular, noisy breathing.

*Rationale*
As the body begins to die, the patient's cardiovascular systems slows, and the skin becomes cold and clammy. Respirations slow, Cheyne Stoke breathing may occur, and secretions accumulate, contributing to alterations in breath sounds and patterns.

*Classification*
Competency Category: Nursing Practice: Alterations in Health
Taxonomic Level: Knowledge/Comprehension

**338. C.** Panic.

*Rationale*
People in panic could initiate the panic reaction in those who appear to be in control. People in panic may not realize that they are injured and require both physical and emotional assessments.

*Classification*
Competency Category: Nursing Practice: Alterations in Health
Taxonomic Level: Critical Thinking

**339. B.** Severe lacerations involving open fractures of major bones.

*Rationale*
Those with open fractures are at an increased risk for severe blood loss if dressings, as indicated, have not yet been applied.

*Classification*
Competency Category: Nursing Practice: Health and Wellness
Taxonomic Level: Critical Thinking

**340. A.** Those with severe head injuries.

*Rationale*
People with severe head injuries are the highest priority because of potential brain damage and spinal cord injury. The other options identified are not life threatening.

*Classification*
Competency Category: Nursing Practice: Alterations in Health
Taxonomic Level: Critical Thinking

**341. B.** "I would like to further discuss your concerns about this. What have you heard about using oxygen at home?"

*Rationale*
Reflecting and clarification are therapeutic techniques. This response encourages exploration of the client's feelings.

*Classification*
Competency Category: Nurse–Person Relationship
Taxonomic Level: Application

**342. C.** Call the physician; report the symptoms; and upon the physician's order, send a blood sample to the laboratory to determine the client's potassium level.

*Rationale*
Furosemide is a potassium-wasting diuretic. A low potassium level may cause weakness and palpitations.

*Classification*
Competency Category: Nursing Practice: Health and Wellness
Taxonomic Level: Critical Thinking

**343. C.** Inhale the mist and quickly exhale.

*Rationale*
The patient should be instructed to hold his or her breath for at least 5 to 10 seconds before exhaling the mist.

*Classification*
Competency Category: Nursing Practice: Health and Wellness
Taxonomic Level: Application

**344. D.** Proportion more fluids during the day than during the night.

*Rationale*
Mr. Tse and nurse should make a fluid schedule, taking into consideration the 1000-mL limitation and additional factors such as periods of wakefulness, number of meals, oral medications, and personal preferences.

*Classification*
Competency Category: Nursing Practice: Health and Wellness
Taxonomic Level: Application

**345. D.** Familiar.

*Rationale*
Familiarity provides a sense of security and promotes safety and may reduce client stress.

*Classification*
Competency Category: Nursing Practice: Health and Wellness
Taxonomic Level: Knowledge/Comprehension

**346. B.** Assess his nausea and sleep interferences; call physiotherapy to cancel or reschedule his appointment.

*Rationale*
Gathering information regarding possible causes of nausea and sleep problems help to identify changes and factors that relate to the changes. Modifying his schedule helps, according to his changed state.

*Classification*
Competency Category: Nursing Practice: Health and Wellness
Taxonomic Level: Critical Thinking

**347. B.** Concerns regarding the cancer and how the surgery will affect her.

*Rationale*
Two primary concerns are the confirmation of cancer and the impending mastectomy.

*Classification*
Competency Category: Nurse–Person Relationship
Taxonomic Level: Application

**348. B.** "This is a very difficult adjustment period for you and your family."

*Rationale*
This response paraphrases the client's concerns about the effect on her family.

*Classification*
Competency Category: Nursing Practice: Health and Wellness
Taxonomic Level: Application

**349. A.** Informing her regarding a Hemovac, pressure dressing, and deep breathing exercises.

*Rationale*
Preoperative teaching related to what she can expect after surgery is important.

*Classification*
Competency Category: Nursing Practice: Alterations in Health
Taxonomic Level: Knowledge/Comprehension

**350. C.** Inform him that she will be going to the recovery room after the operation; they will notify the unit when she is ready to come back.

*Rationale*
Informing him of what to expect will allay his apprehension. He can phone the unit and check for her return.

*Classification*
Competency Category: Nursing Practice: Alterations in Health
Taxonomic Level: Application

**351. D.** Checking for urinary retention and the need to void.

*Rationale*
Return of urinary system after anaesthesia usually takes 6 or more hours, so this assessment is not a priority upon return from the recovery room.

*Classification*
Competency Category: Nursing Practice: Alterations in Health
Taxonomic Level: Application

**352. C.** "I can see you're concerned about this. I could arrange a private place for you to pray."

*Rationale*
This acknowledges the client's concerns and poses a solution to enable him to develop healthy coping strategies to meet his spiritual needs.

*Classification*
Competency Category: Nurse–Person Relationship
Taxonomic Level: Critical Thinking

**353. C.** Infection.

*Rationale*
Infection should be suspected because of the signs of inflammation.

*Classification*
Competency Category: Nursing Practice: Alterations in Health
Taxonomic Level: Critical Thinking

**354. B.** Inspect and palpate the lower abdomen; if it is distended and uncomfortable, insert a straight catheter.

*Rationale*
Conservative measures have been unsuccessful. Eight hours after surgery is enough time for bladder tonus return, so assessment of the distended bladder and catheterization would be appropriate.

*Classification*
Competency Category: Nursing Practice: Alterations in Health
Taxonomic Level: Application

**355. Answers:**

- The publication source is trustworthy.
- The author is reputable and has clinical credibility.
- The research evidence has a methodology and references.
- The publication has a clear layout.
- It is easy to use and has a logical representation.
- The information has purpose and suitability and is current.

*Rationale*
All of the above are criteria that must be considered when evaluating nursing research posted on the Internet.

*Classification*
Competency Category: Professional Practice
Taxonomic Level: Application

**356. Answer:** Nursing informatics is the combination of computer and information science with nursing science.

*Rationale*
Nursing informatics assists in managing and processing nursing data, information, and knowledge in support of nursing practice and the delivery of care. Data, information, and knowledge are the core of informatics.

*Classification*
Competency Category: Professional Practice
Taxonomic Level: Knowledge/Comprehension

**357. Answers:** This may include design, development, and marketing of resources or educational sessions. The nurse may communicate by e-mail or use computerized applications to document patient care, retrieve bibliographic information, and evaluate and use the information for patient teaching.

*Rationale*
Informatics can be implemented in a variety of ways in the nursing practice setting, including patient teaching, patient care, professional development, and as a means of communication between nursing staff.

*Classification*
Competency Category: Professional Practice
Taxonomic Level: Application

**358. Answers:**

- Eliminate redundancies and duplication.
- Enhance quality and reporting of clinical care.
- Standardize common documentation for all patients.
- Automate an ideal clinical documentation workflow.

*Rationale*
Standardized interdisciplinary electronic documentation can help to eliminate redundancies and duplication, enhance patient care, and create consistency in documentation.

*Classification*
Competency Category: Professional Practice
Taxonomic Level: Knowledge/Comprehension

**359. Answers:**

**Passive:** To retain as much joint range of motion as possible and to maintain circulation.
**Active:** To increase muscle strength.
**Resistive:** To provide resistance to increase muscle strength.

*Rationale*
Each of the answers provided describes the purpose of passive, active, and resistive range of motion exercises.

*Classification*
Competency Category: Nursing Practice: Alterations in Health
Taxonomic Level: Application

**360. Answers:**

- The client talks about death and darkness.
- The client starts giving away prized and cherished personal items.
- The client cancels social engagements.
- The client creates a will.

- The client has feelings of hopelessness.
- The client has a loss of interest in activities.
- Client asks about poison, guns, or other lethal objects.

*Rationale*
Common signs of suicidal ideation include talking about death; giving away cherished possessions; withdrawing from social interactions and activities; inquiring about poisons, guns, and other lethal objects; expressing feelings of hopelessness; and creating a will.

*Classification*
Competency Category: Nursing Practice: Alterations in Health
Taxonomic Level: Application

**361. Answer:** 4 g/200 mg $\times$ tablet or 0.4 g = 400 mg = 2 tablets

*Rationale*
This is the correct dose based on the information provided in this question.

*Classification*
Competency Category: Nursing Practice: Alterations in Health
Taxonomic Level: Application

**362. Answers:**

- The patient is able to correctly identify the type of stoma and assess its health.
- The patient is independent in care and is not having problems with skin breakdown, leakage, or odour.
- The patient has returned to previous activities of daily living (e.g., work, sports, sexual relationships).
- The patient identifies problems as they arise and is able to select appropriate assistance (physician, ostomy support group).
- The patient is discriminating about foods that do not interfere with digestive function.
- The patient understands medication intolerances and consults appropriate sources (pharmacist, nurse, physician).
- The patient uses available financial support services.

*Rationale*
A patient who has adapted to having an ostomy is able to assess its health and take appropriate actions when problems arise. The patient is able to implement health teaching into his or her daily

lives. A patient who has adapted to having an ostomy will continue to engage in activities of daily living and recognize the modifications that may be required because of having the ostomy.

*Classification*
Competency Category: Nursing Practice: Alterations in Health
Taxonomic Level: Application

**363. Answers:**

- Administer analgesics before painful procedures or positioning.
- Assess the patient frequently for pain.
- Frequent turning and repositioning of the patient.

*Rationale*
Nurses must assess patients frequently for pain using a valid pain rating scale. Administering analgesics before painful procedures and positioning reduces patients' pain and helps increase their ability to mobilize. Also, frequent turning and repositioning of the patient is essential to prevent the development of pressure ulcers.

*Classification*
Competency Category: Nursing Practice: Alterations in Health
Taxonomic Level: Critical Thinking

**364. Answer:** 25 drops/min.

*Rationale*
This is the correct drop rate based on the information provided in the question. To arrive at the answer, you should perform the following calculation:

$$\frac{\text{Volume to be infused} \times \text{Drop factor}}{\text{Number of hours} \times 60 \text{ minutes}}$$

$$\frac{100 \times 15}{1 \times 60}$$

$$\frac{1500}{60} = 25 \text{ drops/min}$$

*Classification*
Competency Category: Nursing Practice: Alterations in Health
Taxonomic Level: Knowledge/Comprehension

**365. Answers:**

- Given voluntarily.

- Given by a patient who has cognitive capacity to make decisions.
- Given by a patient who is informed about the surgery he or she will be having.

*Rationale*
All of the answers provided are criteria required for consent to surgery to be valid.

*Classification*
Competency Category: Professional Practice
Taxonomic Level: Knowledge/Comprehension

**366. Answer:** Repositioning the patient every 2 hours prevents fluid from collecting in the lung fields. A change in position also relieves pressure and increases activity.

*Rationale*
Fluid collection in the lungs can contribute to infection. Having a patient change position every 2 hours also relieves pressure and increases activity, thereby promoting circulation.

*Classification*
Competency Category: Nursing Practice: Alterations in Health
Taxonomic Level: Knowledge/Comprehension

**367. Answers:**

- Polyuria.
- Diarrhea.
- Vomiting.
- Excessive sweating.

*Rationale*
Polyuria, diarrhea, vomiting, and excessive sweating are all reasons why body fluid losses may exceed fluid intake.

*Classification*
Competency Category: Nursing Practice: Alterations in Health
Taxonomic Level: Critical Thinking

**368. Answers:**

- Red (highly vascular).
- Moist with smooth surfaces (like the inside the mouth).
- It may take up to 6 weeks for swelling to recede and for stoma to achieve its normal size.

*Rationale*
All of the answers provided indicate a healthy stoma.

*Classification*
Competency Category: Nursing Practice: Alterations in Health
Taxonomic Level: Knowledge/Comprehension

## 369. Answers:

- Be sensitive to nonverbal communication.
- If she is able, have her write her responses.
- Use closed questioning techniques.
- Provide a referral to a speech therapist or speech pathologist.
- Explain all measures.
- Provide a supportive and accepting environment.

*Rationale*
All of these answers would be beneficial to enhance communication with Mrs. Evenrude.

*Classification*
Competency Category: Nurse–Person Relationship
Taxonomic Level: Application

## 370. Answers:

| HEALTH TEAM MEMBER | REHABILITATION ROLE |
|---|---|
| Physiotherapist | Preserve functioning of muscles, prevent contractures, help with deep breathing and coughing exercises, prevent hypostatic pneumonia |
| Occupational therapist | Assist in meeting activities of daily living |
| Speech therapist | Assist in regaining speech and pronunciation |
| Recreation therapist | Prevent sensory deprivation |

*Rationale*
Recognizing the roles of various health team members in the rehabilitative process assists the nurse when planning comprehensive care for the client.

*Classification*
Competency Category: Nursing Practice: Health and Wellness
Taxonomic Level: Application

## 371. Answers:

A necrotic stoma:
- Appears within 24 to 72 hours after surgery.
- Has a dark or dusky colour.
- Has a strong, offensive odour.

*Rationale*
The answers provided are all indicative of a necrotic stoma and must be closely monitored by the nurses 24 to 72 hours after surgery.

*Classification*
Competency Category: Nursing Practice: Alterations in Health
Taxonomic Level: Knowledge/Comprehension

## 372. Answers:

- Dysrhythmias.
- Cardiac arrest.
- Arterial oxygen desaturation.
- Bronchoconstriction.
- Decreased arterial oxygen tension.
- Atelectasis.

*Rationale*
The answers provided are all complications that can occur when performing endotracheal suctioning of a patient.

*Classification*
Competency Category: Nursing Practice: Alterations in Health
Taxonomic Level: Application

## 373. Answer: Antiembolism stockings help prevent thrombus formation by facilitating the return of venous blood to the heart.

*Rationale*
Antiembolism stockings help to maintain external pressure on the muscles of the lower extremities and thus may promote venous return and prevent thrombus formation.

*Classification*
Competency Category: Nursing Practice: Health and Wellness
Taxonomic Level: Knowledge/Comprehension

## 374. Answers: Flexion, extension, hyperextension, dorsiflexion, plantarflexion, abduc-

tion, adduction, eversion, inversion, pronation, supination, internal and external rotation, and circumduction.

*Rationale*
These are all joint movements used in range of motion exercises.

*Classification*
Competency Category: Nursing Practice: Alterations in Health
Taxonomic Level: Knowledge/comprehension

### 375. Answers:

- Secure the central line to the chest wall with sutures or Steri-Strips.
- Coil and tape it to the patient's chest.
- Place a tab of tape on the TPN tubing and pin it to the patient's hospital's gown.
- Luerlock all connections and tape them with clear tape.

*Rationale*
The answers provided are all precautions that must be considered to prevent dislodgement or disconnection of a central line.

*Classification*
Competency Category: Nursing Practice: Alterations in Health
Taxonomic Level: Critical Thinking

### 376. Answers:

- Mobilizes respiratory secretions.
- Loosens pulmonary secretions to facilitate their expectoration.
- Promotes a clear airway by draining respiratory secretions toward the oral cavity.

*Rationale*
The purpose of postural drainage is to mobilize respiratory secretions, loosen pulmonary secretions and facilitate their expectoration, and promote a clear airway by draining respiratory secretions toward the oral cavity.

*Classification*
Competency Category: Nursing Practice: Alterations in Health
Taxonomic Level: Application

### 377. Answers:

**Observations seen:** Broken skin, presence of exudate, and signs of infection.

**Treatment objectives:** Protect from mechanical and thermal trauma.
**Manage exudate:** Maintain a most wound environment, prevent infection, prevent further injury, manage related pain, protect from friction and shear, and provide pressure relief.

*Rationale*
When a stage II pressure ulcer is present, treatment plans should focus on maintaining an environment conducive to healing, preventing infection, and promptly managing infection if it arises.

*Classification*
Competency Category: Nursing Practice: Alterations in Health
Taxonomic Level: Application

### 378. Answers:

**Inflammatory phase:** The body's reaction to tissue damage; occurs within minutes of injury.
**Proliferation:** The filling and coverage of the wound bed.
**Remodelling:** Maturation of the wound; may last for more than 1 year.

*Rationale*
Inflammation, proliferation, and remodelling are the three phases of wound healing. The inflammation phase occurs within minutes of tissue injury. Proliferation is the next phase of wound healing when filling and coverage of the wound bed occurs. Remodeling is the final phase of wound healing and occurs with the healing and maturation of the wound.

*Classification*
Competency Category: Nursing Practice: Alterations in Health
Taxonomic Level: Knowledge/Comprehension

### 379. Answers:

- Look after yourself first.
- Think clinically using the priorities of those in need of airway, breathing and circulation interventions.
- Triage and then treat.
- Work within your scope of practice and your own abilities.

*Rationale*
These are all priority actions that must be considered when planning care for a community experiencing a natural disaster such as a tornado.

*Classification*
Competency Category: Nursing Practice: Alterations in Health
Taxonomic Level: Critical Thinking

**380. Answers:** Multi-trauma means that a patient has more than one injury, and multiple casualties means that more than one patient is injured.

*Rationale*
These are the primary differences between multi-trauma and multiple causalities.

*Classification*
Competency Category: Nursing Practice: Alterations in Health
Taxonomic Level: Knowledge/Comprehension

**381. Answers:**

- Suggest a scheduled voiding time.
- Suggest bladder training techniques.
- Assess lifestyle factors that are associated with urinary incontinence.
- Suggest and teach Kegel exercises.

*Rationale*
Nurses can work with clients, suggesting ideas to help them regain control of urinary incontinence. Suggestions may include bladder training techniques and exercises, creating a voiding schedule, and assessing lifestyle factors that may contribute to urinary incontinence.

*Classification*
Competency Category: Nursing Practice: Alterations in Health
Taxonomic Level: Application

**382. Answers:** Cephalic vein, basilic vein, axillary vein, external jugular vein, internal jugular vein, subclavian vein, right and left brachiocephalic veins, and superior vena cava.

*Rationale*
These are all vascular structures used for central venous access.

*Classification*
Competency Category: Nursing Practice: Alterations in Health
Taxonomic Level: Knowledge/Comprehension

**383. Answers:**

- Allergies.

- Coagulation status.
- Diabetes.
- Renal disease.
- Previous central venous catheters.

*Rationale*
These conditions may all create complications when inserting a venous device.

*Classification*
Competency Category: Nursing Practice: Alterations in Health
Taxonomic Level: Critical Thinking

**384. Answers:**

- To remove accumulated air and fluids from the pleural cavity.
- To restore a negative pressure in the pleural cavity.
- To reexpand a collapsed lung.

*Rationale*
Removing accumulated air and fluids from the pleural cavity, restoring negative pressure in the pleural cavity, and reexpanding a collapsed lung are purposes of closed chest drainage.

*Classification*
Competency Category: Nursing Practice: Alterations in Health
Taxonomic Level: Knowledge/Comprehension

**385. Answers:**

- Assess the client's need for feeding.
- Evaluate the client's nutritional status.
- Verify the physician's order.
- Check placement.
- Have all supplies available.
- Auscultate for bowel sounds.

*Rationale*
Assessing the client's need, verifying the physician's order, and checking for placement of the NG tube are all priority actions that the nurse must complete before administering an NG tube feeding.

*Classification*
Competency Category: Nursing Practice: Alterations in Health
Taxonomic Level: Knowledge/Comprehension

**386. Answers:**

- Decompression.
- Gavage.

- Lavage.
- Gastric analysis.

*Rationale*
Decompression, gavage, lavage, and gastric analysis are all reasons a physician may order insertion of a tube.

*Classification*
Competency Category: Nursing Practice: Alterations in Health
Taxonomic Level: Knowledge/Comprehension

**387. Answers:**

- If an IV is already in place, make sure it is an 18/19-gauge needle.
- Prime the IV tubing with 0.9% saline.
- Ask if the patient has received a transfusion before.
- Take baseline vitals.
- Confirm the patient's identity by comparing the patient's armband with the blood product label.

*Rationale*
These are all priority actions that must be considered before administering blood products.

*Classification*
Competency Category: Nursing Practice: Alterations in Health
Taxonomic Level: Critical Thinking

**388. Answer:** Whole blood.

*Rationale*
Whole blood is usually administered with dextrose/lactated Ringer's solution.

*Classification*
Competency Category: Nursing Practice: Alterations in Health
Taxonomic Level: Knowledge/Comprehension

**389. Answers:**

- **Causes:** High concentration of dextrose in solution, infection, fluid infused too fast
- **Signs and symptoms:** Dehydration, nausea, headache, weakness, and thirst
- **Prevention and treatment:** Give solution at the prescribed rate. Check urine for glucose and acetone q4–6h. Give insulin injections to increase metabolisation of the increased glucose.

*Rationale*
Hyperglycemia is caused by high blood sugar. Symptoms include nausea, headache, weakness, and thirst. To prevent hyperglycemia, the client must maintain a balance between insulin and glucose intake. This includes careful monitoring of blood glucose levels and insulin injections to metabolize blood glucose.

*Classification*
Competency Category: Nursing Practice: Alterations in Health
Taxonomic Level: Application

**390. Answers:**

- **Signs and symptoms:** Occipital headaches; cold, clammy skin; dizziness; tachycardia; tingling of the extremities; shaky, blurred vision.
- **Causes:** If TPN is abruptly discontinued or slowed, the individual has too little blood glucose and too much insulin.
- **Prevention and treatment:** The client must have a balance of insulin and glucose. Glucose should be given as soon as possible followed by a meal that includes both protein and carbohydrates. The blood glucose level should then be reassessed.

*Rationale*
Hypoglycemia is caused by low blood sugar. Symptoms include occipital headaches; cold, clammy skin; dizziness; tachycardia; tingling in the extremities; and shaky and blurred vision. To prevent hyperglycemia, the client must maintain a balance between insulin and glucose intake. This includes careful monitoring of blood glucose levels, which includes increased glucose in this scenario.

*Classification*
Competency Category: Nursing Practice: Alterations in Health
Taxonomic Level: Application

**391. Answer:** Central line catheters are more effective for delivery of medication and solutions that are irritating to the veins and are effective for long-term IV therapy.

*Rationale*
Central line catheters result in fewer interstitial IV sites, less irritation to veins, and longer and more permanent IV sites.

*Classification*
Competency Category: Nursing Practice: Alterations in Health
Taxonomic Level: Knowledge/Comprehension

**392. Answers:**

**Bacterial:** Diphtheria, *Mycoplasma pneumonia*, pertussis, pneumonic plague, streptococcus.
**Viral:** Adenovirus, influenza, mumps, parvovirus B19, rubella.

*Rationale*
Different viruses have different modes of transmission. For prevention control, it is important to know the modes of transmission of each virus.

*Classification*
Competency Category: Nursing Practice: Alterations in Health
Taxonomic Level: Knowledge/Comprehension

**393.  Answers:** All of the following are examples of universal precautions:

- Wearing a gown, gloves, and mask when providing patient care.
- Wearing goggles if there is any risk of splashing of patient's body fluids during care (for example, in suctioning).
- Private rooms for patients, with equipment that is not used by other patients.
- Separate handling and disposal of garbage and linens.

*Rationale*
All of these factors protect both the nurse and the patient from exposer to bacteria.

*Classification*
Competency Category: Nursing Practice: Alterations in Health
Taxonomic Level: Application

**394.  Answer:** Policy requires that hand washing occurs both before and after applying gloves to prevent the spread of viruses.

*Rationale*
Because hospital organisms colonizing on health care workers' hands can proliferate in the warm, moist environment provided by gloves, the hands must be thoroughly washed after gloves are removed. Also, reactions to latex may warrant hand washing after gloves are removed.

*Classification*
Competency Category: Nursing Practice: Alterations in Health
Taxonomic Level: Critical Thinking

**395.  Answers:**

- Men: 12–70 U/mL or 55–170 U/L (SI units).
- Women: 10–55 U/mL or 30–135 U/L (SI units).

*Rationale*
Men and women have different CK levels. This is important for nurses to be aware of to ensure that they correctly interpret laboratory value results.

*Classification*
Competency Category: Nursing Practice: Alterations in Health
Taxonomic Level: Knowledge/Comprehension

**396.  Answer:** 6 hours.

*Rationale*
CK levels may increase within 6 hours after damage to these cells. If damage is not persistent, the levels peak at 18 hours after injury and return to normal within 2 to 3 days.

*Classification*
Competency Category: Nursing Practice: Alterations in Health
Taxonomic Level: Knowledge/Comprehension

**397.  Answers:**

- Active bleeding.
- Known bleeding disorder.
- History of hemorrhagic stroke.
- History of intracranial vessel malformation.
- Recent major surgery or trauma.
- Uncontrolled hypertension.
- Pregnancy.

*Rationale*
Thrombolytic therapy is contraindicated in any situation associated with a higher risk of bleeding, as in the situations above.

*Classification*
Competency Category: Nursing Practice: Alterations in Health
Taxonomic Level: Knowledge/Comprehension

**398. Answers:**

- Prolonged diuretic therapy.
- Excessive diaphoresis.
- Insufficient sodium intake.
- Excess water intake.

*Rationale*
These are key causes of hyponatremia.

*Classification*
Competency Category: Nursing Practice: Alterations in Health
Taxonomic Level: Knowledge/Comprehension

**399. Answers:** Dopamine, dobutamine, epinephrine, milrinone, nitroprusside, nitroglycerine, phenylephrine, and methoxamine.

*Rationale*
These are all common vasoactive medication used to treat patients in shock.

*Classification*
Competency Category: Nursing Practice: Alterations in Health
Taxonomic Level: Knowledge/Comprehension

**400. Answers:**

- Low arterial pH.
- Elevated serum $CO_2$ levels.

*Rationale*
With respiratory acidosis, the patient cannot exhale $CO_2$ effectively, resulting in a high $CO_2$ level and a low $O_2$ level. High $CO_2$ and water levels result in a low arterial pH level.

*Classification*
Competency Category: Nursing Practice: Alterations in Health
Taxonomic Level: Knowledge/Comprehension

**401. Answers:**

- Referral to a chronic illness clinic for follow up.
- Need for adequate nutrition, hydration, and moderate exercise.
- Need to take medications as prescribed.
- Need to have the family and patient clearly informed as to the chronic illness and strategies to support wellness.
- Regular flu immunizations.

*Rationale*
Health promotion strategies for assisting clients diagnosed with chronic illnesses include health teaching, acknowledging strengths and abilities, facilitating access to community resources, involving the patient and family in care plan development and implementation, and referring to support group with others experiencing the same condition.

*Classification*
Competency Category: Nursing Practice: Health and Wellness
Taxonomic Level: Knowledge/Comprehension

**402. Answers:** Expresses grief; uses family and friends to work through feelings and issues.

*Rationale*
Grieving is a process that is experienced differently by different people. However, to successfully grieve, it is important for individuals to express and feel their feelings with people who care and support them.

*Classification*
Competency Category: Nursing Practice: Alterations in Health
Taxonomic Level: Knowledge/Comprehension

## ▶ Self-Analysis for Chapter 4

354 Multiple-choice questions × 1 point each = /354 points

\+

48 Short answer questions for a total of 94 points = /94 points

***Total Care of Adults and Older Adults
review questions = 448 points***

## SUPPLEMENTAL RESOURCES

Adams, M., Josephson, D., & Leland, N. (2004). *Pharmacology for nurses: A pathophysiologic approach*. Upper Saddle River, NJ: Pearson Prentice Hall.

Arnold, E., & Boggs, K. (2003). *Interpersonal relationships: Professional communication for nurses* (4th ed.). St. Louis: W.B. Saunders.

Berman, A., Snyder, S., Kozier, B., & Erb, G. (2008). *Kozier and erb fundamentals of nursing* (8th ed.). Upper Saddle River, NJ: Pearson Prentice Hall.

Bickley, L., Hoekelman, R., & Bates, B. (2003). *Bates guide to physical examination and history taking* (8th ed.). Philadelphia: Lippincott Williams & Wilkins.

Canadian Nurses Association. (2005). *The canadian registered nurse examination prep guide*. (4th ed.). Ottawa, ON: Author.

D'Amico, D., & Barbarito, C. (2007) *Health & physical assessment in nursing*. Upper Saddle River, NJ: Pearson Education Health Assessment.

Deglin, J., & Vallerand, A. (2005). *Davis's drug guide for nurses* (9th ed.). Philadelphia: F.A. Davis.

Fischbach, F. (2004). *A manual of lab and diagnostic tests* (7th ed.). Philadelphia: Lippincott Williams & Wilkins.

Hannah, K., Ball, M., & Edwards, M. (2006). *Introduction to nursing informatics* (3rd ed.). New York: Springer.

Hickman, J.S. (2006). *Faith community nursing*. Philadelphia: Lippincott Williams & Wilkins.

Jarvis, C. (2004). *Physical examination and health assessment* (4th ed.). St. Louis: W.B. Saunders.

Lagerquist, S. (ed.) (1996). *Little, Brown's NCLEX-RN exam review*. New York: Addison Wesley Nursing.

LaPorte Matzo, M., Witt Sherman, D., & Matzo, M. (2006). *Palliative care nursing: Quality care to the end of life* (2nd ed.). New York: Springer.

Lewis, S., Heitkemper, M., Dirksen, & O'Brien, P. (2006). *Medical-surgical nursing in Canada*. Toronto, ON: Elsevier Canada.

Lipe, S., & Beasley, S. (2004). *Critical thinking in nursing*. Philadelphia: Lippincott Williams & Wilkins.

Luggen, A., Travis, S., & Meiner, S. (2006). *NGNA core curriculum for gerontological advanced practice nurses*. Thousand Oaks, CA: Sage Publications.

Murray, R., Zentner, J., Pangman, V., & Pangman, C. (2006). *Health promotion strategies through the lifespan* (Canadian edition). Toronto: Pearson Prentice Hall.

Porth, C. (2005). *Pathophysiology: Concepts of altered health states* (7th ed.). Philadelphia: Lippincott Williams & Wilkins.

Robinson-Vollman, A., & Potter, P. (2006 ). In J. Ross-Kerr & M. J. Wood (eds.). *Canadian fundamentals of nursing* (3rd ed.). Toronto, ON: Elsevier Canada.

Ross-Kerr, J., & Wood, M. (2006). *Canadian fundamentals of nursing* (3rd ed.). Toronto: Elsevier.

*Skin and wound care manual, Calgary Health Region*. (2004). Skin Integrity. Calgary, Alberta Canada: Calgary Health Region.

Smeltzer, S., & Bare, B. (2004). *Brunner & Suddarth textbook of medical surgical nursing* (10th ed.). Philadelphia: Lippincott Williams & Wilkins.

Smith, S., Duell, D., & Martin, B. (2008). *Clinical nursing skills: Basics to advanced skills*. Upper Saddle River, NJ: Pearson Prentice Hall.

Stanhope, M., & Lancaster, J. (2004). *Community and public health nursing* (6th ed.). St. Louis: Mosby.

Swearinger, P. (2003). *Manual of medical surgical nursing care*. St. Louis: Elsevier.

Taylor, C., Lillis, C., & LeMone, P. (2005). *Fundamentals of nursing: The art and science of nursing care* (5th ed.). Philadelphia: Lippincott Williams & Wilkins.

Thompson, J., & Manore, M. (2005). *Nutrition: An applied approach*. Boston: Pearson Benjamin Cummings.

Vanetzian, E. (2001). *Critical thinking: An interactive tool for learning medical surgical nursing*. Philadelphia: F.A. Davis.

Veenema, T.G. (2003). *Disaster nursing and emergency preparedness for chemical, biological, and radiological terrorism*. New York: Springer.

Wagner, K., Johnson, K., & Kidd, P. (2006). *High acuity nursing* (4th ed.). Upper Saddle River, NJ: Prentice Hall.

Weinstein (2007). *Plumer's principles and practice of I.V. therapy* (8th ed.). Philadelphia: Lippincott Williams & Wilkins.

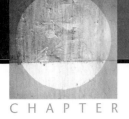

# 5    Child Health Nursing

**Directions:** Below are 200 multiple-choice questions and short answer questions totaling 250 points. These questions will test your knowledge of nursing with a child health population. These questions offer a wide array of case-based and stand-alone questions representing the taxonomies of critical thinking, application, and knowledge/comprehension. Also reflected in these questions are the nursing competencies of health and wellness, alterations in health, professional practice, and nurse–person relationship. After completing these practice questions, check your work in the Answers and Rationales section located at the end of the chapter. Please note the topic areas and types of questions you found difficult and develop a plan to review study sources and increase your knowledge of these areas.

## ▶ Multiple-Choice Questions

1. A 10-month-old child has presented in the emergency department with respiratory compromise. Specific to the pediatric population, which of the following indicates respiratory compromise?

   A. Nasal flaring.
   B. Cyanosis.
   C. Dyspnea.
   D. Tachypnea.

---

*Case Study: An 8-year-old child has a long-standing diagnosis of bronchial asthma. The child presents with an audible expiratory wheeze and intercostal retractions and is quite anxious. The child's parents are in attendance. This is the second visit to the emergency department (ED) this month for these symptoms. Both parents are smokers. Questions 2 to 6 relate to this scenario.*

2. The child's parents require health teaching to address their concern that their child has had two visits to the ED in the past month. The nurse should explain which of the following?

   A. Their environment has little impact on their asthma.
   B. Pediatric patients outgrow asthma.
   C. Pediatric patients readily tolerate asthmatic episodes.
   D. The etiology is often allergens and infection.

3. The child's mother reports that the child experiences symptoms daily and has nighttime symptoms more than once a week. This child's asthma would be classified as which of the following?

   A. Severe persistent asthma.
   B. Moderate persistent asthma.
   C. Moderate intermittent asthma.
   D. Mild intermittent asthma.

4. Which of the following would be a notable characteristic of mucus when this child is having an acute asthma attack?

   A. Coloured.
   B. Copious.
   C. Tenaciousness.
   D. Absent.

5. The nurse would expect this child with full exacerbation of asthmatic symptoms, including $CO_2$ retention, to have which of the following conditions?

   A. Respiratory acidosis.
   B. Respiratory alkalosis.
   C. Metabolic acidosis.
   D. Metabolic alkalosis.

6. From the list below, identify the medication most often prescribed for long-term asthma control.

   A. Oral systemic corticosteroids.
   B. Leukotriene modifiers.
   C. Anticholinergic agents.
   D. Short-acting β-adrenergic agonists.

7. A 12-year-old child is brought to the emergency department and is diagnosed with status asthmaticus. His respiratory rate is 40 breaths/min, and he has decreased breath sounds bilaterally throughout his lung field. After receiving an aerosol bronchodilator, the child sounds worse—his breath sounds are now louder. The nurse knows that this indicates which of the following?

   A. The child's condition is improving.
   B. The child's condition is deteriorating.
   C. The child is about to go into respiratory arrest.
   D. The child does not have asthma.

8. A 3-year-old is brought to the emergency department with an abrupt onset of respiratory illness. The child has a protruding tongue, is making froglike croaking sounds on inspiration, and is having suprasternal and substernal retractions. The child is diagnosed with epiglottitis. Which of the following are clinical observations of epiglottitis?

   A. Absence of spontaneous cough, adventitious breath sounds, and agitation.
   B. Absence of spontaneous cough, rubbing the ear, and agitation.
   C. Spontaneous cough, stridor, and congestion of the lung field.
   D. Absence of spontaneous cough and presence of drooling and agitation.

9. The nurse is caring for a 4-year-old child who has been admitted to hospital with pertussis. It is day 3 of the child's hospitalization. The nurse knows that the child will be placed under:

   A. Contact precautions.
   B. Airborne precautions.
   C. Droplet precautions.
   D. No precautions.

10. A nurse is conducting a respiratory assessment on a 3-year-old patient who is not showing any signs of distress. She would expect to find a respiratory rate of:

    A. 12–20 breaths/min.
    B. 11–22 breaths/min.
    C. 20–33 breaths/min.
    D. 30–60 breaths/min.

11. A 12-year-old child with cystic fibrosis is admitted to the floor with increased respiratory compromise secondary to an upper respiratory tract infection. Identify the immediate priority nursing diagnosis.

    A. Risk for infection related to bacterial growth and impaired body defenses.
    B. Ineffective airway clearance related to thick, tenacious mucus production.
    C. Risk for imbalanced nutrition (less than body requirements) related to impaired absorption of nutrients.
    D. Compromised family coping related to the child's chronic illness.

12. Which of the following describes the etiology of cystic fibrosis?

    A. It is inherited as an autosomal dominant trait.
    B. It is inherited as an autosomal recessive trait.
    C. Its inheritance is affected by the newborn's gestational age.
    D. Its inheritance is affected by the child's gender.

13. Cystic fibrosis is a generalized dysfunction of the:

    A. Endocrine glands.
    B. Pituitary gland.
    C. Exocrine glands.
    D. Adrenal glands.

14. Which of the following is a classic clinical manifestation of cystic fibrosis?

    A. Steatorrhea.
    B. Hyponatremia.
    C. Urinary tract infections.
    D. Integumentary compromise.

15. Identify the health teaching a nurse would include for a parent whose 4-month-old child has been newly diagnosed with cystic fibrosis (CF).

    A. It is okay to only breastfeed your child for nutrition.
    B. Your child will probably have a poor appetite at feeding times.
    C. Your child will need to take a pancreatic enzyme before every meal.
    D. You will not have to modify your home environment for your child.

16. A 16-year-old male patient presents with extreme lethargy, retractions of the intercostal spaces, a persistent expiratory wheeze, diminished breath sounds, and signs of tachycardia and tachypnea. Based on the

following arterial blood gas results: pH, 7.10:
$PCO_2$ 80; $PO_2$, 35, $HCO_3$, 29, this patient is in:

A. Respiratory acidosis.
B. Respiratory alkalosis.
C. Metabolic acidosis.
D. Metabolic alkalosis.

17. What significant assessment finding would a
    nurse anticipate when caring for an adolescent
    with a spontaneous pneumothorax?

    A. Asymmetrical chest movement.
    B. Hemoptysis.
    C. Tachycardia.
    D. Respiratory arrest.

18. An RN is caring for a pediatric oncology patient.
    The child's parents have expressed concern that
    they will develop the same type of cancer. In
    preparation for health teaching, the nurse
    should be aware that the biggest difference in
    pediatric cancers compared with adult cancers is
    that they:

    A. Are diagnosed during dormant growth
       periods.
    B. Usually involve epithelial tissue.
    C. Have a short latency period.
    D. Are usually slow growing.

19. A nurse is providing health teaching to the
    parents of a 4-year-old child who has been diag-
    nosed with benign febrile seizures. The nurse
    should explain to the parents that:

    A. Their child will become developmentally
       delayed.
    B. This diagnosis will progress to one of
       epilepsy.
    C. The seizures will continue throughout the
       child's life.
    D. An acute respiratory or ear infection is
       usually present.

_____

**Case Study:** *A nurse is assessing a 17-year-old adolescent with a previous head injury. The parents
inform the nurse of drastic personality changes with
aggressive behaviour since the injury. Questions 20
and 21 relate to this scenario.*

20. Based on the parents' report of drastic personal-
    ity changes, the nurse can determine that the
    injury was in which lobe of the brain?

    A. Frontal.
    B. Occipital.
    C. Temporal.
    D. Parietal.

21. On further assessment of this teen 1 hour later,
    the nurse identifies apnea, bradycardia, and a
    widening pulse pressure. What is occurring at
    this time?

    A. The teen's condition is stabilizing.
    B. The intracranial pressure is increasing.
    C. The teen likely has a bladder infection.
    D. The teen has received too much pain
       medication.

22. A 12-year-old girl is admitted to the floor after
    falling off her bike and striking her head on the
    pavement. She was not wearing a helmet and
    sustained loss of consciousness for 2 minutes.
    What is the priority nursing assessment for the
    client with a head injury?

    A. Papillary changes.
    B. Alterations in vital signs.
    C. Orientation to person, time, and place.
    D. Headache and vomiting.

23. A 14-year-old boy jumps off a school building,
    landing on his feet before falling to the ground.
    He has temporary paralysis and no visible
    damage to the spinal cord. The nurse identifies
    the following mechanism of injury responsible
    for this spinal cord injury.

    A. Hyperextension.
    B. Compression.
    C. Overrotation.
    D. Axial loading.

24. You are the RN caring for an infant who had a
    head injury 24 hours ago. The injury was
    sustained after a fall from an upper floor
    window onto a patio. The child is NPO and
    receiving IV fluid administration. What type of
    IV solution would contribute to the
    deterioration of a child with increased intracra-
    nial pressure?

    A. Total parental nutrition.
    B. Isotonic solution.
    C. Hypertonic solution.
    D. Hypotonic solution.

25. A 16-year-old teen has had a basal skull fracture
    in a motor vehicle accident. The teen has increas-
    ing drowsiness and is febrile. What is the teen
    most at risk for developing?

    A. Meningitis.
    B. Pneumonia.
    C. Renal failure.
    D. Paralytic ileus.

26. A 12-year-old child has pain, numbness, and tin-
    gling of his feet and lower legs. A diagnosis of

Guillain-Barré syndrome is made. With this diagnosis, what is the patient now predisposed to?

A. Orthostatic hypotension.
B. Descending paralysis and ascending resolution.
C. Gradual onset of autoimmune response.
D. Asymmetric paralysis.

27. What cranial nerve is being assessed when the nurse asks the child to repeat a whispered word?

A. I.
B. IV.
C. VIII.
D. X.

28. Of the following, which is the least likely cause of a neural tube defect?

A. Maternal exposure to virus or bacteria.
B. Predisposed genetic influence.
C. Exposure to radiation during the third trimester.
D. Deficiency of folic acid during the first 6 weeks of pregnancy.

29. Congenital hydrocephalus is:

A. The absence of functional brain activity.
B. An abnormal accumulation of cerebrospinal fluid (CSF) within the cranial vault.
C. A defect in the closure of the vertebral column.
D. Spinal cord and nerves protruding through the vertebrae.

*Case Study:* A 12-year-old girl patient is brought to the emergency department (ED) complaining of severe right lower quadrant pain. Her pulse and respirations are elevated, and she has localized tenderness and sluggish bowel sounds. Questions 30 to 32 relate to this scenario.

30. After being attended to in the ED, the child states that the pain has suddenly resolved and she feels better. Which of the following would the nurse suspect?

A. A ruptured appendix.
B. Gastroenteritis.
C. Celiac disease.
D. Food allergies.

31. What would be the priority treatment at this point?

A. Preparation for emergency surgery.
B. Initiation of antibiotic therapy.
C. Referral for dietary revision.
D. Modification of pain management strategies.

32. The child has been prescribed a 3-day course of treatment of gentamicin sulfate while recuperating. Which of the following manifestations would indicate that the child is developing gentamicin toxicity?

A. Electrolyte disturbances.
B. Decreased renal output.
C. Joint discomfort.
D. Visual disturbances.

*Case Study:* You are caring for a 9-month-old child with severe diarrhea that has lasted 3 days. The child has poor skin turgor and dry mucous membranes. Questions 33 to 35 relate to this scenario.

33. Poor skin turgor and dry mucous membranes suggest which of the following?

A. Anemia.
B. Jaundice.
C. Dehydration.
D. Hyponatremia.

34. Identify the priority nursing diagnosis for this child.

A. Risk for impaired skin integrity.
B. Fluid volume deficit.
C. Risk for impaired parenting.
D. Risk for infection.

35. After initial rehydration therapy, which of the following is the expected therapeutic management for this child?

A. Water, breast milk, and lactose-free formula.
B. Fruit juices, carbonated soft drinks, and gelatin.
C. Chicken or beef broth.
D. BRAT diet.

*Case Study:* A 5-year-old child had a hernia repair yesterday. The child is vomiting, has a nasogastric (NG) tube to low Gomco intermittent suction, and has diarrhea. Questions 36 and 37 relate to this scenario.

36. Based on this information, which of the following is the child likely to experience?

A. Hypokalemia.
B. Hyperkalemia.
C. Hypernatremia.
D. Hypocalcemia.

37. The NG tube is removed, but the child starts vomiting again and is still not feeding well. To provide nutrition, another NG tube is reinserted

as ordered by the physician. Its position has been verified by radiography. Identify the priority nursing action before starting NG feeds on this child.

A. Check the physician's order.
B. Check the NG tube for placement.
C. Aspirate the stomach contents.
D. Start infusion of the nutrition source.

38. What is the most common cause of an electrolyte imbalance in a child who is vomiting and being cared for at home?

A. Withholding food in a child who has vomited.
B. Feeding the child after each episode of vomiting.
C. Withholding fluid for several hours after the child has vomited.
D. Using herbal remedies in a child who has vomited.

39. The mother of an infant is concerned that her child may have diarrhea. The nurse explains that one of the signs of diarrhea includes:

A. Passing one to three stools a day.
B. Passing stool that is yellow in color.
C. Little effort required moving the bowels.
D. Odorless stool.

40. A nurse is providing an inservice to unregulated assistive personnel participating in the care of pediatric patients who have gastroesophageal reflux. The nurse realizes that these personnel need to review prior teaching when one them states:

A. "I usually lay the child flat after feeding."
B. "I feed the child thickened foods."
C. "I place the child in an upright position during feeding."
D. "I don't rush the child while feeding him or her."

41. A nurse is providing an inservice to the community focusing on preventing the incidence of hepatitis in children. Which type of hepatitis could a child contract from a contaminated diaper changing table?

A. Hepatitis D.
B. Hepatitis B.
C. Hepatitis C.
D. Hepatitis A.

42. A 16-year-old adolescent has right upper quadrant pain, brown urine, jaundiced sclerae, and pruritus. What type of hepatitis is this adolescent likely to be diagnosed with?

A. Hepatitis A.
B. Hepatitis B.

C. Hepatitis C.
D. Hepatitis D.

43. When educating adolescents about hepatitis, which of the following would be significant?

A. Hepatitis immunization is not necessary in this age group.
B. Intravenous drug users are at low risk for transmission.
C. Hepatitis B is a sexually transmitted disease.
D. Hepatitis is curable with medical management.

44. Identify the developmental group most at risk for accidental injuries in the listed pediatric populations.

A. Infants.
B. Toddlers.
C. School-aged children.
D. Newborns.

45. A nurse is assessing the family of a 1-month-old infant and observes that the parents are argumentative and appear fatigued. They indicate that the baby is not breastfeeding well and cries through the night. What would be the nurse's priority nursing diagnosis for this infant?

A. Altered nutrition (less than body requirements) related to difficulty sucking.
B. Parental sleep pattern disturbance related to the baby's feeding schedule.
C. Knowledge deficit related to normal infant growth and development.
D. Altered role performance related to new responsibilities within the family.

46. During the initial shift assessment on a 2-year-old child diagnosed with otitis media, the nurse finds the child restless, diaphoretic, and hot to the touch. The priority action is to check the child's core body temperature. What is the best route to assess core body temperature in this child?

A. Rectal route.
B. Axillary route.
C. Oral route.
D. Tympanic route.

47. A 12-year-old patient is scheduled for surgery in 1 hour to repair a fracture. The child's preoperative vital signs show him to be febrile. What is the priority action at this time?

A. Inform the surgeon.
B. Record the temperature only.
C. Administer oral antipyretics.
D. Place cool compresses on the child.

48. The nurse is assessing a fresh postoperative 7-year-old boy for pain and finds him playing in bed with his toys. The nurse should understand which of the following?

    A. Nurses can accurately estimate children's pain from their physical appearance or activity.
    B. A child who resumes his or her usual play activity is not experiencing pain.
    C. Some children distract themselves with play while in pain.
    D. Narcotic analgesics are too dangerous for young children.

49. An 8-year-old girl is complaining of stomach pains and headache and is not sleeping well. She has also started bedwetting again. In the pediatric population, what are these often signs of?

    A. Food allergies.
    B. Stress and anxiety.
    C. Attention seeking.
    D. Dislike of school.

50. The nurse is aware that toddlers are prone to temper tantrums, partly because of their inability to express themselves verbally. From the following, what is the most realistic approach in dealing with a hospitalized child's temper tantrum?

    A. Offer material or emotional bribes.
    B. Offer disapproval and then ignore the tantrum.
    C. Punish the child after the tantrum.
    D. Get angry at the child during the tantrum.

51. A nurse is caring for a 4-year-old child on complete bed rest. What would be a priority nursing diagnosis when caring for this child?

    A. Diversionary activity deficit related to lack of appropriate toys and peers.
    B. Sleep pattern disturbance related to routines of hospitalization.
    C. Risk of altered nutrition (less than body requirements) related to lack of appetite.
    D. Risk of altered growth and development related to the effects of illness.

52. A common character trait of adolescents involves feeling that their experiences and feelings are unique and that no one has ever felt as they do. What is this called?

    A. Invulnerability.
    B. Egocentrism.
    C. Imaginary audience.
    D. Personal fable.

53. The parents of a pregnant adolescent are outraged that they are being refused medical information about their daughter's condition. What is the best response by the RN to address their anger?

    A. "Your daughter's medical information is considered confidential, and you aren't entitled to it just because you are her parents."
    B. "I'm not supposed to tell you, but she's pregnant and will need your support."
    C. "I can appreciate your concerns. If we obtain permission from your daughter, we can include you in our discussions."
    D. "Your daughter will now have to be responsible for her own health."

54. Improvements in prenatal care, diagnostic testing, and treatment modalities have decreased infant mortality rates. Which of the following statement remains true?

    A. Congenital anomalies continue to be a leading cause of infant mortality.
    B. There is a no definitive relationship between birth weight and mortality.
    C. Although children and infants are smaller in size than adults, they are the same physiologically.
    D. Death rates for infants are not significant compared with rates in the general population.

55. A nurse is conducting a cardiac assessment for a 3-year-old patient who is not showing any signs of cardiac compromise. She would expect to find a normal heart rate range of:

    A. 60–100 bpm.
    B. 70–110 bpm.
    C. 80–130 bpm.
    D. 100–170 bpm.

56. A nurse is continuing the cardiac assessment on the 3-year-old child who is not showing any signs of cardiac compromise and is auscultating the child's chest. Which of the following heart sounds is abnormal in children?

    A. S1.
    B. S2.
    C. S3.
    D. S4.

57. Which of the following is an indicator of early compensation in a child with cardiac compromise?

    A. Hypotension.
    B. Bradycardia.
    C. Tachycardia.
    D. Severe metabolic acidosis.

**58.** A 4-year-old patient has been identified as having a cardiac arrhythmia. The nurse assesses the child and finds her febrile, in pain, and anxious with an elevated WBC. What arrhythmia is most associated with these clinical manifestations?

A. Bradycardia.
B. Tachycardia.
C. Atrial flutter.
D. Heart block.

**59.** When beginning a shift on a pediatric unit, which of the following is the priority nursing action after receiving shift report on your patients?

A. Confirm correct IV fluids and rates.
B. Review medical orders.
C. Review patient history.
D. Confirm that allergy bands are on patients who need them.

*Case Study:* *You are caring for a 5-year-old girl who has a history of multiple admissions for fractures and cuts. The mother explains that the child fractured her femur by falling but does not give any further details. The child indicates that the mother's boyfriend was with her when the injury occurred, and her recollection of the event conflicts with her mother's explanation. Questions 60 to 61 relate to this scenario.*

**60.** The nurse's immediate responsibility is to:

A. Collect forensic specimens for laboratory analysis.
B. Keep the child safe and assess for abuse.
C. Call the police department and report abuse.
D. Restrict family who are visiting the child.

**61.** The nurse is aware that an adult who sexually or physically abuses a child:

A. Is most likely a stranger to the child.
B. Is most likely known to the child.
C. Is doing so with the knowledge of the parents.
D. Was not abused him- or herself as a child.

**62.** A 6-year-old child has been newly diagnosed with a peanut allergy. What is potentially the biggest threat to this child's health?

A. Anaphylaxis.
B. Hives.
C. Pruritus.
D. Urticaria.

**63.** A child is born with spina bifida (myelomeningocele). The nurse is aware that this child is most at risk for what kind of allergy?

A. Pet allergies.
B. Food allergy.

C. Environmental allergy.
D. Latex allergy.

**64.** A physician has ordered a referral for skin testing on a child suspected of having allergies. The nurse is aware that all of the following are true of skin testing *except*:

A. It is done to isolate an allergen to which the child is sensitive.
B. Systemic antihistamines are given before testing.
C. A wheal will appear at the site of the test for a positive reaction.
D. The test is read within 20 minutes of administration.

**65.** A nurse is providing health teaching to the mother of a child recently diagnosed with allergies. It is clear that more teaching sessions are required when the mother states:

A. "I gave my children allergies when I breastfed them."
B. "We need to plan family vacations when the pollen count is low."
C. "My husband will have to smoke in the garage now."
D. "I won't be able to wear perfume anymore."

**66.** A 7-year-old child has gastrointestinal symptoms, urticaria, and atopic dermatitis. The symptoms appeared 2 hours after the child ate dinner. The nurse suspects which of the following allergies?

A. Environmental allergy.
B. Pet allergies.
C. Food allergy.
D. Drug allergy.

**67.** You have just admitted a 10-year-old child with a spinal cord injury and facial lacerations. The child was sitting in the front passenger seat of a car that was rear ended by another vehicle. The driver of the car had three drinks in 5 hours before the accident. There were four other passengers in the car. Identify the most significant factor that contributed to the child's injuries.

A. Being rear ended by another vehicle.
B. Multiple passengers.
C. Sitting in the front seat.
D. The driver's alcohol consumption.

**68.** A 7-year-old patient has a penicillin allergy. The nurse is aware that all of the following are true of penicillin allergies *except*:

A. Urticaria occurs 1 to 72 hours after initiation of the drug.

B. Urticaria resolves within 1 to 2 days after discontinuation of the drug.

C. It is related to known pharmacologic actions of the drug.

D. It is safe to give cephalosporins to this child.

69. A child who fell though ice and was submerged for longer than 1 minute is admitted to the emergency department diagnosed with hypothermia near drowning. At which point will you best be able to determine the child's outcome?

A. Three days after the incident.

B. As soon as CPR is successfully initiated.

C. As soon as the patient is warmed.

D. After the parents' initially visit.

70. Which of the following would be the appropriate choice for a pediatric patient requiring an isotonic IV solution?

A. Lactated Ringer's solution.

B. D5W/lactated Ringer's solution.

C. D5W/0.45% NaCl.

D. 0.33% NaCl.

71. A nurse is aware that the normal serum osmolarity of an isotonic solution is within which of the following ranges?

A. 130–150 mmol/L.

B. 150–240 mmol/L.

C. 240–340 mmol/L.

D. 340–380 mmol/L.

72. A 13-year-old young woman has been admitted to your floor with bradycardia. She has a history of eating binges and then purging. She also exercises 3 hours each day. Her resting heart rate is currently 50 bpm. When planning care for this patient, the priority focus should be:

A. Anorexia nervosa.

B. A healthy weight.

C. Athletic training.

D. Bulimia.

73. The period in which physical changes relating to sexual maturation take place is called:

A. Identity diffusion.

B. Adolescent turmoil.

C. Pubescence.

D. The maturational stage.

74. A 17-year-old young man is admitted to your floor for a second course of treatment for acute lymphoblastic leukemia. He was scheduled to travel with the school basketball team this weekend and is extremely angry and withdrawn. The nurse realizes that this

adolescent's anger has most likely arisen from which of the following?

A. Impact on social interactions.

B. Conflict with parents.

C. Fears.

D. Material things.

---

*Case Study:* A 15-year-old young man, John, is brought to the emergency department in a coma. He is well known to the hospital for multiple prior admissions of uncontrolled type 1 diabetes. He currently has 500 cc/hr urine output, blood pressure of 82/66 mm Hg, and a pulse of 135 bpm and has been diagnosed with diabetic ketoacidosis. Questions 75 and 76 relate to this scenario.

75. Based on the information above, what is the patient most at risk for?

A. Hypocalcemia.

B. Hypernatremia.

C. Metabolic alkalosis.

D. Shock from dehydration.

76. John has stabilized and has been put on a pediatric medical unit. Which of the following should be the priority focus for the nurse when preparing health teaching for John?

A. Relocating closer to the hospital.

B. Coping with a chronic disease.

C. Risk for injury and readmission.

D. Management of the therapeutic regimen.

77. A nurse is caring for a 14-year-old young man with type 1 diabetes. The health teaching has focused on reviewing the signs and symptoms of hypoglycemia. The nurse determines that the adolescent needs further teaching when he says:

A. "If my blood sugar is low, I will be able to deal with it."

B. "If my blood sugar is low, I will feel sweaty and anxious."

C. "If my blood sugar is low, my heart rate will speed up."

D. "If my blood sugar is low, my blood pressure will increase."

78. Which of the following would be the priority focus for health teaching by the nurse for a child recently diagnosed with type 1 diabetes and her family?

A. The signs and symptoms of hyperglycemia.

B. The importance of rotating insulin injection sites.

C. The signs and symptoms of hypoglycemia.

D. The importance of balanced nutrition.

79. Which of the following would a nurse emphasize to Rachelle during the initial health teaching?

    A. Activity levels rarely determine insulin requirements.
    B. Meal sizes are not usually considered when determining insulin needs.
    C. The need for insulin always decreases when strenuous sports are played.
    D. Insulin is always administered subcutaneously.

80. Despite continuous health teaching, Rachelle will only use her left thigh for insulin administration. The nurse is aware this is happening because:

    A. The child is exerting control over the situation.
    B. This an adolescent attention-seeking behaviour.
    C. Repeatedly using the same site is less painful.
    D. The child is afraid of scarring and bruising.

81. A 10-year-old child diagnosed with type 1 diabetes has the following order: "Regular insulin 8 U ordered 15 to 30 minutes ac and hs." After verifying the insulin order, what is the next step the RN should take?

    A. Draw up the insulin.
    B. Have the insulin cosigned.
    C. Administer the insulin.
    D. Check the blood glucose level.

82. From the following, what type of insulin is being prescribed?

    Onset: Reaches the blood within 30 minutes after injection
    Peak time: 2 to 4 hours later
    Duration: 4 to 8 hours

    A. Rapid-acting insulin.
    B. Short-acting insulin.
    C. Intermediate-acting insulin.
    D. Long-acting insulin.

83. What must the RN consider when teaching a family how to administer insulin to a newly diagnosed child?

    A. Keeping track of the rotation schedule for sites used.
    B. The insulin absorption rate varies in different parts of the body.

C. Some insulin injection sites are easier to access than others.
D. The importance of maintaining the schedule at school.

84. Which of the following statements is true when administering medication to pediatric patients?

    A. There are no choice restrictions with drug selection.
    B. There are no concerns when using the oral route.
    C. Age, weight, and growth and development should be considered.
    D. The deltoid muscle is the first site choice for intramuscular injections.

85. What is a pharmacokinetic consequence nurses must consider when administering medication to neonates and infants younger than age 1 year?

    A. Slowed excretion of drugs eliminated by the kidneys.
    B. Decreased absorption of topical drugs by neonates.
    C. Decreased distribution of drugs into the central nervous system.
    D. Protein-binding capacity in neonates is fully developed.

86. Which of the following clinical manifestations would the nurse anticipate in a 2-year-old patient with a *Clostridium difficile* infection?

    A. Diarrhea.
    B. Vomiting.
    C. Headaches.
    D. Productive cough.

87. Which of the following would a nurse most likely chose as an IV site for an 11-month-old child?

    A. Antecubital.
    B. Forearm.
    C. Upper arm.
    D. Scalp.

88. A nurse is assessing a 4-year-old patient's peripheral IV line because it is not infusing. In this population, what is the most common cause of this?

    A. The IV bag is empty.
    B. The pump has not been turned on.
    C. The position of the child's extremity is incorrect.
    D. The height of the IV bag is incorrect.

89. A nurse is providing health teaching to the mother of a young child who requires oral medication administration after discharge. Which of

the following statements indicates to the nurse that the child's mother requires further teaching?

A. "I will store all the medications out of our children's reach."
B. "I will have the poison control center number close to the phone."
C. "I will get my child to take the medication by telling her it's candy."
D. "I will mix the medication with fruit puree to make it taste better."

90. Which of the following would be the least effective method of administering medication to a 4-year-old child?

A. Crushing medication and mixing it with food.
B. Play-acting to give a sick doll some medication.
C. Having the child's parents present in the room.
D. Providing detailed explanations of the procedure.

91. You are the RN caring for a 17-year-old oncology patient who is an intelligent and informed patient about his medical condition and treatment. He has refused his morning medications and says he intends to refuse all future medications. The nurse is aware that the patient is expressing which of the following ethical principles?

A. Beneficence.
B. Autonomy.
C. Veracity.
D. Nonmaleficence.

92. An RN has made a medication error. The patient is a 5-kg baby, and the order was for morphine 3 mg IV push. The nurse administered morphine 3 mg IV push at the prescribed time to the correct patient. Identify which of the following was incorrect and resulted in this medication error.

A. Right drug.
B. Right time.
C. Right dose.
D. Right patient.

---

*Case Study:* A 7-year-old boy is admitted to the unit with suspected spinal cord injury. He was riding with his father on an all-terrain vehicle when the accident occurred. A rigid cervical collar is in place. Questions 93 to 95 relate to this scenario.

93. What is the most probable reason for the injury?

A. Not wearing a seatbelt.
B. The father was driving too fast.
C. Bad weather conditions.
D. Not wearing a helmet.

94. When a child is involved in a motor vehicle accident, which of the following protective restraints, if worn, is most likely to prevent a spinal cord injury?

A. A helmet with face shield.
B. A lap seatbelt.
C. A lap and shoulder belt.
D. Forward-facing car seats.

95. The child is diagnosed with a spinal cord compression, and his condition has stabilized. Identify the most likely cause of secondary injury in this scenario.

A. Ischemia and edema.
B. Improper positioning.
C. Orthostatic hypotension.
D. Renal failure.

96. A nurse is working in a group home specifically developed for pediatric patients with cognitive impairment. On this particular shift, the nurse is feeling completely overwhelmed with the workload assignment. The personal support worker offers to help the nurse finish administering medications to the rest of the clients to help her catch up. From the following, which would be the correct option?

A. The personal support worker can safely administer medications to the clients.
B. The nurse can accept the offer and assist the personal support worker.
C. The nurse can delegate a nursing activity to anyone he or she determines to be appropriate.
D. The nurse is legally accountable for the medication administration.

97. A nurse is providing a community-based inservice to mothers related to preventing accidental injury in children. In comparison between Canada and the United States, what is the primary cause of accidental injuries among US children?

A. Improper use of firearms.
B. Scalding burns caused by hot bath water.
C. Poisoning from household cleansers.
D. Suffocation from plastic bags.

98. A public health nurse has been asked to provide an inservice to parents at a community health inservice regarding feeding and nutrition for toddlers. Which of the following would the nurse include in this inservice?

A. "Make dessert and give it to your child as a reward for good eating habits."
B. "The total amount eaten per meal is more important that the amount eaten each day."

C. "Toddlers often eat one food for days on end."

D. "Let children choose what to eat and when they want to eat it."

99. A nurse is aware that the ability to demonstrate empathy is key in pediatric nursing. Identify which of the following choices best describes empathy.

A. It is a quality of projecting sincerity.

B. It is best demonstrated with a gentle tone of voice.

C. It is the ability to put yourself in another person's place.

D. It is the distance at which you position yourself from others.

100. Which of the following is an effective therapeutic communication technique when working with pediatric clients?

A. Silence.

B. Using technical terminology.

C. Using clichés.

D. Negative feedback.

101. A nurse is caring for a 7-year-old hospitalized patient who is extremely angry and has been yelling at the nursing staff. Identify the best strategy in dealing with this child.

A. Thoroughly explain all details of care you will be providing.

B. Limit the number of trips into the child's room.

C. Mirror the child's behaviour back to the child.

D. Keep your tone gentler and quieter than the child's.

102. A 7-year-old boy states to his nurse, "I'm not worried about the needles I have to get. My friend at school gets needles all the time, and he's okay. If he's okay, then I'm going to be okay, right?" The nurse's response is, "You are saying you're not worried, but you look very nervous. Are you a little worried?" By responding in this manner, the nurse is using which of the following therapeutic communication techniques?

A. Clarifying.

B. Paraphrasing.

C. Perception checking.

D. Reflecting.

103. Identify the stage of development of a pediatric patient who would be frightened of intrusive

procedures such as assessing temperatures and blood pressures.

A. Toddler.

B. Preschool.

C. School age.

D. Adolescent.

104. Identify the stage of development of a pediatric patient who will learn a health procedure best if broken down into several brief stages.

A. Toddler.

B. Preschool.

C. School age.

D. Adolescent.

105. Identify the stage of development of a pediatric patient who has minimal regard for the long-term consequences of his or her actions when receiving health teaching.

A. Toddler.

B. Preschool.

C. School age.

D. Adolescent.

106. Identify the stage of development of a pediatric patient who is most receptive to the use of puppets and dolls for explanation of his or her illness or surgery.

A. Toddler.

B. Preschool.

C. School age.

D. Adolescent.

107. A 4-year-old boy is admitted for minor elective surgery and is frightened and anxious. Which of the following has the greatest influence on the child's reaction to the hospital experience?

A. The health teaching of the nurse.

B. Parental reinforcement.

C. Meeting the doctor.

D. The child's cognitive level.

108. What is the purpose of measuring head circumference in a child during the first 1 to 2 years of life?

A. To measure brain growth.

B. To measure nutritional status.

C. To measure bone fusion.

D. To measure bonnet size.

109. A nurse is assessing a 5-year-old child who is rubbing his eye and frequently blinking. The

eyelids and eyelashes indicate erythema. The nurse suspects which of the following?

A. Strabismus.
B. Conjunctivitis.
C. Esotropia.
D. Exotropia.

110. Which of the following could potentially be considered a normal finding in examining the eyes of a newborn?

A. Pale conjunctiva.
B. Congenital cataract.
C. Consensual constriction.
D. Subconjunctival hemorrhage.

111. Identify the correct position to examine the ear canal of an 18-month-old child.

A. Pulling the pinna up and back.
B. Pulling the pinna up and forward.
C. Pulling the pinna down and back.
D. Pulling the pinna down and forward.

112. The nurse is aware that the eliciting of the gag reflex is part of a mouth assessment. Which of the following conditions would contraindicate assessment of a gag reflex?

A. Croup.
B. Dental caries.
C. Epiglottitis.
D. Pneumonia.

113. When auscultating cardiac sounds of school-age children and adolescents, what is a common finding?

A. Sinus arrhythmia.
B. Ventricular tachycardia.
C. Asystole.
D. Atrial fibrillation.

114. What is the greatest challenge when conducting a cardiothoracic assessment on newborns, infants, and toddlers?

A. The child's crying.
B. The child's body size.
C. The child's cooperation.
D. The size of the equipment.

115. A nurse is aware that a 4-year-old child who has unintelligible speech is most likely to also have which of the following concerns?

A. Poor parental influence.
B. A nutritional deficit.
C. A hearing deficit.
D. Being an only child.

116. A 16-year-old young man is playing with friends at a construction site and steps on a rusty nail. The physician orders a tetanus shot. What type of immunity will be provided to this client who is receiving the tetanus shot?

A. Naturally acquired active immunity.
B. Artificially acquired active immunity.
C. Naturally acquired passive immunity.
D. Artificially acquired passive immunity.

117. Which of the following presents the greatest risk to newborn infants?

A. Fluid and electrolyte imbalances.
B. Age-specific disease.
C. Inability to monitor their own care.
D. Inability to communicate.

118. Identify the stage of development of a pediatric patient who is most likely to be affected by separation anxiety while hospitalized and separated from his or her primary caregiver.

A. Newborn.
B. Toddler.
C. School age.
D. Adolescent.

119. Which of the following is a realistic way to address issues of separation anxiety when working with pediatric clients?

A. Canceling diagnostic procedures.
B. Promoting open parental visiting.
C. Restricting visits from other family members.
D. Having all child care performed by nursing staff.

120. A 5-year-old hospitalized patient is admitted for observation after falling out of a second story window and is placed on strict head injury protocol with neural assessment every 2 hours for 48 hours. Initially, the child is quiet and playing quietly in bed. The next day, the child is anxious, crying, and irritable. Identify the priority nursing diagnoses for this situation from those listed below.

A. Disturbed sleep pattern.
B. Risk for imbalanced nutrition.
C. Interrupted family process.
D. Knowledge deficit.

121. Which of the following interventions would help minimize sleep deprivation in pediatric patients?

A. Encouraging naps during the day.
B. Giving the child a glass of water before bed.
C. Removing all toys from the bed.
D. Clustering patient care.

**Case Study:** *A 2-week-old infant has been presented to the physician's office with complaints from both parents related to difficulty feeding. The baby is currently experiencing tachycardia and tachypnea and was difficult to resuscitate at birth. The physician suspects a congenital heart defect. Questions 122 and 123 relate to this scenario.*

122. From the following list, what is the least likely cause of congenital heart defects in children?

    A. Intrauterine infection.
    B. Maternal nutrition.
    C. Maternal medication.
    D. Maternal alcohol consumption.

123. What priority health teaching should the nurse offer to the parents of this infant?

    A. It is dangerous to let your child cry.
    B. Frequent small feeds throughout the day are preferred.
    C. It is okay to roughhouse with your child.
    D. No precautions are required for future trips to the dentist.

124. Identify one characteristic you would expect to see in an older child diagnosed with a congenital heart defect.

    A. Capillary refill < 3 seconds.
    B. Pale colour of the extremities.
    C. Clubbing of fingers.
    D. Boundless energy.

125. Identify the ratio of ventilations to compressions used for resuscitating a 10-year-old child.

    A. 1:5.
    B. 2:10.
    C. 2:15.
    D. 2:20.

126. A nurse is providing health teaching to the parents of a 5-year-old child recently diagnosed with a congenital heart defect. The nurse reviews the concepts of cardiopulmonary arrest and resuscitation and actions required of the parents in case such an event occurs. The nurse recognizes that more health teaching is required when the child's father states:

    A. "The chance of my child arresting is unlikely."
    B. "I have to use compressions to circulate the blood."
    C. "I will give one breath for every five compressions."

    D. "As soon as my child responds, he can hear what's happening."

**Case Study:** *Jill, age 7 years, is brought to the emergency department by her parents. She has a variety of nonspecific symptoms, including lethargy, fatigue, and a low-grade fever. Questions 127 and 128 relate to this scenario.*

127. Upon initial assessment, which stage of the infection process is Jill presenting with?

    A. Incubation period.
    B. Prodromal period.
    C. Active illness.
    D. Convalescent period.

128. Jill is placed in an isolation room, and masks are to be worn by all persons in the room (with the exception of the patient). A surgical mask must be placed on the patient if she is to be moved from the room. What type of isolation precautions are being applied?

    A. Standard precautions.
    B. Airborne precautions.
    C. Droplet precautions.
    D. Contact precautions.

129. Indicate from the list below the child most at risk for acquiring a nosocomial infection.

    A. A child who has been hospitalized less than 24 hours.
    B. A child who is immunosuppressed.
    C. A child who has not had antibiotic therapy.
    D. A child who is ill at home.

130. An 8-year-old girl is presented to the physician's office febrile with a headache. The child is generally lethargic. She has a reddened lesion on her cheek that looks like she has been slapped. Which of the following infections would the nurse suspect?

    A. Erythema infectiosum (fifth disease).
    B. Measles (rubeola).
    C. Chickenpox (varicella).
    D. Pityriasis rosea.

131. A hospitalized young child is crying and saying that her mouth is sore. The nurse assesses and finds white plaque on the surface of the tongue that does not scrap off and suspects thrush (oral candidal infection). Identify the causative agent category.

    A. Virus.
    B. Bacteria.

C. Parasite.

D. Fungus.

132. A 12-year-old boy presents to the physician's office in the summer with a rash on his left knee that is round with a raised border. He is complaining of knee pain. He cannot remember hurting his leg but spends most of his time outdoors playing in the forest with his friends. The nurse suspects which of the following?

   A. Tetanus.
   B. Lyme disease.
   C. Pin worms.
   D. Diphtheria.

---

*Case Study:* Brittany, a 14-year-old young woman, has fever, chills, and a headache. She complains of extreme fatigue and a lack of energy that has lasted "a while." On assessment, the nurse finds that Brittany has enlarged tonsils and swollen lymph nodes. Questions 133 and 134 relate to this scenario.

---

133. The nurse suspects which of the following infections?

   A. Mumps (epidemic parotitis).
   B. Infectious mononucleosis.
   C. Scarlet fever.
   D. Herpes simplex.

134. Brittany is placed on bed rest through the acute phase of the infection, which has lasted 8 days. Why has bed rest been prescribed during this time?

   A. To prevent spreading the infection.
   B. To prevent further fatigue.
   C. To prevent rupture of the spleen.
   D. To prevent immunosuppression.

---

*Case Study:* A nurse is assessing Mohamed, a 1-year-old child, who appears pale, anorexic, and irritable and has diarrhea and a beefy-red tongue. Questions 135 and 136 relate to this scenario.

---

135. From the above information, what disorder does Mohamed most likely have?

   A. Pernicious anemia.
   B. Sickle cell anemia.
   C. Aplastic anemia.
   D. Iron deficiency anemia.

136. Mohamed has been diagnosed with pernicious anemia. The nurse is aware that the health teaching prepared for Mohamed's parents must include:

   A. The cause is related to an inadequate intake of dietary iron.
   B. The child will be placed on a diet of meat, eggs, and green vegetables.
   C. A dietary intake of large amounts of milk products is a contributing factor.
   D. The child will require lifelong monthly injections of vitamin B12.

137. At what age are infants with low birth weight often diagnosed with iron deficiency anemia?

   A. 3 months of age.
   B. 6 months of age.
   C. 2 years of age.
   D. 3 years of age.

138. What are the risk factors for developing iron deficiency anemia in a child older than age 2 years?

   A. Maternal iron deficiency anemia.
   B. Gastroesophageal reflux.
   C. Pyloric stenosis.
   D. Chronic blood loss.

139. A 30-kg infant is prescribed ferrous sulfate for severe iron deficiency anemia. The dosage prescribed is 6 mg/kg/day. If the child received this dosage t.i.d., what would be the correct amount to be administered for each dose?

   A. 30 mg.
   B. 50 mg.
   C. 60 mg.
   C. 90 mg.

140. Which of the following statements is correct regarding children being presented to hospital with iron deficiency anemia?

   A. They generally do not drink milk.
   B. They have decreased hemoglobin levels.
   C. They have a ruddy appearance.
   D. They have increased hematocrit levels.

141. The nurse is aware that children diagnosed with iron deficiency anemia are encouraged to eat foods high in iron. From the following, which would be the most appropriate food recommendation for a child diagnosed with iron deficiency anemia?

   A. Meat.
   B. Milk.
   C. Bananas.
   D. Pasta.

---

*Case Study:* Dieon is a 3-year-old African Canadian child who has been feeling ill over the past month. His parents make an appointment and bring him to

---

*the doctor's office for further investigation.*
*Questions 142 to 147 relate to this scenario.*

142. Dieon is brought to the physician's office with a protruding abdomen and icteric sclera and is febrile. The nurse suspects which of the following?

    A. Iron deficiency anemia.
    B. Sickle cell anemia.
    C. Pernicious anemia.
    D. Aplastic anemia.

143. Dieon requires a blood transfusion. His current weight is 15 kg. The commonly accepted rate for transfusions is 10 mL/kg/hr. The physician's order is written to infuse red blood cells at 15 mL/kg over 2 hours. The nurse realizes:

    A. Clarification is needed because the order is unsafe.
    B. The transfusion administered will be run as ordered.
    C. The transfusion must be run slower than ordered.
    D. The transfusion must be run faster than ordered.

144. With administering blood products to Dieon, what type of solution must also be infused with the blood transfusion?

    A. Hypotonic.
    B. Hypertonic.
    C. Isotonic.
    D. TPN.

145. After 10 minutes of receiving the blood transfusion, Dieon begins to complain of headache and back pain and is hypotensive. What should the nurse suspect?

    A. Anxiety.
    B. An anaphylactic reaction.
    C. Sickle cell crisis.
    D. Boredom.

146. Based on Dieon's complaints of headache and back pain and his hypotensive symptoms, what is the nurse's priority action?

    A. Try to relieve the child's anxiety.
    B. Distract the child with activity.
    C. Slow the transfusion rate.
    D. Discontinue the transfusion.

147. It is now 2 months after the blood transfusion, and Dieon is brought to the physician's office febrile, jaundiced, and lethargic. The nurse now suspects which of the following?

    A. Hepatitis.
    B. Sickle cell disease.
    C. Influenza.
    D. Renal failure.

148. A young male infant is brought to the physician's office for a scheduled circumcision. His parents call the telehealth nurse after the physician's office has closed reporting that their infant is bleeding profusely and has been for the past 3 hours. The telehealth nurse suspects which of the following?

    A. Poor sterile technique
    B. Intravascular coagulation.
    C. Polycythemia.
    D. Hemophilia A.

149. Hemophilia A is best identified as a disease with:

    A. Increased vessel permeability.
    B. A sex-linked recessive trait.
    C. A hemorrhagic rash.
    D. A decrease in the number of circulating platelets.

150. Identify the clinical manifestation most indicative of a child with hemophilia A.

    A. Purpural rash on the buttocks.
    B. Miniature petechiae.
    C. Painful bleeding into the joints.
    D. Cyanotic fingers and toes.

151. From the list below, what is the priority topic for health teaching a nurse would emphasize with parents of a child newly diagnosed with hemophilia A?

    A. Dietary changes.
    B. Vitamin B12 replacement.
    C. Hygiene restrictions.
    D. Injury prevention.

152. A child with hemophilia A is actively bleeding. What is the best treatment option to control the bleeding?

    A. Administration of platelets.
    B. Administration of red blood cells.
    C. Administration of concentrated factor VIII.
    D. Administration of white blood cells.

153. A nurse is taking a health history of a 10-year-child and discovers that the child has difficulties in urinary control during the day. What is this condition called?

    A. Nocturnal enuresis.
    B. Diurnal enuresis.
    C. Primary enuresis.
    D. Secondary enuresis.

**154.** What is a common risk factor contributing to the development of diurnal enuresis?

    A. Female gender.
    B. Increased bladder capacity.
    C. Urinary tract infections.
    D. Character of the child.

**155.** What is a long-term complication of urinary tract infections in the children?

    A. Fever.
    B. Increased frequency of urination.
    C. Renal scarring.
    D. Toilet training anxiety.

**156.** Which of the following predisposes pediatric clients to urinary tract infections?

    A. Being uncircumcised (boys).
    B. Wearing cloth diapers.
    C. Scheduled toileting.
    D. Constipation.

**157.** A school health nurse is providing an inservice on preventing urinary tract infections in the children. Identify the information that should be included in this inservice.

    A. Teaching young girls to wipe from front to back after going to the bathroom.
    B. Encouraging children to hold their urine until they really feel they have to go.
    C. Teaching parents to only purchase undergarments made of synthetic fabrics.
    D. Stressing the importance of restricting the consumption of fluids throughout the day.

**158.** A nurse attending the inservice states, "There is no research to justify wiping front to back. It really makes no difference." What response would best support evidence-based practice?

    A. "Our community newspaper just ran an article on this topic supporting this technique."
    B. "Current professional research indicates that this technique is key in preventing infections."
    C. "Would you like to share the basis of your comments with the group?"
    D. "Could you share with the group your techniques for preventing infection?"

**159.** Identify a common therapeutic technique for treatment of a urinary tract infection in the pediatric population.

    A. Offering large quantities of cranberry juice.
    B. Restricting fluid intake for 48 hours.
    C. Offering large quantities of any kind of fluid.
    D. Encouraging the child to sit in a bubble bath.

**160.** Sharon is a nurse caring for the child with a urinary tract infection and is 1 hour late administering the child's prescribed antibiotic therapy and pain medication even though the child's mother has repeatedly asked for it. Liz, the charge nurse, challenges Sharon about the lateness of the medications. Sharon responds, "It's no big deal; at least he got the medication." What is the best course of action for Liz to take?

    A. No course of action because the nurse is working on a busy floor.
    B. Reassign responsibility of this patient to another nurse.
    C. Speak to the unit manager so he or she can handle the situation.
    D. Speak to the unit manager and fill out a medication error form.

**161.** The parents of the child diagnosed with a polycystic kidney state: "This is our fault. We gave this to our child." What response might the nurse make that would be the most therapeutic?

    A. "It's true that you gave this to your child and will to any future children you might have."
    B. "Although this is an inherited disease, you were not aware of it, so it's not your fault."
    C. "Can you tell me more about how you're feeling?"
    D. "It sounds like you're feeling responsible for the illness. Can we talk about that?"

**162.** A nurse is attempting to measure blood pressure in an infant and is confused about which cuff size to select. Identify the most serious consequence of an incorrect cuff size.

    A. A wider cuff than necessary gives a higher reading.
    B. A narrower cuff than necessary gives a higher reading.
    C. Too much pressure may be applied to the arm.
    D. It will take considerably longer to read the blood pressure.

**163.** When planning care for a visually impaired child, the health care team would include:

    A. Maintaining a tidy environment around the child.
    B. Enrolling the child in sign language interpretation classes.
    C. Using visual aids to facilitate communication.
    D. Limiting verbal communication to avoid startling the child.

**164.** Identify appropriate terminology to use when describing a diagnostic procedure to school-age children.

  A. Use the word "test" to describe a procedure.
  B. Use the phrase "I'm going to take your blood."
  C. Use the phrase "this won't hurt a bit."
  D. Use the phrase "the x-ray machine is like a big camera."

**165.** Jan, a new graduate nurse, is assigned to care for a pediatric patient with advanced bone cancer who requires multiple dressing changes and pharmacologic interventions. Jan is finding the assignment extremely challenging and is considering requesting a different patient assignment. Which of the following would be a reasonable solution to this situation?

  A. Refusing the patient assignment and leaving the unit to go home.
  B. Keeping her concerns to herself and continuing to care for the child.
  C. Telling the charge nurse she is sick and leaving during the shift.
  D. Suggesting a shared assignment with a senior nurse.

**166.** The parents of a child who has received high doses of antibiotics ask the nurse to explain the term "ototoxicity." The nurse is aware that ototoxicity describes a potential consequence of medications having an adverse effect on:

  A. The organs of urination.
  B. The organs of hearing.
  C. Bone formation.
  D. The organs of vision.

**167.** Which of the following patients is at greatest risk for drug-induced hearing loss?

  A. A child with congenital heart disease receiving long-term dioxin therapy.
  B. A child with uncontrolled asthma receiving high-dose corticosteroids.
  C. A child with diabetes receiving long-term insulin therapy.
  D. A child with a chronic infection receiving high-dose gentamycin therapy.

**168.** A 5-year-old child who has autism is admitted to the nursing unit. When caring for this child, the nurse notices the child is repeating her words back to her. What is the name of this symptom of autism?

  A. Labile mood.
  B. Echolalia.
  C. Dyslexia.
  D. Hyperactivity.

**169.** A nurse is conducting a community inservice focused on attention deficit hyperactivity disorder (ADHD). Identify appropriate information that should be included.

  A. Girls with ADHD show more aggression than boys with ADHD.
  B. Diagnosis usually occurs before the child reaches school age.
  C. Sleep disturbances are common for children with ADHD.
  D. The child will fatigue from the increased activity level.

**170.** Identify which of the following is a priority nursing diagnosis when working with a family caring for their chronically ill child at home.

  A. Knowledge deficit related to a newly diagnosed disease.
  B. Anxiety related to changes in health status.
  C. Caregiver role strain related to the demands of the child's care.
  D. Risk for social isolation related to the disease process.

**171.** A 16-year-old young woman presents to the school nurse describing an incident at a school dance on the weekend. After returning from the bathroom and continuing drinking her punch, the student became drowsy and disoriented and woke up in the back of a stranger's car hours later. The nurse suspects the young woman ingested which of the following?

  A. Gravol.
  B. Rohypnol.
  C. Ritalin.
  D. Ramipril.

**172.** A common anxiety-producing event in the adolescent population is the presence of acne. A school health nurse is supporting a 15-year-old young woman who is experiencing acne. What is a common myth related to acne often perpetuated in adolescent populations?

  A. Diet plays a significant role in acne production.
  B. Do not pick or squeeze acne lesions because it will just increase symptoms.
  C. Excessive face washing is not necessary to prevent lesions from forming.
  D. Makeup may increase lesion formation.

**173.** What is the most appropriate health teaching that can be provided to prevent head injuries among preschool children?

  A. Do not allow children to ride bicycles.
  B. Do not allow children to approach strange animals.

C. Children should always wear helmets when riding bicycles.

D. Preschoolers should be taught that not all people are friends.

174. What is the most common reason why some children become bullies?

    A. Their parents are overprotective.
    B. They are being bullied themselves.
    C. They don't like their victims.
    D. Their parents are very strict.

175. What potentially is the most effective method a nurse can deliver sex education to school-age children?

    A. Providing a sex education course that includes films and discussions.
    B. Using booklets that children take home and instructing them to ask questions after reading.
    C. Delivering coeducation sex education classes.
    D. Reading sex education pamphlets with the children.

176. A nurse is providing suggestions to the parents of a 5-year-old child who stutters. What of the following could have a further negative impact on the child's language skills?

    A. In the child's presence, discussing the difficulty he is having with speech.
    B. Resisting the urge to interrupt the child or fill in the word.
    C. Resisting the urge to instruct the child to speak slowly.
    D. Ensuring that members of the family don't refer to the child as a "stutterer."

177. One of the most influential determinants of childhood obesity is:

    A. Health influences.
    B. Age.
    C. Environmental factors.
    D. Social pressures.

178. A community nurse is conducting home visits to families with newborn babies. What is a priority focus of the visit in relation to newborn preventive health?

    A. Introducing screening tests.
    B. Testing suck reflexes.
    C. Testing grasp reflexes.
    D. Measuring sleep patterns.

179. A hospitalized 7-year-old patient is sitting in bed repeatedly using profanity while blinking his eyes and jerking his neck. The nurse suspects the child has what disorder?

    A. Childhood schizophrenia.
    B. Childhood depression.
    C. Tourette's syndrome.
    D. Pica.

180. Methylphenidate hydrochloride (Ritalin) has been prescribed for a 6-year-old child with attention deficit hyperactivity disorder. Health teaching for parents should include which of the following statements?

    A. "You will see a positive response to Ritalin in approximately 8 weeks."
    B. "You should give the dose to your child right before his evening bedtime."
    C. "Extended-release tablets may be crushed or chewed."
    D. "If discontinued, Ritalin must be tapered off slowly."

181. Which of the following would be a priority nursing diagnosis for an autistic child hospitalized for diagnostic testing?

    A. Impaired social interaction related to the developmental disability.
    B. Knowledge deficit related to the developmental disability.
    C. Chronic low self-esteem related to altered perceptions.
    D. Risk for injury related to a lack of understanding of environmental hazards.

182. The family of a child who is cognitively challenged is concerned about fostering independence in their child. For this family, health teaching should emphasize all of the following except:

    A. Teach your child with a group of other children.
    B. Teach one step at a time to facilitate your child's short-term memory.
    C. Use generous praise as a reward for learning.
    D. Limit principles and abstract concepts in the teaching.

183. The nurse realizes the grandmother of a child with a cognitive impairment requires more health teaching when she states:

    A. "I will have to watch for illness in my granddaughter because she won't be able to tell me."
    B. "I won't be able to treat my granddaughter based on her chronological age."
    C. "My granddaughter will never be able to attend school."

D. "My granddaughter may need speech therapy later in life."

184. Identify the priority nursing diagnosis for a child who has had a gastrostomy tube inserted for feedings.

A. Pain related to the procedure.
B. Imbalanced nutrition related to the inability to swallow.
C. Anxiety related to hospitalization.
D. Altered body image related to placement of the gastrostomy tube.

185. A nurse has received an order to insert a nasogastric (NG) tube in an 8-month-old infant to facilitate enteral feeds. Which of the following is correct regarding inserting an NG tube in an infant?

A. Measure the space from the bridge of the nose to the earlobe to the xiphoid process.
B. Children younger than 1 year old require a number 8 feeding tube.
C. Children older than 1 year of age require a number 10 feeding tube.
D. Measure the space from the bridge of the nose to the earlobe to a point halfway between the xiphoid process and the umbilicus.

186. The side of the finger and the lateral aspect of the heel are anatomic sites most appropriate for which specimen collection?

A. Venipuncture.
B. Capillary puncture.
C. Arterial blood gases.
D. Oxygen saturation.

187. Which determinant has the most impact on the experience of a child admitted to a hospital for diagnostic procedures?

A. Developmental stage of the child.
B. Weight of the child.
C. Parental presence.
D. Actual procedure being performed.

*Case Study:* A 1-year-old child, Jenny, is admitted to the nursing unit with a congenital condition that relates directly to increased intraocular pressure in the eye globe. Questions 188 to 190 relate to this scenario.

188. The nurse is aware that the child's diagnosis is:

A. Glaucoma.
B. Cataract.
C. Conjunctivitis.
D. Foreign body injury.

189. Jenny's mother is questioning the necessity to treat the congenital glaucoma and asks, "Does she really need to be treated for this? Why don't we just wait and see if she grows out of it?" At this point, what should health teaching focus on?

A. Calming the mother's fears by agreeing with her.
B. Sharing that if left untreated, the condition will destroy the optic nerve.
C. Sharing that if left untreated, Jenny will also redevelop glaucoma when she is elderly.
D. Suggesting that the mother seek a second opinion.

190. Mary, RN, is working with Jenny and is providing health teaching to her family. The secondary nurse, Lori, listens to a conversation Mary has with Jenny's family and feels compelled to speak with Mary about the accuracy of the information that she has provided to the family. What statement concerned Lori?

A. "Congenital glaucoma accounts for approximately 10% of children with visual impairment."
B. "Congenital glaucoma is usually a unilateral condition."
C. "Congenital glaucoma is caused by a recessive gene inheritance pattern."
D. "Symptoms are usually noticeable by 1 year of age."

*Case Study:* A nurse is conducting a physical examination of Paul, age 4 months. Upon assessing his pupils, the nurse notes a white pupil opening. Questions 191 and 192 relate to this scenario.

191. Paul is unable to grasp objects that are placed near him and does not respond to facial expressions. The nurse suspects:

A. Glaucoma.
B. Foreign body injury.
C. Conjunctivitis.
D. Cataract.

192. Paul is scheduled for surgical removal of the cloudy lens and insertion of an intraocular lens. What is the greatest concern for Paul after surgery?

A. Vomiting.
B. Pain.
C. Eye patching.
D. Bleeding.

193. An 11-year-old girl is brought to the clinic complaining of difficulty reading the blackboard in her classroom, yet she has no difficulty reading her laptop screen or reading books. The nurse is

aware that the child is presenting with which of the following?

A. Myopia.
B. Strabismus.
C. Photophobia.
D. Hyperopia.

194. A nurse is caring for a 10-year-old child who has a visual impairment. Identify the correct information to incorporate in the nursing care of this child.

A. It is important to speak loudly when communicating with visually impaired children.
B. It is important to touch visually impaired children before speaking to them.
C. It is important to make sure that visually impaired children hear you before touching them.
D. It is important to remember that visually impaired children are usually cognitively challenged.

*Case Study: Kelly, age 6 years, is seen in clinic with severe ear pain of the left ear. The mother states that he just "got over a bad cold but seemed better." He recently started pulling at his ear and has become increasingly irritable. Kelly's temperature is currently 38.2°C. A diagnosis of acute otitis media is made. Questions 195 to 197 relate to this scenario.*

195. What would be an expected finding upon examination of Kelly?

A. Impacted cerumen in the external canal.
B. Increased discomfort on manipulation of the auricle.
C. A red tympanic membrane.
D. A shiny tympanic membrane.

196. What health teaching will be necessary for Kelly's mother?

A. Temporary conductive loss in the child is not expected.
B. A full prescribed course of antibiotics is necessary.
C. There is no risk of permanent damage to hearing.
D. Exposure to cigarette smoke is not a concern.

197. While sitting on the examining table, Kelly states that his ear doesn't hurt anymore. Which of the following is likely occurring?

A. The tympanic membrane has spontaneously ruptured.
B. The infection is resolving, and the ear is getting better.

C. The child is distracted by all the stimuli.
D. The blockage in the ear has resolved.

198. What is the primary reason a myringotomy tube would need to be inserted into a child's ear?

A. To provide a channel for the cerumen to drain.
B. To provide air to the middle ear.
C. To provide clear visual access to the structures.
D. To decrease inflammation of the tonsils.

199. The nurse is planning health teaching for parents after insertion of myringotomy tubes in their children. When planning these teaching sessions, she would include all of the following *except*:

A. Baths are preferable to showers.
B. The child should use ear plugs for swimming.
C. The child should sit in a seat in the front of the class.
D. This is a short-term problem.

200. A 16-year-old young man patient with juvenile arthritis states, " I'm tired of not being able to play sports with my friends, and these medications make me feel sick to my stomach. That's it! I'm done with these meds. I'm going to live like a regular kid from now on, not some freak!" Identify the best response for the nurse.

A. "That's simply not possible. You have to follow the doctor's orders."
B. "Stop yelling. You're waking up all of the other patients."
C. "I'm going to review some choices you have regarding your care."
D. "If you stop taking your medications, you won't be able to walk."

▶ **Short Answer Questions**

201. Identify two reasons why breathing exercises are important for children diagnosed with cystic fibrosis. (2 points)

202. Identify two potential causes for increased intracranial pressure in the pediatric population. (3 points)

203. Describe how the nurse would measure the function of cranial nerve X in a child. (1 point)

204. Identify the most common reason for a first-time seizure in an 8-year-old child compared with a first-time seizure in an adult. (2 points)

205. A nurse is inserting a nasogastric (NG) tube into an unconscious pediatric patient. Identify the most serious risk associated with this procedure. (1 point)

206. A nurse is sharing health teaching with the parents of a child who has chronic diarrhea. The child has received home remedies, including herbal medicine. Identify one important directive that the nurse should share with the parents regarding home remedies. (1 point)

207. A nurse is providing health teaching to a 14-year-old adolescent who is newly diagnosed with celiac disease. The focus of this teaching session is to provide information related to dietary changes that will enable the adolescent to maintain a healthy state. Identify two of the grains this adolescent will have to remove from his diet. (3 points)

208. Identify a common side effect from immunization for pediatric clients. (1 point)

209. Identify three factors that influence a child's response to pain. (4 points)

210. Identify the leading cause of cardiac arrest among children and infants. (1 point)

211. A nurse is speaking to a small group of parents who have had children diagnosed with congenital heart disease. One of the parents asks for a description of congestive heart failure. What is the best response to this question? (1 point)

212. Explain why parents of a child diagnosed with congenital heart disease would also be asking about congestive heart failure. (1 point)

213. Identify a primary goal of therapeutic management for the parents of a child diagnosed with allergies. (1 point)

214. What medication is prescribed as the antidote for morphine? (1 point)

215. Children with congenital heart disease tend to display abnormal positions, including frequent squatting or knee-to-chest positions. Explain why these children assume these positions. (1 point)

216. An 8-year-old child is placed on a liquid preparation of ferrous sulfate therapy for the treatment of iron deficiency anemia and is told to use a straw when drinking the elixir. Explain why using the straw is emphasized. (1 point)

**217.** The child is also directed to take the ferrous sulfate elixir with citrus juice. Explain this directive. (1 point)

*Case Study:* *A nurse is caring for a 15-year-old pregnant adolescent. She lives at home with her parents and has a boyfriend who is also 15 years old. Both adolescents attend high school, neither is currently working, and they both have plans for higher education. Questions 224 to 227 relate to this scenario.*

**218.** Identify the most common pathogen that causes urinary tract infections in the pediatric population. (1 point).

**224.** Identify two physiologic risks to the adolescent mother as a direct result of not receiving prenatal care. (2 points)

**219.** Identify the most likely course of medical treatment in a pediatric patient with a urinary tract infection. (1 point)

**225.** Identify two physiologic risks to the baby as a direct result of the adolescent mother's not receiving prenatal care. (2 points)

**220.** A nurse is providing health teaching to a group of adolescent girls focusing on urinary tract infections. Included in the information is a condition called honeymoon cystitis. Briefly describe this condition. (1 point)

**226.** Identify three psychological risks to the adolescent mother as a direct result of not receiving prenatal care. (3 points)

**227.** Identify three risk factors contributing to an unplanned teen pregnancy. (3 points)

**221.** Identify two signs of a urinary tract infection in children ages 10 to 16 years. (3 points)

**222.** Identify two signs of a urinary tract infection in children ages 3 to 8 years. (3 points)

**228.** Identify three physical indicators of a child who is being neglected. (3 points)

**229.** Identify a potential challenge a nurse would anticipate when removing a cast from a 5-year-old child. (1 point)

**223.** Dave, a 17-year-old young man, is an active sports enthusiast and attends high school. Identify and explain the leading cause of accidental death for individuals this age and gender. (1 point)

# ▶ Answers and Rationales

**1. A.** Nasal flaring.

*Rationale*
Nasal flaring refers to the enlargement of the opening of the nostrils during breathing. Nasal flaring is seen primarily in infants and younger children. Any condition that causes the infant to work harder to obtain enough air can cause nasal flaring. Although many causes of nasal flaring are not serious, some can be life threatening. In young infants, nasal flaring can be a very important sign of respiratory distress. All of the other choices could potentially be seen in both adult and pediatric populations.

*Classification*
Competency Category: Nursing Practice: Alterations in Health
Taxonomic Level: Knowledge/Comprehension

**2. D.** The etiology is often allergens and infection.

*Rationale*
Because the child has long-standing asthma, the nurse would assess the parents' level of understanding about the disease before offering information. Given that both parents are smokers, allergen-triggered asthma is a probable cause or at least an aggravator.

Respiratory tract infections cause epithelial damage and stimulate the production of IgE antibodies directed toward the viral antigens. They also increase airway responsiveness to other asthma triggers that may persist for weeks beyond the original infection (smoking is a main allergen). Usual triggers of bronchial asthma in children are allergies that initiate the inflammatory response. As few as 50% of children will remain asymptomatic for the remainder of their lives. As many as one in two children who had childhood asthma who are asymptomatic at 18 years of age are likely to have recurrent, symptomatic disease by age 26 years. Asthma usually persists as a low-grade, subclinical condition. Asthmatic episodes may be life threatening in all age groups.

*Classification*
Competency Category: Nurse–Person Relationship
Taxonomic Level: Critical Thinking

**3. B.** Moderate persistent asthma.

*Rationale*
In severe persistent asthma, symptoms are continual symptoms combined with frequent nighttime symptoms. Moderate persistent asthma involves daily symptoms with nighttime symptoms more than one night per week. Symptoms of mild persistent asthma occur more than two times a week but no more than one time per day with nighttime symptoms more than twice per month. Finally, symptoms of mild intermittent asthma occur less than twice per week with nighttime symptoms less than two times per month.

*Classification*
Competency Category: Nursing Practice: Alterations in Health
Taxonomic Level: Knowledge/Comprehension

**4. C.** Tenaciousness.

*Rationale*
The smaller diameter of the airways in young children and the tenaciousness of mucus are characteristics of pediatric clients experiencing an asthma attack.

*Classification*
Competency Category: Nursing Practice: Alterations in Health
Taxonomic Level: Knowledge/Comprehension

**5. A.** Respiratory acidosis.

*Rationale*
This patient has an elevated $PaCO_2$ and decreased $PaO_2$ with decreased pH. Respiratory acidosis caused by mucus filling the lung bases has resulted in impaired gas exchange in the alveoli.

*Classification*
Competency Category: Nursing Practice: Alterations in Health
Taxonomic Level: Knowledge/Comprehension

**6. B.** Leukotriene modifiers.

*Rationale*
Leukotriene modifiers are the only long-term medications listed. They block inflammatory and bronchospasm effects and are not used to treat acute episodes. Oral systemic corticosteroids are used to treat moderate to severe exacerbations. They prevent progression and relapses to gain control of severe persistent asthma (3- to 10-day course). Anticholinergic agents block efferent vagal pathways that cause bronchoconstriction, and β-adrenergic agonists are short-acting agents used to treat patients with acute attacks but are not recommended for daily use.

*Classification*
Competency Category: Nursing Practice: Health and Wellness
Taxonomic Level: Application

**7. A.** The child's condition is improving.

*Rationale*
The child's condition is improving. Louder breath sounds mean that more air is moving throughout the lung field.

*Classification*
Competency Category: Nursing Practice: Alterations in Health
Taxonomic Level: Application

**8. D.** Absence of spontaneous cough and presence of drooling and agitation.

*Rationale*
The child is drooling because of their difficulty swallowing and excessive secretions. This child will also appear extremely restless and anxious. The inflammation is not in the lung field, so adventitious breath sounds are not detected. Ear rubbing is indicative of otitis media, not epiglottitis. Spontaneous cough is not evident in clients with epiglottitis.

*Classification*
Competency Category: Nursing Practice: Alterations in Health
Taxonomic Level: Knowledge/Comprehension

**9. C.** Droplet precautions.

*Rationale*
Pertussis is spread via droplet transmission, so droplet precautions are necessary for the first 5 days after the child has begun medical treatment.

*Classification*
Competency Category: Nursing Practice: Alterations in Health
Taxonomic Level: Application

**10. C.** 20–33 breaths/min.

*Rationale*
Normal respiration rates in the pediatric population are as follows:

    Newborns: 30–60 breaths/min.
    3 years old: 20–30 breaths/min.
    6–10 years old: 11–22 breaths/min.
    17 years old: 12–20 breaths/min.

*Classification*
Competency Category: Nursing Practice: Health and Wellness
Taxonomic Level: Knowledge/Comprehension

**11. B.** Ineffective airway clearance related to thick, tenacious mucus production.

*Rationale*
The nurse's first priority is to assess the child's respiratory status and to maintain patency of the airway. All other options would then be addressed.

*Classification*
Competency Category: Nursing Practice: Alterations in Health
Taxonomic Level: Critical Thinking

**12. B.** It is inherited as an autosomal recessive trait.

*Rationale*
Cystic fibrosis is an inherited autosomal recessive trait. This disease does not occur unless two genes for the disease are present. The gender of the child is unimportant in terms of inheritance, and the disease is not curable.

*Classification*
Competency Category: Nursing Practice: Alterations in Health
Taxonomic Level: Knowledge/Comprehension

**13. C.** Exocrine glands.

*Rationale*
Cystic fibrosis is a generalized dysfunction of the exocrine glands.

*Classification*
Competency Category: Nursing Practice: Alterations in Health
Taxonomic Level: Knowledge/Comprehension

**14. A.** Steatorrhea.

*Rationale*
Steatorrhea is a condition in which the stools are large, foul smelling, bulky, and frothy as a result of a lack of pancreatic enzymes to aid in the digestion of fats, proteins, and some sugars.

*Classification*
Competency Category: Nursing Practice: Alterations in Health
Taxonomic Level: Knowledge/Comprehension

**15. C.** Your child will need to take a pancreatic enzyme before every meal.

*Rationale*
Children with CF are unable to effectively absorb nutrients from their diet. As a result, pancreatic enzymes must be given before meals. These enzymes are available in liquid and capsule form. The liquid form eases administration to infants, toddlers, and children who are unable to swallow caplets.

Regarding the other choices, children with CF require supplemental protein because breast milk does not contain enough protein to meet their needs. Extra protein is required because these children cannot absorb all of the protein they ingest. Mothers that choose to breastfeed should be informed that they can supplement their breast milk with formula in conjunction with enzymes to meet the child's dietary protein needs; children with CF often have a ravenous appetite. The home environment may need to be modified to accommodate for home oxygen and chest physiotherapy equipment.

*Classification*
Competency Category: Nurse–Person Relationship
Taxonomic Level: Critical Thinking

**16. A.** Respiratory acidosis.

*Rationale*
Based on the results of these blood gases, this patient is in respiratory acidosis.

*Classification*
Competency Category: Nursing Practice: Alterations in Health
Taxonomic Level: Application

**17. A.** Asymmetrical chest movement.

*Rationale*
If a pneumothorax is large or if a tension pneumothorax is present, it may push the mediastinum toward the unaffected lung, causing asymmetrical chest movement.

*Classification*
Competency Category: Nursing Practice: Alterations in Health
Taxonomic Level: Knowledge/Comprehension

**18. C.** Have a short latency period.

*Rationale*
A unique feature of childhood cancers is the short period of latency, which contrasts sharply with the long latency period that is common in adults. Carcinomas (epithelial tissue) almost never occur in children because these cancers most commonly result from environmental carcinogens and require a long latency period from exposure to the appearance of the carcinoma. Children have not lived long enough to be affected. Childhood cancers are most often diagnosed during peak periods of physical and maturation and in general are extremely fast growing (80% metastases at diagnosis).

*Classification*
Competency Category: Nursing Practice: Alterations in Health
Taxonomic Level: Knowledge/Comprehension

**19. D.** An acute respiratory or ear infection is usually present.

*Rationale*
Benign febrile seizures occur most frequently between the ages of 6 months and 5 years. An acute respiratory or ear infection usually is present, with no evidence of central nervous system infection or inflammation. The interictal electrocardiogram is normal during benign febrile seizures, so there is no evidence to support a developmental impact. The seizure does not usually recur during the same infection; rather, there is a pattern of one seizure per febrile illness. Each seizure is usually short in duration (≤15 minutes).

*Classification*
Competency Category: Nursing Practice: Alterations in Health
Taxonomic Level: Critical Thinking

**20. A.** Frontal.

*Rationale*
The frontal lobe regulates personality and judgment. The occipital lobe regulates vision, the temporal lobe regulates hearing, and the parietal lobe regulates sensation.

*Classification*
Competency Category: Nursing Practice: Alterations in Health
Taxonomic Level: Application

**21. B.** The intracranial pressure is increasing.

*Rationale*
Cushing's triad (apnea, bradycardia, and widening pulse pressure) is a hallmark of increasing intracranial pressure, which indicates that the teen's condition is deteriorating.

*Classification*
Competency Category: Nursing Practice: Alterations in Health
Taxonomic Level: Critical Thinking

**22. C.** Orientation to person, time, and place.

*Rationale*
Any change in level of consciousness, including confusion, is the first sign that the patient's neural status is changing.

*Classification*
Competency Category: Nursing Practice: Alterations in Health
Taxonomic Level: Knowledge/Comprehension

**23. B.** Compression.

*Rationale*
Compression injuries occur as a result of force from above or below. There is generally temporary neural dysfunction without visible damage to the spinal cord.

*Classification*
Competency Category: Nursing Practice: Alterations in Health
Taxonomic Level: Knowledge/Comprehension

**24. D.** Hypotonic solution.

*Rationale*
Hypotonic solution has a lower concentration and is more dilute than body fluids and serum. Fluid is osmotically pulled into the cells, causing them to burst or swell and would further increase intracranial pressure. Hypertonic solution has a greater concentration than body fluids and pulls water out of cells so that cells shrink.

*Classification*
Competency Category: Nursing Practice: Alterations in Health
Taxonomic Level: Knowledge/Comprehension

**25. A.** Meningitis.

*Rationale*
Head trauma and fractures place an individual at high risk for meningitis. A patient who is febrile with increasing drowsiness should be investigated for post-traumatic meningitis.

*Classification*
Competency Category: Nursing Practice: Alterations in Health
Taxonomic Level: Knowledge/Comprehension

**26. A.** Orthostatic hypotension.

*Rationale*
Orthostatic hypotension is very common with sudden position changes.

*Classification*
Competency Category: Nursing Practice: Alterations in Health
Taxonomic Level: Knowledge/Comprehension

**27. C.** VIII.

*Rationale*
Cranial nerve VIII measures equilibrium and hearing. Hearing is assessed by asking the child to repeat a whispered word.

*Classification*
Competency Category: Nursing Practice: Alterations in Health
Taxonomic Level: Knowledge/Comprehension

**28. C.** Exposure to radiation during the third trimester.

*Rationale*
A neural tube defect is a failure of the tube to close during the first trimester of development. Therefore, exposure in the third trimester would not be related to a neural tube defect. All other choices listed are possible causes.

*Classification*
Competency Category: Nursing Practice: Alterations in Health
Taxonomic Level: Knowledge/Comprehension

**29. B.** An abnormal accumulation of cerebrospinal fluid (CSF) within the cranial vault.

*Rationale*
Congenital hydrocephalus is an accumulation of excessive amounts of CSF within the ventricles of the brain. The faulty drainage of CSF from the ventricles often results in malformation of the skull and an abnormal development of cognitive or language skills and psychomotor skills.

*Classification*
Competency Category: Nursing Practice: Alterations in Health
Taxonomic Level: Knowledge/Comprehension

**30. A.** A ruptured appendix.

*Rationale*
When a child with severe right lower quadrant pain has a sudden relief of pain, a ruptured appendix should be suspected.

*Classification*
Competency Category: Nursing Practice: Alterations in Health
Taxonomic Level: Critical Thinking

**31. A.** Preparation for emergency surgery.

*Rationale*
Preparing for emergency surgery is the priority action at this point in time. Antibiotic therapy would be

initiated after surgery in addition to addressing pain control and dietary revision.

*Classification*
Competency Category: Nursing Practice: Alterations in Health
Taxonomic Level: Critical Thinking

**32. B.** Decreased renal output.

*Rationale*
Gentamicin sulfate is an antibiotic that can cause ototoxicity and nephrotoxicity. Therefore, a decrease in renal output would be concerning.

*Classification*
Competency Category: Nursing Practice: Alterations in Health
Taxonomic Level: Application

**33. C.** Dehydration.

*Rationale*
Signs of dehydration include poor skin turgor, lack of tearing, and dry mucous membranes.

*Classification*
Competency Category: Nursing Practice: Alterations in Health
Taxonomic Level: Knowledge/Comprehension

**34. B.** Fluid volume deficit.

*Rationale*
Initial treatment should focus on the child's fluid and electrolyte balance and rehydrating the child. Subsequent measures to identify the possible microorganisms responsible and resting the gastrointestinal tract should also be addressed.

*Classification*
Competency Category: Nursing Practice: Alterations in Health
Taxonomic Level: Application

**35. A.** Water, breast milk, and lactose-free formula.

*Rationale*
Water, breast milk, and lactose-free formula are low-sodium fluids that are often used during maintenance fluid therapy. Fruit juices, carbonated soft drinks, and gelatin have a high carbohydrate content, very low electrolyte content, and high osmolarity, so they are not used to manage diarrhea. Caffeinated soda is a mild diuretic, so its use may lead to increased loss of water and sodium. Chicken or beef broth has excessive sodium and inadequate carbohydrate con-

tent. The BRAT (bananas, rice, applesauce, and toast or tea) diet has little nutritional value.

*Classification*
Competency Category: Nursing Practice: Alterations in Health
Taxonomic Level: Critical Thinking

**36. A.** Hypokalemia.

*Rationale*
Vomiting, diarrhea, and NG to low Gomco suction are all common causes of hypokalemia. Diuretic therapy can also contribute to hypokalemia.

*Classification*
Competency Category: Nursing Practice: Alterations in Health
Taxonomic Level: Application

**37. B.** Check the NG tube for placement.

*Rationale*
The priority nursing action before initiating an NG feed is to check the tube for placement.

*Classification*
Competency Category: Nursing Practice: Alterations in Health
Taxonomic Level: Critical Thinking

**38. B.** Feeding the child after each episode of vomiting.

*Rationale*
The most optimum treatment for vomiting is to withhold food and fluid from the stomach for approximately 3 to 6 hours. The child will not vomit if the stomach is empty. Food and fluids should then be reintroduced gradually. If a child is fed after a vomiting incident, the child will vomit again, which prolongs the vomiting cycle and increases the risk of electrolyte imbalances.

*Classification*
Competency Category: Nursing Practice: Alterations in Health
Taxonomic Level: Knowledge/Comprehension

**39. C.** Little effort required moving the bowels.

*Rationale*
A bowel movement for a child with diarrhea is effortless and may be explosive. In passing normal stool, some effort or pushing may be involved on the child's part. All other descriptors describe normal characteristics of stool in an infant.

*Classification*
Competency Category: Nursing Practice: Alterations in Health
Taxonomic Level: Knowledge/Comprehension

**40. A.** "I usually lay the child flat after feeding."

*Rationale*
Children need to remain upright for 1 hour after feeding. The force of gravity assists in preventing reflux.

*Classification*
Competency Category: Nursing Practice: Health and Wellness
Taxonomic Level: Critical Thinking

**41. D.** Hepatitis A.

*Rationale*
The mode of transmission of hepatitis A in children includes exposure to contaminated changing tables and ingestion of fecally contaminated water or shellfish.

*Classification*
Competency Category: Nursing Practice: Health and Wellness
Taxonomic Level: Critical Thinking

**42. B.** Hepatitis B.

*Rationale*
These clinical manifestations are suggestive of hepatitis B. Hepatitis B in the pediatric population is seen more in adolescents than younger children because of lifestyle choices. Although it is generally not possible to differentiate the type of hepatitis from the clinical manifestations, the symptoms of hepatitis B are more marked and extreme than other forms of hepatitis.

*Classification*
Competency Category: Nursing Practice: Alterations in Health
Taxonomic Level: Knowledge/Comprehension

**43. C.** Hepatitis B is a sexually transmitted disease.

*Rationale*
Hepatitis B can be transmitted through semen in addition to blood plasma.

*Classification*
Competency Category: Nursing Practice: Health and Wellness
Taxonomic Level: Knowledge/Comprehension

**44. B.** Toddlers.

*Rationale*
Increased mobility and the exploratory nature of toddlers increase the risk of falls and injuries.

*Classification*
Competency Category: Nursing Practice: Health and Wellness
Taxonomic Level: Application

**45. A.** Altered nutrition (less than body requirements) related to difficulty sucking.

*Rationale*
The nurse's initial priority should be to address the caloric intake of the baby through health teaching and support of the parents to ensure that the baby will meet age-appropriate growth and development milestones.

*Classification*
Competency Category: Nursing Practice: Alterations in Health
Taxonomic Level: Application

**46. A.** Rectal route.

*Rationale*
Core body temperatures are measured at the tympanic or rectal sites. The tympanic site should not be used for clients who may have drainage from or an infection in the ear. Surface body temperatures are measured at the oral and axillary sites.

*Classification*
Competency Category: Nursing Practice: Alterations in Health
Taxonomic Level: Critical Thinking

**47. A.** Inform the surgeon.

*Rationale*
The surgeon must be informed immediately to decide whether to proceed with the surgery. A child scheduled for surgery in 1 hour would be NPO, so oral antipyretics would not be an option. Although cool compresses might relieve some discomfort, the priority action is to notify the physician.

*Classification*
Competency Category: Professional Practice
Taxonomic Level: Critical Thinking

**48. C.** Some children distract themselves with play while in pain.

*Rationale*
Some children distract themselves with play or music while in pain and may sleep as a result of exhaustion. Nurses commonly underestimate children's pain when they do not rely on children's self-reports. Narcotics can be used safely with children.

*Classification*
Competency Category: Nursing Practice: Alterations in Health
Taxonomic Level: Application

**49. B.** Stress and anxiety.

*Rationale*
Bedwetting, altered sleep patterns, and somatic complaints by a child can all result from stress.

*Classification*
Competency Category: Nursing Practice: Health and Wellness
Taxonomic Level: Knowledge/Comprehension

**50. B.** Offer disapproval and then ignore the tantrum.

*Rationale*
Stating one's disapproval and then ignoring the tantrum generally results in a quick resolution of the tantrum. Offering material or emotional bribes may actually increase the frequency of tantrums. Punishing the child does not decrease the frequency of tantrums because the tantrums are generated by an inability to express their feelings. Mirroring the tantrum behaviour reinforces that style of communication.

*Classification*
Competency Category: Nurse–Person Relationship
Taxonomic Level: Application

**51. A.** Diversionary activity deficit related to lack of appropriate toys and peers.

*Rationale*
Ill children are at risk for sensory deprivation because of bed rest and confinement to a hospital room, where little sensory stimulation is provided. Hospitalized children tend to watch television for numerous hours, providing little interaction with others. There is nothing in the scenario to suggest sleep deprivation. Actual diagnoses always take priority over "risk of" diagnoses.

*Classification*
Competency Category: Nursing Practice: Alterations in Health
Taxonomic Level: Application

**52. D.** Personal fable.

*Rationale*
Although each of these choices is relevant to adolescents, personal fable is the most appropriate answer because it is a feeling that no one understands what they are going through. Egocentrism refers to the perception that their perspective of the world is the most realistic. Adolescents also believe that that they are being watched constantly. This is referred to as having an imaginary audience. Invulnerability refers to an illusion that misfortune or accidents only happen to others.

*Classification*
Competency Category: Nurse–Person Relationship
Taxonomic Level: Knowledge/Comprehension

**53. C.** "I can appreciate your concerns. If we obtain permission from your daughter, we can include you in our discussions."

*Rationale*
The reality of this situation is that the parents may be included in the exchange of medical information but only with the daughter's consent. Sharing that fact with the parents clearly identifies that the decision is the daughter's to make and that she is entitled to make it. The nurse must support the client's right to privacy and confidentiality.

*Classification*
Competency Category: Professional Practice
Taxonomic Level: Critical Thinking

**54. A.** Congenital anomalies continue to be a leading cause of infant mortality.

*Rationale*
Congenital anomalies continue to be a leading cause of infant mortality. Birth weight is considered the major determinant of neonatal mortality in technologically developed countries. Children and infants are not only smaller than adults but are also significantly different physiologically and therefore respond differently to diseases and treatment. The number of deaths in the first year of life is proportionately high compared with death rates at other ages. In the United States, the death rate for infants younger than 1 year of age is greater than the rate for individuals age 1 through 54 years. It is not until age 55 years and over that the death rate begins to exceed the rate for infants.

*Classification*
Competency Category: Nursing Practice: Health and Wellness
Taxonomic Level: Application

**55. B.** 70–110 bpm.

*Rationale*
The following are normal heart rates in the pediatric population:

> Newborns: 100–170 bpm.
> Infants to 2 years old: 80–130 bpm.
> 2–6 years old: 70–110 bpm.
> 10–16 years old: 60–100 bpm.

*Classification*
Competency Category: Nursing Practice: Health and Wellness
Taxonomic Level: Knowledge/Comprehension

**56. D.** S4.

*Rationale*
S4 is the only heart sound of the choices that is abnormal in children. It is indicative of an atrial gallop. S1 and S2 are normal heart sounds, and S3 may be normal in children.

*Classification*
Competency Category: Nursing Practice: Alterations in Health
Taxonomic Level: Knowledge/Comprehension

**57. C.** Tachycardia.

*Rationale*
Tachycardia is an early compensatory sign of cardiac compromise. All of the other choices are late signs.

*Classification*
Competency Category: Nursing Practice: Alterations in Health
Taxonomic Level: Knowledge/Comprehension

**58. B.** Tachycardia.

*Rationale*
Fever, pain, anxiety, hypovolemia, hypoxia, acidosis, infection, and sympathomimetics drugs often induce tachycardia.

*Classification*
Competency Category: Nursing Practice: Alterations in Health
Taxonomic Level: Knowledge/Comprehension

**59. A.** Confirm correct IV fluids and rates.

*Rationale*
Confirming correct IV fluids and rates is a priority action at the beginning of a shift. This ensures that appropriate steps can be taken to correct it early in the shift, thus minimizing potential complications. Reviewing the physician's orders, patient history, and allergy bands are appropriate before pouring and administering medications.

*Classification*
Competency Category: Nursing Practice: Health and Wellness
Taxonomic Level: Application

**60. B.** Keep the child safe and assess for abuse.

*Rationale*
The assessment for risk is the priority nursing action. This would include verbalizing your concerns to the most immediate supervisor and involving hospital social workers and the medical team. These initial steps need to be implemented, and then the appropriate authorities must be alerted.

*Classification*
Competency Category: Professional Practice
Taxonomic Level: Application

**61. B.** Is most likely known to the child.

*Rationale*
Adult abusers are most often known to the child and family and are often in a position of trust.

*Classification*
Competency Category: Nursing Practice: Alterations in Health
Taxonomic Level: Knowledge/Comprehension

**62. A.** Anaphylaxis.

*Rationale*
Anaphylaxis is an acute clinical syndrome. It is a severe and life-threatening reaction that is immediate upon exposure to an antigen.

*Classification*
Competency Category: Nursing Practice: Health and Wellness
Taxonomic Level: Knowledge/Comprehension

**63. D.** Latex allergy.

*Rationale*
Latex allergies pose serious health hazard to 80% of children with spina bifida because of their repeated exposure to latex products during surgery, multiple bladder catheterizations, and disease-associated factors.

*Classification*
Competency Category: Nursing Practice: Alterations in Health
Taxonomic Level: Knowledge/Comprehension

**64. B.** Systemic antihistamines are given before testing.

*Rationale*
Systemic antihistamines would suppress the sensitivity response, and the test would not provide an accurate assessment of the child's allergies. There is a potential for false-negative results if antihistamines are administered before testing.

*Classification*
Competency Category: Nursing Practice: Alterations in Health
Taxonomic Level: Application

**65. A.** "I gave my children allergies when I breastfed them."

*Rationale*
The longer the duration of exclusive breastfeeding, the less likely the baby will have childhood allergies.

*Classification*
Competency Category: Nursing Practice: Health and Wellness
Taxonomic Level: Critical Thinking

**66. C.** Food allergy.

*Rationale*
Symptoms of food allergies usually occur within 2 hours of ingestion.

*Classification*
Competency Category: Nursing Practice: Alterations in Health
Taxonomic Level: Application

**67. C.** Sitting in the front seat.

*Rationale*
Children younger than age 12 years should not sit in the front seat of any vehicle that has airbags. They can sustain serious or fatal injuries from the deployed airbags.

*Classification*
Competency Category: Nursing Practice: Alterations in Health
Taxonomic Level: Critical Thinking

**68. D.** It is safe to give cephalosporins to this child.

*Rationale*
Cephalosporins should be avoided in children with proven penicillin sensitivity because they may also be sensitive to these.

*Classification*
Competency Category: Nursing Practice: Alterations in Health
Taxonomic Level: Application

**69. C.** As soon as the patient is warmed.

*Rationale*
You cannot determine the neural or hemodynamic status of the child until the child's body temperature is increased.

*Classification*
Competency Category: Nursing Practice: Alterations in Health
Taxonomic Level: Knowledge/Comprehension

**70. A.** Lactated Ringer's solution.

*Rationale*
Lactated Ringer's solution is an isotonic solution, D5W/lactated Ringer's solution is a hypertonic solution, D5W/0.45% NaCl is a hypertonic solution, and 0.33% NaCl is a hypotonic solution.

*Classification*
Competency Category: Nursing Practice: Alterations in Health
Taxonomic Level: Knowledge/Comprehension

**71. C.** 240–340 mmol/L.

*Rationale*
130–150 mmol/L is hypotonic.
150–240 mmol/L is hypotonic.
240–340 mmol/L is isotonic.
340–380 mmol/L is hypertonic.

*Classification*
Competency Category: Nursing Practice: Health and Wellness
Taxonomic Level: Knowledge/Comprehension

**72. D.** Bulimia.

*Rationale*
Bulimia is an eating disorder marked by recurrent episodes of binge eating, self-induced vomiting, excessive exercising, and an exaggerated concern about body shape and weight.

*Classification*
Competency Category: Nursing Practice: Alterations in Health
Taxonomic Level: Critical Thinking

**73. C.** Pubescence.

*Rationale*
Pubescence is the stage in which physical changes related to sexual maturation take place.

*Classification*
Competency Category: Nursing Practice: Health and Wellness
Taxonomic Level: Knowledge/Comprehension

**74. A.** Impact on social interactions.

*Rationale*
This young man is most likely reacting to the social isolation of his peers because of missing out on interaction with his friends.

*Classification*
Competency Category: Nursing Practice: Alterations in Health
Taxonomic Level: Knowledge/Comprehension

**75. D.** Shock from dehydration.

*Rationale*
Dehydration results from the osmotic diuresis associated with hyperglycemia and polyuria. The patient is at risk for shock from dehydration.

*Classification*
Competency Category: Nursing Practice: Alterations in Health
Taxonomic Level: Critical Thinking

**76. D.** Management of the therapeutic regimen.

*Rationale*
The priority immediately after recovery is therapy management, including reviewing that the interruption of insulin administration may result in diabetic ketoacidosis. The multiple admissions implies that the adolescent either does not understand the consequences of his disease or is making choices that are not consistent with the health teaching. This is an opportunity to review those choices.

*Classification*
Competency Category: Nurse–Person Relationship
Taxonomic Level: Critical Thinking

**77. A.** "If my blood sugar is low, I will be able to deal with it."

*Rationale*
Hypoglycemia also causes confusion and hallucinations. Patients may not always be able to respond appropriately to remedy the situation. All other options are true of hypoglycemia.

*Classification*
Competency Category: Nurse–Person Relationship
Taxonomic Level: Critical Thinking

**78. C.** The signs and symptoms of hypoglycemia.

*Rationale*
The priority would be the signs and symptoms hypoglycemia because it is the only option on the list that is potentially life threatening.

*Classification*
Competency Category: Nursing Practice: Alterations in Health
Taxonomic Level: Critical Thinking

**79. D.** Insulin is always administered subcutaneously.

*Rationale*
The goal of the session is "self-administration," so the information related to actually administering insulin is prioritized (i.e., information that insulin is always self-administered subcutaneously). Too much information at one session will confuse the client. A separate session should be dedicated to the actual insulin concerns, which are the other three choices.

*Classification*
Competency Category: Nurse–Person Relationship
Taxonomic Level: Knowledge/Comprehension

**80. C.** Repeatedly using the same site is less painful.

*Rationale*
Repeatedly injecting the same site causes scar tissue (lipohypertrophy) to form, and little or no pain is felt with subsequent injections. It also decreases insulin absorption. Scarring is more likely to occur with same-site injection rather than with rotating injection sites.

*Classification*
Competency Category: Nursing Practice: Health and Wellness
Taxonomic Level: Critical Thinking

**81. D.** Check the blood glucose level.

*Rationale*
Insulin is never administered without first checking the blood glucose level.

*Classification*
Competency Category: Nursing Practice: Health and Wellness
Taxonomic Level: Application

**82. B.** Short-acting insulin.

*Rationale*
Rapid-acting insulin has an onset of 15 minutes, a peak that lasts for 30 to 60 minutes, and a duration of 5 hours.
Short-acting insulin has an onset of 30 to 60 minutes, a peak of 2 to 4 hours, and a duration of 4 to 8 hours.
Intermediate-acting insulin has an onset of 1 to 6 hours, a peak of 8 to 12 hours, and a duration of 18 to 24 hours.
Long-acting insulin has an onset of 4 to 8 hours, a peak of 14 to 24 hours, and a duration of 36 hours.

*Classification*
Competency Category: Nursing Practice: Health and Wellness
Taxonomic Level: Knowledge/Comprehension

**83. B.** The insulin absorption rate varies in different parts of the body.

*Rationale*
The insulin absorption varies in different parts of the body. It is very important to methodically use one anatomic area and then move to another to minimize variation in absorption rates. An example of this is using the abdomen for the morning injection and the arm for the evening injection.

*Classification*
Competency Category: Nursing Practice: Alterations in Health
Taxonomic Level: Critical Thinking

**84. C.** Age, weight, and growth and development should be considered.

*Rationale*
Age, weight, and growth and development must be considered because safe dose ranges are calculated on these considerations. There are numerous drug restrictions for the pediatric population. Not all drugs used in adults are transferable to children. Using the oral route with a resistant child may lead to aspiration. When administering intramuscular injections, the thigh muscle is generally the first site choice. The deltoid muscle is usually quite small in most children and adolescents. The gluteal muscle us acceptable in older children but is not a developed muscle in children who do not walk.

*Classification*
Competency Category: Nursing Practice: Alterations in Health
Taxonomic Level: Application

**85. A.** Slowed excretion of drugs eliminated by the kidneys.

*Rationale*
Neonates and infants younger than age 1 year have slowed excretion of drugs eliminated by the kidneys because of their decreased glomerular filtration rate. Renal function development is mature by age 1 year. The skin of infants and neonates is thick and permeable, so topical absorption is increased. Infants and neonates have an immature blood–brain barrier, so they have increased distribution of drugs into the central nervous system.

Plasma protein binding is reduced until approximately age 1 year, so there may be a greater proportion of unbound medication and greater risks of adverse drug effects.

*Classification*
Competency Category: Nursing Practice: Alterations in Health
Taxonomic Level: Application

**86. A.** Diarrhea.

*Rationale*
Characteristics of a *C. difficile* infection include watery diarrhea.

*Classification*
Competency Category: Nursing Practice: Alterations in Health
Taxonomic Level: Knowledge/Comprehension

**87. D.** Scalp.

*Rationale*
Scalp or feet veins are the first choice in this age group. In late toddlerhood, peripheral sites become an option.

*Classification*
Competency Category: Nursing Practice: Health and Wellness
Taxonomic Level: Knowledge/Comprehension

**88. C.** The position of the child's extremity is incorrect.

*Rationale*
The most likely reason for difficulty running an IV in this age group is a positional issue of the patient or extremity because of the child's activity level.

*Classification*
Competency Category: Nursing Practice: Health and Wellness
Taxonomic Level: Knowledge/Comprehension

**89. C.** "I will get my child to take the medication by telling her it's candy."

*Rationale*
If a child thinks the medication is candy, she may try to access it on her own and potentially poison herself or other children.

*Classification*
Competency Category: Nursing Practice: Health and Wellness
Taxonomic Level: Application

**90. D.** Providing detailed explanations of the procedure.

*Rationale*
A detailed explanations of the procedure will increase the child's anxiety and prolong the situation. A brief explanation and quick medication administration is the most effective method.

*Classification*
Competency Category: Nursing Practice: Health and Wellness
Taxonomic Level: Knowledge/Comprehension

**91. B.** Autonomy.

*Rationale*
Autonomy is an individual's freedom to make informed decisions. Beneficence is nursing care for the good of the patient, veracity is the moral obligation to tell the truth, and nonmaleficence is an obligation to not harm patients.

*Classification*
Competency Category: Professional Practice
Taxonomic Level: Knowledge/Comprehension

**92. C.** Right dose.

*Rationale*
The dose is too high for a child who only weighs 5 kg. It is the responsibility of the nurse to verify that medications are within safe pediatric dose ranges before giving any medication to a pediatric patient.

*Classification*
Competency Category: Professional Practice
Taxonomic Level: Critical Thinking

**93. A.** Not wearing a seatbelt.

*Rationale*
If safety restraints such as seatbelts are not used in motor vehicle accidents, the child becomes a projectile and is at high risk for injury if thrown from the vehicle.

*Classification*
Competency Category: Nursing Practice: Alterations in Health
Taxonomic Level: Application

**94. C.** A lap and shoulder belt.

*Rationale*
A combination lap and shoulder belt is the safest restraint choice of those listed. Using a lap seatbelt places the child at greater risk of spinal cord injury, as does using a forward-facing car seat.

*Classification*
Competency Category: Nursing Practice: Alterations in Health
Taxonomic Level: Knowledge/Comprehension

**95. A.** Ischemia and edema.

*Rationale*
The primary cause of injury was the motor vehicle accident. Secondary injury is most likely to be caused by ischemia and edema of the spinal cord or column.

*Classification*
Competency Category: Nursing Practice: Alterations in Health
Taxonomic Level: Critical Thinking

**96. D.** The nurse is legally accountable for the medication administration.

*Rationale*
When an RN delegates a nursing responsibility to someone who is not licensed to practice nursing, the RN remains responsible and legally accountable for the care provided. It would not under any circumstances be acceptable to delegate medication administration to an unlicensed personal support worker.

*Classification*
Competency Category: Professional Practice
Taxonomic Level: Application

**97. A.** Improper use of firearms.

*Rationale*
Although accidental injuries are common in both countries, improper use of firearms is much less a factor in Canada than in the United States. Other injuries affecting children in Canada include neglect, bicycling accidents, and pedestrian accidents. Preventing injury is the best strategy for improving survival.

*Classification*
Competency Category: Nursing Practice: Health and Wellness
Taxonomic Level: Critical Thinking

**98. C.** "Toddlers often eat one food for days on end."

*Rationale*
It is common and not harmful for toddlers to have food jags, eating one food for days on end. Making dessert a reward makes vegetables and other foods seem less desirable. It is an unreasonable expectation to let the child choose his or her own food at this age.

*Classification*
Competency Category: Nursing Practice: Health and Wellness
Taxonomic Level: Application

**99. C.** It is the ability to put yourself in another person's place.

*Rationale*
Empathy is the ability to put oneself in another's place and experience a feeling as that person is experiencing it. This way, you can anticipate a child's actions and fears.

*Classification*
Competency Category: Nurse–Person Relationship
Taxonomic Level: Critical Thinking

**100. A.** Silence.

*Rationale*
Silence offers an opportunity for the child to answer spontaneously and cautiously. More information is usually forthcoming if the nurse gives the child the opportunity to respond. All other choices are considered factors that could potentially interfere with communication in the pediatric population.

*Classification*
Competency Category: Nurse–Person Relationship
Taxonomic Level: Critical Thinking

**101. D.** Keep your tone gentler and quieter than the child's.

*Rationale*
By keeping your tone gentler and quieter than the child's, you are not reacting to the tone of or force of the child's anger. This may also calm the child.

*Classification*
Competency Category: Nurse–Person Relationship
Taxonomic Level: Application

**102. C.** Perception checking.

*Rationale*
Perception is documenting a feeling or emotion. The nurse is asking for the child to validate the perception of his feelings. Paraphrasing includes documenting a statement or fact. Clarifying includes repeating back to the child the exact statement. Reflecting involves repeating back to the child the last word he said.

*Classification*
Competency Category: Nurse–Person Relationship
Taxonomic Level: Application

**103. B.** Preschool.

*Rationale*
Preschool children often have an overactive imagination and associate unreal characteristics to inanimate objects. As a result they may fear intrusive procedures and the equipment required for these procedures such as a thermometer and blood pressure cuff.

*Classification*
Competency Category: Nurse–Person Relationship
Taxonomic Level: Application

**104. C.** School age.

*Rationale*
School-age children learn best with short, separate procedures rather than one long procedure. Too much information is overwhelming for them.

*Classification*
Competency Category: Nurse–Person Relationship
Taxonomic Level: Application

**105. D.** Adolescent.

*Rationale*
Adolescent patients retain new information best if they can see how it will immediately affect them. Long-term benefits have little meaning for them.

*Classification*
Competency Category: Nurse–Person Relationship
Taxonomic Level: Application

**106. B.** Preschool.

*Rationale*
Preschoolers believe that puppets and dolls are actually talking to them, so using puppets is a common teaching method in many children's hospitals.

*Classification*
Competency Category: Nurse–Person Relationship
Taxonomic Level: Application

**107. B.** Parental reinforcement.

*Rationale*
Positive parental reinforcement has the greatest impact on a child and provides reassurance and comfort to face potentially frightening experiences.

*Classification*
Competency Category: Nursing Practice: Alterations in Health
Taxonomic Level: Application

**108. A.** To measure brain growth.

*Rationale*
Measuring head circumference is an important determinant of brain growth and potential neurologic function.

*Classification*
Competency Category: Nursing Practice: Health and Wellness
Taxonomic Level: Knowledge/Comprehension

**109. B.** Conjunctivitis.

*Rationale*
Conjunctivitis is an infection of the conjunctiva that covers the eye. It is suspected in this case because erythema suggests an infection.

*Classification*
Competency Category: Nursing Practice: Alterations in Health
Taxonomic Level: Knowledge/Comprehension

**110. D.** Subconjunctival hemorrhage.

*Rationale*
A subconjunctival hemorrhage may be common in newborns because of the high pressures experienced during vaginal delivery. This kind of hemorrhage usually resolves within approximately 7 days.

*Classification*
Competency Category: Nursing Practice: Alterations in Health
Taxonomic Level: Critical Thinking

**111. C.** Pulling the pinna down and back.

*Rationale*
Pulling the pinna down and back best facilitates visualization for examining the ear canal of a child younger than 2 years old.

*Classification*
Competency Category: Nursing Practice: Health and Wellness
Taxonomic Level: Knowledge/Comprehension

**112. C.** Epiglottitis.

*Rationale*
An inflamed epiglottis will rise with the pressure of a tongue blade and potentially obstruct the airway.

*Classification*
Competency Category: Nursing Practice: Alterations in Health
Taxonomic Level: Knowledge/Comprehension

**113. A.** Sinus arrhythmia.

*Rationale*
This population may have a noticeable increase in heart rate during inhalation and a decrease in heart rate during exhalation.

*Classification*
Competency Category: Nursing Practice: Alterations in Health
Taxonomic Level: Application

**114. A.** The child's crying.

*Rationale*
It is extremely difficult to auscultate and evaluate heart and lung sounds in a crying child, and this is often the greatest obstacle.

*Classification*
Competency Category: Nursing Practice: Alterations in Health
Taxonomic Level: Application

**115. C.** A hearing deficit.

*Rationale*
Speech problems are directly related to hearing problems because the child is unable to actually hear the sounds or words to repeat them.

*Classification*
Competency Category: Nursing Practice: Alterations in Health
Taxonomic Level: Application

**116. D.** Artificially acquired passive immunity.

*Rationale*
A tetanus shot provides artificially acquired passive immunity and is given for rapid, temporary immunity.

*Classification*
Competency Category: Nursing Practice: Alterations in Health
Taxonomic Level: Application

**117. A.** Fluid and electrolyte imbalances.

*Rationale*
The extracellular fluid volume of a newborn is 40% of his or her total body water. Any incidence of vomiting or diarrhea can leave newborns at risk for a potentially serious situation of fluid and electrolyte imbalances.

*Classification*
Competency Category: Nursing Practice: Alterations in Health
Taxonomic Level: Knowledge/Comprehension

**118. B.** Toddler.

*Rationale*
Separation anxiety starts as early as 5 months old and is most evident in toddlers and preschoolers.

*Classification*
Competency Category: Nursing Practice: Health and Wellness
Taxonomic Level: Knowledge/Comprehension

**119. B.** Promoting open parental visiting.

*Rationale*
Most young children need to have their primary care-giver with them whenever possible. Many pediatric institutions have embraced open visiting hours for parents, including rooming-in, to facilitate minimizing the anxiety of both the child and the parents. Many health care professionals also encourage the primary caregiver to participate in the child's care while the child is hospitalized.

*Classification*
Competency Category: Nurse–Person Relationship
Taxonomic Level: Application

**120. A.** Disturbed sleep pattern.

*Rationale*
This child has a disturbed sleep pattern because of being frequently awakened during the night for neural assessments.

*Classification*
Competency Category: Nursing Practice: Alterations in Health
Taxonomic Level: Application

**121. D.** Clustering patient care.

*Rationale*
Clustering patient care minimizes the numbers of interruptions that are placed on a child who is resting. It is important for the nurse to organize tasks and responsibilities so that the number of disturbances to the child is minimized and as much care as possible can be clustered or completed at the same time. All of the other options provided could potentially disturb and interrupt a child's sleep pattern and contribute to sleep deprivation.

*Classification*
Competency Category: Nursing Practice: Alterations in Health
Taxonomic Level: Knowledge/Comprehension

**122. D.** Maternal alcohol consumption.

*Rationale*
Although maternal alcohol consumption places the fetus at considerable risk for many problems, a congenital heart defect is unlikely. All other choices listed are more likely to contribute to a congenital heart defect.

*Classification*
Competency Category: Nursing Practice: Alterations in Health
Taxonomic Level: Knowledge/Comprehension

**123. B.** Frequent small feeds throughout the day are preferred.

*Rationale*
Because these children fatigue so quickly, frequent small meals are suggested to ensure that the child receives his or her nutritional needs. Roughhousing would be considered too physically demanding on the child. Allowing child to set his or her own activity level works best. All future trips to the dentist will require prophylactic antibiotic therapy before the child has any procedures because the mouth contains bacteria that can be lethal in the form of infectious endocarditis if it enters the bloodstream.

*Classification*
Competency Category: Nurse–Person Relationship
Taxonomic Level: Critical Thinking

**124. C.** Clubbing of fingers.

*Rationale*
Clubbing of fingers is a change in the angle between the fingernail and the nail bed. It is seen because of the increased capillary growth in the fingertips that occurs while the body tries to supply more oxygen routes to distal body cells. It is a sign or cardiac or respiratory disease. Capillary refill is usually above 5 seconds in children with congenital heart defects, and most children with congenital heart disease tend to have a reddened complexion because of the polycythemia produced in attempt to oxygenate body cells. Children with congenital health defects are easily fatigued and often tired.

*Classification*
Competency Category: Nursing Practice: Alterations in Health
Taxonomic Level: Knowledge/Comprehension

**125. C.** 2:15.

*Rationale*
A ratio of two breaths per 15 compressions is used in older children, and one breath per five

compressions is used for infants and children younger than 8 years old.

*Classification*
Competency Category: Nursing Practice: Alterations in Health
Taxonomic Level: Knowledge/Comprehension

**126. A.** "The chance of my child arresting is unlikely."

*Rationale*
Children with any kind of heart disease are at high risk for a cardiopulmonary arrest, so this statement indicates that the father requires more health teaching.

*Classification*
Competency Category: Nursing Practice: Health and Wellness
Taxonomic Level: Application

**127. B.** Prodromal period.

*Rationale*
The prodromal stage includes nonspecific symptoms that are generally vague. This stage is short and proceeds to specific symptoms and illness.

*Classification*
Competency Category: Nursing Practice: Alterations in Health
Taxonomic Level: Knowledge/Comprehension

**128. C.** Droplet precautions.

*Rationale*
The restrictions placed identify droplet precautions. Coughing, sneezing, and talking are most likely to spread infection via droplet spores. Airborne precautions also include airflow requirements of the isolation room so that the air in the room is not circulated to the rest of the facility and the requirement that the room have a door that is closable, preferably with double-door access.

*Classification*
Competency Category: Nursing Practice: Alterations in Health
Taxonomic Level: Knowledge/Comprehension

**129. B.** A child who is immunosuppressed.

*Rationale*
An immunosuppressed child is at highest risk for developing a nosocomial infection because of a depressed immune system. Generally, the risk for nosocomial infections increases if the child is

hospitalized longer than 72 hours and has been receiving multiple courses of antibiotic therapy. A child who is ill at home is not at risk for developing a hospital-acquired infection.

*Classification*
Competency Category: Nursing Practice: Alterations in Health
Taxonomic Level: Knowledge/Comprehension

**130. A.** Erythema infectiosum (fifth disease).

*Rationale*
The presentation of fifth disease includes an age group of 2 to 12 years, fever, headache, malaise, and an intensely red rash on the face that gives the child a "slapped face" appearance.

*Classification*
Competency Category: Nursing Practice: Alterations in Health
Taxonomic Level: Knowledge/Comprehension

**131. D.** Fungus.

*Rationale*
Thrush is a fungal infection that presents with white plaques on the surface of the tongue and on the buccal membrane. The child will complain of pain and difficulty eating.

*Classification*
Competency Category: Nursing Practice: Alterations in Health
Taxonomic Level: Knowledge/Comprehension

**132. B.** Lyme disease.

*Rationale*
Lyme disease is transmitted by ticks and is seen in summer and early fall. Children who play in the forest are at risk.

*Classification*
Competency Category: Nursing Practice: Alterations in Health
Taxonomic Level: Knowledge/Comprehension

**133. B.** Infectious mononucleosis.

*Rationale*
This adolescent is presenting with symptoms indicating infectious mononucleosis.

*Classification*
Competency Category: Nursing Practice: Alterations in Health
Taxonomic Level: Application

**134. C.** To prevent rupture of the spleen.

*Rationale*

In patients with infectious mononucleosis, the spleen enlarges, and the individual is at risk for a spontaneous rupture with any trauma to the area. The child is placed on bed rest during the acute phase of illness, which usually lasts about 7 to 10 days, to prevent this complication.

*Classification*

Competency Category: Nursing Practice: Alterations in Health
Taxonomic Level: Application

**135. A.** Pernicious anemia.

*Rationale*

Pernicious anemia is caused by a vitamin B12 deficiency. The most frequent cause is an inability to use vitamin B12 with a lack of intrinsic factor. Symptoms usually appear the first 2 years of life, and the child is pale, anorexic, and irritable with chronic diarrhea. The beefy-red tongue is caused by papillary atrophy. Sickle cell anemia is the presence of abnormally shaped red blood cells, and aplastic anemia is a depression of hematopoietic activity in the bone marrow.

*Classification*

Competency Category: Nursing Practice: Alterations in Health
Taxonomic Level: Knowledge/Comprehension

**136. D.** The child will require lifelong monthly injections of vitamin B12.

*Rationale*

Pernicious anemia requires lifelong monthly intramuscular injections of vitamin B12. All other choices refer to iron deficiency anemia.

*Classification*

Competency Category: Nursing Practice: Health and Wellness
Taxonomic Level: Knowledge/Comprehension

**137. B.** 6 months of age.

*Rationale*

Iron stores develop near the end of gestation, so babies with low birth weight have fewer iron stores. Complicating this is the fact that babies with low birth weight also grow rapidly and their demand for red blood cells increases. Presentation is typically around the 6-month period when they have depleted all maternal stores.

*Classification*

Competency Category: Nursing Practice: Alterations in Health
Taxonomic Level: Knowledge/Comprehension

**138. D.** Chronic blood loss.

*Rationale*

Chronic blood loss is the most common cause in this age group. All other options listed and their complications would be seen much earlier in infants.

*Classification*

Competency Category: Nursing Practice: Alterations in Health
Taxonomic Level: Knowledge/Comprehension

**139. C.** 60 mg.

*Rationale*

6 mg × 30 kg = 180 mg/24 hours.
The dose is to be administered three times every 24 hours, resulting in 180 mg/3 = 60 mg/dose.

*Classification*

Competency Category: Nursing Practice: Alterations in Health
Taxonomic Level: Application

**140. B.** They have decreased hemoglobin levels.

*Rationale*

The altered hemoglobin level is caused by improper hemoglobin formation as a consequence of decreased iron stores in the body. The majority of the iron in the body is incorporated in hemoglobin.

*Classification*

Competency Category: Nursing Practice: Alterations in Health
Taxonomic Level: Knowledge/Comprehension

**141. A.** Meat.

*Rationale*

From the list, meat is the food source with the highest iron content.

*Classification*

Competency Category: Nursing Practice: Health and Wellness
Taxonomic Level: Knowledge/Comprehension

**142. B.** Sickle cell anemia.

*Rationale*

Sickle cell anemia occurs almost exclusively in people of African descent. The typical presentation is a protruding abdomen from an enlarged spleen and liver and yellow sclerae from chronic destruction of the sickled cells.

*Classification*
Competency Category: Nursing Practice: Alteration in Health
Taxonomic Level: Knowledge/Comprehension

**143. B.** The transfusion administered will be run as ordered.

*Rationale*
This order will require 112 mL/hr, which is safe and can be administered as ordered.

*Classification*
Competency Category: Nursing Practice: Alteration in Health
Taxonomic Level: Application

**144. C.** Isotonic.

*Rationale*
The blood must be infused with a solution that is as isotonic as possible. Normal saline is the correct choice.

*Classification*
Competency Category: Nursing Practice: Alteration in Health
Taxonomic Level: Application

**145. B.** An anaphylactic reaction.

*Rationale*
If these symptoms start immediately after a blood transfusion has begun, an anaphylactic reaction is occurring.

*Classification*
Nursing Practice: Alteration in Health
Taxonomic Level: Application

**146. D.** Discontinue the transfusion.

*Rationale*
The blood transfusion should be discontinued immediately and the attending physician contacted and informed of Dieon's current symptoms.

*Classification*
Competency Category: Nursing Practice: Alteration in Health
Taxonomic Level: Application

**147. A.** Hepatitis.

*Rationale*
It is likely that the child may have contracted hepatitis from a contaminated blood transfusion.

*Classification*
Competency Category: Nursing Practice: Alteration in Health
Taxonomic Level: Knowledge/Comprehension

**148. D.** Hemophilia A.

*Rationale*
Hemophilia A is suspected. Young infants do not have many injuries until they start moving and independently walking. A procedure such as circumcision may be the first opportunity to see the profuse bleeding associated with this disease.

*Classification*
Competency Category: Nursing Practice: Alteration in Health
Taxonomic Level: Application

**149. B.** A sex-linked recessive trait.

*Rationale*
Hemophilia A is best described as a disease caused by deficiency of the clotting factor VIII and is transmitted as a sex-linked recessive trait.

*Classification*
Competency Category: Nursing Practice: Alteration in Health
Taxonomic Level: Knowledge/Comprehension

**150. C.** Painful bleeding into the joints.

*Rationale*
Children present with bruising of the extremities, soft tissue bleeding, and painful hemorrhaging into the joints, which are injuries sustained when the child starts walking. A purpural rash on the buttocks may indicate Henoch-Schonlein syndrome. Whereas miniature petechiae may indicate idiopathic thrombocytopenic purpura, cyanotic fingers and toes may indicate disseminated intravascular coagulation.

*Classification*
Competency Category: Nursing Practice: Alteration in Health
Taxonomic Level: Knowledge/Comprehension

**151. D.** Injury prevention.

*Rationale*
Injury prevention is the priority focus for the health teaching. A priority focus when teaching parents is on how to prevent bleeding episodes and what to do when a bleed occurs.

*Classification*
Competency Category: Nursing Practice: Health and Wellness
Taxonomic Level: Critical Thinking

**152. C.** Administration of concentrated factor VIII.

*Rationale*
Hemophilia A is a deficiency of factor VIII, which is a coagulation component. Therefore, even minor bleeding episodes need to be controlled by administering factor VIII.

*Classification*
Competency Category: Nursing Practice: Health and Wellness
Taxonomic Level: Knowledge/Comprehension

**153. B.** Diurnal enuresis.

*Rationale*
Diurnal enuresis is urinary incontinence that occurs during the day. Nocturnal enuresis is urinary incontinence that occurs during the night. Children with primary enuresis never have a period of dryness. Children with secondary enuresis have had a 6- to 12-month period of dryness after a period of wetting.

*Classification*
Competency Category: Nursing Practice: Health and Wellness
Taxonomic Level: Knowledge/Comprehension

**154. C.** Urinary tract infections.

*Rationale*
Urinary tract infections are a common risk factor for enuresis and generally occur more commonly in boys than in girls. In addition, decreased bladder capacity is a common risk factor for urinary tract infections.

*Classification*
Competency Category: Nursing Practice: Health and Wellness
Taxonomic Level: Knowledge/Comprehension

**155. C.** Renal scarring.

*Rationale*
In addition to hypertension and decreased renal function, renal scarring is a potential long-term complication of urinary tract infections in children.

*Classification*
Competency Category: Nursing Practice: Alterations in Health
Taxonomic Level: Knowledge/Comprehension

**156. D.** Constipation.

*Rationale*
Constipation can cause pressure on the bladder and inhibit complete bladder emptying, resulting in

urinary stasis. Urinary stasis puts the child at risk for a urinary tract infection.

*Classification*
Competency Category: Nursing Practice: Alterations in Health
Taxonomic Level: Knowledge/Comprehension

**157. A.** Teaching young girls to wipe from front to back after going to the bathroom.

*Rationale*
Teaching young girls to wipe front to back takes germs away from the opening that leads to the urinary system and decreases the risk of developing urinary tract infections.

*Classification*
Competency Category: Nursing Practice: Health and Wellness
Taxonomic Level: Knowledge/Comprehension

**158. B.** "Current professional research indicates that this technique is key in preventing infections."

*Rationale*
Although sharing information and learning are encouraged in the nursing profession, it is the obligation of the nurse facilitating the inservice to correct misinformation that may be shared with the group.

*Classification*
Competency Category: Professional Practice
Taxonomic Level: Critical Thinking

**159. C.** Offering large quantities of any kind of fluid.

*Rationale*
A large quantity of any kind of fluid the child will drink will help flush the infection out of the urinary tract.

*Classification*
Competency Category: Nursing Practice: Alterations in Health
Taxonomic Level: Knowledge/Comprehension

**160. D.** Speak to the unit manager and fill out a medication error form.

*Rationale*
Nurses are expected to demonstrate professional conduct, including safely administering medication. Administering scheduled medication 1 hour late is a medication error and should be identified to the unit manager to speak directly with the nurse as per her job responsibilities.

*Classification*
Competency Category: Professional Practice
Taxonomic Level: Critical Thinking

**161. D.** "It sounds like you're feeling responsible for the illness. Can we talk about that?"

*Rationale*
Polycystic kidney disease is an inherited disorder. Restating or clarifying the parents' concerns and then giving them an opportunity to expand on them is the most therapeutic option available when communicating with the parents.

*Classification*
Competency Category: Nurse–Person Relationship
Taxonomic Level: Critical Thinking

**162. B.** A narrower cuff than necessary gives a higher reading.

*Rationale*
The cuff should be no more than two thirds and not less than half the length of the upper arm. A wider cuff will give a lower reading, and a narrower cuff will give a higher reading.

*Classification*
Competency Category: Nursing Practice: Alterations in Health
Taxonomic Level: Knowledge/Comprehension

**163. A.** Maintaining a tidy environment around the child.

*Rationale*
Visually impaired children explore their environment by feel. A tidy and organized environment can support this and promote the child's safety. It is a priority to make sure all items that could potentially injure the child are removed from the environment. This includes dinner trays and supplies for procedures.

*Classification*
Competency Category: Nursing Practice: Health and Wellness
Taxonomic Level: Critical Thinking

**164. D.** Use the phrase "the x-ray machine is like a big camera."

*Rationale*
This phrase helps the child associate what you are describing with something he or she is already familiar with. Using the term "test" implies that the child could either pass or fail the procedure. A school-age child will think you are taking all of his or her blood if the phrase "I want to take your blood" is used. Telling a child a procedure will not hurt usually leads

to a loss of trust. Even noninvasive procedures can be perceived as painful by a child who is anxious.

*Classification*
Competency Category: Nurse–Person Relationship
Taxonomic Level: Critical Thinking

**165. D.** Suggesting a shared assignment with a senior nurse.

*Rationale*
Suggesting a shared assignment shows collaboration and uses the experience and skills of colleagues. It would never be wise to continue with an assignment that was too difficult for the skill set and experience of the graduate nurse.

*Classification*
Competency Category: Professional Practice
Taxonomic Level: Application

**166. B.** The organs of hearing.

*Rationale*
Ototoxic drugs have an adverse effect on the organs of hearing.

*Classification*
Competency Category: Nursing Practice: Alterations in Health
Taxonomic Level: Knowledge/Comprehension

**167. D.** A child with a chronic infection receiving high-dose gentamycin therapy.

*Rationale*
Of the pharmacologic choices listed, high-dose antibiotic therapy is the most likely to potentially have an ototoxic effect.

*Classification*
Competency Category: Nursing Practice: Alterations in Health
Taxonomic Level: Critical Thinking

**168. B.** Echolalia.

*Rationale*
Echolalia describes the behaviour of repetitive words or phrases spoken by others. It is also described as compulsive parroting of what is said.

*Classification*
Competency Category: Nursing Practice: Alterations in Health
Taxonomic Level: Knowledge/Comprehension

**169. C.** Sleep disturbances are common for children with ADHD.

*Rationale*
Sleep disturbances are common for children with ADHD. The diagnosis is commonly made after the child starts attending school and is unable to display attentive behaviour in class.

*Classification*
Competency Category: Nursing Practice: Health and Wellness
Taxonomic Level: Critical Thinking

**170. C.** Caregiver role strain related to the demands of the child's care.

*Rationale*
The families of children with chronic illness require considerable support to manage the stress and challenges of caring for the child at home. These families are at high risk for caregiver role strain. Nursing support is needed to help families learn new adaptation skills to manage the child's care.

*Classification*
Competency Category: Nursing Practice: Health and Wellness
Taxonomic Level: Critical Thinking

**171. B.** Rohypnol.

*Rationale*
Rohypnol is a date rape drug. It is colorless, odorless, and tasteless. The effects are drowsiness, impaired motor skills, and amnesia.

*Classification*
Competency Category: Nursing Practice: Health and Wellness
Taxonomic Level: Application

**172. A.** Diet plays a significant role in acne production.

*Rationale*
Diet does not actually influence the development of acne lesions; rather, acne is caused by the changes in puberty, specifically the rapid increase in androgen secretion, which causes the sebaceous glands to become active.

*Classification*
Competency Category: Nursing Practice: Health and Wellness
Taxonomic Level: Knowledge/Comprehension

**173. C.** Children should always wear helmets when riding bicycles.

*Rationale*
Although some of the options provided are valid health teaching measures to prevent accidents in preschoolers, only one option realistically addresses head injury.

*Classification*
Competency Category: Nursing Practice: Health and Wellness
Taxonomic Level: Critical Thinking

**174. B.** They are being bullied themselves.

*Rationale*
Children who are bullies are generally lashing out with violence because they are being bullied themselves.

*Classification*
Competency Category: Nursing Practice: Health and Wellness
Taxonomic Level: Critical Thinking

**175. D.** Reading sex education pamphlets with the children.

*Rationale*
Reading the pamphlets with the children shows that you are available to answer their questions and can prompt specific discussion as you read together. Films rarely answer all of the questions this age group may have, and a question and answer period at the end is intimidating for youngsters, who rarely ask questions in front of their peers. Sex education classes are most beneficial if they are same-sex classes, which fosters a safer environment for asking questions. Giving school-age children pamphlets to read out of the presence of the nurse is ineffective because the children will rarely seek out the nurse to ask questions at another time.

*Classification*
Competency Category: Nursing Practice: Health and Wellness
Taxonomic Level: Critical Thinking

**176. A.** In the child's presence, discussing the difficulty he is having with speech.

*Rationale*
Discussing the child's speech difficulty in front of him will only make him more conscious of his speech patterns and probably aggravate the situation.

*Classification*
Competency Category: Nursing Practice: Health and Wellness
Taxonomic Level: Critical Thinking

**177. C.** Environmental factors.

*Rationale*
The greatest determinant of childhood obesity is environmental factors, which include parental diet choices and influence. Children of obese parents are inclined to obesity based on the food served in the family home.

*Classification*
Competency Category: Nursing Practice: Health and Wellness
Taxonomic Level: Knowledge/Comprehension

**178. A.** Introducing screening tests.

*Rationale*
Introducing screening tests is a part of preventive health because they may identify the presence of a health condition before symptoms are evident.

*Classification*
Competency Category: Nursing Practice: Health and Wellness
Taxonomic Level: Critical Thinking

**179. C.** Tourette's syndrome.

*Rationale*
Tourette's syndrome is an inherited disorder in which the individual displays a combination of vocal and motor tics as described in the stem of the question.

*Classification*
Competency Category: Nursing Practice: Alterations in Health
Taxonomic Level: Application

**180. D.** "If discontinued, Ritalin must be tapered off slowly."

*Rationale*
Ritalin must never be stopped abruptly and requires tapering of the dose as directed by a physician. Parents who see an improvement in the child may think the child no longer needs to take the medication, so information specific to the need to taper Ritalin is very important to share.

*Classification*
Competency Category: Nurse–Person Relationship
Taxonomic Level: Critical Thinking

**181. A.** Impaired social interaction related to the developmental disability.

*Rationale*
Autism is a disorder that involves abnormalities of communication and social interaction. The initial pri-

ority nursing diagnosis should focus on the child's impaired social interaction.

*Classification*
Competency Category: Nurse–Person Relationship
Taxonomic Level: Critical Thinking

**182. A.** Teach your child with a group of other children.

*Rationale*
Teaching a cognitively challenged child within a group of other children may lead to distraction and unsuccessful learning. Children with cognitively challenges need to be in an environment with little extra stimuli so they can focus on learning.

*Classification*
Competency Category: Nursing Practice: Health and Wellness
Taxonomic Level: Critical Thinking

**183. C.** "My granddaughter will never be able to attend school."

*Rationale*
Children with cognitive impairments are not restricted from attending school. They may need more individualized programs, but it is very important for them to attend school to learn how to socialize.

*Classification*
Competency Category: Nurse–Person Relationship
Taxonomic Level: Application

**184. B.** Imbalanced nutrition related to the inability to swallow.

*Rationale*
Gastrostomy tubes are inserted if a child cannot swallow or for medical conditions that include esophageal atresia, severe gastroesophageal reflux, and esophageal structures. Imbalanced nutrition would be a priority nursing diagnosis.

*Classification*
Competency Category: Nursing Practice: Alterations in Health
Taxonomic Level: Critical Thinking

**185. D.** Measure the space from the bridge of the nose to the earlobe to a point halfway between the xiphoid process and the umbilicus.

*Rationale*
This identifies the correct measurement for placement of an NG tube for a child younger than age

1 year. Answer A identifies the correct measurement for placement of an NG tube for a child older than age 1 year.

*Classification*
Competency Category: Nursing Practice: Health and Wellness
Taxonomic Level: Application

**186. B.** Capillary puncture.

*Rationale*
These anatomic sites are best used for capillary puncture.

*Classification*
Competency Category: Nursing Practice: Health and Wellness
Taxonomic Level: Knowledge/Comprehension

**187. A.** Developmental stage of the child.

*Rationale*
The developmental stage of the child determines the starting point with respect to how the child interprets the experience. All procedures, invasive or otherwise, produce stress for the child and perhaps also the parents. The presence of the parents may help settle a child but does not remove all anxiety and fear, particularly after a procedure has started.

*Classification*
Competency Category: Nurse–Person Relationship
Taxonomic Level: Knowledge/Comprehension

**188. A.** Glaucoma.

*Rationale*
Congenital glaucoma is an inner eye condition that involves increased intraocular pressure in the eye globe. Generally, this condition is a result of inadequate or blocked drainage of the aqueous humor. Congenital glaucoma is related to a developmental anomaly in the angle of the anterior chamber that prevents proper drainage at the canal of Schlemm.

*Classification*
Competency Category: Nursing Practice: Alterations in Health
Taxonomic Level: Application

**189. B.** Sharing that if left untreated, the condition will destroy the optic nerve.

*Rationale*
If left untreated, the pressure in the eye globe will continue to increase and eventually destroy the optic nerve. It is imperative that the child have therapeutic management initiated immediately.

*Classification*
Competency Category: Nurse–Person Relationship
Taxonomic Level: Critical Thinking

**190. B.** "Congenital glaucoma is usually a unilateral condition."

*Rationale*
Congenital glaucoma is usually bilateral. To share information that the condition is usually unilateral implies that the child has normal, unaffected vision in one eye. This inaccurate information would be cause for concern.

*Classification*
Competency Category: Nurse–Person Relationship
Taxonomic Level: Application

**191. D.** Cataract.

*Rationale*
Leukocoria is evident in a child suspected of having a cataract. The pupil opening appears to be white. In addition, subsequent blurred vision would be suspected in an infant who was not responding to the facial expressions of others and who could not grasp objects or toys placed near him or her.

*Classification*
Competency Category: Nursing Practice: Alterations in Health
Taxonomic Level: Knowledge/Comprehension

**192. A.** Vomiting.

*Rationale*
Vomiting is the greatest concern after surgery because it increases intraocular pressure, which may then put additional strain on the suture line.

*Classification*
Competency Category: Nursing Practice: Alterations in Health
Taxonomic Level: Critical Thinking

**193. A.** Myopia.

*Rationale*
Myopia is nearsightedness. The light rays focus at a point in front of the retina, and the individual is able to clearly see objects directly in front of him or her but is unable to see at a distance.

*Classification*
Competency Category: Nursing Practice: Alterations in Health
Taxonomic Level: Application

**194. C.** It is important to make sure that visually impaired children hear you before touching them.

*Rationale*
It is important that all members of the health care team understand that it is best to speak to a visually impaired child before touching him or her. It is not necessary to speak loudly because the child's hearing is not generally impaired nor is his or her cognitive ability.

*Classification*
Competency Category: Nursing Practice: Alterations in Health
Taxonomic Level: Knowledge/Comprehension

**195. C.** A red tympanic membrane.

*Rationale*
An unaffected tympanic membrane is shiny and pearl gray in color. A red or bulging tympanic membrane indicates an infection.

*Classification*
Competency Category: Nursing Practice: Alterations in Health
Taxonomic Level: Knowledge/Comprehension

**196. B.** A full prescribed course of antibiotics is necessary.

*Rationale*
A full course of antibiotic therapy is necessary to ensure that the infection has been completely eradicated.

*Classification*
Competency Category: Nurse–Person Relationship
Taxonomic Level: Critical Thinking

**197. A.** The tympanic membrane has spontaneously ruptured.

*Rationale*
A sudden resolution of ear pain often indicates that the tympanic membrane has spontaneously ruptured, and the relief of the buildup of pressure has resolved the pain.

*Classification*
Competency Category: Nursing Practice: Alterations in Health
Taxonomic Level: Critical Thinking

**198. B.** To provide air to the middle ear.

*Rationale*
A myringotomy tube is placed into a child's ear to provide air to the middle ear to prevent otitis media with effusion. If the source of air to the middle ear is cut off, the epithelial cells of the ear change in function and become secretory cells, and the ear fills with secretions. The placement of the myringotomy tube for 6 to 12 months generally stops the secretory process of the middle ear.

*Classification*
Competency Category: Nursing Practice: Alterations in Health
Taxonomic Level: Critical Thinking

**199. D.** This is a short-term problem.

*Rationale*
The course of otitis media with effusion is long term in most children. Parents and children need continued support and encouragement throughout the duration of myringotomy tube insertion.

*Classification*
Competency Category: Nursing Practice: Alterations in Health
Taxonomic Level: Critical Thinking

**200. C.** "I'm going to review some choices you have regarding your care."

*Rationale*
Reviewing choices and options provides patients with a sense of control over their own health situation and empowers them to make choices. It is likely that this adolescent is actually striving to have more control over his chronic illness rather than feeling controlled by it.

*Classification*
Competency Category: Nursing Practice: Health and Wellness
Taxonomic Level: Critical Thinking

## ▶ Short Answer Questions

**201. Answer:**

- Children with cystic fibrosis generally display ineffective breathing patterns. Therefore, breathing exercises would be a priority for the following two reasons: to develop full lung capacity and strengthen lung tissue.

*Rationale*
Children with cystic fibrosis generally display ineffective breathing patterns that do not expand full lung capacity. This leaves them predisposed to frequent respiratory infections.

*Classification*
Competency Category: Nurse–Person Relationship
Taxonomic Level: Critical Thinking

**202. Answers:**

- Coughing.
- Bearing down to pass stool.
- Pain.
- Agitation.

*Rationale*

Chronic constipation and straining to pass stool, persistent and frequent coughing, pain, and being agitated are all potential causes for an increased intracranial pressure in the pediatric population.

*Classification*

Competency Category: Nursing Practice: Alterations in Health

Taxonomic Level: Knowledge/Comprehensions

**203. Answers:**

- By asking the child to swallow.
- By eliciting a gag reflex by pressing a tongue blade on the posterior surface of the tongue.

*Rationale*

Cranial nerve X (i.e., the vagus nerve) measures swallowing and the gag reflex. The answers provided identify how a nurse would assess the patient if cranial nerve X were intact.

*Classification*

Competency Category: Nursing Practice: Alterations in Health

Taxonomic Level: Knowledge/Comprehension

**204. Answers:**

- When a child experiences a seizure for the first time, it indicates epilepsy or a true seizure disorder.
- When an adult experiences a seizure for the first time, it indicates a structural cause such as a space-occupying lesion, tumor, stroke, or trauma.

*Rationale*

The answers provided represent the significant differences between initial onset of seizures in children versus adults.

*Classification*

Competency Category: Nursing Practice: Alterations in Health

Taxonomic Level: Critical Thinking

**205. Answer:** Mistakenly inserting the NG into the lung field because no cough or gag reflex is intact when the patient is unconscious.

*Rationale*

When inserting an NG tube into an unconscious child, a serious risk is mistakenly inserting the NG tube into the lung field. Because the child is unconscious, the child's cough or gag reflex is no longer intact.

*Classification*

Competency Category: Nursing Practice: Alterations in Health

Taxonomic Level: Knowledge/Comprehension

**206. Answer:** If a family is using herbal remedies at home to treat a child's illness, this information must be shared with health care professionals.

*Rationale*

The most important information related to home herbal remedies is to make sure the parents are sharing this information with medical professionals. This is to ensure that the child does not receive two different forms of the same drug or drugs that may counteract the home remedy.

*Classification*

Competency Category: Nurse–Person Relationship

Taxonomic Level: Knowledge/Comprehension

**207. Answers:**

- Celiac disease is a sensitivity to the gluten factor of protein found in grains.
- Specific grains to be removed from the diet include wheat, rye, oats, and barley.

*Rationale*

Children diagnosed with celiac disease have a sensitivity to the gluten factor of protein found in grains. Children diagnosed with this disease and their families must be instructed about diet and diet modifications. Specific grains to be removed from the diet include wheat, rye, oats, and barley.

*Classification*

Competency Category: Nursing Practice: Health and Wellness

Taxonomic Level: Knowledge/Comprehension

**208. Answers:**

- Low-grade fever.
- Complaints of pain at the injection site.

*Rationale*

Low-grade fever and complaints of pain at the injection site are common side effects of injection among children.

*Classification*

Competency Category: Nursing Practice: Health and Wellness

Taxonomic Level: Knowledge/Comprehension

**209. Answers:**

- Personality traits.
- Parental presence.
- Meaning of pain.
- Developmental level.
- Culture.
- Past experiences.

*Rationale*
Personality traits, the presence of the child's parents, the developmental level of the child, personal meanings of pain, culture, and past experiences can influence a child's response to pain.

*Classification*
Competency Category: Nursing Practice: Alterations in Health
Taxonomic Level: Knowledge/Comprehension

**210. Answer:** Respiratory failure is the leading cause of cardiac arrest in children because of the diameter of the airway and obstruction.

*Rationale*
Respiratory failure is the leading cause of cardiac arrest among children and infants. Because of the small diameter of children's airways, obstruction can occur.

*Classification*
Competency Category: Nursing Practice: Alterations in Health
Taxonomic Level: Knowledge/Comprehension

**211. Answer:** Congestive heart failure is a process that indicates that the heart is unable to maintain cardiac function to meet the metabolic demands of the heart. Cardiac output is insufficient.

*Rationale*
When speaking with parents of children with congenital heart disease, a concise description should be provided.

*Classification*
Competency Category: Nurse–Person Relationship
Taxonomic Level: Knowledge/Comprehension

**212. Answers:**

- Congestive heart failure is generally the first consequence seen in a child with congenital heart disease and is often diagnosed first.
- It can also remain an ongoing complication.

*Rationale*
Parents of children with congenital heart disease also need information about congestive heart failure because congestive heart failure is generally the first consequence seen in a child with congenital heart disease. It is often the primary diagnosis and can remain an ongoing complication.

*Classification*
Competency Category: Nursing Practice: Alterations in Health
Taxonomic Level: Knowledge/Comprehension

**213. Answers:**

- Reduce the child's exposure to the allergen.
- Reduce the child's response to the allergen with pharmacologic intervention.

*Rationale*
The primary goal of therapeutic management for the parents of a child diagnosed with allergies includes reducing the child's exposure to the allergen and response to the allergen with pharmacologic intervention.

*Classification*
Competency Category: Nursing Practice: Health and Wellness
Taxonomic Level: Critical Thinking

**214. Answer:** Narcan.

*Rationale*
Narcan is an opioid antagonist that is given as an antidote for morphine. An antidote is an agent that neutralizes a poison or counteracts its effects.

*Classification*
Competency Category: Nursing Practice: Alterations in Health
Taxonomic Level: Knowledge/Comprehension

**215. Answer:** The child squats or assumes a knee-to-chest position to trap blood in the lower extremities because of the hyperflexion of the knee and hip.

*Rationale*
Children with congenital heart disease squat or assume a knee-to-chest position to trap blood in the lower extremities. This allows them to more easily oxygenate the blood remaining in the upper body.

*Classification*
Competency Category: Nursing Practice: Alterations in Health
Taxonomic Level: Knowledge/Comprehension

**216. Answer:** The straw prevents staining of the teeth from the ferrous sulfate.

*Rationale*
Drinking from a straw helps minimize staining of the teeth. This can be a side effect noted when ferrous sulfate is taken in liquid form.

*Classification*
Competency Category: Nursing Practice: Health and Wellness
Taxonomic Level: Application

**217. Answer:** Vitamin C enhances absorption of the elixir.

*Rationale*
The child is directed to take the ferrous sulfate elixir with citrus juice because vitamin C enhances the absorption of the elixir.

*Classification*
Competency Category: Nursing Practice: Alterations in Health
Taxonomic Level: Knowledge/Comprehension

**218. Answer:** *Escherichia coli,* a gram-negative pathogen commonly spread through stool.

*Rationale*
*Escherichia coli* is a gram-negative pathogen that is commonly spread through stool.

*Classification*
Competency Category: Nursing Practice: Alterations in Health
Taxonomic Level: Knowledge/Comprehension

**219. Answer:** Oral administration of antibiotics specific to the pathogen.

*Rationale*
Oral administration of antibiotics specific to the pathogen would be the most likely course of medical treatment in a child with a urinary tract infection.

*Classification*
Competency Category: Nursing Practice: Alterations in Health
Taxonomic Level: Knowledge/Comprehension

**220. Answers:**

- It is a lower urinary tract infection seen in some young adolescent women after their first sexual intercourse experience.
- These urinary tract infections occur because of inflammation and local irritation caused by sexual activity.

*Rationale*
These urinary tract infections occur because of inflammation and local irritation caused by sexual activity.

*Classification*
Competency Category: Nurse–Person Relationship
Taxonomic Level: Critical Thinking

**221. Answers:**

- Pain on urination.
- Burning.
- Hematuria.
- Frequency.

*Rationale*
The answers provided are all common symptoms of urinary tract infections in children ages 10 to 16 years.

*Classification*
Competency Category: Nursing Practice: Alterations in Health
Taxonomic Level: Knowledge/Comprehension

**222. Answers:**

- Fever.
- Abdominal pain.
- Enuresis.
- Malaise.

*Rationale*
The answers provided are all common symptoms of urinary tract infections in children ages 3 to 8 years.

*Classification*
Competency Category: Nursing Practice: Alterations in Health
Taxonomic Level: Knowledge/Comprehension

**223. Answer:** Motor vehicle accidents.

*Rationale*
Motor vehicle accidents are the leading cause of death among adolescents because of their poor decision-making skills, inexperience, risk-taking behaviours, and immaturity. Recent research suggests that the frontal lobe of the brain is not fully developed in adolescents, so their poor decision-making skills are influenced by biology (see http://www.waldorflinbrary.org/Articles/Adolesce2.pdf).

*Classification*
Competency Category: Nursing Practice: Health and Wellness
Taxonomic Level: Application

**224. Answers:**

Physiologic Risks:

- Iron deficiency anemia.
- Preeclampsia (a complication of pregnancy characterized by increasing hypertension, proteinuria, and edema).
- Cephalopelvic disproportion.

*Rationale*

Many teenage girls have an iron deficiency because of their low protein intake from an inability to balance the amount of iron lost with the menstrual flow. Pregnancy compounds iron deficiency anemia because the teenager must supply enough iron for fetal growth and her increasing blood volume. Iron supplements should be taken during pregnancy and would likely be addressed during prenatal care sessions. Preeclampsia and edema are most likely to occur in primiparas younger than 20 years of age.

Monitoring blood pressure is another component of prenatal assessments. Cephalopelvic disproportion occurs because of the still immature development of the adolescent body. A predetermined disproportion detected during prenatal care sessions offers the opportunity for appropriate planning rather than a long, exhausting birthing process in which the baby is not descending.

*Classification*
Competency Category: Nursing Practice: Health and Wellness
Taxonomic Level: Application

**225. Answers:**

- Preterm birth.
- Baby with low birth weight.
- Increased rates of smoking in pregnant adolescent females (refer to http://www.hc-sc.gc.ca/hl-vs/pubs/tobac-tabac/ssbs-peda/ags-at_e.html).
- Risk for inadequate nutrition because of adolescent dietary habits.
- Possibly poor weight gain in an effort to minimize appearance of being pregnant.

*Rationale*

A preterm baby (one born before the end of 37 weeks gestation) is at risk for multiple medical complications, depending on the gestational age. A baby with low birth weight may be a full-term infant but one who will have difficulty maintaining core body temperature, have a wasted appearance, and

have multiple other medical challenges. The infant is also at risk for inadequate nutrition because of adolescent dietary habits and possibly poor weight gain because of the mother's effort to minimize her appearance of being pregnant.

*Classification*
Competency Category: Nursing Practice: Health and Wellness
Taxonomic Level: Application

**226. Answers:**

- Interruption of developmental tasks.
- Increased psychological load and stress.
- Fears of rejection by peers and parents.
- Conflict in parental and own value systems.
- Financial dependence on parents.

*Rationale*

All of the answers provided are psychological risks of an adolescent mother as a direct result of not receiving prenatal care.

*Classification*
Competency Category: Nursing Practice: Health and Wellness
Taxonomic Level: Application

**227. Answers:**

- Living in poverty.
- Having low educational achievement.
- Living in a dysfunctional family.
- Engaging in high-risk behaviours
- Having low self-esteem.
- Having a sense of immorality.
- Having a belief that pregnancy could never happen to oneself.

*Rationale*

Young women may try to use a pregnancy to escape a poor living situation. Those with low education and literacy levels may not possess the knowledge or information needed to protect themselves from unwanted pregnancies. Also, young women living in family situations with few rules or boundaries may be at increased risk for unwanted pregnancy. Adolescents may have little regard for the consequences of having unprotected sex. Additionally, a young woman with low self-esteem may be pressured into a sexual relationship, resulting in an unwanted pregnancy. In addition, adolescents often have a belief that pregnancy could never happen to them and therefore neglect to use contraceptives.

*Classification*
Competency Category: Nursing Practice: Health and Wellness
Taxonomic Level: Critical Thinking

## 228. Answers:

* Inadequate weight gain.
* Failure to thrive.
* Poor growth pattern.
* Constant hunger.
* Seasonally unsuitable clothes.
* Poor hygiene.
* Developmental delays.
* Thin hair.
* Muscle weakness.
* Poor stamina.

*Rationale*
All of the answers provided are possible indicators that a child is being neglected.

*Classification*
Competency Category: Nursing Practice: Alterations in Health
Taxonomic Level: Knowledge/Comprehension

## 229. Answer: Fear of the electric cast cutter.

*Rationale*
Children at this age often have a strong fear of the electronic cast cutter. They are afraid that the cast cutter will cut their limb as well.

*Classification*
Competency Category: Nursing Practice: Alterations in Health
Taxonomic Level: Critical Thinking

## ▶ Self-Analysis for Chapter 5

> 200 Multiple-choice questions × 1 point each = /200 points
> +
> 29 Short answer questions for a total of 50 points = /50 points
>
> ***Total Child Health Nursing review questions = /250 points***

## SUPPLEMENTAL RESOURCES

Adams, M., Josephson, D., & Holland, L. (2005). *Pharmacology for nurses: A pathophysiologic approach.* Upper Saddle River, NJ: Pearson Education.

Bindler, R., & Ball, J. (2003). *Clinical skills manual for pediatric nursing* (3rd ed.). Upper Saddle River, NJ: Prentice Hall.

Hatfield, N. (2004). *Introducing pediatric nursing* (6th ed.). Philadelphia: Lippincott Williams & Wilkins.

Ignatavicius, D., & Workman, L. (2006). *Medical-surgical nursing: Critical thinking for collaborative care* (5th ed.). St. Louis: Elsevier.

Leifer, G. (2004). *Introduction to maternity and pediatric nursing* (4th ed.). St. Louis: Elsevier.

Karch, A. (2006). *2006 Nursing drug guide.* Philadelphia: Lippincott Williams & Wilkins.

London, M., Ladewig, P., Ball, J., & Bindler, R. (2005). *Maternal–newborn & child nursing: Family centered care.* Upper Saddle River, NJ: Prentice Hall.

McCance, K., & Huether, S. (2004). Pathophysiology: *The biologic basis for disease in adults and children* (5th ed.). St. Louis: Mosby.

Newsham, D. (2000). Parental non-concordance with occlusion therapy. *British Journal of Ophthalmology, 84*(9), 957–962.

Pillitteri, A. (2003). *Maternal & child health nursing: Care of the childbearing and childbearing families* (4th ed.). Philadelphia: Lippincott Williams & Wilkins.

Porth, C. (2005). *Pathophysiology: Concepts of altered health states* (7th ed.). Philadelphia: Lippincott Willliams & Wilkins.

Taylor, C., Lillis, C., & LeMone, P. (2005). *Fundamentals of nursing: The art and science of nursing care* (5th ed.). Philadelphia: Lippincott Williams & Wilkins.

Wong, D., Perry, S., Hockenberry, M., & Lowdermilk, D.L. (2006). *Maternal child nursing care* (3rd ed.). St. Louis: Mosby.

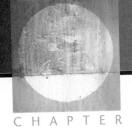
# 6 Maternal–Child Health Nursing

**Directions:** Below are 200 multiple-choice questions and short answer questions totaling 250 points. These questions will test your knowledge of nursing with a maternal child health population. These questions offer a wide array of case-based and stand-alone questions representing the taxonomies of critical thinking, application, and knowledge/comprehension. Also reflected in these questions are the nursing competencies of health and wellness, alterations in health, professional practice, and nurse–person relationship. After completing these practice questions, check your work in the Answers and Rationales section located at the end of the chapter. Please note the topic areas and types of questions you found difficult and develop a plan to review study sources and increase your knowledge of these areas.

## ▶ Multiple-Choice Questions

1. A nurse orienting a new staff member for the shift asks if he can be assigned the least complex intrapartum case to give him time to review documentation. Which of the following intrapartum factors places the fetus at least risk?

    A. Placenta previa.
    B. Cord compression.
    C. Abruptio placenta.
    D. Early fetal heart decelerations.

2. Which of the following statements about the viral disease toxoplasmosis in pregnancy is appropriate for nurses to teach pregnant women in prenatal classes?

    A. The infant may present with central nervous system anomalies, rhinitis, and rash on the palms and soles of the feet.
    B. The infected newborn will secrete this virus for many years.

    C. The infant is usually asymptomatic at birth with symptoms, such as chronic diarrhea, recurrent infections, and neurologic dysfunction, emerging over the first 2 years of life.
    D. The condition is contracted from raw meat and cat feces.

3. A nurse is teaching newborn care to a group of new mothers. Which of the following will the nurse identify as the predominant methods of heat loss in newborns?

    A. Sweating and peripheral vasoconstriction.
    B. Transepidermal water loss and radiative and convective losses.
    C. Loss through urine and feces.
    D. Sweating and conductive losses.

4. Jessica McCourt is in her second trimester of pregnancy. The nurse observes large brown spots on Jessica's cheeks. Jessica asks the nurse about other skin changes that she might expect during her pregnancy. Which of the following responses about skin changes in pregnancy is appropriate?

    A. Lightening of the nipples and breast areolas.
    B. Decrease in sweating.
    C. Noticeable decrease in the growth of hair.
    D. Darkened line in the midline of the abdomen.

5. When performing Leopold's maneuvers, the nurse feels a firm, round, movable part in the fundal portion of the uterus and a long, smooth surface in the mother's right side close to the midline. What is the likely position of the fetus?

    A. ROA.
    B. LSA.
    C. RSA.
    D. LOA.

6. Rhonda, age 23 years, is a long-distance runner and is 8 weeks pregnant with her first baby.

Rhonda tells the nurse that she would like to continue running throughout the pregnancy and asks the nurse if there are any safety risks because of changes in her musculoskeletal system. Which response by the nurse correctly identifies musculoskeletal changes in pregnancy that may be a safety risk to Rhonda?

A. All muscles are weakened.
B. The long bones increase in density.
C. The spinal column flattens.
D. The joints of the pelvis relax.

7. Madeline Brown is in her third trimester of pregnancy. Upon assessment, the nurse observes that Madeline has diastasis recti. Which of the following is the best description of this term?

A. Numbness and tingling of the hands associated with pressure on the brachial plexus.
B. Separation of the central muscle, allowing the abdominal contents to protrude from the midline.
C. Edema involving the peripheral nerves during the last trimester.
D. Softening of connective and collagen tissue from circulating sex hormones.

8. A triage nurse is completing an initial assessment of the women in the waiting room. Which of the following statements helps the nurse to correctly recognize that a woman is in true labour?

A. "I passed some thick, red-tinged mucus when I urinated this morning."
B. "My baby dropped, and I have to urinate more frequently now."
C. "The contractions in my uterus are getting stronger and closer now."
D. "My bag of waters just broke."

9. Which of the following situations does the nurse recognize as having the greatest risk for the fetus?

A. A fundal height of 27 cm at 32 weeks gestation.
B. A fetal heart rate of 170 bpm with fetal movements.
C. A breech lie.
D. A gestational age of 37 weeks.

10. The physician has left instructions for the nurse to call when the client is in the second stage of labour. Which of the following does the nurse identify as a sure sign that the second stage of labour has begun?

A. The amniotic membranes rupture.
B. The cervix cannot be felt during a vaginal examination.

C. The woman experiences a strong urge to bear down.
D. The presenting part is below the ischial spines.

*Case Study:* Helen Jones, a 19-year-old primigravida, is 40 weeks pregnant with her first baby. She is admitted in early labour. She tells you that she is frightened about her labour and birth. Helen's partner, Josh, is sitting in the waiting room. Questions 11 to 15 relate to this scenario.

11. Which of the following actions is correct when using palpation to assess the characteristics and pattern of Helen's uterine contractions?

A. Place your hand on her abdomen below the umbilicus and palpate the uterine tone with your fingertips.
B. Determine the frequency by timing from the end of one contraction until the end of the next contraction.
C. Evaluate the intensity by pressing your fingertips into the fundus.
D. Assess uterine contractions every 30 minutes throughout the first stage of labour.

12. Helen reports that her contractions are "less painful." The nurse assesses that Helen's contractions are mild and irregular. Which of the following suggestions by the nurse for changing position would be most appropriate to promote efficient uterine contractions?

A. Sitting or standing.
B. Lying supine.
C. Lying prone.
D. Sidelying.

13. As Helen's labour progresses, she asks you if she could use the warm-water tub bath on the unit. Which of the following responses by the nurse would be most appropriate?

A. "No. No one is allowed to tub bathe during labour."
B. "Yes, as long as your membranes are not ruptured."
C. "Yes, as long as the warm water doesn't raise your temperature."
D. "No, because warm water can diminish labour contractions."

14. Helen would like to have an epidural anesthesia and asks about the risks of the procedure. Which of the following responses would be most appropriate?

A. The risks include hypotension and a prolonged second stage of labour.

B. The risks include severe headache and coldness in the lower extremities.

C. The risks include continued back pain and a short first stage of labour.

D. The risks include hypertension and a reduced red blood cell count.

15. Josh tells the nurse that he will remain in the waiting room while Helen is in labour. Helen's sister has been chosen to be her birth companion. Which of the following nurse's responses would be most appropriate?

A. Encourage Josh to stay with his wife because, as the father, he is the best birth companion.

B. Tell Josh that he will receive updates of his wife's progress and be called as soon as the baby is born.

C. Inform Helen and Josh that only fathers can stay in the birthing room.

D. Asks Helen if she agrees with Josh's desire to stay in the waiting room.

16. Tobias, one of the participants in a prenatal class, inquires about the role of a doula in labour. Which of the following responses would be most appropriate?

A. Doulas time contractions and keep them from becoming too lengthy.

B. Doulas perform vaginal examinations and abdominal assessment during labour.

C. Doulas can serve as a support person and coach during labour.

D. The doula replaces the husband as a woman's support person.

17. In planning resources for the community, the nurse recognizes which of the following family forms as the most socially vulnerable?

A. Blended family.

B. Extended family.

C. Nuclear family.

D. Single-parent family.

18. A nurse is preparing to write a research paper on prenatal care and overall health in industrialized nations. Which of the following indicators will provide the most information on the adequacy of prenatal care and overall health in industrialized nations?

A. Incidence of specific infections such as tuberculosis and AIDS.

B. Infant mortality rate.

C. Maternal mortality rate.

D. Incidence of low-birth-weight infants.

19. Jennifer Adams works on the antenatal unit and has been asked to cover in the fetal assessment unit for a few hours. The client Jennifer is caring for is ordered a contraction stress test (CST), and Jennifer is uncertain how to perform the procedure. Which of the following actions by Jennifer would be most appropriate?

A. Refer to the AWHONN (2006) guidelines for professional practice and follow the printed guidelines.

B. Consult the agency procedure book and follow the printed guidelines.

C. Consult with a senior nurse on the unit.

D. Do not proceed with the procedure.

---

*Case Study:* Millie is a 45-year-old divorced white woman. She is also a pediatric nurse at the children's hospital. Her youngest child is now 25 years old. She has been experiencing unusually heavy periods for the past 6 months and then no period for the past 3 months. During these 3 months, Millie has been fatigued and experiencing nausea and vomiting. Despite feeling unwell, she has gained 3 kg in the past 3 months.

Millie comes to the clinic to obtain information on menopause and to find out why she has been feeling so sick. Her pregnancy test result is positive. Millie appears to be in disbelief. The physical examination confirms a uterus enlarged to a 15-week size, and fetal heart tones are heard. Millie is spotting. Questions 20 to 23 relate to this scenario.

20. Which of the following does the nurse identify as a risk associated with Millie's pregnancy?

A. Hypotension.

B. Pregnancy loss.

C. Obesity.

D. Phenylketonuria.

21. Which of the following appropriately identifies the screening test for congenital anomalies?

A. Chorionic villa sampling.

B. Triple test for alpha fetoprotein.

C. Amniocentesis.

D. Doppler test.

22. Millie has just completed a series of hepatitis B vaccine. Which of the following responses by the nurse would be appropriate regarding the risks of this vaccine to the fetus?

A. Neurologic defects.

B. Congenital heart defects.

C. Macrosomia.

D. No risks.

23. Millie tells the nurse she stopped taking her birth control pills because she thought she was in menopause. Which of the following nurse's statements is appropriate?

    A. "You usually need to have been without a period for 6 month to be sure you will not get pregnant."
    B. "Menopause is never predictable, and until you are 50-years-old, you are capable of getting pregnant."
    C. "A woman should continue her method of birth control until she has not had a period for 1 year."
    D. "You should always use protection to prevent STIs. As a nurse, you should know this risk."

24. Constance had a cesarean section with her first pregnancy and is hoping to have a vaginal birth with this pregnancy. She begins to cry at her 38-week visit when she realizes that her baby is a breech presentation. She says, "I just know it's going to be horrible again. I won't be able to breastfeed my baby. It will be painful." Which of the following nurse's response is appropriate?

    A. "Tell me about your previous baby's birth."
    B. "Don't worry. We will be here to help you through this."
    C. "A cesarean section is always done for breech presentation."
    D. "It is safer to have a cesarean section than a VBAC."

25. A new mother is distraught over the unusual shape of her baby's head. Which of the following is an accurate response from the nurse when explaining about caput succedaneum?

    A. It is a subcutaneous collection of blood between the cranial bone and the periosteum.
    B. It is from patent anterior and posterior fontanels.
    C. It is caused by swelling of the tissues over or under the fetal scalp during labour.
    D. It is asymmetrical overriding of cranial bones caused by birth.

26. Which of the following does the nurse identify is the most important component of the Apgar score?

    A. Heart rate.
    B. Respiratory rate.
    C. Color.
    D. Muscle tone.

27. Which of the following Apgar scores does the nurse appropriately recognize as indicating the need for stimulation of the newborn?

    A. 0 to 3.
    B. 4 to 6.
    C. 7 to 9.
    D. 8 to 10.

28. Baby Garm is observed for episodes of rapid respirations, gagging, and regurgitation of mucus during reactivity periods. Which of the following is the nurse's best explanation for when reactivity periods occur?

    A. When the infant becomes chilled.
    B. During the first two or three feedings.
    C. At 4 to 6 hours of life.
    D. After the baby cries.

29. A new mother questions the nurse about when her colostrum will be replaced with "real milk." Which of the following is the most appropriate nurse's response?

    A. 12 hours after birth.
    B. Days 1 to 2.
    C. Days 2 to 5.
    D. 1 week.

30. While working in the newborn nursery, a nurse appropriately identifies which of the following as the most appropriate nursing action to prevent neonatal infection?

    A. Good hand washing.
    B. Isolation of infected infants.
    C. Universal precautions.
    D. Separate gown technique.

31. During the first postpartum day after a vaginal birth, the nurse notices that the mother is talkative but is hesitant to make decisions about the baby. According to Reva Rubin (1984), which of the following is the appropriate phase the woman is experiencing?

    A. Having trouble attaching to her baby.
    B. The taking-in phase.
    C. The taking-hold phase.
    D. The letting-go phase.

32. Which of the following is an accurate statement about hemodynamic changes occurring in the postpartum period?

    A. Increase in hematocrit.
    B. Transient tachycardia.
    C. Decrease in circulatory blood volume.
    D. Increase in cardiac output.

33. The nurse correctly identifies which of the following as the hormone that plays a central role in the preparation of the breast for lactation?

    A. Estrogen.
    B. Prolactin.
    C. Oxytocin.
    D. Progesterone.

34. When teaching a group of new mothers, the nurse correctly identifies the following as the time when physiologic jaundice may be found in the newborn:

    A. During the first 24 hours of life.
    B. Between 2 and 4 days of life.
    C. After 5 days postpartum.
    D. Often with formula-fed babies.

35. Billie is concerned about how long to nurse her newborn each time. Which of the following responses is an appropriate response from the nurse?

    A. She should nurse for 5 to 10 minutes.
    B. She should nurse for 10 to 20 minutes.
    C. She should nurse for 20 to 30 minutes.
    D. The duration of breastfeeding should be determined by the newborn's signs of satiety.

36. Mrs. Dassouki has a puerperal infection. Which of the following is one of the initial signs of a puerperal infection in a postpartum woman?

    A. Pain.
    B. Malaise.
    C. Foul-smelling lochia.
    D. Fever.

37. The nurse appropriately identifies which of the following as one of the signs or symptoms of a pulmonary embolus in a postpartum woman?

    A. Sudden intense back pain.
    B. Unusual apprehension.
    C. Hypertension.
    D. Bradycardia.

38. Which of the following is an appropriate nursing intervention for treatment of thrombophlebitis in a postpartum woman?

    A. Leg massage.
    B. Restriction of fluid intake.
    C. Elevation of the affected leg.
    D. Discouragement of mobility.

39. A new mother asks the nurse why her baby's hands and feet are bluish in color. Which of the following is the nurse's best response for the name of this condition?

    A. Erythema toxicum.
    B. Vernix caseosa.
    C. Acrocyanosis.
    D. Harlequin color.

40. The nurse correctly recognizes which of the following trends are occurring within the childbearing population in Canada?

    A. Increase in cesarean section rate.
    B. More natural births with less medical interventions.
    C. Increase in public funds for using midwives.
    D. Increase in VBACS (vaginal births after cesarean sections).

41. Which of the following does the World Health Organization (WHO) recommend as the duration for *exclusive* breastfeeding from birth?

    A. 3 to 4 months.
    B  4 to 6 months.
    C. 6 months.
    D. 1 year.

42. What is the correct initiation rate for breastfeeding for Canadian women today?

    A. 55%.
    B. 65%.
    C. 75%.
    D. 85%.

43. Currently, how many Canadian women still breastfeed at 6 months?

    A. 30%.
    B. 40%.
    C. 50%.
    D. 60%.

44. The nurse appropriately identifies which of the following factors that has influenced the trend in Canada toward shorter hospital stays after delivery?

    A. Research validating the safety of shorter stays.
    B. Efforts to contain health care costs.
    C. Cooperative efforts between caregivers and families.
    D. The need to improve access to quality care.

45. A client questions the nurse about how long her postpartum flow will last. Which of the following is the nurse's most appropriate response?

    A. 5 to 7 days.
    B. 1 to 3 weeks.

C. 2 to 6 weeks.

D. 7 to 12 weeks.

46. A client, Ruby, would like to attend a new mothers' group that meets in her community. Her mother tells her that she shouldn't go out for at least 30 days after the baby's birth. Ruby is unhappy about this and asks the nurse if she can go. What is the nurse's most appropriate response?

A. Reassure her that leaving the house before 30 days postpartum is not prohibitive.

B. Discuss the differences between beliefs among cultures.

C. Discuss what her mother's concerns are.

D. Discuss Ruby's wants and desires.

47. Which of the following nurse's statements is accurate about postpartum depression in postpartum women?

A. It occurs within 3 to 5 days postpartum.

B. It is more prevalent in our North American culture.

C. It occurs in 10% to 15% of all postpartum women.

D. It is easy to recognize.

48. Which of the following *protective* factor(s) decreases the incidence of postpartum depression in postpartum women?

A. Early discharge from hospital.

B. Supportive relationship with the primary care provider.

C. Ongoing relationships with other mothers with young children.

D. Passive coping behaviours.

49. Which of the following amounts of blood loss within 24 hours does the nurse appropriately classify as a vaginal postpartum hemorrhage?

A. 500 mL.

B. 750 mL.

C. 1000 mL.

D. 1500 mL.

50. Signs and symptoms the nurse would observe with a late postpartum hemorrhage include which of the following?

A. Backache.

B. Lochia alba.

C. Boggy uterus.

D. Need for the peripad to be changed every 4 hours for moderate amounts of lochia.

51. Two days after her delivery, Juniata is given a shot of RhoGAM. At the postpartum home visit, Juniata asks the nurse why she needed RhoGAM. The most appropriate response from the nurse of why women are given RHOGAM is which of the following?

A. To suppress antibody formation in a woman with Rh-positive blood after giving birth to an Rh-negative baby.

B. To suppress antibody formation in a woman with Rh-negative blood after giving birth to an Rh-positive baby.

C. To suppress antibody formation in a woman with Rh positive-blood after giving birth to an Rh-positive baby.

D. To suppress antibody formation in a woman with RH-negative blood after giving birth to an Rh-negative baby.

52. When asked by a student nurse what complications can occur after an episiotomy, the nurse knows which of the following is the most appropriate response?

A. Difficulty with voiding.

B. Perineal discomfort.

C. Mobility difficulties.

D. Difficulty with breastfeeding.

53. When asked by a new mother when she can stop giving her infant formula and start giving him cow's milk, which of the following is the most appropriate response from the nurse?

A. 4 to 6 months old.

B. 6 to 9 months old.

C. 9 to 12 months old.

D. After 12 months old.

54. A new father asks the nurse about supplementation of vitamin D for his newborn. Which of the following is the most appropriate response from the nurse?

A. "Your baby will receive vitamin D when he starts solid foods."

B. "Newborns in Canada do not need a supplement of vitamin D because of exposure to large amounts of sunshine."

C. "Your baby needs 200 IU per day when being breastfed."

D. "Your baby needs 400 IU per day when being breastfed."

55. Cassie tells the nurse she would like to breastfeed for the first month postpartum and then switch her baby to cow's milk. The nurse knows which of the following nutritional information about cow's milk?

A. Cow's milk lacks adequate protein.

B. Cow's milk is an acceptable alternative.

C. Cow's milk should not be used with infants younger than 9 months of age.

D. Cow's milk has higher amounts of iron.

56. When asked by a father to compare the feeding habits between formula-fed and breastfed infants, which of the following is the correct response from the nurse about formula-fed infants?

A. They experience shorter periods between feeds.

B. They digest their milk more rapidly.

C. They wish to feed every 1.5 to 3 hours.

D. They usually feed every 3 to 4 hours.

57. Melissa calls a public health nurse at 3 weeks postpartum to tell her that her infant, who is breastfed, is not gaining weight as rapidly as her friend's newborn, who is the same age and is formula fed. Which of the following is the most appropriate response from the nurse?

A. "All babies gain weight at different times. It is important to not make comparisons."

B. "You need to bring your baby into the office because she may be ill."

C. "Formula-fed babies generally gain weight faster than breastfed babies."

D. "Your friend may be overfeeding her baby."

58. A nurse is scheduling a phenylketonuria (PKU) metabolic screening test for a newborn. The nurse knows that the most appropriate time to perform the heel stick is which of the following?

A. No later than 12 hours after birth.

B. At least 24 hours after birth.

C. Before the baby has been breastfed or received formula.

D. Immediately after the first feed of glucose and water.

59. A new father asks a nurse how to know if he is using good bottle-feeding technique. The most appropriate response from the nurse would be which of the following?

A. Prop the bottle on a rolled towel.

B. Point the nipple at the infant's tongue.

C. Keep the nipple full of formula throughout the feeding.

D. Burp the newborn only after he or she has finished the bottle.

*Case Study:* A community health unit is analyzing data to determine program and service needs for the population that she is serving. Questions 60 to 62 relate to this scenario.

60. The nurse is providing the results of a community assessment to her colleagues. Which of the following determinants of health does she know is most influential on the outcomes of the postpartum families living within this community?

A. Income and social status.

B. Education and literacy.

C. Social support networks.

D. Physical environment.

61. The community nurse is working with local agencies and businesses to find space to provide a free parenting group for low-income women. Which of the principles of primary health care will she use when finding space in the women's own community?

A. Using appropriate technology.

B. Increasing accessibility.

C. Encouraging community participation.

D. Prevention and health promotion.

62. The nurse acquires space in a community hall and establishes a support group for low-income postpartum women in the neighborhood. This is an example of which of the following Ottawa Charter strategies for health promotion?

A. Creating supportive environments.

B. Strengthening community action.

C. Developing personal skills.

D. Building healthy public policy.

*Case Study:* Baby Tran develops a yellowish tinge to his trunk and face within the first 24 hours after birth. The nurse is providing care for him in the newborn nursery. Questions 63 to 65 relate to this scenario.

63. Baby Tran becomes lethargic and has difficulty breastfeeding. The nurse is aware that the most likely condition the baby is experiencing is which of the following?

A. Pathologic jaundice.

B. Physiologic jaundice.

C. Breastfeeding jaundice.

D. Bile duct blockage.

64. The nurse reflects on Baby Tran's change in skin color. Which of the following is the most appropriate nursing response?

A. Do nothing because the jaundice will resolve as the liver matures.

B. Keep an eye on the change in skin color over the next 24 hours.

C. Notify Baby Tran's primary caregiver as soon as possible.

D. Advise the mother to stop breastfeeding and offer formula instead.

65. When Baby Tran's parents notice his skin color, they ask the nurse if their baby has "that deadly liver disease." The most appropriate nursing response would be which of the following?

A. "We will be isolating your baby for a few days until his skin is no longer yellow. He has a condition known as jaundice."

B. "This has nothing to do with your baby's liver."

C. "I can tell you are worried about your baby. Let's talk about this change in your baby's skin color."

D. "You let us worry about your baby. This is a pretty critical time for him."

*Case Study: Jasmine complains to her colleague about the heavy client assignments. Jasmine tells her colleague that she is currently providing care for three women in labour at the same time. Jasmine's colleague advises her to "hang in there; it will get better soon!" Questions 66 to 69 relate to this scenario.*

66. Despite cutting her lunch and coffee breaks short, Jasmine confides that she still does not have enough time to provide good nursing care to her clients. Which of the following best describes the minimum "standard of care" required of registered nurses?

A. The minimum number of registered nurses required to provide safe care.

B. Nursing care as described in policy and procedure manuals.

C. The care that a reasonable, prudent nurse would provide in a comparable situation.

D. The minimum number of total nursing time required for safe nursing practice.

67. One of the women Jasmine is caring for requires a cesarean section for labour dystocia. The woman's husband signs the consent form for the cesarean section. Which of the following individuals is responsible for obtaining the informed consent before a cesarean section?

A. The primary care provider.

B. The admitting nurse.

C. A senior staff nurse.

D. Jasmine.

68. Jasmine answers the call bell in one of her assigned birthing rooms. The client and her husband are very distressed and complain that Jasmine has been negligent in providing care during the woman's labour. Which of the following is Jasmine's best defense against an accusation of negligence?

A. She was acting on the advice of an experienced nurse.

B. She is certified in all competencies required for nursing care.

C. She met the national standards of practice.

D. She followed the primary care provider's written orders.

69. As a novice nurse, Jasmine is frustrated by the increased workload on the nursing staff. Which of the following best describes the attributes of experienced nurses?

A. They spend more time giving direct care to women in labour.

B. They know more about the physiology of labour and birth.

C. They are more aware of the subtle cues that indicate changes during labour and birth.

D. They require less supervision in managing complex cases.

*Case Study: Farrah, para 3, gravida 4, is admitted to the birth centre in labour early on Sunday morning. She has been living in Canada for 9 years and is fluent in English. Farrah is accompanied by her mother-in-law. Questions 70 to 74 relate to this scenario.*

70. Although Farrah is fluent in English, she defers to her mother-in-law when asked to sign the hospital consent forms. Which of the following factors contributes to the challenges the nurse faces in obtaining consent?

A. Patterns of verbal communication.

B. Religious beliefs.

C. Influence of the extended family.

D. Gender identity.

71. Farrah's husband, Hameed, arrives at the birth centre with two family members. The family is distressed to discover that the on-call physician is a man. Hameed forbids the physician from providing care for his wife. What is the nurse's best strategy in which to provide care in labour and birth when confronted with a cultural conflict?

A. Tell the family they are compromising the well-being of the baby.

B. Ask the mother to talk to her husband and convince him that it is okay.

C. Try to educate the family about the physician's on-call schedule.

D. Try to respect the cultural limitations in each situation.

**72.** The nurse is reviewing Farrah's prenatal history. Which of the following is a significant factor in anticipating complications in labour and birth?

A. History of postpartum hemorrhage (PPH).

B. Urinary tract infection at 16 weeks gestational age.

C. Para 3, gravida 4.

D. Amniocentesis performed at 14 weeks gestational age.

**73.** The nurse completes the maternal and fetal assessments. Farrah is experiencing contractions every 3 minutes, ROP position, intact membranes, and a moderate amount of bloody show. The quality of the tracing on the external fetal monitor is poor, and the nurse would like to place an internal fetal scalp electrode (FSE) to better assess the baby. Which of the following prevents the nurse from being able to complete this activity?

A. The moderate amount of bloody show.

B. The frequency of the uterine contractions.

C. The intact membranes.

D. The position of the baby.

**74.** The fetal heart rate (FHR) shows a baseline of 120 bpm with variability present. Which of the following is the range for normal fetal heart rate?

A. 110 to 160 bpm.

B. 110 to 180 bpm.

C. 120 to 160 bpm.

D. 100 to 180 bpm.

---

*Case Study:* William and Lilly are visiting family members in Canada. They are Chinese citizens expecting their first baby in 6 weeks. Lilly has been experiencing nausea and backache for the past 12 hours. The nurse quickly discovers that William and Lilly do not read or write English. Questions 75 to 79 relate to this scenario.

**75.** The primary care provider has ordered a biophysical profile (BPP) test. Which of the following is the best way for the nurse to obtain the couple's consent for the test?

A. Read the information on the consent form slowly in English and instruct Lilly to sign the consent.

B. Allow the primary care provider to deal with the situation. Assume that William and Lilly will understand what will happen.

C. Locate a bilingual staff member or an interpreter to translate before the couple signs the consent.

D. Use nonverbal language (pictures or gestures) to explain what will happen and ensure that the couple understands.

**76.** The BPP test is performed, and the score is 6. The primary care provider orders an induction of labour (IOL) with Pitocin. The nurse identifies the most significant factor behind Lilly's induction of labour is which of the following?

A. The reassuring BPP score.

B. The family wants their baby to be Canadian.

C. The suspicious BPP score.

D. The family is unable to afford long-term hospitalization in Canada.

**77.** Lilly is becoming more vocal and is moaning with her regular uterine contractions. The nurse performs a fetal and maternal assessment. Based on the assessment findings, the nurse discontinues the Pitocin. Which of the following is the correct indication for discontinuing the IV Pitocin?

A. The uterine contractions exceed 80 seconds in duration.

B. The uterine contractions are more frequent than every 1 to 2 minutes.

C. The uterus does not relax between uterine contractions.

D. Lilly is complaining of increasing discomfort.

**78.** The nurse notes that Lilly's temperature is elevated and her mucous membranes are becoming dry. Lilly is refusing ice and sips of water. Which is the most appropriate nursing action at this time?

A. Encourage Lilly to drink the ice and water.

B. Notify the primary care provider.

C. Increase the IV Pitocin to 125 mL/hr for hydration.

D. Offer Lilly hot beverages.

**79.** Lilly is restless and moving frequently in bed. She appears to be more uncomfortable with the contractions but refuses pain medication when offered. William leaves the room to stretch his legs. Which of the following nurse's response is most helpful?

A. Stand silently at the back of the room.

B. Stand next to her at the side of the bed.

C. Turn up the volume of the music playing in the room.

D. Turn on the television as a focal point.

**Case Study:** *Lisa and Mark arrive to at the hospital stating that the uterine contractions began 4 hours ago. As they are walking into the fetal assessment unit, Mark tells the nurse that this is Lisa's fourth pregnancy. Questions 80 to 84 relate to this scenario.*

80. What is the most immediate question for the nurse to ask Lisa and Mark during the immediate assessment?

    A. "When is your baby due?"
    B. "Have you taken prenatal classes?"
    C. "Do you have any known allergies?"
    D. "Do you have a birth plan?"

81. The assessment reveals that Lisa is 5 cm dilated, 60% effaced, 0 station, vertex presenting in the LOP position. From this data, which of the following can the nurse expect while providing care in labour and birth?

    A. Precipitous labour and birth.
    B. Braxton Hicks contractions.
    C. Vaginal breech birth.
    D. Back labour.

82. Lisa's baby is currently at 38 6/7 weeks gestational age. If the baby is born today, which of the following terms accurately describes the gestational age of the newborn?

    A. Premature.
    B. Postterm.
    C. Preterm.
    D. Term.

83. Mark provides the nurse with the birth plan that they wish to follow, if possible. Mark is coaching Lisa through the contractions. What is the best way for the nurse to meet this family's needs during labour and birth?

    A. Enter the birthing room as few times as possible to do the required assessments.
    B. Enter the birthing room only when requested.
    C. Stay in the room as much as possible because they will likely require support.
    D. Contact the primary care provider to discuss the birth plan.

84. Lisa's membranes rupture, and the nurse notes that the amniotic fluid is meconium stained. Which of the following activities should the nurse immediately perform?

    A. Administer oxygen at 4 L/min.
    B. Change the client to the left lateral position.

    C. Inform the primary care provider that birth is imminent.
    D. Begin continuous fetal heart rate monitoring.

**Case Study:** *Holly is 6 weeks pregnant after many fertility treatments. While at work, she experiences mild cramping and has a gush of bright red vaginal bleeding. Questions 85 to 89 relate to this scenario.*

85. Holly calls the 24-hour nurse hotline in great distress. She is soaking a maxi pad in less than 1 hour with fresh blood. What is the most appropriate response from the nurse?

    A. Tell her that it is nothing to worry about because many women have bleeding during their pregnancies.
    B. Tell her to lie down and call her health care provider tomorrow if the symptoms continue.
    C. Do nothing because she is likely miscarrying.
    D. Have her seek immediate attention from her primary care provider.

86. Holly and her husband Jeff wonder if the bleeding has been caused by Holly's working long hours in a stressful work environment. What is the most appropriate response from the nurse?

    A. "Your spontaneous bleed is not work related."
    B. "It is hard to know why a woman bleeds during early pregnancy."
    C. "I can understand your need to find an answer about what caused this. Let's talk about this further."
    D. "There must have been something wrong with the pregnancy."

87. A student nurse asks the nurse how common miscarriages are within all pregnancies. How many clinically recognized pregnancies end in miscarriage?

    A. 5% to 10%.
    B. 10% to 20%.
    C. 20% to 30%.
    D. 30% to 40%.

88. Holly does not miscarry and is advised to be on moderate bed rest until the bleeding subsides. Holly is concerned about missing work, as well as not being able to do any housework or cooking. What is the most appropriate response from the nurse?

    A. "Let's talk about what you can do while on bed rest to still meet these needs."
    B. "You don't want to do anything to jeopardize this pregnancy."

C. "Who can help you in this regard?"
D. "It is only for a brief period of time during your pregnancy."

89. Holly is experiencing muscle cramps and pain in her legs while on bed rest. What is an appropriate recommendation from the nurse?

A. Do passive ROM exercises.
B. Do gentle exercises of the legs.
C. Walk around the room a few times every hour.
D. Limit all activity.

*Case Study:* Trina, a 42-year-old primigravida, is 22 weeks pregnant with twins after many years of trying to conceive. Questions 90 to 94 relate to this scenario.

90. Trina is experiencing uterine cramping with light activity. She does not have any backache or bloody show. She is quite concerned about the cramping and asks the nurse what is happening. The most appropriate response from the nurse would be which of the following?

A. "You are showing the early signs of preterm labour."
B. "You are probably experiencing Braxton Hicks contractions."
C. "You are likely miscarrying."
D. "These cramps are nothing to worry about."

91. Based on the assessment that the nurse makes regarding Trina's cramping, which of the following recommendations is appropriate from the nurse?

A. She should change her activity.
B. She should call her primary care provider.
C. She should go to an emergency room for an urgent assessment.
D. She should do nothing and wait to see if her symptoms progress.

92. Trina has not been drinking many liquids for the past few days. The nurse recommends she drink 8 to 10 glasses of water because hydration will:

A. Flush toxins from Trina's system.
B. Increase blood flow to the placenta.
C. Decrease uterine contractility.
D. Decrease vaginal infections.

93. Trina gets very agitated with the situation and tells the nurse that she can't cope with anything else happening in her pregnancy. Which of the

following immediate responses is most appropriate from the nurse?

A. "You are coping just fine. Look how far you have made it in your pregnancy!"
B. "You have been through a lot already with your pregnancy. Let's talk about this further."
C. "Do you have anyone to talk to about this? You seem really stressed."
D. "I know you are upset. However, you need to put this in perspective for the sake of the pregnancy."

94. Two days later, Trina tells the nurse that her husband George blames her for the cramping, telling her that she is not taking good care of herself. Which of the following is the most appropriate response from the nurse?

A. "What do you think, Trina? Did you do anything you shouldn't have?"
B. "Your husband is wrong. You didn't do anything to cause this."
C. "Let's talk about how this cramping occurs so we can help you understand what causes it."
D. "It is natural to blame one another when things become difficult."

*Case Study:* Cayley, a 36-year-old multipara, is at 20 weeks gestation and comes to the prenatal clinic in distress. The nurse is going in to assess her status. Questions 95 to 99 relate to this scenario.

95. Cayley has been experiencing swelling of her lower extremities and headaches two to three times a week. She is worried about her baby and her own health. What is an appropriate response from the nurse?

A. "Your symptoms are normal for your gestation. You have nothing to worry about."
B. "I am glad you came in! We need to assess you further."
C. "I am sending you to your primary care provider this afternoon."
D. "Well, you are pregnant, so we can expect some symptoms."

96. Cayley tells the nurse she has been to see her primary care provider but does not feel like he is taking her symptoms seriously. Which of the following is the most appropriate response from the nurse?

A. "Try not to take it personally."
B. "You are right to be upset with him."
C. "Have you thought of switching providers?"
D. "Tell me more about your experience with your primary care provider and how this made you feel."

**97.** Cayley's baseline blood pressure before pregnancy was 112/72 mm Hg, and today it is 153/83 mm Hg. There is no protein in Cayley's urine. The nurse believes Cayley is likely experiencing which of the following prenatal conditions?

   A. Mild preeclampsia.
   B. Hypotension of pregnancy.
   C. Mild eclampsia.
   D. Hypertension.

**98.** Cayley calls the nurse at 22 weeks gestation to report that she is experiencing some swelling of her face and hands, with puffiness in her eyelids in the morning. What is an appropriate response from the nurse?

   A. Tell her that this is a normal finding during pregnancy.
   B. Tell her to lie in a lateral recumbent position.
   C. Tell her to monitor her symptoms for 24 hours.
   D. Refer her to her primary care provider.

**99.** Cayley tells the nurse that her in-laws are coming to stay for a long holiday and they have not changed their plans, even with Cayley experiencing complications in her pregnancy. Cayley's husband gets defensive when she tries to discuss it with him. The most appropriate response from the nurse is which of the following?

   A. "It is inappropriate that they are coming for a visit at this time."
   B. "Tell me what you are most worried about regarding their visit, and we can go from there."
   C. "Why is your husband defensive? He should stand up for the two of you."
   D. "I think you can manage with them here and be on bed rest."

---

*Case Study: Ruth is 38 years old and is pregnant with twins. She has an appointment at the prenatal clinic. Questions 100 to 104 relate to this scenario.*

**100.** Ruth asks the nurse what risks are associated with having twins. What is an appropriate response from the nurse?

   A. Hypotension and bradycardia.
   B. Fetal macrosomia.
   C. Oligohydramnios.
   D. Low birth weight.

**101.** The student nurse asks the nurse what the risk for preterm labour is for women who are carrying multiple fetuses. The most appropriate response from the nurse is which of the following?

   A. 35%.
   B. 40%.
   C. 45%.
   D. 55%.

**102.** When asked by a student which population of women is at *highest* risk for spontaneous preterm birth, which of the following is the most appropriate response from the nurse?

   A. Those of low socioeconomic status.
   B. Those who smoke.
   C. Those with a multi-fetal pregnancy.
   D. Those who are unusually fatigued.

**103.** Within 1 month, Ruth is placed on bed rest within the antenatal care program and has a nurse visit her on a regular basis at home. Which of the following recommendations should the nurse suggest to her about her position in bed?

   A. She should lie on her right side as much as possible.
   B. She should lie on her left side as much as possible.
   C. She should lie on her back as much as possible.
   D. She can lie in whichever position is comfortable.

**104.** Ruth's husband approaches the nurse after the prenatal appointment and expresses his concern about how the family will cope with twins. What is an appropriate response from the nurse?

   A. "You will do fine. Families have been having twins a long time!"
   B. "Can you afford to get someone to help in the home?"
   C. "Let's talk about what is concerning you."
   D. "Have you contacted your local twin and triplet club for further support?"

---

*Case Study: A nurse is facilitating a series of early pregnancy childbirth education classes in the community for single parents. Questions 105 to 109 relate to this scenario.*

**105.** The nurse knows that the childbirth education classes meet which of the following determinants of health for the parents in the community?

   A. Community participation.
   B. Social support networks.

C. Prevention and health promotion.

D. Accessibility.

106. The nurse receives word from her nursing manager that because of budget cuts, the childbirth education classes will no longer be subsidized for parents. The nurses in the health unit begin to lobby their health department and provincial government for funding to keep the subsidies available. This is an example of which value within the Canadian Nurses Association (CNA) 2002 Code of Ethics?

A. Accountability.

B. Justice.

C. Dignity.

D. Health and well-being.

107. The nurse facilitating the childbirth education classes does a "needs assessment" with the group of parents on the first day of class. This teaching strategy is best used for which of the following reasons?

A. To assess the parents' readiness and interest in learning.

B. To identify strategies for change.

C. To create an environment conducive to learning.

D. To evaluate the learning process.

108. A mother approaches the nurse to discuss which childbirth education classes she should take. Which of the following responses is the most appropriate from the nurse?

A. "Is this your first pregnancy?"

B. "What do you want to learn about?"

C. "What classes are available at the centre?"

D. "What can you afford?"

109. After class one week, a group of concerned mothers approaches the nurse to tell her that one of the nurse facilitators has been sharing their personal stories with other parents outside of the group. Which behaviours within the therapeutic relationship are not being demonstrated?

A. Accountability.

B. Confidentiality.

C. Advocacy.

D. Responsibility.

*Case Study:* Madison has delivered a dead fetus at 36 weeks gestation. Madison and her husband are overwhelmed with disbelief and confusion. Questions 110 to 114 relate to this scenario.

110. The nurse knows that the correct term for losing a fetus at this time is which of the following?

A. Miscarriage.

B. Neonatal death.

C. Stillbirth.

D. Abortion.

111. Two hours after giving birth, Madison turns to the nurse and asks, "What do you think caused my baby to die? What did I do wrong?" Which of the following nurse's responses would be most appropriate?

A. The nurse is silent and stays present with Madison.

B. "It is hard to know why a baby at this age would die."

C. "Do you want me to get the hospital chaplain?"

D. "I can understand your need to find an answer about what caused this. Let's talk about this further."

112. The nurse is aware that which of the following factors affects Madison and her husband's response to this loss?

A. Previous experience with children.

B. Expectation of a healthy birth outcome.

C. Support from a spiritual leader.

D. Assigned meaning to the event.

113. In assisting Madison and her husband to deal with their loss, which of the following actions would be most appropriate from the nurse?

A. Control his or her emotions so as to not upset the parents.

B. Remind them that everything happens for a reason and there must have been something wrong with the baby.

C. Provide an early opportunity for the couple to see their child if they desire.

D. Leave the parents alone as much as possible in their grief.

114. Madison asks the nurse about the "triple marker test" done in pregnancy. Which of the following nurse's response is correct?

A. The test assesses for Down syndrome.

B. The test assesses for spina bifida.

C. The test assesses for anencephaly.

D. The test assesses for a congenital cardiac anomaly.

115. Ruby and Clarence show the nurse their birth plan. The nurse inquires about their specific choices and wishes for the birth of their first baby. Which of the following best describes why

the nurse is asking questions about the family's birth plan?

A. Establishing rapport with the family.
B. Acting as an advocate for the family.
C. Attempting to correct any misinformation the family may have received.
D. Recognizing the family as active participants in their care.

116. A woman's membranes have ruptured and the amniotic fluid is meconium stained. The nurse inserts an internal fetal scalp electrode (FSE). What is the nurse's best explanation for why the woman requires internal fetal monitoring?

A. Assure her that the baby is fine.
B. The baby has had a bowel movement that indicates severe fetal distress.
C. The baby needs to be observed more closely.
D. The FSE has been ordered by the primary care provider.

117. Which of the following does the nurse recognize as a non-reassuring fetal heart rate pattern?

A. Accelerations with contractions.
B. Early decelerations with contractions.
C. Variable decelerations.
D. Late decelerations with minimal variability.

118. Brandi, age 15 years, is 4 cm dilated and 100% effaced and is in active labour with her first baby. The nurse contacts the primary care provider to communicate her findings of fetal heart rate decelerations, thick meconium in the amniotic fluid, and low fetal scalp pH results. What is the most appropriate nursing action at this time?

A. Encourage Brandi to get into the right lateral position.
B. Increase the oxygen to 7 L/min.
C. Prepare Brandi for an assisted or cesarean birth.
D. Contact the social worker to inform him or her of imminent birth.

119. Which of the following is the most common cause for late decelerations?

A. Maternal position.
B. Prematurity.
C. Placental insufficiency.
D. Cord compression.

120. Beth and Douglas arrive to the hospital stating that Beth's contractions started 3 hours ago. As they are walking into the room, Beth tells the nurse that this is their fifth baby. What is the

nurse's first priority while performing the admission?

A. Review Beth's obstetrical history.
B. Assess Beth's coping skills in labour.
C. Ensure that Beth will have a support person in labour.
D. Assess the imminence of birth.

121. Karen, a multiparous 26-year-old woman, has been in labour for several hours and is becoming anxious and distressed with her frequent strong contractions. The nurse observes a moderate amount of bloody show and performs a vaginal examination to assess the progress of labour. What does the nurse anticipate Karen's cervical dilatation will be at this time?

A. 1 to 2 cm.
B. 3 to 4 cm.
C. 5 to 7 cm.
D. 8 to 10 cm.

122. A nurse responds to the call bell in the room of Bertha, a multiparous woman who has been in labour for 2 hours. Bertha tells the nurse that she feels "the baby coming." The nurse observes the baby's head crowning. Which of the following is the nurse's most immediate response?

A. Instruct the woman to push through the pain.
B. Return to the nurse's station to phone the primary care provider.
C. Tell the woman not to push.
D. Instruct the woman to pant so the nurse can support the baby's head as it crowns.

123. A nurse has been providing care to a woman in labour for the past 9 hours. The father remains at the bedside while his partner is sleeping with the epidural block in situ. Which of the following is the most appropriate nursing action?

A. Encourage the father to take a break for 1 hour.
B. Instruct the father to contact another support person to take his place because he is exhausted.
C. Offer to remain with the woman while he takes a short break.
D. Suggest that he goes home to sleep for a few hours.

124. Maxine is a primigravida in early labour. She asks the nurse for pain medication. Which of the following is the nurse's most appropriate response?

A. No; narcotics cause fetal depression.
B. No; narcotics may lead to maternal hypotension.

C. Yes; narcotics are very effective in early labour.

D. No; narcotics prolong labour.

**125.** Jane is experiencing difficulties coping with her frequent and strong uterine contractions. The vaginal examination reveals that Jane's cervix is 4 to 5 cm dilated and 80% effaced. The nurse suggests the use of a narcotic analgesic to make her more comfortable, but Jane is frightened the medication will hurt the baby. What is the nurse's most appropriate response?

A. "This medication does not cross the placenta, so your baby will not receive any of the medication."

B. "Some of the medication crosses the placenta, but your baby will not experience serious side effects."

C. "Some of the medication crosses the placenta, but it should be out of the baby's system by the time of birth."

D. "Some of the medication crosses the placenta, but is quickly excreted by the fetus."

**126.** Delphine states that she doesn't want any pain medication during labour. She tells the nurse that she wants something for the "burning pain when the baby comes out." Which of the following is the nurse's best suggestion to help Delphine meet her goal during labour and birth?

A. General anesthesia.

B. IV narcotic analgesia.

C. IM narcotic analgesia.

D. Pudendal block.

*Case Study:* Gretchen and Xavier are expecting their third baby. Xavier tells the nurse that the contractions started 5 hours ago and are now coming every 3 minutes and lasting for 60 seconds. Questions 127 to 130 relate to this scenario.

**127.** The nurse performs the initial assessment and reports the following findings to the primary care provider: The fetal heart rate is 152 bpm, cervix is 100% effaced and 5 cm dilated, the membranes are intact, and the presenting part is well applied to the cervix and is at -1 station. The nurse recognizes that Gretchen is in which stage of labour?

A. Second.

B. Latent.

C. Active.

D. Third.

**128.** The nurse determines that Gretchen has an antenatal or intrapartum risk score of 2. Based on this information, which activity level should the nurse recommend to Gretchen during labour?

A. Bathroom privileges only.

B. Ambulate ad lib.

C. Up in the chair at the side of the bed.

D. Complete bed rest with IV hydration.

**129.** The nurse performs another assessment 4 hours later. Gretchen's contractions continue to be 1:3 for 60 seconds duration and of mild intensity. Her cervix remains at 5 cm dilated and 100% effaced. Based on these findings, which of the following procedures will Gretchen most likely experience during this labour and birth?

A. Oxytocin induction.

B. Biophysical profile.

C. Oxytocin augmentation.

D. Amnioinfusion.

**130.** The primary care provider arrives at the hospital and decides that Gretchen will require a cesarean section. What is the final assessment the nurse should make in the birthing room immediately before Gretchen is transported to the operating theatre?

A. Vaginal examination.

B. Abdominal palpation.

C. Fetal heart tones.

D. Maternal temperature.

*Case Study:* Mrs. Ballal, age 19 years, para 0, gravida 1, term pregnancy, was discharged home last evening in false labour. Questions 131 to 135 relate to this scenario.

**131.** Mrs. Ballal returns to the hospital complaining of strong contractions for the past 2 hours. Which of the following assessments will indicate to the nurse that she is in true labour?

A. Progressive cervical dilatation and effacement.

B. Mucousy pink show.

C. Increased fetal activity.

D. 1:5 uterine contractions.

**132.** The nurse assesses Mrs. Ballal's contractions. Which of the following methods will the nurse use to measure the duration of the 1:5 uterine contractions?

A. The beginning of one contraction to the beginning of the next contraction.

B. The acme of one contraction to the acme of the next contraction.

C. The beginning of one contraction to the end of the same contraction.

D. The end of one contraction to the end of the next contraction.

133. Mrs. Ballal is experiencing severe back pain and asks the nurse why this is happening. Which of the following is the nurse's best explanation for the cause of the back pain in labour?

A. Displacement of the bladder.

B. Uterine distention.

C. Referred pain from the uterus.

D. Contractions start in the lower lumbar region.

134. Mrs. Ballal asks the nurse when she can have an epidural. Which of the following is the nurse's best explanation for when Mrs. Ballal may have the epidural anesthesia?

A. Whenever she wants the epidural.

B. Epidural anesthesia is contraindicated in cases of severe back pain.

C. When she is in active labour.

D. Within 2 to 4 hours of birth.

135. Mrs. Ballal enters the phase of transitional labour. She is thrashing in bed and appears to be very distressed. She screams at her husband and the nurse to "leave me alone." What is the most appropriate nursing response at this time?

A. Leave the room immediately.

B. Tell Mrs. Ballal that she is demonstrating abusive behaviour that will not be tolerated.

C. Ask her husband to leave the room immediately because he is annoying his wife.

D. Stand quietly at the back of the room.

136. The nurse gives Mrs. Smith 10 mg IV morphine to promote comfort during labour. Which of the following is not associated with the administration of morphine in the intrapartum period?

A. Maternal and fetal respiratory depression.

B. Decreased fetal heart rate variability.

C. Decreased maternal heart rate.

D. Increased maternal comfort.

---

**Case Study:** *Lim and Huang are expecting their first baby. While performing the admission history, the nurse notes several new and old bruises on Lim's neck and body. Lim is silent and withdrawn. Huang answers all of the questions. Questions 137 to 139 relate to this scenario.*

137. Based on her observations, the nurse suspects partner abuse. Which of the following is the most appropriate nursing intervention at this time?

A. Contact the primary care provider and communicate your suspicions of abuse.

B. Ask Lim if she would like Huang to wait outside in the lobby.

C. Encourage Lim to leave Huang because she is at risk for further abuse when the baby is born.

D. Tell Huang to wait outside in the lobby while Lim is being examined.

138. Which of the following is true regarding partner abuse in pregnancy in Canada?

A. It occurs most frequently in Asian families.

B. Partner abuse in pregnant women is rare.

C. Partner abuse may increase during pregnancy.

D. It occurs in approximately 3% to 5% of pregnant women.

139. Lim tells the nurse that she has been beaten by Huang for the past 6 years. Which of the following emotional reactions will the nurse expect to observe in women who are physically abused?

A. Mania.

B. Anger.

C. Apathy toward the husband.

D. Ambivalence toward the husband.

140. Lisa, a 22-year-old primigravida, approaches the nurse during the prenatal clinic and states that her boyfriend is saying hurtful things about her weight gain. "He even told me I repulse him!" What is the most appropriate response from the nurse?

A. "It is important that you gain a certain amount of weight during your pregnancy."

B. "How much weight have you gained?"

C. "What do you think of your changing shape?"

D. "That comment sounds like it upset you. Tell me how you are feeling about your boyfriend's comments."

141. A pregnant woman's hepatitis B report reads "HBsAg = positive." Which of the following correctly describes the woman's hepatitis B status?

A. Susceptible.

B. Infected.

C. Immune.

D. A carrier.

142. A woman's hepatitis B report reads "HBsAg = positive, HBeAg = positive, and IgM anti-HBc = positive." Which of the following correctly describes the woman's current hepatitis B status?

   A. Acutely infected.
   B. Chronically infected.
   C. Of a low infection level.
   D. Not infectious.

---

**Case Study:** *Shelley works as a staff nurse on a busy antenatal unit in a tertiary care centre. Questions 143 to 144 relate to this scenario.*

143. Shelley learns that one of her nursing colleagues has called in "sick" for the shift. Shelley has been assigned 13 high-risk antenatal clients rather than the usual workload of six clients. What is the most appropriate nursing action to resolve this situation?

   A. Call the emergency department and tell them that you are unable to admit any more antenatal women to the unit.
   B. Work with the available nurses that are currently on the unit.
   C. Reassess the workload with the charge nurse and request assistance.
   D. Contact the nurse who called in sick and ask her to reconsider coming in to work.

144. A nursing attendant comes to help on the unit. What information should the nurse know before delegating tasks to the attendant?

   A. All nursing activities performed by the attendant should be directly supervised by a registered nurse.
   B. Some nursing activities performed by the attendant should be directly supervised by a registered nurse.
   C. The attendants' level of knowledge and comfort level in performing specific nursing activities should be considered.
   D. The attendant has previously completed and practiced the delegated activities.

145. A woman is hospitalized for gestational hypertension. A nursing attendant reports that the woman's blood pressure is "extremely high." What is the most appropriate nursing action at this time?

   A. Ask the nursing attendant to recheck the woman's blood pressure in 15 minutes.
   B. Ask the nursing attendant to repeat the woman's blood pressure immediately.

   C. Notify the hospital supervisor immediately.
   D. Notify the primary care provider immediately.

146. The condition of the woman with gestational hypertension is rapidly deteriorating. The primary care provider orders a loading dose of IV magnesium sulfate ($MgSO_4$), increased surveillance, and increased nursing interventions. What is the most appropriate nursing action to resolve this situation?

   A. Ask the nursing attendant to provide one-on-one care to the woman and reassign the other clients.
   B. Inform the primary care provider that as a nursing attendant you are unable to commence the IV $MgSO_4$ and provide the level of care the woman requires.
   C. Meet with nursing colleagues and reassign the woman to an RN.
   D. Notify the hospital supervisor immediately.

---

**Case Study:** *A nurse and a nursing student are visiting expectant and new mothers in the community. Questions 147 to 150 relate to this scenario.*

147. The nurse tells the student that they will be visiting a family that experienced a stillbirth at 38 weeks gestation. The student begins to cry and says, "I can't possibly participate in the visit. I just found out I am pregnant. I can't deal with the thought of losing a baby in pregnancy." What is the nurse's most appropriate response to the student?

   A. Tell the student it is okay to cry and encourage her to talk about the way she is feeling.
   B. Tell the student to take the day off and spend time with her other children.
   C. Tell the student that her behaviour is unprofessional and that participating in the visit is a valuable part of her clinical experience.
   D. Tell the student to go home and forget about the experience.

148. The preceptor overhears the student talking to the grieving parents about her own pregnancy. The student also makes arrangements with the mother to pick up her maternity clothes and baby furniture on the weekend. What is the nurse's most appropriate response to the student?

   A. Say nothing because this appears to be a mutually convenient arrangement.
   B. Discuss the situation with the nursing student after the visit has ended.

C. Tell the grieving woman that she should not give away her baby furniture in case she needs it in the future.

D. Immediately report the incident to the nursing association.

149. They drive to the home of a client with postpartum depression and discover her and her baby completely naked in the backyard. The woman is unable to communicate in an effective manner. They are both cold and crying. What is the nurse's most appropriate response to resolve this situation?

A. Contact the woman's husband to come home from work and immediately take her to the emergency department.

B. Ask the woman if she is thinking of harming herself or her baby.

C. Contact the nursing supervisor to clarify the appropriate actions in this acute mental health situation.

D. Ask the nursing student to stay with the woman while the nurse performs the last home visit in the community.

150. The student asks the preceptor how to apply the portable external fetal monitor (EFM) in the home setting. What is the best way for the preceptor to teach the new procedure?

A. Instruct the student to read about the procedure in the regional policy and procedure manual.

B. Demonstrate for 1 week and then supervise the student performing the procedure for 1 week.

C. Demonstrate once and then supervise the student while she performs the procedure.

D. Encourage the student to learn the skill in labour and delivery so that she can work more independently in the home setting.

151. Rajinder, RN, meets her neighbor and new baby at the local market. The neighbor tells Rajinder that she received outstanding nursing care from one of her colleagues during her labour and childbirth. What is the best way for Rajinder to recognize her nursing colleague's professional efforts?

A. Place a birth announcement on the regional web site with special thanks to the nursing colleague.

B. Send your colleague an anonymous card in the mail from "a special admirer."

C. Share the feedback with the nursing colleague.

D. It is a breech of confidentiality to share this information with the colleague.

152. The nurse makes a medication error when administering $MgSO_4$. She administers a 50-g loading dose instead of a 5-g dose. What should be the nurse's immediate action?

A. Complete an incident report as per the institutional policy.

B. Contact the hospital supervisor.

C. Assess the client and contact the primary care provider.

D. Assess the client and seek the advice of an experienced colleague.

153. Alyssa is admitted and treated for premature labour at 30 weeks gestation. She has not experienced any uterine activity for the past 48 hours and is discharged home. Alyssa tells the nurse that she "does not want to go home." Which of the following is the nurse's most appropriate response?

A. Ask Alyssa why she does not want to go home.

B. Inform the primary care provider that Alyssa does not want to go home.

C. Instruct Alyssa to return to the hospital if she experiences 1:5 uterine contractions.

D. Ask Alyssa if she has any support in the home.

154. A nurse's colleague is talking about a local celebrity's girlfriend in the cafeteria during a lunch break. The colleague says, "She has several tattoos and piercings." Which of the following is the nurse's most appropriate response?

A. Discuss the colleague's behaviour in private.

B. Confront the colleague immediately to prevent her from causing more harm.

C. Ignore the comment because it is not considered harmful.

D. Report the colleague's behaviour to the nurse manager.

155. Brenda Thomas is hospitalized for severe preeclampsia. Her husband tells the nurse that he is frustrated to have been waiting for 4 hours for the physician to discuss his wife's deteriorating condition. What is the nurse's most appropriate response?

A. Reassure Mr. Thomas that this is very unusual behaviour for the physician.

B. Tell Mr. Thomas to return home and the physician will contact him later.

C. Notify the physician that Mr. Thomas has been waiting to discuss his wife's condition.

D. Reassure Mr. Thomas that his wife's condition is stable at present.

156. The nurse is preparing an inservice on hyperemesis gravidarum for a regional education day. Which of the following is true of perinatal nursing research?

    A. Research findings always contribute to changing perinatal nursing practice.
    B. Research findings do not always change perinatal nursing practice.
    C. Quantitative research yields the most useful findings for perinatal nursing practice.
    D. Randomized clinical trials yield the most useful research findings for perinatal nursing practice.

157. Which of the following ethical principles supports expectant mothers when conflicts between maternal and fetal rights arise during childbirth?

    A. Autonomy.
    B. Justice.
    C. Nonmaleficence.
    D. Jurisprudence.

158. Which of the following supports the concept of woman-centred care in childbirth?

    A. Birth without medications or interventions.
    B. Birth without an external fetal monitor attached during labour.
    C. Birth with the father and siblings present in the room.
    D. Birth with the father and doula present.

159. Yvonne and Bert have just experienced the loss of their first baby. The nurse enters the birthing room to assess Yvonne's pain level and observes the couple embraced together in the same bed. What is the nurse's most appropriate response?

    A. Tell Bert he must get out of the bed so that you can provide nursing care.
    B. Tell Bert that you are not comfortable providing care for Yvonne with the couple in bed.
    C. Tell Bert that his behaviour is not appropriate for a medical institution.
    D. Ensure their privacy.

160. Mr. and Mrs. Waters constantly complain about the care Mrs. Waters is receiving on the antenatal unit. They have spent the past 15 minutes complaining to the nurse about the care Mrs. Waters is receiving today. What is the most appropriate response by the nurse?

    A. Explain that the unit is short staffed and you are doing the best you can.
    B. Explain that this frustration may cause the uterine contractions to start.

    C. Encourage them to talk for 10 more minutes and then remind them that you have other tasks to perform on the unit.
    D. Encourage the family to identify their frustrations and fears.

161. A newspaper journalist calls the unit to ask the nurse for information regarding the increasing cesarean section rates in Canada. Which of the following is the most common cause of primary cesarean section?

    A. Cephalopelvic disproportion (CPD).
    B. Placenta previa.
    C. Prolonged latent stage of labour.
    D. Cost to the health care system.

162. Nury is HIV positive and in active labour. What should the nurse wear to protect herself from the HIV virus during birth?

    A. Masks and a gown.
    B. Eye protection, shoe covers, and a mask.
    C. A surgical cap.
    D. Eyewear, gloves, and a gown.

---

***Case Study:*** *Barbara is admitted to the birthing suite in active labour accompanied by her husband Robert. She is a primigravida at 40 weeks gestation and has intact membranes, a bloody show, and 1:3 uterine contractions. The fetal heart rate is 145 bpm. Vaginal examination reveals that the cervix is fully effaced and 6 cm dilated and the presenting part is at -4 station. Questions 163 to 165 relate to this scenario.*

163. The nurse is concerned about prolapse of the umbilical cord. She tells Barbara and Robert to inform her immediately when spontaneous rupture of the membranes occurs. When is a prolapse of the cord most likely to occur?

    A. When the fetal heart rate is at or above 145 bpm.
    B. During the first stage of labour.
    C. When the presenting part is not engaged on the cervix.
    D. When the membranes are intact.

164. Robert uses the call bell to tell the nurse that Barbara's membranes have ruptured and "something is hanging out on the bed!" What is the primary goal of the emergency care when prolapse of the umbilical cord occurs?

    A. Prevent or relieve pressure on the umbilical cord.
    B. Prevent drying of the cord while it is still pulsating.

C. Prevent cold air from stimulating vasoconstriction.

D. Restore circulation by stimulating the cord with a sterile glove.

165. The nurse should encourage Barbara into which position to relieve pressure on the umbilical cord?

A. Sidelying.
B. Knee–chest.
C. Squatting.
D. Semi-Fowler's.

166. Which of the following conditions is the leading cause of neonatal death in Canada?

A. NEC.
B. Congenital heart disease.
C. Respiratory distress syndrome.
D. Prematurity.

---

*Case Study:* Suzette, a 31-year-old primipara, gave birth 36 hours ago to a healthy girl and will be discharged later today from the hospital. The nurse is providing breastfeeding education. Questions 167 to 171 relate to this scenario.

167. Which of the following behaviours does the nurse recognize as an effective latch during breastfeeding?

A. Dimpling of the baby's cheeks.
B. Audible suck–swallow cycles.
C. The entire nipple is in the baby's mouth.
D. The baby is easily removed from the breast.

168. Suzette's nipples are red and bruised, and a small crack is visible on the right nipple. What is likely causing this problem?

A. An incorrect latch.
B. This is normal for a few days and will heal.
C. The baby's mouth is too small for the mother's large breast.
D. The mother is fair skinned, and her nipples need to toughen up.

169. Which of the following would be the best long-term recommendation from the nurse to relieve Suzette's nipple discomfort while breastfeeding?

A. Give her a nipple shield.
B. Remove the baby from the breast and reposition her.
C. Have Suzette breastfeed only from the nipple that is not injured.
D. Have Suzette pump her breast milk until her nipples heal and give breast milk from the bottle.

170. Suzette asks the nurse how she will know that her baby is getting enough breast milk. Which of the following is the best indicator that baby is receiving enough milk?

A. The baby is sleeping well.
B. The baby has six to eight heavy, wet diapers a day from day 4 onward.
C. The baby feeds frequently.
D. The breasts feel less heavy after feeds.

171. Suzette is exhibiting signs of early engorgement, but her milk is still flowing easily. Which of the following suggestions would the nurse give to Suzette to treat engorgement?

A. Restricting fluid intake.
B. Feeding on both breasts with every feed.
C. Applying ice packs before a feed.
D. Taking a warm shower.

---

*Case Study:* Antononia, gravida 2, para 2, had an emergency cesarean birth after 24 hours of labour. She was discharged home from the hospital after 72 hours. The nurse is visiting her in her home the day after her hospital discharge. Questions 172 to 175 relate to this scenario.

172. Antononia is complaining of her fear of having a bowel movement after surgery. Which of the following recommendations from the nurse is most appropriate?

A. Take a warm shower.
B. Increase her consumption of foods rich in fibre.
C. Decrease her pain medication.
D. Take a laxative.

173. The nurse completes Antononia's postpartal assessment. Which of the following assessments are not initiated by the nurse?

A. Lochia assessment.
B. Involution of the uterus.
C. Perineal assessment.
D. Treatment of pain.

174. Antononia complains to the nurse that she needs to change her maxi pad after 3 hours. Which of the following is an appropriate response from the nurse?

A. Do nothing because this is a normal finding.
B. Notify her primary health care provider.
C. Palpate her uterus.
D. Check her vaginal pad again before completing the visit.

175. Antononia tells the nurse that she is experiencing abdominal cramps whenever she nurses her baby. The most appropriate explanation that the nurse could provide would be which of the following?

    A. The sympathetic nervous system is stimulated when the baby nurses.
    B. Oxytocin is released when the baby sucks, which causes the uterus to contract.
    C. The cramps will decrease if Antononia massages her uterus before nursing her baby.
    D. The cramps will stop after her body has expelled all blood clots from her uterus.

---

*Case Study: Bhindu is 21 days postpartum and calls the health unit crying. She is experiencing a breastfeeding problem and needs the nurse to see her. The nurse in the community arrives that afternoon at Bhindu's home. Questions 176 to 180 relate to this scenario.*

176. The nurse notes that Bhindu's left breast nipple is cracked and bleeding slightly. Her left breast is sore to touch, and an area under the breast is firm, painful, red, and warm to touch. She has a fever of 39°C. Bhindu says she is feeling unwell and is wondering how she is going to manage over the next 24 hours. What is likely causing this breastfeeding problem?

    A. Plugged breast duct.
    B. Mastitis.
    C. Engorgement.
    D. Thrush infection.

177. What is the most appropriate nurse's recommendation in light of Bhindu's symptoms?

    A. Advise her to stop breastfeeding because of transfer of infection to the baby.
    B. Advise her to pump her breasts and discard this milk.
    C. Advise her to see her primary care provider as soon as possible.
    D. Advise her to continue to breastfeed but on the left side only.

178. Bhindu tells the nurse that she and her husband had an argument before he left for work in the morning. He was up all night not able to sleep with the baby crying, and he wants her to give the baby formula. Bhindu starts to cry and says she wants to continue to breastfeed. What is the most appropriate immediate response from the nurse?

    A. "I know an excellent support group for breastfeeding."

B. "Let's talk about this further. What you are feeling right now?"
    C. "Have you considered offering breast milk and formula?"
    D. "I will come back in a few days and talk to your husband."

179. The nurse returns to Bhindu's home after several days to assess how she is managing and to do a breastfeeding assessment. Bhindu informs the nurse that she is now taking Cloxacillin PO qid for 10 days. She asks the nurse if she can continue to breastfeed. What is the nurse's most appropriate response to Bhindu?

    A. "You need to stop breastfeeding for the full 10 days."
    B. "You need to pump your breasts and discard the milk to keep up your milk supply."
    C. "You need to continue to breastfeed, and the antibiotics will protect your baby from infection."
    D. "Give formula now and then breastfeed after completing your antibiotics."

180. Bhindu asks the nurse how to prevent further breastfeeding episodes such as the one she has just experienced. What is the most appropriate recommendation from the nurse?

    A. Feed the baby on the right side only for the next few feeds.
    B. Massage the milk ducts while feeding on both sides of the breast.
    C. Avoid using a breast pump to reduce breast trauma.
    D. Feed the baby on a schedule to allow breast tissue to heal.

---

*Case Study: Cyndie is a 17-year-old single mother who has given birth after a difficult 20-hour labour. She has few visitors during her short hospital stay. Questions 181 to 184 relate to this scenario.*

181. On her first postpartum day, Cyndie seems overwhelmed with her new baby and asks the nurse how she is supposed to interact with her baby when all the baby does is eat and sleep. Which of the following actions would be most effective for the nurse to use to facilitate mother–infant attachment?

    A. Encourage Cyndie to pay attention to her baby.
    B. Demonstrate different positions for holding the baby.

C. Encourage Cyndie to watch a video on attachment.

D. Show Cyndie how the baby initiates interaction with her and attends to her.

**182.** To further facilitate parent–infant interaction between Cyndie and her baby, what information would the nurse point out to Cyndie about cues the baby is transmitting?

A. Cues are not always purposeful.

B. Cues are not always meaningful.

C. Cues are frequently nonverbal and behavioural.

D. Cues occur randomly.

**183.** The student nurse who is caring for Cyndie questions the nurse about attachment. Which of the following behaviours would the nurse list that might indicate that Cyndie is having difficulty attaching to her newborn?

A. Describing the baby's likeness to her family members.

B. Talking at length about her difficult labour and birth.

C. Holding the baby in the enface position.

D. Letting the baby cry to get to sleep.

**184.** On the second postpartum day, the nurse observes that Cyndie becomes agitated when her baby cries during breastfeeding. Which of the following is the most appropriate response from the nurse?

A. Refer Cyndie to a lactation consultant.

B. Demonstrate ways that Cyndie can comfort her infant.

C. Leave the crying baby with Cyndie so they can get better acquainted before discharge.

D. Tell Cyndie that her baby is hungry and that she needs to breastfeed.

*Case Study: A community health nurse visits a new postpartal family the day after discharge from the hospital. Questions 185 to 188 relate to this scenario.*

**185.** The community nurse introduces herself to the family and outlines the purpose of her home visit. She asks permission before sitting down in the home. These behaviours demonstrate which elements of the therapeutic relationship?

A. Accountability.

B. Choice.

C. Respect.

D. Genuineness.

**186.** The community nurse works with the family to answer their questions on baby care. The nurse does not disclose her home address or accept an invitation to stay for lunch. This demonstrates which of the following behaviours within the therapeutic relationship?

A. Maintaining boundaries.

B. Ensuring confidentiality.

C. Building trust and rapport.

D. Displaying professional communication.

**187.** When the student nurse asks why care is provided for postpartum families in the home, which of the following is the nurse's most appropriate response?

A. It provides for more control over the practice environment.

B. It gives more opportunity to teach self and infant care.

C. It provides the ability to assess the physical and psychological condition of the mother and baby.

D. It allows the nurse to interact with the family in their own natural setting.

**188.** As the nurse returns to visit the family 2 days later, she hears shouting and swearing between the mother and father and several loud crashes just as she is going to knock on the door. What is the most appropriate response from the nurse?

A. Knock on the door and wait to see if someone answers.

B. Try the door to see if it is open and go in to protect the baby.

C. Knock on the door and shout, "It is the nurse. Can I help you?"

D. Return to her car and call for backup or security from her health unit.

*Case Study: Mai has been discharged home with her baby boy, Pong. She is 72 hours postpartum and has been exclusively breastfeeding. The nurse is visiting the family in their home. Questions 189 to 193 relate to this scenario.*

**189.** Baby Pong has a yellowish tinge to his face and trunk when the nurse blanches his skin. Which physiologic reason has caused the jaundice?

A. Inability of the liver to bind bilirubin for excretion.

B. An enzyme in the breast milk.

C. Blood incompatibility.

D. Bile duct blockage.

**190.** Baby Pong has been lethargic and has to awakened for feeds. He has lost 9% of his weight since birth. Which of the following recommendations does the nurse discuss with his mother, Mai?

    A. Readmitting the baby back in to the hospital because of the large weight loss.

    B. Calling the baby's primary care practitioner for advice.

    C. Breastfeeding the baby eight to 12 times in 24 hours and waking him for feeds.

    D. Offering the baby formula to increase his weight gain.

**191.** The nurse assesses Pong's caloric intake. What guideline does she recommend in determining the appropriate number and color of stools for Pong at 72 hours postpartum?

    A. A minimum of one to three green to yellow stools.

    B. A minimum of one dark and sticky stool.

    C. A minimum of four to five stools that are loose, seedy, and easily passed.

    D. Assessing stools in infants is not an accurate measurement of hydration.

**192.** The nurse recommends that Mai express or pump her breasts to increase her milk supply in addition to offering her breast to her baby. Mai has a manual breast pump. Which of the following recommendations does the nurse offer around pumping her breasts?

    A. Pump eight times a day.

    B. Pump after feedings.

    C. Pump for 30 minutes at a time.

    D. Purchase or rent an electric pump for more efficiency.

**193.** The nurse returns in 2 days. Mai's mother is staying with the family for 3 months to help with child care. She encourages Mai to offer formula for Pong's night feeds so she can get some rest. Mai asks the nurse if this will lessen her milk supply. Which of the following is the most appropriate response from the nurse?

    A. Encourage Mai to teach the baby to sleep through the night.

    B. Tell her that it is important to breastfeed at least once at night to release the hormone prolactin.

    C. Tell her that offering formula at night will not interfere with her milk supply.

    D. Tell her that she needs her rest more than she needs to breastfeed her infant.

*Case Study:* Carrie, age 33 years, delivered a healthy baby boy 5 days ago. Her husband calls the after-hours nursing line to say he is worried about his wife. Questions 194 to 198 relate to this scenario.

**194.** Carrie is experiencing insomnia and weepiness lasting several minutes to several hours every day. Which of the following factors or conditions does the nurse believe is causing this experience?

    A. Postpartum baby blues.

    B. Postpartum anxiety.

    C. Postpartum reaction.

    D. Postpartum depression.

**195.** Carrie's husband asks the nurse what is wrong with his wife and why she isn't more joyful about the birth of their child. Which of the following is the most appropriate response from the nurse?

    A. "I am concerned about her as well. I will refer her to her primary care provider ASAP."

    B. "Many mothers are a little weepy and depressed for the first few days after giving birth."

    C. "Your wife is at risk for postpartum depression."

    D. "Your wife needs some sleep."

**196.** Carrie asks the nurse if she is at risk for developing postpartum depression. Based on Carrie's history, the nurse knows which factor puts Carrie at risk?

    A. Previous history of postpartum depression.

    B. Multiparity.

    C. Her age.

    D. Length of time between pregnancies.

**197.** The nurse phones Carrie after several weeks into the postpartum period to conduct a postpartum depression screen. Carrie complains that she doesn't feel love toward her baby. In fact, she says she resents the baby because of the attention he receives from her husband. She has been unable to complete household tasks and care of her baby. What is the most appropriate immediate action from the nurse?

    A. Refer her to her primary care provider as soon as possible.

    B. Refer her to a local postpartum support service as soon as possible.

    C. Ask her if she has any thoughts of hurting herself or her baby.

D. Call her husband and say you are concerned about her.

**198.** Carrie is now 3 months postpartum and asks the nurse about using condoms for sexual intercourse. Which of the following is the most appropriate response from the nurse?

A. "Condoms should be used by unmarried women in the postpartum period."
B. "Women at risk for acquiring sexually transmitted infections should use condoms."
C. "Condoms should be used by women at risk of acquiring candidiasis."
D. "Sexual intercourse should not be resumed until 4 to 6 months postpartum."

**199.** Margaret is attending her first prenatal appointment. She states that she drank beer throughout her last pregnancy to "build iron" in her blood. Margaret asks the nurse if it is okay to have a few drinks with this current pregnancy. Which of the following responses by the nurse would be most appropriate?

A. "It is not safe to consume alcohol during pregnancy."
B. "It is safe to consume one or two drinks per week in the first trimester."
C. "It is safe to consume wine and beer in moderation during pregnancy."
D. "It is safe to consume one or two drinks per week in the third semester."

**200.** A nurse completes the initial assessment of a newborn. According to the due date (EDC) on the antenatal record, the baby is 12 days postmature. Which of the following physical findings does not confirm that this newborn is 12 days postmature?

A. Meconium aspiration.
B. Absence of lanugo.
C. Hypoglycemia.
D. Increased amounts of vernix.

## ▶ Short Answer Questions

**Case Study:** *Ulanda is 34 weeks gestational age and is experiencing heavy vaginal bleeding. She is on her way to the hospital in an ambulance. Questions 201 to 204 relate to this scenario.*

**201.** What is the definition of antepartum hemorrhage (APH), and what are two determining factors of the condition? (3 points)

**202.** Identify four causes of antepartum hemorrhage. (3 points)

**203.** What are five clinical manifestations of abruptio placenta? (3 points)

**204.** What are three possible *fetal* complications associated with antepartum hemorrhage? (3 points)

**Case Study:** *Rosie is a 16-year-old obese pregnant high school student. She is visiting her aunt in another province for the summer vacation. Neither Rosie's parents nor her aunt know that she is pregnant. Rosie has had no prenatal care. Questions 205 to 207 relate to this scenario.*

**205.** Rosie wakes up with a "stomach ache" one morning. She takes a handful of antacid tablets and walks 20 minutes to the mall. At the mall, Rosie calls her aunt to pick her up, complaining that her "stomach ache is getting worse." They drive to the hospital emergency room. Rosie is immediately taken to an assessment room because she is hysterical and thrashing in pain. The nurse helps Rosie take off her baggy clothes as Rosie begins to push and the membranes rupture. What are five nursing priorities for the Rosie during this precipitous birth? (5 points)

**206.** Within the next 2 minutes, the nurse delivers a 5-lb baby with Apgar scores of 9 at 1 minute and 10 at 5 minutes. The baby is pink and crying and appears to be approximately 36 weeks gestational age by physical examination. What are three nursing priorities for the baby during a precipitous birth? (3 points)

**207.** What are five nursing priorities when caring for Rosie in the immediate postpartum period? (3 points)

**208.** What are five contraindications for performing a vaginal examination? (4 points)

---

**Case Study:** *Sally is 25 years old, para 0, gravida 1, and is at 41 weeks gestation. She is admitted to the perinatal clinic for a nonstress test. Sally's pregnancy has progressed past her due date. Questions 209 to 211 relate to this scenario.*

**209.** What are two major consequences of a pregnancy continuing past the established due date? (2 points)

**210.** The resident physician inserts prostaglandin E2 gel that evening to "ripen" Sally's cervix and increase readiness for induction of labour in the morning. After 3 hours, Sally is experiencing mild to moderate contractions every 5 minutes and states that they are "really starting to hurt now." Sally requests something for the pain but is not sure what she wants. List eight

nonpharmacologic comfort measures that the nurse can offer to Sally. (4 points)

**211.** Sally's contractions begin to decrease in frequency and intensity. She is advised to rest overnight and is scheduled for an induction of labour with Pitocin in the morning. What is the difference between Pitocin induction and Pitocin augmentation? (3 points)

---

**Case Study:** *A nurse receives a discharge summary from the hospital on a postpartum family whose baby was born 48 hours earlier. She prepares to visit them that morning. Questions 212 to 214 relate to this scenario.*

**212.** List five activities the nurse would focus on during the home visit. (5 points)

**213.** What are five important areas of the physical assessment the nurse should complete on the new mother during the postpartal home visit? (3 points)

**214.** What five areas of the psychosocial assessment should the nurse complete with the new mother during the postpartal home visit? (3 points)

---

**Case Study:** *The nurse is instructing a group of new parents about feeding their infants. The topic of today's class is breastfeeding. Question 215 relates to this scenario.*

**215.** List five benefits to infants from breastfeeding. (3 points)

## ▶ Answers and Rationales

**1. D.** Early fetal heart decelerations.

*Rationale*
Placenta previa (placenta covering cervical os), cord compression (obstruction of the umbilical cord), and abruption placenta (separation of the placenta from the uterine wall) are high-risk, life-threatening hypoxic conditions for the fetus during labour and birth. Early fetal heart decelerations indicate head compression as the fetus descends through the maternal pelvis. Although fetal heart decelerations may be nonreassuring, this condition is not a high-risk intrapartum factor.

*Classification*
Competency Category: Nursing Practice: Alterations in Health
Taxonomic Level: Knowledge/Comprehension

**2. D.** The condition is contracted from raw meat and cat feces.

*Rationale*
Toxoplasmosis in pregnancy is contracted from raw meat and cat feces. Manifestations in newborns may be lethal.

*Classification*
Competency Category: Nursing Practice: Health and Wellness
Taxonomic Level: Knowledge/Comprehension

**3. B.** Transepidermal water loss and radiative and convective losses.

*Rationale*
Heat loss in newborns occurs primarily by evaporation, radiation, and convection.

*Classification*
Competency Category: Nursing Practice: Health and Wellness
Taxonomic Level: Knowledge/Comprehension

**4. D.** "Darkened line in the midline of the abdomen."

*Rationale*
The linea nigra is a pigmented line extending in the symphysis pubis to the top of the fundus in the midline.

*Classification*
Competency Category: Nursing Practice: Health and Wellness
Taxonomic Level: Application

**5. C.** RSA.

*Rationale*
Fetal health assessment includes using Leopold's maneuvers to identify fetal presentation, lie, and position. Upon palpation, a round, firm, movable part in the fundus (top of uterus) indicates the fetal head. This is a longitudinal lie, breech presentation with the fetal spine on the right side of midline. The presenting part is the sacrum. The likely position of the fetus is RSA (right sacrum anterior).

*Classification*
Competency Category: Nursing Practice: Health and Wellness
Taxonomic Level: Critical Thinking

**6. D.** The joints of the pelvis relax.

*Rationale*
Slight relaxation and increased mobility of the pelvis are normal during pregnancy and are caused by the ovarian hormone relaxin. This may cause the pregnant woman to feel "unstable" while walking, which has definite safety implications for a long-distance runner.

*Classification*
Competency Category: Nursing Practice: Health and Wellness
Taxonomic Level: Application

**7. B.** Separation of the central muscle, allowing the abdominal contents to protrude from the midline.

*Rationale*
Diastasis recti are caused by separation of the abdominal muscles, allowing abdominal contents to protrude at midline.

*Classification*
Competency Category: Nursing Practice: Health and Wellness
Taxonomic Level: Knowledge/Comprehension

**8. C.** "The contractions in my uterus are getting stronger and closer now."

*Rationale*
True labour is defined as the onset of regular uterine contractions that increase in frequency, intensity, and duration.

*Classification*
Competency Category: Nursing Practice: Alterations in Health
Taxonomic Level: Knowledge/Comprehension

**9. A.** A fundal height of 27 cm at 32 weeks gestation.

*Rationale*
Optimal fetal growth and development during pregnancy are assessed with fundal height measurement. Fundal height, measured in centimeters, should equal gestational weeks throughout the pregnancy (e.g., fundal height of 27 cm should occur at 27 weeks gestation). A fundal height of 27 cm at 32 weeks gestation is a very ominous finding that requires immediate attention and investigation.

*Classification*
Competency Category: Nursing Practice: Alterations in Health
Taxonomic Level: Application

**10. B.** The cervix cannot be felt during a vaginal examination.

*Rationale*
The second stage of labour begins when the cervix is fully dilated and effaced and when the cervix cannot be felt during a vaginal examination.

*Classification*
Competency Category: Nursing Practice
Taxonomic Level: Application

**11. A.** Place your hand on her abdomen below the umbilicus and palpate the uterine tone with your fingertips.

*Rationale*
This is the correct technique to assess uterine contractions using palpation.

*Classification*
Competency Category: Nursing Practice: Health and Wellness
Taxonomic Level: Knowledge/Comprehension

**12. A.** Sitting or standing.

*Rationale*
Sitting or standing facilitates the progress of labour because it uses the principle of gravity.

*Classification*
Competency Category: Nursing Practice: Alterations in Health
Taxonomic Level: Application

**13. C.** "Yes, as long as the warm water doesn't raise your temperature."

*Rationale*
The temperature of the water should be constantly maintained at body temperature (i.e., 37°C or lower) to prevent hyperthermia.

*Classification*
Competency Category: Nursing Practice: Alterations in Health
Taxonomic Level: Application

**14. A.** The risks include hypotension and a prolonged second stage of labour.

*Rationale*
Hypotension and a prolonged second stage of labour are risks associated with epidural anesthesia.

*Classification*
Competency Category: Nursing Practice: Alterations in Health
Taxonomic Level: Knowledge/Comprehension

**15. B.** Tell Josh that he will receive updates of his wife's progress and be called as soon as the baby is born.

*Rationale*
This statement respects the decision of the family and facilitates open communication between the nurse, Helen, and Josh during labour and birth.

*Classification*
Competency Category: Nurse–Person Relationship
Taxonomic Level: Critical Thinking

**16. C.** Doulas can serve as a support person and coach during labour.

*Rationale*
The role of the doula in labour and birth is to provide support. Doulas do not assist with the birth process and do not replace the husband or partner.

*Classification*
Competency Category: Nursing Practice: Health and Wellness
Taxonomic Level: Knowledge/Comprehension

**17. D.** Single-parent family.

*Rationale*
Single-parent families tend to be the most socially and economically vulnerable, creating an unstable and deprived environment for the growth potential of children.

*Classification*
Competency Category: Nursing Practice: Health and Wellness
Taxonomic Level: Application

**18. B.** Infant mortality rate.

*Rationale*
The infant mortality rate, which is the number of deaths of infants younger than 1 year of age per 1000 births, reflects the adequacy of prenatal care and the overall health of the nation.

*Classification*
Competency Category: Nursing Practice: Health and Wellness
Taxonomic Level: Knowledge/Comprehension

**19. B.** Consult the agency procedure book and follow the printed guidelines.

*Rationale*
According to the Canadian Nurses Association (CNA) Code of Ethics, if a nurse is uncertain how to perform a procedure, the guidelines printed in the agency procedure book should be followed.

*Classification*
Competency Category: Professional Practice
Taxonomic Level: Critical Thinking

**20. B.** Pregnancy loss.

*Rationale*
Millie's advanced maternal age (i.e., 45-years-old) puts her at increased risk for pregnancy loss.

*Classification*
Competency Category: Nursing Practice: Alterations in Health
Taxonomic Level: Application

**21. C.** Amniocentesis.

*Rationale*
Amniocentesis to screen for congenital anomalies can be done starting at 14 weeks gestation; thus, it is appropriate for Millie at this stage. This procedure carries a risk of spontaneous abortion, infection, and placental abruption.

*Classification*
Competency Category: Nursing Practice: Health and Wellness
Taxonomic Level: Application

**22. D.** No risks.

*Rationale*
There are no known risks to the fetus with hepatitis B vaccine during pregnancy.

*Classification*
Competency Category: Nursing Practice: Health and Wellness
Taxonomic Level: Application

**23. C.** "A woman should continue her method of birth control until she has not had a period for 1 year."

*Rationale*
Evidence-based practice recommends continuing with birth control method until the woman has not had a period for 1 year. Nurses should never be critical or judgmental.

*Classification*
Competency Category: Nursing Practice: Health and Wellness
Taxonomic Level: Knowledge/Comprehension

**24. A.** "Tell me about your previous baby's birth."

*Rationale*
Constance appears to be afraid of having another cesarean section. The nurse needs to allow Constance to express her fears and also needs to listen to what problems she experienced last time so she is able to address each one. This kind of open-ended question facilitates effective and therapeutic communication.

*Classification*
Competency Category: Professional Practice
Taxonomic Level: Affective: Application

**25. C.** It is caused by swelling of the tissues over or under the fetal scalp during labour.

*Rationale*
Caput succedaneum is swelling or edema occurring in or under the fetal scalp during labour. The edema that crosses the suture lines is gradually absorbed and disappears around the third day of life.

*Classification*
Competency Category: Nursing Practice: Alterations in Health
Taxonomic Level: Knowledge/Comprehension

**26. A.** Heart rate.

*Rationale*
The heart rate is auscultated or palpated at the junction of the umbilical cord and skin. This is the most important assessment of the Apgar score.

*Classification*
Competency Category: Nursing Practice: Health and Wellness
Taxonomic Level: Knowledge/Comprehension

**27. B.** 4 to 6.

*Rationale*
An Apgar score between 4 and 6 indicates moderate difficulty and the need for stimulation.

*Classification*
Competency Category: Nursing Practice: Alterations in Health
Taxonomic Level: Knowledge/Comprehension

**28. C.** At 4 to 6 hours of life.

*Rationale*
The newborn usually shows a predictable pattern of behaviour during the first several hours after birth characterized by two periods of reactivity. The first period is 30 minutes after birth. The second period occurs around 4 to 6 hours of life. During the second period, the newborn is awake and alert; the heart and respiratory rates increase; production of respiratory and gastric mucus increases; and the newborn responds by gagging, choking, and regurgitating if swallows milk incorrectly.

*Classification*
Competency Category: Nursing Practice: Health and Wellness
Taxonomic Level: Knowledge/Comprehension

**29. C.** Days 2 to 5.

*Rationale*
Colostrum production begins early in pregnancy and may last for several days after birth. In most cases, colostrum is replaced by transitional milk within 2 to 5 days after birth. Transitional milk is then produced until approximately 2 weeks postpartum.

*Classification*
Competency Category: Nursing Practice: Health and Wellness
Taxonomic Level: Knowledge/Comprehension

**30. A.** Good hand washing.

*Rationale*
The caregiver should wash his or her hands before and after each client contact. For population health measures, hand washing remains the most important control procedure for contact with all newborns. The other actions are not necessary in most situations (e.g., isolation of infected infants is not usually present).

*Classification*
Competency Category: Nursing Practice: Health and Wellness
Taxonomic Level: Knowledge/Comprehension

**31. B.** The taking-in phase.

*Rationale*
The taking-in phase is the period after birth characterized by the woman's dependency and passivity with others. Maternal needs are dominant, and talking about the birth is an important task. The new mother follows suggestions, is hesitant about making decisions, and is still preoccupied with her needs.

*Classification*
Competency Category: Nursing Practice: Health and Wellness
Taxonomic Level: Application

**32. A.** Increase in hematocrit.

*Rationale*
Hemoglobin and erythrocyte values vary during the early postpartum period, but they should approximate or exceed prelabour values within 2 to 6 weeks. As extracellular fluid is excreted, hemoconcentration occurs, with a concomitant increase in hematocrit.

*Classification*
Competency Category: Nursing Practice: Health and Wellness
Taxonomic Level: Knowledge/Comprehension

**33. B.** Prolactin.

*Rationale*
Prolactin is a pituitary hormone that triggers and sustains milk production.

*Classification*
Competency Category: Nursing Practice: Health and Wellness
Taxonomic Level: Knowledge/Comprehension

**34. B.** Between 2 and 4 days of life.

*Rationale*
Physiologic jaundice occurs 48 hours or more after birth, peaks at the fifth to seventh day, and disappears between the seventh and tenth day postpartum.

Physiologic jaundice is caused by the normal reduction of red blood cells and occurs in both breast-fed and bottle-fed babies. It is more common with poorly established hydration, which is more likely associated with breastfed babies.

*Classification*
Competency Category: Nursing Practice: Health and Wellness
Taxonomic Level: Knowledge/Comprehension

**35. D.** The duration of breastfeeding should be determined by the newborn's signs of satiety.

*Rationale*
Although many older babies can take in the majority of their milk in the first 5 to 10 minutes, this cannot be generalized to all babies. Newborns, who are learning to nurse and are not always efficient at sucking, often need much longer to feed. The ability to take in milk is also subject to the mother's let-down response. Although many mothers may let down immediately, some may not. Some may eject their milk in small batches several times during a nursing session. Rather than guess, it is best to allow baby to suck until he or she shows signs of satiety such as self-detachment and relaxed hands and arms.

*Classification*
Competency Category: Nursing Practice: Health and Wellness
Taxonomic Level: Knowledge/Comprehension

**36. D.** Fever.

*Rationale*
Puerperal infection is any clinical infection of the genital canal that occurs within 28 days of childbirth. Classification continues to be the presence of a fever of 38°C on 2 consecutive days within the first 10 days postpartum (not counting the first 24 hours after birth).

*Classification*
Competency Category: Nursing Practice: Alterations in Health
Taxonomic Level: Knowledge/Comprehension

**37. B.** Unusual apprehension.

*Rationale*
One important sign of a pulmonary embolism is apprehension and a sense of impending catastrophe.

*Classification*
Competency Category: Nursing Practice: Alterations in Health
Taxonomic Level: Knowledge/Comprehension

**38. C.** Elevation of the affected leg.

*Rationale*
Measures to prevent thromboembolic disease encourage increasing blood flow and decreasing venous stasis. This includes elevation of the legs while sitting.

*Classification*
Competency Category: Nursing Practice: Alterations in Health
Taxonomic Level: Application

**39. C.** Acrocyanosis.

*Rationale*
Acrocyanosis is a blue color of hands and feet appearing in most infants at birth. It may persist for 7 to 10 days.

*Classification*
Competency Category: Nursing Practice: Health and Wellness
Taxonomic Level: Knowledge/Comprehension

**40. A.** Increase in cesarean section rate.

*Rationale*
Cesarean sections accounted for 22.5% of all in-hospital deliveries during 2001 and 2002, a jump from 15% of all deliveries in 1979 and 1980. The number of cesarean sections performed in Canada has reached an all-time high.

*Classification*
Competency Category: Nursing Practice: Health and Wellness
Taxonomic Level: Knowledge/Comprehension

**41. C.** 6 months

*Rationale*
The WHO currently recommends breastfeeding exclusively to the age of about 6 months and then continuing breastfeeding and complementary foods for up to 2 years of age or beyond.

*Classification*
Competency Category: Nursing Practice: Health and Wellness
Taxonomic Level: Knowledge/Comprehension

**42. C.** 75%.

*Rationale*
The duration of breastfeeding has decreased since 1960. Recent Canadian statistics show that although almost 75% of mothers begin

breastfeeding in the hospital, only 60% and 30% are still exclusively breastfeeding at 3 and 6 months, respectively.

*Classification*
Competency Category: Nursing Practice: Health and Wellness
Taxonomic Level: Knowledge/Comprehension

**43. A.** 30%.

*Rationale*
The duration of breastfeeding has decreased since 1960. Recent Canadian statistics show that although almost 75% of mothers begin breastfeeding in the hospital, only 60% and 30% are still exclusively breastfeeding at 3 and 6 months, respectively.

*Classification*
Competency Category: Nursing Practice: Health and Wellness
Taxonomic Level: Knowledge/Comprehension

**44. B.** Efforts to contain health care costs.

*Rationale*
The average length of stay in Canada decreased during the early 1990s in an effort to contain health care costs.

*Classification*
Competency Category: Nursing Practice: Professional Practice
Taxonomic Level: Knowledge/Comprehension

**45. C.** 2 to 6 weeks.

*Rationale*
In breastfeeding women, lochia usually continues to 6 weeks postpartum.

*Classification*
Competency Category: Nursing Practice: Health and Wellness
Taxonomic Level: Application

**46. D.** Discuss Ruby's wants and desires.

*Rationale*
This response further explores Ruby's feelings so the nurse can assist her.

*Classification*
Competency Category: Nurse–Person Relationship
Taxonomic Level: Affective

**47. C.** It occurs in 10% to 15% of all postpartum women.

*Rationale*
Approximately 10% to 15% of women experience postpartum depression.

*Classification*
Competency Category: Nursing Practice: Alterations in Health
Taxonomic Level: Knowledge/Comprehension

**48. C.** Ongoing relationships with other mothers with young children.

*Rationale*
Other mothers with young children offer valuable kinds of support because women need to talk about their feelings with others who understand them. The women's partners often do not understand postpartum depression and are not as supportive as other mothers.

*Classification*
Competency Category: Nursing Practice: Alterations in Health
Taxonomic Level: Application

**49. A.** 500 mL.

*Rationale*
Postpartum hemorrhage has been traditionally defined as the loss of more than 500 mL of blood after a vaginal birth and 1000 mL after a cesarean birth.

*Classification*
Competency Category: Nursing Practice: Alterations in Health
Taxonomic Level: Knowledge/Comprehension

**50. A.** Backache.

*Rationale*
With a late postpartum hemorrhage, which is often related to subinvolution of the placental site, the fundal height is greater than expected. The lochia fails to normally progress from rubra to serosa to alba. Some women report irregular, heavy bleeding. Leukorrhea, backache, and foul-smelling lochia may occur if infection is a cause.

*Classification*
Competency Category: Nursing Practice: Alterations in Health
Taxonomic Level: Application

**51. B.** To suppress antibody formation in a woman with Rh-negative blood after giving birth to an Rh-positive baby

*Rationale*

RhoGAM is indicated to suppress antibody formation in women with Rh-negative blood after birth, miscarriage or pregnancy termination, abdominal trauma, ectopic pregnancy, or amniocentesis.

*Classification*

Competency Category: Nursing Practice: Health and Wellness

Taxonomic Level: Application

**52. B.** Perineal discomfort.

*Rationale*

Complications associated with an episiotomy are blood loss, infection, pain, and perineal discomfort that may continue for days or weeks after giving birth.

*Classification*

Competency Category: Nursing Practice: Alterations in Health

Taxonomic Level: Application

**53. C.** 9 to 12 months old.

*Rationale*

If an infant is not breastfed or is partially breastfed, commercial formulas are the most acceptable alternative to breast milk until the baby is 9 to 12 months of age.

*Classification*

Competency Category: Nursing Practice: Health and Wellness

Taxonomic Level: Knowledge/Comprehension

**54. D.** "Your baby needs 400 IU per day when being breastfed."

*Rationale*

It is recommended that all breastfed, healthy, term infants in Canada receive a daily vitamin D supplement of 10 µg (400 IU). Supplementation should begin at birth and continue until the infant's diet includes at least 10 µg (400 IU) per day of vitamin D from other dietary sources or until the breastfed infant reaches 1 year of age.

*Classification*

Competency Category: Nursing Practice: Health and Wellness

Taxonomic Level: Knowledge/Comprehension

**55. C.** Cow's milk should not be used with infants younger than 9 months of age.

*Rationale*

The quality and quantity of nutrients in cow's milk differs greatly from those of human milk, and cow's milk does not contain many of the various growth and immunologic factors found in human milk. Cow's milk also contains great amounts of protein and minerals and smaller amounts of essential fatty acids than human milk. Cow's milk has a low iron content, and the iron is poorly absorbed. To lower the risk of iron deficiency anemia, drinking cow's milk is not recommended for babies younger than 9 to 12 months of age.

*Classification*

Competency Category: Nursing Practice: Health and Wellness

Taxonomic Level: Knowledge/Comprehension

**56. D.** They usually feed every 3 to 4 hours.

*Rationale*

Formula is harder to digest than breast milk, so formula-fed babies typically feed less frequently than breastfed babies (every 3 to 4 hours instead of every 2 to 3 hours).

*Classification*

Competency Category: Nursing Practice: Health and Wellness

Taxonomic Level: Application

**57. A.** "All babies gain weight at different times. It is important to not make comparisons."

*Rationale*

Babies gain weight at different times. As long as babies are gaining weight within the acceptable weight gain guidelines used by public health practitioners, they are considered to have normal weight gain.

*Classification*

Competency Category: Nursing Practice: Health and Wellness

Taxonomic Level: Application

**58. B.** At least 24 hours after birth.

*Rationale*

The PKU screening test needs to be done after the infant is older than 24 hours of age and no later than 7 days of age. The timing of the screening test is determined by the age of the infant.

*Classification*

Competency Category: Nursing Practice: Health and Wellness

Taxonomic Level: Application

**59. C.** Keep the nipple full of formula throughout the feeding.

*Rationale*

The bottle should be held so that fluid fills the nipple and less air in the bottle is able to enter the nipple.

*Classification*
Competency Category: Nursing Practice: Health and Wellness
Taxonomic Level: Application

**60. A.** Income and social status.

*Rationale*
Strong and growing evidence suggests that higher social and economic status is associated with better health. In fact, these factors seem to be the most important determinants of health. The other determinants are important but are not the most influential on the outcomes of health.

*Classification*
Competency Category: Nursing Practice: Health and Wellness
Taxonomic Level: Critical Thinking

**61. B.** Increasing accessibility.

*Rationale*
Increasing accessibility is important because people should have reasonable access to essential health services with no financial or geographical barriers.

*Classification*
Competency Category: Professional Practice
Taxonomic Level: Critical Thinking

**62. B.** Strengthening community action.

*Rationale*
Community development draws on existing human and material resources to enhance self-help and social support and to develop flexible systems for strengthening public participation in and direction of health matters.

*Classification*
Competency Category: Professional Practice
Taxonomic Level: Critical Thinking

**63. A.** Pathologic jaundice.

*Rationale*
Jaundice that appears before 24 hours of age is considered to be pathologic and warrants immediate attention.

*Classification*
Competency Category: Nursing Practice: Alterations in Health
Taxonomic Level: Critical Thinking

**64. C.** Notify Baby Tran's primary caregiver as soon as possible.

*Rationale*
Jaundice that appears before 24 hours of age is considered to be pathologic and warrants immediate attention.

*Classification*
Competency Category: Nursing Practice: Alterations in Health
Taxonomic Level: Critical Thinking

**65. C.** "I can tell you are worried about your baby. Let's talk about this change in your baby's skin color."

*Rationale*
This response further explores the parents' feelings so the nurse can assist them.

*Classification*
Competency Category: Nursing Practice: Alterations in Health
Taxonomic Level: Affective

**66. C.** The care that a reasonable, prudent nurse would provide in a comparable situation.

*Rationale*
The minimum standard of care required of nursing practice is the care that a reasonable, prudent nurse would provide in a comparable situation.

*Classification*
Competency Category: Professional Practice
Taxonomic Level: Knowledge/Comprehension

**67. A.** The primary care provider.

*Rationale*
The primary care provider is responsible for obtaining the informed consent from the client, guardian, or designate before a cesarean section is done.

*Classification*
Competency Category: Professional Practice
Taxonomic Level: Application

**68. C.** She met the national standards of practice.

*Rationale*
Following the recognized national standards of practice (i.e., from the Association of Women's Health, Obstetric and Neonatal Nurses) helps protect nurses from accusations of negligence.

*Classification*
Competency Category: Professional Practice
Taxonomic Level: Application

**69. C.** They are more aware of the subtle cues that indicate changes during labour and birth.

*Rationale*

Experienced nurses are able to view individual client situations more holistically. It has been demonstrated that experienced nurses are more aware of subtle maternal and fetal cues that indicate changes during labour and birth.

*Classification*

Competency Category: Professional Practice
Taxonomic Level: Application

**70. C.** Influence of the extended family.

*Rationale*

The influence of the extended family is the cultural factor that is causing the nurse's dilemma. It is common for English-speaking women to defer to an extended family member in both formal and informal decision-making situations.

*Classification*

Competency Category: Nursing Practice: Alterations in Health
Taxonomic Level: Application

**71. D.** Try to respect the cultural limitations in each situation.

*Rationale*

The nurse knows she must make every effort to respect and work within the cultural limitations in each client situation.

*Classification*

Competency Category: Professional Practice
Taxonomic Level: Critical Thinking

**72. A.** History of postpartum hemorrhage (PPH).

*Rationale*

Women who have a history of PPH are at higher risk for a PPH in subsequent pregnancies. This is a significant factor for the nurse to know in planning and being prepared for the birth of the baby because this is the woman's fourth labour and birth.

*Classification*

Competency Category: Nursing Practice: Alterations in Health
Taxonomic Level: Critical Thinking

**73. C.** The intact membranes.

*Rationale*

An FSE may not be applied with intact amniotic membranes. An amniotomy must be performed instead.

*Classification*

Competency Category: Nursing Practice: Alterations in Health
Taxonomic Level: Critical Thinking

**74. A.** 110 to 160 bpm.

*Rationale*

The range for normal fetal heart rate is 110 to 160 bpm.

*Classification*

Competency Category: Alterations in Health
Taxonomic Level: Critical Thinking

**75. C.** Locate a bilingual staff member or an interpreter to translate before the couple signs the consent.

*Rationale*

With the increase in immigration in Canada over the past 10 years, many non–English-speaking families are entering the health care system. Health regions and institutions offer the services of interpreters or cultural health brokers to assist in translating services to facilitate effective communication and obtaining informed consent. It is prudent to identify a staff member or hospital visitor who may be fluent in the client's language. Consent must be obtained in the client's language of origin.

*Classification*

Competency Category: Professional Practice
Taxonomic Level: Critical Thinking

**76. C.** The suspicious BPP score.

*Rationale*

BPP scoring is based on five assessment criteria. The low BPP score, 6 of 10, is considered suspicious and indicates that the well-being of the baby may be compromised. The decision to induce labour increases the risks related to prematurity of birth because Lilly is only at 34 weeks gestation.

*Classification*

Competency Category: Nursing Practice: Alterations in Health
Taxonomic Level: Critical Thinking

**77. C.** The uterus does not relax between uterine contractions.

*Rationale*

One of the nursing responsibilities with the administration of an oxytocic, such as Pitocin, is to assess for uterine hyperstimulation (as per institutional policy, e.g., every 15 minutes). Uterine hyperstimulation is defined as a uterus that does not relax between uterine contractions or uterine contractions that occur more frequently than 1:2, exceed 90 seconds in duration, and are strong in intensity.

*Classification*
Competency Category: Nursing Practice: Alterations in Health
Taxonomic Level: Critical Thinking

**78. D.** Offer Lilly hot beverages.

*Rationale*
It is common for Asian women in labour to drink only hot beverages because of a birth philosophy related to yin and yang. Offering the woman hot beverages that are available on the unit is culturally sensitive and will achieve the goal of hydration.

*Classification*
Competency Category: Nursing Practice: Alterations in Health
Taxonomic Level: Critical Thinking

**79. B.** Stand next to her at the side of the bed.

*Rationale*
The client is alone and is progressing well in labour as evidenced by her restless behaviours. She is refusing analgesia but will benefit from the one-on-one nursing care model if she is aware that the nurse is attending her at the bedside.

*Classification*
Competency Category: Nurse–Person Relationship
Taxonomic Level: Application

**80. A.** "When is your baby due?"

*Rationale*
This is Lisa's fourth pregnancy, and she has been labouring for 4 hours, so knowing when the baby is due is the priority because the birth may be imminent. This client has had three previous childbirth experiences and knows when to present to the hospital to give birth. The nurse must be prepared for a preterm, term, or postterm infant. The nurse is not aware of the quality of the uterine contractions at this time.

*Classification*
Competency Category: Nursing Practice: Alterations in Health
Taxonomic Level: Critical Thinking

**81. D.** Back labour.

*Rationale*
Posterior positions generally cause more discomfort for the labouring woman because the rotation of the fetal head puts pressure on the sacral nerves, causing sharp pain.

*Classification*
Competency Category: Nursing Practice: Alterations in Health
Taxonomic Level: Application

**82. D.** Term.

*Rationale*
A term infant is born after the beginning of week 38 and before week 42 of pregnancy.

*Classification*
Competency Category: Nursing Practice: Health and Wellness
Taxonomic Level: Knowledge/Comprehension

**83. A.** Enter the birthing room as few times as possible to do the required assessments.

*Rationale*
The birth plan is a vehicle for communicating to the health care providers the family's desires regarding the birth attendant; birth setting; support person; and activities during labour, birth, and the postpartum period. The nurse should collaborate with the couple to respect their plans and achieve the goals of safe childbirth.

*Classification*
Competency Category: Nurse–Person Relationship
Taxonomic Level: Affective

**84. D.** Begin continuous fetal heart rate monitoring.

*Rationale*
Meconium staining in the amniotic fluid is not always a sign of fetal distress but is correlated with its occurrence. It reveals that the fetus has had an episode of loss of sphincter control. This clinical situation requires further investigation with fetal heart rate monitoring.

*Classification*
Competency Category: Alterations in Health
Taxonomic Level: Critical Thinking

**85. D.** Have her seek immediate attention from her primary care provider.

*Rationale*
Holly should be advised to immediately report any spotting or bleeding that occurs during pregnancy to her primary health provider so that a thorough assessment can be performed.

Classification
Competency Category: Nursing Practice: Alterations in Health
Taxonomic Level: Knowledge

**86. C.** "I can understand your need to find an answer about what caused this. Let's talk about this further."

*Rationale*
The woman and her family may search for a cause for a spontaneous early bleed so they can plan knowledgeably for future pregnancies. However, even with modern technology and medical advances, a direct cause cannot usually be determined. This response further explores Holly and Jeff's feelings so the nurse can assist them.

*Classification*
Competency Category: Nurse–Person Relationship
Taxonomic Level: Application

**87. B.** 10% to 20%.

*Rationale*
About 10% to 20% of all clinically recognized pregnancies end in miscarriage.

*Classification*
Competency Category: Nursing Practice: Alterations in Health
Taxonomic Level: Knowledge/Comprehension

**88. A.** "Let's talk about what you can do while on bed rest to still meet these needs."

*Rationale*
When a client is prescribed bed rest, the nurse needs to emphasize how the woman can maintain some sense of personal control and have some personal choices open to her.

*Classification*
Competency Category: Professional Practice
Taxonomic Level: Application

**89. B.** Do gentle exercises of the legs.

*Rationale*
Gentle exercises, such as circling the feet or gently tensing and relaxing the leg muscles, improve muscle tone and circulation and provide a sense of well-being.

*Classification*
Competency Category: Professional Practice
Taxonomic Level: Application

**90. B.** "You are probably experiencing Braxton Hicks contractions."

*Rationale*
Braxton Hicks contractions are irregular, generally painless, and occur intermittently throughout pregnancy, often beginning around 16 weeks gestation. The contractions facilitate uterine blood flow.

*Classification*
Competency Category: Nursing Practice: Health and Wellness
Taxonomic Level: Critical Thinking

**91. A.** She should change her activity.

*Rationale*
Braxton Hick's contractions stop with a change in activity.

*Classification*
Competency Category: Nursing Practice: Alterations in Health
Taxonomic Level: Critical Thinking

**92. C.** Decrease uterine contractility.

*Rationale*
Dehydration may increase uterine contractility by decreasing uterine blood flow and increasing pituitary secretion of antidiuretic hormone and oxytocin.

*Classification*
Competency Category: Nursing Practice: Health and Wellness
Taxonomic Level: Critical Thinking

**93. B.** "You have been through a lot already with your pregnancy. Let's talk about this further."

*Rationale*
This response acknowledges Trina's experience and provides the opportunity to explore her feelings further so the nurse can assist her.

*Classification*
Competency Category: Nurse–Person Relationship
Taxonomic Level: Affective

**94. C.** "Let's talk about how this cramping occurs so we can help you understand what causes it."

*Rationale*
This response further explores Trina's feelings so the nurse can assist her.

*Classification*
Competency Category: Nurse–Person Relationship
Taxonomic Level: Affective

**95. B.** "I am glad you came in! We need to assess you further."

*Rationale*
Cayley's symptoms need to be explored further to rule out hypertension and other possible complications of pregnancy. Her symptoms are not urgent enough at this point to refer her to her primary care provider until after the nurse has assessed her further.

*Classification*
Competency Category: Nursing Practice–Alterations in Health
Taxonomic Level: Application

**96. D.** "Tell me more about your experience with your primary care provider and how this made you feel."

*Rationale*
This response further explores Cayley's feelings so the nurse can assist her.

*Classification*
Competency Category: Nurse–Person Relationship
Taxonomic Level: Affective

**97. D.** Hypertension.

*Rationale*
Based on the above rationale, Cayley has an increase in her blood pressure, which should be monitored but is not high enough to be considered hypertension.

*Classification*
Competency Category: Nursing Practice: Alterations in Health
Taxonomic Level: Critical Thinking

**98. D.** Refer her to her primary care provider.

*Rationale*
With preeclampsia, edema begins to accumulate in the upper part of the body rather than just the typical ankle edema of pregnancy. With severe preeclampsia, the edema is present in the woman's hands and face as puffiness and is not responsive to 12 hours of bed rest. A primary care provider needs to be seen to determine the appropriate treatment.

*Classification*
Competency Category: Nursing Practice: Alterations in Health
Taxonomic Level: Critical Thinking

**99. B.** "Tell me what you are most worried about regarding their visit, and we can go from there."

*Rationale*
This response further explores Cayley's feelings so the nurse can assist her.

*Classification*
Competency Category: Nurse–Person Relationship
Taxonomic Level: Application

**100. D.** Low birth weight.

*Rationale*
Preterm birth is more than 5.9 times higher with multiple fetal pregnancies than singleton pregnancies. The complication of infant prematurity and low birth weight is associated with preterm birth.

*Classification*
Competency Category: Nursing Practice: Alterations in Health
Taxonomic Level: Knowledge/Comprehension

**101. D.** 55%.

*Rationale*
The rate of preterm birth for twins increased from 40.9% in 1981 to 55% in 1997 in the United States and Canada.

*Classification*
Competency Category: Nursing Practice: Alterations in Health
Taxonomic Level: Knowledge/Comprehension

**102. C.** Those with a multi-fetal pregnancy.

*Rationale*
The cause of preterm labour is unknown and is assumed to be multifactorial. Low socioeconomic status, smoking, and unusual fatigue during pregnancy are risk factors for preterm birth but alone do not carry the same high risk as multi-fetal pregnancy. The risk of preterm birth is substantially higher for women with multi-fetal pregnancy (55% risk).

*Classification*
Competency Category: Nursing Practice: Alterations in Health
Taxonomic Level: Application

**103. B.** She should lie on her left side as much as possible.

*Rationale*
Lying in the left lateral recumbent position decreases pressure on the vena cava, increasing venous return, circulatory volume, and placental and renal perfusion. Improved renal blood flow helps decrease angiotension II levels, promotes dieresis, and lowers blood pressure.

*Classification*
Competency Category: Nursing Practice: Health and Wellness
Taxonomic Level: Application

**104. C.** "Let's talk about what is concerning you."

*Rationale*
This response allows exploration of the husband's experience so the nurse can assist him.

*Classification*
Competency Category: Nurse–Person Relationship
Taxonomic Level: Application

**105. B.** Social support networks.

*Rationale*
Support from families, friends, and the community is associated with better health. Such social support networks may be very important in helping people solve problems and deal with adversity, as well as in maintaining a sense of mastery and control over their life circumstances. The caring and respect that occur in social relationships and the resulting sense of satisfaction and well-being seem to act as buffers against health problems.

*Classification*
Competency Category: Nursing Practice: Health and Wellness
Taxonomic Level: Knowledge/Comprehension

**106. B.** Justice.

*Rationale*
The value of justice is practiced when nurses assist persons in receiving a share of health services and resources proportionate to their needs and in promoting social justice. In this case, the nurses are advocating for this population's equitable share of health services.

*Classification*
Competency Category: Nursing Practice: Professional Practice
Taxonomic Level: Application

**107. A.** To assess the parents' readiness and interest in learning.

*Rationale*
A "needs assessment" determines what the parents already know and what they are interested in learning about. They will be more open to participate if topics they show an interest in are discussed.

*Classification*
Competency Category: Nurse–Person Relationship
Taxonomic Level: Application

**108. B.** "What do you want to learn about?"

*Rationale*
To be client centered, the nurse needs to determine what this mother's learning needs are. Other barriers, such as finances and access to classes, should be part of the nurse's role to work with the parents to overcome if the nurse is practicing within a primary health care and CNA Code of Ethics philosophy.

*Classification*
Competency Category: Nurse–Person Relationship
Taxonomic Level: Application

**109. B.** Confidentiality.

*Rationale*
Confidentiality is safeguarding information learned in the context of a professional relationship and ensuring it is shared outside the health care team only with the person's informed consent, as may be legally required, or when the failure to disclose it would cause significant harm.

*Classification*
Competency Category: Nursing Practice: Professional Practice
Taxonomic Level: Application

**110. C.** Stillbirth.

*Rationale*
A stillbirth is the birth of a baby after 20 weeks gestation and 1 day that does not show any signs of life.

*Classification*
Competency Category: Nursing Practice: Alterations on Health
Taxonomic Level: Knowledge/Comprehension

**111. D.** "I can understand your need to find an answer about what caused this. Let's talk about this further."

*Rationale*
This response attends to Madison and further explores her feelings so the nurse can help her express her grief.

*Classification*
Competency Category: Nurse–Person Relationship
Taxonomic Level: Affective

**112. D.** Assigned meaning to the event.

*Rationale*
It is important to gain some understanding of the parents' perception of their unique loss. The meaning of the loss is determined by the parents' familial and cultural systems.

*Classification*
Competency Category: Nursing Practice: Health and Wellness
Taxonomic Level: Application

**113. C.** Provide an early opportunity for the couple to see their child if they desire.

*Rationale*
Seeing the baby helps parents face the reality of the loss, reduces painful fantasies, and offers an opportunity for closure. The wishes of the parents should be respected whether or not they want to see their baby.

*Classification*
Competency Category: Nurse–Person Relationship
Taxonomic Level: Critical Thinking

**114. A.** The test assesses for Down syndrome.

*Rationale*
The triple marker test is performed at 16 to 18 weeks gestation and uses three maternal serum markers in combination with maternal age to calculate the risk score. Down syndrome is associated with lower-than-normal levels of the maternal serum markers.

*Classification*
Competency Category: Nursing Practice: Alterations in Health
Taxonomic Level: Knowledge/Comprehension

**115. D.** Recognizing the family as active participants in their care.

*Rationale*
The nurse recognizes the family as active participants in their care by discussing and inquiring about their birth plans. The nurse is then able to advocate for the family throughout the labour and birth experience.

*Classification*
Competency Category: Nurse–Person Relationship
Taxonomic Level: Affective

**116. C.** The baby needs to be observed more closely.

*Rationale*
It is not ethical to tell this woman that her baby is "fine." The passage of meconium indicates that the fetus has experienced a stressor in the intrauterine environment. The well-being of the fetus is not yet known and requires further observation and evaluation with the internal FSE.

*Classification*
Competency Category: Nursing Practice: Alterations in Health
Taxonomic Level: Application

**117. D.** Late decelerations with minimal variability.

*Rationale*
Late decelerations are periodic uniform changes in the fetal heart rate that are associated with uterine contractions. They are also associated with metabolic acidemia when paired with absent short-term variability and decreased long-term variability.

*Classification*
Competency Category: Nursing Practice: Alterations in Health
Taxonomic Level: Critical Thinking

**118. C.** Prepare Brandi for an assisted or cesarean birth.

*Rationale*
Fetal heart decelerations, thick meconium, and low fetal scalp pH indicate severe fetal distress. Because the woman is a primigravida and in early labour at 4 cm cervical dilatation, it is unlikely that the baby will tolerate further labour and a vaginal birth. The baby will be delivered immediately, so it is prudent for the nurse to begin preparing the client for an assisted or operative birth.

*Classification*
Competency Category: Nursing Practice: Alterations in Health
Taxonomic Level: Critical Thinking

**119. C.** Placental insufficiency.

*Rationale*
The presence of late decelerations indicates that the fetus is affected by placental insufficiency. There is decreased blood flow and oxygen available during the

contraction when the uterine blood vessels are compressed during a contraction.

*Classification*
Competency Category: Nursing Practice: Alterations in Health
Taxonomic Level: Knowledge/Comprehension

**120. D.** Assess the imminence of birth.

*Rationale*
Because this is their fifth baby and the woman has been in labour for 3 hours, it is essential for the nurse to assess for the imminence of birth. After this has been established, the nurse will know how much time he or she has to review the obstetrical history, assess Beth's coping skills, and ensure the presence of a support person for the labour and birth.

*Classification*
Competency Category: Nursing Practice: Health and Wellness
Taxonomic Level: Application

**121. D.** 8 to 10 cm.

*Rationale*
The woman is multiparous and likely to be in transitional labour as evidenced by her increasing anxiety and distress. She has been in labour for several hours, and the uterine contractions are strong and frequent. The amount of bloody show indicates remarkable cervical changes. Her cervical dilatation will most likely be 8 to 10 cm.

*Classification*
Competency Category: Nursing Practice: Alterations in Health
Taxonomic Level: Critical Thinking

**122. D.** Instruct the woman to pant so the nurse can support the baby's head as it crowns.

*Rationale*
These methods should be used during the second stage of labour as the fetal head is crowning. Less intense pushing may facilitate a slow delivery of the head and avoids tears and the need for episiotomy. Encouraging the woman to pant through the contractions will distract her and help her use breathing techniques.

*Classification*
Competency Category: Nursing Practice: Alterations in Health
Taxonomic Level: Critical Thinking

**123. C.** Offer to remain with the woman while he takes a short break.

*Rationale*
It is possible that the father is reluctant to leave his partner alone during this time. It is appropriate, if possible, for the nurse to offer to stay with his partner while he goes for a break. He will be able to take a break and know that his partner is not alone at the time.

*Classification*
Competency Category: Nurse–Person Relationship
Taxonomic Level: Application

**124. D.** No; narcotics prolong labour.

*Rationale*
Narcotics may decrease uterine activity if given in early labour.

*Classification*
Competency Category: Nursing Practice: Alterations in Health
Taxonomic Level: Knowledge/Comprehension

**125. C.** "Some of the medication crosses the placenta, but it should be out of the baby's system by the time of birth."

*Rationale*
The medication (i.e., narcotic analgesia) crosses the placenta, but it should be out of the baby's system by the time of birth. The woman is at 4 to 5 cm cervical dilatation and not fully effaced. Because she is a primigravida, she most likely has 5 hours of labour before the baby's birth.

*Classification*
Competency Category: Nursing Practice: Alterations in Health
Taxonomic Level: Application

**126. D.** Pudendal block.

*Rationale*
A pudendal block is administered during the second stage of labour to relive pain in the lower vagina, vulva, and perineum. A pudendal block must be administered 10 to 20 minutes before anesthesia is required.

*Classification*
Competency Category: Nursing Practice: Alterations in Health
Taxonomic Level: Application

**127. C.** Active.

*Rationale*
Because the cervix is dilating (i.e., 5 cm) and has fully effaced (100%), the woman appears to be in active labour. The regular uterine contractions are effective

in facilitating fetal descent through the pelvis because the presenting part is well applied on the cervix and is at -1 station.

*Classification*
Competency Category: Nursing Practice: Health and Wellness
Taxonomic Level: Application

**128. B.** Ambulate ad lib.

*Rationale*
The woman should be encouraged to ambulate as desired during labour and birth.

*Classification*
Competency Category: Nursing Practice: Health and Wellness
Taxonomic Level: Critical Thinking

**129. C.** Oxytocin augmentation.

*Rationale*
The woman's progress in labour over the past 4 hours is unsatisfactory. Augmentation of labour, which is the simulation of uterine contractions after labour has started spontaneously, will most likely be ordered.

*Classification*
Competency Category: Nursing Practice: Alterations in Health
Taxonomic Level: Critical Thinking

**130. C.** Fetal heart tones.

*Rationale*
The incidence of cesarean birth is increasing in Canada to the highest reported rates ever. The purpose of a cesarean section is to preserve the life or health of the mother and her fetus. It may be the best choice for birth when there is evidence of maternal and fetal complications. The final assessment the nurse should make in the birthing room before transporting the client to the operating theatre is to assess fetal heart tones. This information should be communicated to the theatre staff so they are aware of the presence or absence of fetal distress.

*Classification*
Competency Category: Alterations in Health
Taxonomic Level: Critical Thinking

**131. A.** Progressive cervical dilatation and effacement.

*Rationale*
True labour is defined as the onset of regular uterine contractions that cause progressive cervical dilatation and effacement.

*Classification*
Competency Category: Nursing Practice: Alterations in Health
Taxonomic Level: Application

**132. C.** The beginning of one contraction to the end of the same contraction.

*Rationale*
The duration of the uterine contraction is measured in seconds by timing the onset of the contraction to the end of the same contraction.

*Classification*
Competency Category: Nursing Practice: Alterations in Health
Taxonomic Level: Knowledge/Comprehension

**133. C.** Referred pain from the uterus.

*Rationale*
Referred pain is pain that originates in the uterus and radiates to the abdominal wall, lumbosacral areas of the back, iliac crest, gluteal area, and thighs. This pain may occur with contractions or in between contractions.

*Classification*
Competency Category: Nursing Practice: Alterations in Health
Taxonomic Level: Application

**134. C.** When she is in active labour.

*Rationale*
Epidural anesthesia is the most commonly used method of pain relief for labour in Canada. It is imperative that the epidural be administered when the woman is in active labour.

*Classification*
Competency Category: Nursing Practice: Alterations in Health
Taxonomic Level: Application

**135. D.** Stand quietly at the back of the room.

*Rationale*
It is unsafe to leave the woman unattended in the room when she is in transitional labour and birth is imminent. Standing at the back of the room allows the nurse to provide safe care during labour and birth and lets the woman know that the nurse is still present in the room.

*Classification*
Competency Category: Nursing Practice: Alterations in Health
Taxonomic Level: Critical Thinking

**136. C.** Decreased maternal heart rate.

*Rationale*
Maternal heart rate is not affected by the administration of a narcotic analgesic.

*Classification*
Competency Category: Nursing Practice: Alterations in Health
Taxonomic Level: Application

**137. D.** Tell Huang to wait outside in the lobby while Lim is being examined.

*Rationale*
It is common for abusers to isolate their partners to maintain control. Pregnancy and birth are trigger points for intimate partner abuse because the abuser may experience a sense of loss of control. The time in hospital may be the only time the victim has to communicate with others. It is important to assess the woman away from the potential abuser to further explore the suspicions of abuse. Asking the potential abuser to wait in another room helps the nurse achieve this goal.

*Classification*
Competency Category: Nursing Practice: Alterations in Health
Taxonomic Level: Application

**138. C.** Partner abuse may increase during pregnancy.

*Rationale*
Pregnancy and birth are trigger points for intimate partner abuse because the abuser may experience a sense of loss of control. This is especially true if abuse occurred before the pregnancy. During pregnancy, the mother and baby take priority, and the abuser attempts to maintain or regain control by abusing the woman.

*Classification*
Competency Category: Nursing Practice: Alterations in Health
Taxonomic Level: Knowledge/Comprehension

**139. D.** Ambivalence toward the husband.

*Rationale*
Women who are abused by their intimate partners appear hopeless. They often exhibit behaviours that demonstrate depression and ambivalence toward their abuser.

*Classification*
Competency Category: Nursing Practice: Alterations in Health
Taxonomic Level: Application

**140. D.** "That comment sounds like it upset you. Tell me how you are feeling about your boyfriend's comments."

*Rationale*
This response allows Lisa to express her feelings so the nurse can assist her.

*Classification*
Competency Category: Nurse–Person Relationship
Taxonomic Level: Affective

**141. B.** Infected.

*Rationale*
The presence of HBsAg in serum (i.e., HBsAg = positive) identifies an infected person in either an acute or chronic carrier state.

*Classification*
Competency Category: Nursing Practice: Alterations in Health
Taxonomic Level: Application

**142. A.** Acutely infected.

*Rationale*
HBeAg and anti-HBe are investigated when HBsAg is found. They are prognostic indicators of infection. The presence of the marker IgM identifies acute infection within the past 4 to 6 months.

*Classification*
Competency Category: Nursing Practice: Alterations in Health
Taxonomic Level: Application

**143. C.** Reassess the workload with the charge nurse and request assistance.

*Rationale*
Reassessing the client assignment will bring the issue of the unsafe workload to the charge nurse's attention. After this has been established, it is reasonable to request assistance.

*Classification*
Competency Category: Professional Practice
Taxonomic Level: Critical Thinking

**144. C.** The attendants' level of knowledge and comfort level in performing specific nursing activities should be considered.

*Rationale*
RNs are responsible for providing and delegating safe nursing care. They remain responsible when

delegating nursing tasks to other members of the health care team. The nurse should delegate tasks in collaboration with the nursing attendant.

*Classification*
Competency Category: Professional Practice
Taxonomic Level: Critical Thinking

**145. D.** Notify the primary care provider immediately.

*Rationale*
Because of the markedly high blood pressure and the diagnosis, it is imperative that the primary care provider is notified immediately.

*Classification*
Competency Category: Professional Practice
Taxonomic Level: Critical Thinking

**146. C.** Meet with nursing colleagues and reassign the woman to an RN.

*Rationale*
Collaborating with colleagues is essential in this case. Reassigning the woman to an RN will provide the appropriate level of nursing care to the woman in this situation.

*Classification*
Competency Category: Professional Practice
Taxonomic Level: Critical Thinking

**147. A.** Tell the student it is okay to cry and encourage her to talk about the way she is feeling.

*Rationale*
Encouraging the nursing student to cry and express her feelings about perinatal death will help her identify her fears in a caring, supportive, and nonjudgmental manner.

*Classification*
Competency Category: Professional Practice
Taxonomic Level: Critical Thinking

**148. B.** Discuss the situation with the nursing student after the visit has ended.

*Rationale*
The nurse has a professional responsibility to discuss this situation with the nursing student in private. The student needs to know that these actions are insensitive to the grieving parents and are unprofessional. The actions do not value therapeutic boundaries between health care providers and their clients in the community.

*Classification*
Competency Category: Professional Practice
Taxonomic Level: Critical Thinking

**149. C.** Contact the nursing supervisor to clarify the appropriate actions in this acute mental health situation.

*Rationale*
The nurse should contact the immediate nursing supervisor to clarify or guide the correct nursing actions in this acute mental health situation. Community mental health services may be available that could visit the home and assess and intervene in this situation. The nurse should help the mother and baby inside and stay with them until the supervisor advises how best to manage the situation.

*Classification*
Competency Category: Professional Practice
Taxonomic Level: Critical Thinking

**150. C.** Demonstrate once and then supervise the student while she performs the procedure.

*Rationale*
This method of instruction facilitates preceptor learning by demonstration. The preceptor is accountable for delegating nursing interventions to student learners.

*Classification*
Competency Category: Professional Practice
Taxonomic Level: Critical Thinking

**151. C.** Share the feedback with the nursing colleague.

*Rationale*
Sharing the feedback with her colleague will recognize the value of the colleague's professional efforts and accomplishments.

*Classification*
Competency Category: Professional Practice
Taxonomic Level: Critical Thinking

**152. C.** Assess the client and contact the primary care provider.

*Rationale*
An accurate client assessment should be performed, and the primary care provider should be contacted immediately. The nurse should anticipate orders for changes to the management of care in this situation.

*Classification*
Competency Category: Professional Practice
Taxonomic Level: Critical Thinking

**153. A.** Ask Alyssa why she does not want to go home.

*Rationale*
It is important for the nurse to identify Alyssa's concerns and reasons for staying in hospital.

*Classification*
Competency Category: Nurse–Person Relationship
Taxonomic Level: Critical Thinking

**154. A.** Discuss the colleague's behaviour in private.

*Rationale*
This behaviour is unprofessional and breaches client confidentiality as per the Canadian Nurses Association Code of Ethics. The nurse is obligated to approach the colleague and discuss her inappropriate behaviours. Discussing this in private demonstrates professional conduct.

*Classification*
Competency Category: Professional Practice
Taxonomic Level: Critical Thinking

**155. C.** Notify the physician that Mr. Thomas has been waiting to discuss his wife's condition.

*Rationale*
Because of the wife's severe and deteriorating condition, the nurse is obligated to advocate for the family and notify the physician of the husband's request for a meeting and information.

*Classification*
Competency Category: Professional Practice
Taxonomic Level: Critical Thinking

**156. B.** Research findings do not always change perinatal nursing practice.

*Rationale*
Research findings may or may not contribute to changes in nursing practice.

*Classification*
Competency Category: Professional Practice
Taxonomic Level: Application

**157. A.** Autonomy.

*Rationale*
The principle of autonomy supports conflicts between maternal and fetal rights. The woman has the right to choose for herself what she believes to be in her best interests versus the well-being of the fetus. This is the concept of self-determination, of being in charge of one's person.

*Classification*
Competency Category: Professional Practice
Taxonomic Level: Application

**158. C.** Birth with the father and siblings present in the room.

*Rationale*
Woman-centred birth is the philosophy that recognizes the value of the woman's beliefs, values, and desires within the context of the family.

*Classification*
Competency Category: Professional Practice:
Taxonomic Level: Knowledge/Comprehension

**159. D.** Ensure their privacy.

*Rationale*
Coping with grief may be an overwhelming experience for the woman and her partner. The nurse needs to encourage and support the couple to maintain their relationship and keep open the channels of communication after the loss of their baby. Maintaining the couple's privacy is the appropriate method of responding in this situation because immediate nursing care is not required.

*Classification*
Competency Category: Nurse–Person Relationship
Taxonomic Level: Critical Thinking

**160. D.** Encourage the family to identify their frustrations and fears.

*Rationale*
This response will assist the family to identify their frustrations and fears so the nurse can work toward resolving their issues.

*Classification*
Competency Category: Nurse–Person Relationship
Taxonomic Level: Application

**161. A.** Cephalopelvic disproportion (CPD).

*Rationale*
In Canada, CPD is the most common indication for primary cesarean section.

*Classification*
Competency Category: Professional Practice
Taxonomic Level: Knowledge/Comprehension

**162. D.** Eyewear, gloves and a gown.

*Rationale*
The nurse should use universal precautions, including wearing eyewear, gloves, and a gown. All of these items protect the nurse's vulnerable areas, which may transmit the HIV virus from the contact with body fluids that may occur during birth.

*Classification*
Competency Category: Professional Practice
Taxonomic Level: Critical Thinking

**163. C.** When the presenting part is not engaged on the cervix.

*Rationale*
Prolapse of the umbilical cord is a serious perinatal emergency. It occurs when the umbilical cord comes down along the side of the presenting part or precedes the presenting part. It occurs in about 5% of pregnancies and is likely to occur when the fetal presenting part is high in the pelvis (e.g., -4 station).

*Classification*
Competency Category: Professional Practice
Taxonomic Level: Critical Thinking

**164. A.** Prevent or relieve pressure on the umbilical cord.

*Rationale*
A vaginal examination should be immediately performed with the purpose of lifting the presenting part off the cord.

*Classification*
Competency Category: Professional Practice
Taxonomic Level: Critical Thinking

**165. B.** Knee–chest.

*Rationale*
The knee–chest position is the only position that will relieve pressure on the umbilical cord.

*Classification*
Competency Category: Professional Practice
Taxonomic Level: Application

**166. D.** Prematurity.

*Rationale*
Prematurity is the leading cause of death and is responsible for nearly two thirds of neonatal deaths in Canada. Prematurity is correlated with teenage pregnancy, lack of prenatal care, nonwhite mothers, and chronic disease.

*Classification*
Competency Category: Professional Practice
Taxonomic Level: Application

**167. B.** Audible suck–swallow cycles.

*Rationale*
Audible suck–swallow cycles indicate that the nipple is at the back of the baby's palate and the baby is swallowing milk, quickly at first and then more slowly, as his or her appetite is satisfied. When the baby begins to receive milk, his or her jaw will work all the way back to the ear.

*Classification*
Competency Category: Health and Wellness
Taxonomic Level: Application

**168. A.** An incorrect latch.

*Rationale*
A good latch will be comfortable and should not cause redness, bruising, or cracks.

*Classification*
Competency Category: Nursing Practice: Alterations in Health
Taxonomic Level: Application

**169. B.** Remove the baby from the breast and reposition her.

*Rationale*
The baby has a poor latch, so the best response for long-term success with breastfeeding is to reposition the baby and assist Suzette to see and feel what a good latch is like.

*Classification*
Competency Category: Nursing Practice: Alterations in Health
Taxonomic Level: Critical Thinking

**170. B.** The baby has six to eight heavy, wet diapers a day from day 4 onward.

*Rationale*
This is the indicator for adequate hydration with breastfed babies over a 24-hour period.

*Classification*
Competency Category: Nursing Practice: Health and Wellness
Taxonomic Level: Critical Thinking

**171. D.** Taking a warm shower.

*Rationale*
Using warm compresses or a taking warm shower with water flowing over the breasts will soften the breast tissue before a feed.

*Classification*
Competency Category: Nursing Practice: Alteration in Health
Taxonomic Level: Critical Thinking

**172. B.** Increase her consumption of foods rich in fibre.

*Rationale*
Antononia's diet needs to be high in roughage and fibre to promote normal bowel elimination.

*Classification*
Competency Category: Nursing Practice: Health and Wellness
Taxonomic Level: Critical Thinking

**173. B.** Involution of the uterus.

*Rationale*
The uterus should not be palpated on a postpartal home visit because of discomfort from the cesarean birth.

*Classification*
Competency Category: Nursing Practice: Health and Wellness
Taxonomic Level: Critical Thinking

**174. A.** Do nothing because this is a normal finding.

*Rationale*
Lochia should not exceed a moderate amount, such as four to eight partially saturated perineal pads daily. The amount of lochia reported by Antononia is within these parameters.

*Classification*
Competency Category: Nursing Practice: Health and Wellness
Taxonomic Level: Critical Thinking

**175. B.** Oxytocin is released when the baby sucks, which causes the uterus to contract.

*Rationale*
Afterpains, which are intermittent cramping of the uterus, tend to be noticed by multiparas rather than primiparas. In this situation, the uterus must contract more forcefully to regain its prepregnancy size. These sensations are noticed most intensely while breastfeeding because the infant's sucking causes a release of oxytocin from the posterior pituitary, increasing the strength of the contractions.

*Classification*
Competency Category: Nursing Practice: Health and Wellness
Taxonomic Level: Application

**176. B.** Mastitis.

*Rationale*
Mastitis is a localized inflammation of the breast that occurs from milk that has not drained from the breast. It can progress to an infection and presents with fever and chills, which may develop quickly.

*Classification*
Competency Category: Nursing Practice: Alterations in Health
Taxonomic Level: Application

**177. C.** Advise her to see her primary care provider as soon as possible.

*Rationale*
Bhindu needs to see her primary care provider as soon as she can to treat the infection.

*Classification*
Competency Category: Nursing Practice: Alterations in Health
Taxonomic Level: Critical Thinking

**178. B.** "Let's talk about this further. What you are feeling right now?"

*Rationale*
This response further explores Bhindu's feelings so the nurse can assist her.

*Classification*
Competency Category: Nurse–Person Relationship
Taxonomic Level: Affective

**179. C.** "You need to continue to breastfeed, and the antibiotics will protect your baby from infection."

*Rationale*
The antibiotics will protect or treat the baby as well as the mother. Also, continuing to breastfeed helps mastitis to resolve more quickly.

*Classification*
Competency Category: Nursing Practice: Alterations in Health
Taxonomic Level: Critical Thinking

**180. B.** Massage the milk ducts while feeding on both sides of the breast.

*Rationale*
The breasts need to be massaged while feeding to clear the ducts during feeding and to prevent further episodes of mastitis.

*Classification*
Competency Category: Nursing Practice: Alterations in Health
Taxonomic Level: Application

**181. D.** Show Cyndie how the baby initiates interaction with her and attends to her.

*Rationale*
Teaching Cyndie how her baby comes prepared to interact with her will help her see that they are in a reciprocal relationship. This will help Cyndie to identify in the future other cues the baby is giving to communicate with her and increases the opportunities for attachment.

*Classification*
Competency Category: Nursing Practice: Health and Wellness
Taxonomic Level: Critical Thinking

**182. C.** Cues are frequently nonverbal and behavioural.

*Rationale*
Cues are nonverbal and behavioural in nature. They provide a means for the baby to interact with his or her parents.

*Classification*
Competency Category: Nursing Practice: Health and Wellness
Taxonomic Level: Knowledge/Comprehension

**183. D.** Letting the baby cry to get to sleep.

*Rationale*
Not responding to the needs of the newborn may indicate that the mother is not attaching to her infant.

*Classification*
Competency Category: Nursing Practice: Alterations in Health
Taxonomic Level: Application

**184. B.** Demonstrate ways that Cyndie can comfort her infant.

*Rationale*
Cyndie may need the nurse to demonstrate how to comfort the baby. She has not had a lot of visitors and may not have had this role modeling.

*Classification*
Competency Category: Nursing Practice: Health and Wellness
Taxonomic Level: Critical Thinking

**185. C.** Respect.

*Rationale*
The nurse is a guest in the family's home and needs to respect their time and space.

*Classification*
Competency Category: Nurse–Person Relationship
Taxonomic Level: Application

**186. A.** Maintaining boundaries.

*Rationale*
The nurse needs to demonstrate her professional boundaries, which includes not disclosing personal information or accepting a meal.

*Classification*
Competency Category: Nurse–Person Relationship
Taxonomic Level: Critical Thinking

**187. D.** It allows the nurse to interact with the family in their own natural setting.

*Rationale*
Community settings do not allow the family to be in their own home environment, where they are usually the most relaxed. In the home environment, the nurse can better assess how the family interacts and copes within their own surroundings.

*Classification*
Competency Category: Nurse–Person Relationship
Taxonomic Level: Application

**188. D.** Return to her car and call for backup or security from her health unit.

*Rationale*
The nurse needs to consider her own personal safety in this situation and how she will be of the most help to this family. She needs to get some backup support before entering the house because of the potential for violence. She should not go into the home if her safety is in danger.

*Classification*
Competency Category: Nursing Practice: Health and Wellness
Taxonomic Level: Critical Thinking

**189. C.** Blood incompatibility.

*Rationale*
Physiologic jaundice is caused by accelerated destruction of fetal red blood cells, impaired conjugation of bilirubin, and increased bilirubin reabsorption from the intestinal tract. The condition does not have pathologic basis; rather, it is a normal response of the newborn.

*Classification*
Competency Category: Nursing Practice: Alterations in Health
Taxonomic Level: Knowledge/Comprehension

**190. C.** Breastfeeding the baby 8 to 12 times in 24 hours and waking him for feeds.

*Rationale*
A 9% weight loss is within the normal parameters for weight loss during the first 3 to 4 days postpartum. However, it is on the high end of normal. The baby is also displaying signs of further weight loss and poor feeding because of lethargy and sleeping through feeds. Breastfeeding him 8 to 12 times in 24 hours and waking him for feeds is the most immediate response to increase his intake and to maintain his mother's milk supply.

*Classification*
Competency Category: Nursing Practice: Alterations in Health
Taxonomic Level: Critical Thinking

**191. A.** A minimum of one to three green to yellow stools.

*Rationale*
Because feeding practices, ineffective sucking, and other problems may diminish the mother's milk supply or prevent the baby from receiving an adequate portion of hindmilk, it is possible for a baby to be adequately hydrated yet have an inadequate calorie intake. Frequent urination remains one valid indicator of adequate newborn hydration from foremilk intake. Multiple daily stooling is an indicator of adequate newborn calorie intake from hindmilk. Both factors are needed to fully assess neonatal breastfeeding. Because a lack of daily stooling may be associated with inadequate newborn calorie intake, it is also a predictor of poor infant weight gain. Early detection of this situation

can be crucial for the baby's health and the continuation of breastfeeding.

*Classification*
Competency Category: Nursing Practice: Health and Wellness
Taxonomic Level: Application

**192. B.** Pump after feedings.

*Rationale*
It is best to pump after breastfeeding when the milk has already "let down" and is accessible.

*Classification*
Competency Category: Nursing Practice: Alterations in Health
Taxonomic Level: Application

**193. B.** Tell her that it is important to breastfeed at least once at night to release the hormone prolactin.

*Rationale*
Breastfeeding is important at night to release the hormone prolactin, which will sustain the overall milk supply.

*Classification*
Competency Category: Nursing Practice: Health and Wellness
Taxonomic Level: Critical Thinking

**194. A.** Postpartum baby blues.

*Rationale*
Postpartum baby blues occurs in up to 70% of women after the birth of a child. This condition is a mild depression, but the woman's functioning is usually not impaired. It usually begins on days 3 to 10 postpartum.

*Classification*
Competency Category: Nursing Practice: Alterations in Health
Taxonomic Level: Application

**195. B.** "Many mothers are a little weepy and depressed for the first few days after giving birth."

*Rationale*
This response is an accurate description of the postpartum baby blues.

*Classification*
Competency Category: Nursing Practice: Alterations in Health
Taxonomic Level: Critical Thinking

**196. A.** Previous history of postpartum depression.

*Rationale*
A history of a previous postpartum depression is the most significant risk factor for developing it again in future pregnancies.

*Classification*
Competency Category: Nursing Practice: Alterations in Health
Taxonomic Level: Application

**197. C.** Ask her if she has any thoughts of hurting herself or her baby.

*Rationale*
While conducting the postpartum depression screen, the nurse needs to determine client's risk of suicide and the potential for harm toward her baby because she has identified resentment toward the baby. Assessment of suicide risk reflects the standard of care. This assessment will not increase the client's risk but may save her life or her infant's life. Carrie's response to this question will determine how much risk she is under and what next steps are required.

*Classification*
Competency Category: Nursing Practice: Alterations in Health
Taxonomic Level: Critical Thinking

**198. B.** "Women at risk for acquiring sexually transmitted infections should use condoms."

*Rationale*
Condoms are classified as "barrier" contraception in that they create a physical barrier to prevent the transmission of sexually transmitted infections. They are an appropriate choice for women at risk of acquiring infections.

*Classification*
Competency Category: Nursing Practice: Health and Wellness
Taxonomic Level: Application

**199. A.** "It is not safe to consume alcohol during pregnancy."

*Rationale*
Complete abstinence from alcohol use during pregnancy is recommended. A safe level of alcohol consumption during pregnancy has not yet been established.

*Classification*
Competency Category: Nursing Practice: Health and Wellness
Taxonomic Level: Knowledge/Comprehension

**200. D.** Increased amounts of vernix.

*Rationale*
Vernix caseosa is a whitish substance that serves as a protective covering over the fetal body throughout the pregnancy. Vernix usually disappears by term gestation. It is highly unusual for a 12-day postmature baby to have increased amounts of vernix. A discrepancy between EDC and gestational age by physical examination must have occurred.

*Classification*
Competency Category: Nursing Practice: Alterations in Health
Taxonomic Level: Critical Thinking

**201. Answer:** Vaginal bleeding is a deviation from normal that may occur at any point during pregnancy. APH is vaginal bleeding between 20 weeks and the birth of the baby. APH occurs in 3% to 5% of all pregnancies in Canada. Classifications of APH include placenta previa, placenta abruption, unclassified, and genital tract lesions.

*Rationale*
Vaginal bleeding is a deviation from normal that may occur at any point during pregnancy. APH is defined as vaginal bleeding between 20 weeks and the birth of the baby. APH occurs in 3% to 5% of all pregnancies in Canada. Classifications of APH include placenta previa, placenta abruption, unclassified, and genital tract lesions.

*Classification*
Competency Category: Nursing Practice: Alterations in Health
Taxonomic Level: Knowledge/Comprehension

**202. Answers:**
- Contact bleeding: intercourse, Pap smear, examination, cervical polyp.
- Inflammation and infection.
- Dilatation and effacement or incompetent cervix.
- Abruptio placenta.
- Placenta previa.
- Vasa previa.
- Sinus rupture.

*Rationale*
Bleeding in the second and third trimesters can be caused by contact bleeding, trauma, coitus, placental complications, or cervical changes.

## Classification
Competency Category: Nursing Practice: Alterations in Health
Taxonomic Level: Application

### 203. Answers:

- Bleeding may be concealed (not visible) or external (visible) per the vagina.
- Abdominal pain or backache.
- Uterine irritability or contractions.
- Normal fetal presentation.
- Anemia and level of shock exceeding apparent blood loss.
- Uterine tenderness and increased uterine tone.
- Coagulopathy.

### Rationale
Premature separation of the placenta occurs when the placenta begins to separate from the uterus and bleeding results. This occurs in approximately 10% of pregnancies and is a frequent cause of fetal death. At the time of the separation, the woman may experience sharp, stabbing abdominal pain or backache. Heavy bleeding usually occurs with the separation, but blood can pool under the placenta and be hidden from view. The uterus may become irritable. Signs of shock usually occur rapidly because of the blood loss. The uterus becomes tense and feels rigid to the touch. If bleeding is excessive, blood fibrinogen may be depleted, and disseminated intravascular coagulation can occur.

### Classification
Competency Category: Nursing Practice: Alterations in Health
Taxonomic Level: Application

### 204. Answers:

- Death.
- Intrauterine growth retardation.
- Anemia.
- Malpresentation.

### Rationale
Premature separation of the placenta occurs when the placenta begins to separate from the uterus and bleeding results. This is an emergency situation that occurs in approximately 10% of pregnancies and is a frequent cause of fetal death. Fetal outcome is contingent on the extent of placental separation and the degree of fetal hypoxia. Intrauterine growth retardation, fetal anemia, and malpresentations are associated with antepartum hemorrhage.

### Classification
Competency Category: Nursing Practice: Alterations in Health
Taxonomic Level: Critical Thinking

### 205. Answers:

- Prevent perineal tearing.
- Prevent blood loss.
- Provide emotional support.
- Ensure that bladder is empty to decrease the risk of postpartum hemorrhage.
- Monitor blood pressure.

### Rationale
Rosie is at a higher risk for birth trauma with a precipitous delivery. Supporting the perineum and encouraging the mother to push gently is important to decrease the incidence of perineal tears. Rosie will require a great deal of emotional support to deal with her denial of the pregnancy. The absence of prenatal care means that her physical status is unknown. She is also at risk for anemia and blood pressure disorders because of her age and weight.

### Classification
Competency Category: Nursing Practice: Alterations in Health
Taxonomic Level: Critical Thinking

### 206. Answers:

- Warmth (drying the baby well, covering the head, placing the baby skin to skin on the mother's dry abdomen).
- Clearing the airway (suction nose and mouth).
- Sterile clamping of the cord (sterility is more important than speed).

### Rationale
This is an unexpected and precipitous birth, likely without any instruments or warm blankets present for the baby. Loss of temperature occurs very quickly in neonates, so warmth is a high priority. The nurse also needs to find suction to clear the baby's mouth and nose (if required) to maintain a patent airway. Having a sterile cord clamp ready is also a high priority.

### Classification
Competency Category: Nursing Practice: Alterations in Health
Taxonomic Level: Critical Thinking

**207. Answers:**

- Monitor vital signs.
- Monitor lochia.
- Observe for vaginal bleeding.
- Ensure that the uterus is well contracted.
- Ensure that the bladder is empty.
- Encourage bonding with the baby.
- Provide emotional support.

*Rationale*
Nursing priorities for Rosie are similar to those for any postpartum mother and include monitoring vital signs and lochia, observing for vaginal bleeding, ensuring that the uterus is well contracted and the bladder is kept empty, establishing lactation (if desired), encouraging bonding with the baby, and providing emotional support.

*Classification*
Competency Category: Nursing Practice: Health and Wellness
Taxonomic Level: Application

**208. Answers:**

- Placenta previa.
- Ruptured membranes at term; not in labour.
- Preterm labour.
- Active genital herpes.
- Undiagnosed third trimester bleeding.

*Rationale*
Vaginal examination provides health care providers with maternal and fetal assessment information that is important in determining the progress of care and management of labour. It is important for caregivers to know when a vaginal examination should and should not be performed.

*Classification*
Competency Category: Nursing Practice: Alterations in Health
Taxonomic Level: Critical Thinking

**209. Answers:**

- Decreased nourishment to the fetus.
- Decreased respiratory function for the fetus.

*Rationale*
There is an increased risk for stillbirth in pregnancies that progress past the confirmed due date. The major consequence of postdates is the decreased ability of the placenta to nourish and provide respiratory function for the fetus.

*Classification*
Competency Category: Nursing Practice: Alterations in Health
Taxonomic Level: Knowledge/Comprehension

**210. Answers:**

Cutaneous strategies:

- Counterpressure.
- Therapeutic touch and massage.
- Walking.
- Rocking.
- Changing position.
- Application of heat and cold.
- TENS.
- Acupressure.
- Hydrotherapy.

Sensory strategies:

- Aromatherapy.
- Breathing techniques.
- Music.
- Imagery.
- Use of focal points.

Cognitive strategies:

- Hypnosis.
- Biofeedback.

*Rationale*
Sally is experiencing contractions from the prostaglandin E2 gel. Because she is a primigravida, the contractions will most likely dissipate over time. It is appropriate to offer Sally a nonpharmacologic option for pain relief at this time. If Sally continues into established labour, it is appropriate to offer a stronger form of pain relief (i.e., pharmacologic analgesia or anesthesia).

*Classification*
Competency Category: Nursing Practice: Alterations in Health
Taxonomic Level: Critical Thinking

**211. Answers:**

- Induction refers to labour that has not started on its own.
- Augmentation occurs when labour has started but is not effective and needs to be enhanced with Pitocin.

*Rationale*

Pitocin is the most commonly used medication administered to women during childbirth. Pitocin's tocolytic effect stimulates the uterus to contract. It is imperative to assess the uterus for contractions before Pitocin is administered. Separate policies are used for the administration of Pitocin for augmentation and induction of labour.

*Classification*

Competency Category: Nursing Practice: Alterations in Health

Taxonomic Level: Application

**212. Answers:**

- Conduct a physical assessment of the mother and newborn.
- Assess the infant's feeding and weight gain.
- Evaluate maternal psychosocial adjustment, bonding, and attachment.
- Evaluate parental behaviour, coping skills, and care of the newborn.
- Determine environmental strengths and risk factors.
- Provide client and family teaching.
- Consult with the primary care provider, lactation consultant, or other appropriate resource(s).
- Refer the family to appropriate community resources
- Schedule follow-up care with home visits or telephone contact.

*Rationale*

Nursing care in the home provides both physical and psychosocial support and links the family to the larger health systems. The postpartal home visit is conducted by a registered nurse who is experienced in postpartal maternal and newborn care. The visit is conducted within 24 to 48 hours of discharge and is designed to provide assistance to the family as they deal with questions or concerns that may arise as they begin caring for their infant.

*Classification*

Competency Category: Nursing Practice: Health and Wellness

Taxonomic Level: Critical Thinking

**213. Answers:**

- Vital signs: Blood pressure, pulse, respirations, temperature.

- Breasts: Breastfeeding or not breastfeeding, condition of the nipples and breast tissue, milk supply.
- Involution of the uterus: Fundal height, firmness of the uterus.
- Bladder: Urine output (frequency, dysuria, odor).
- Bowel: Bowel pattern.
- Perineum: Swelling, bruising, episiotomy.
- Lochia: Amount, color, odor.
- Legs: Swelling, edema, hot spots, pain, mobility.

*Rationale*

The nurse needs to follow through on a complete postpartum physical assessment as the woman is recovering from childbirth and may be breastfeeding. Because the length of stay in the hospital remains relatively short for mothers to recover and assimilate the knowledge they need to appropriately care for themselves and their newborns, this assessment is crucial.

*Classification*

Competency Category: Nursing Practice: Health and Wellness

Taxonomic Level: Application

**214. Answers:**

- Attachment.
- Coping skills.
- Parental role attainment.
- Sociocultural considerations.
- Learning needs.
- Financial resources.
- Interaction between the couple.
- Interaction with the baby.
- Ability to meet the newborn's needs.
- Social supports.

*Rationale*

The home setting provides an opportunity for the nurse and family to interact in a more relaxed environment, one where the family has control over the setting. It also provides an invaluable opportunity for the nurse to assess the psychosocial aspects of parenting in the setting where the family will grow and develop.

*Classification*

Competency Category: Nursing Practice: Health and Wellness

Taxonomic Level: Application

**215. Answers:**

- Provides protection against gastrointestinal infections.
- Provides protection against respiratory and ear infections.
- Contains growth factors and hormones to help with growth and development.
- May help prevent or delay the start of allergies.
- Provides a decreased risk of sudden infant death syndrome.
- Provides protective effects against childhood lymphoma, leukemia, and insulin-dependent diabetes.
- Enhances jaw development, decreasing problems with malocclusions and malalignment of the teeth.
- Changes to meet the baby's growing needs.
- Decreases the risk of childhood obesity.
- Is always fresh and at the right temperature.
- Human milk is made for human babies.

*Rationale*

Breastfeeding is the optimal method for feeding infants because it is made for humans and is tailored to the specific infant.

*Classification*

Competency Category: Nursing Practice: Health and Wellness

Taxonomic Level: Knowledge/Comprehension

## ▶ Self-Analysis for Chapter 6

> 200 Multiple-choice questions × 1 point each = /200 points
> +
> 15 Short answer questions for a total of 50 points = /50 points
>
> *Total Maternal–Child Health Nursing review questions =/250 points*

## SUPPLEMENTAL RESOURCES

Arnold, J., & Boggs, S. (2002). *Interpersonal relationships: Professional communications skills for nurses.* Philadelphia: Saunders.

Association of Women's Health, Obstetric and Neonatal Nurses. (2003). *Fetal heart monitoring principles and practice.* Dubuque, IA: Kendall Hunt.

Beck, C.T. (2002). Revision of the postpartum depression predictor's inventory. *Journal of Obstetric, Gynecologic and Neonatal Nursing, 31*(4), 394–402.

Beck, C.T., & Driscoll, J.W. (2005). *Postpartum mood and anxiety disorders.* Boston: Jones and Bartlett.

Blackburn, S.T. (2003). *Maternal, fetal and neonatal physiology: A clinical perspective.* St. Louis: Saunders.

Briggs, G.G., Freeman, R.K., & Yaffe, S.J. (2005). *Drugs in pregnancy and lactation.* Philadelphia: Lippincott Williams & Wilkins.

Canadian Institute for Health Information (2004). *Giving birth in Canada: Providers of maternity and infant care.* Ottawa, ON: Author.

Canadian Nurses Association (2002). *Code of ethics.* Ottawa, ON: Author.

Condon, M.C. (2004). *Women's health: An integrated approach to wellness and illness.* Upper Saddle River, NJ: Prentice Hall.

Cunningham, F., Leveno, K., Bloom, S., Hauth, J., Gilstrap, L., & Wenstrom, K. (2005). *Williams obstetrics.* New York: McGraw-Hill.

Enkin, M., Kierse, M., Neilson, J., Crowther, C., Duley, L., Hodnett, E., & Hofmeyer, J. (2000). *A guide to effective care in pregnancy and childbirth.* Oxford, NY: Oxford University Press.

Freda, M.C. (2002). *Perinatal patient education: A practical guide with education handouts of patients.* Philadelphia: Lippincott Williams & Wilkins.

Health Canada. (2004). *Vitamin D supplementation for breast-fed infants: 2004 health Canada recommendation.* Ottawa, ON: Author.

Health Canada. (2005). *Alternate milks.* Ottawa, ON: Author.

Health Canada. (2006). *Primary health care.* Ottawa, ON: Author.

Hodnett, E., Gates, S., Hofmeyer, G., & Sakala, C. (2003). Continuous support for women during childbirth. *The Cochrane database of systemic reviews,* 2006 (3). Chichester, UK: John Wiley & Sons.

Hughes, S.C., Levinson, G., & Rosen, M.A. (2002). *Anesthesia for obstetrics.* Philadelphia: Lippincott Williams & Wilkins.

Klaus, M., Kennell, J., & Klaus, P. (1996). *Bonding: Building the foundations of secure attachment and independence.* New Jersey: Addison Wesley.

Lowdermilk, D., & Perry, S. (2007). *Maternity and women's health care.* Philadelphia: Mosby.

Lowe, N. (2002). The nature of labour pain. *American Journal of Obstetrics and Gynecology, 186*(5), S16–S24.

Martin, J. (2002). *Intrapartum management modules.* Philadelphia: Lippincott Williams & Wilkins.

Mauthner, N. (1998). Reassessing the importance and role of the marital relationship in postnatal depression. Methodological and theoretical implications. *Journal of Reproductive and Infant Psychology, 16*(3), 157–176.

Merenstein, G.B., & Gardner, S.L. (2002). *Handbook of neonatal intensive care.* St. Louis: Mosby.

Mohrbacher, N., Stock, J., & La Leche League International. (2003). *The breastfeeding answer book.* Schaumburg, IL: La Leche League International.

Olds, S., London, M., Ladewig, P., & Davidson, M. (2004). *Maternal newborn nursing and women's health care.* Upper Saddle River, NJ: Pearson.

Orshan, S.A. (2008). *Maternity, newborn, and women's health nursing: Comprehensive care across the lifespan.* Philadelphia: Lippincott Williams & Wilkins.

Pillitteri, A. (2004). *Maternal and child health nursing.* Philadelphia: Lippincott Williams & Wilkins.

Porth, C.M. (2005). *Pathophysiology: Concepts of altered health states.* Philadelphia: Lippincott Williams & Wilkins.

Public Health Agency of Canada. (2006). *What determines health?* Ottawa, ON: Author.

Simkin, P. (2002). Supportive care during labour: A guide for busy nurses. *Journal of Obstetric, Gynecologic and Neonatal Nursing, 31*(6), 721–732.

Tucker, S. (2004). *Pocket guide to fetal monitoring and assessment.* St. Louis: Mosby.

Willis, C.E., & Livingstone, V.H. (1995). Infant insufficient milk syndrome associated with maternal postpartum hemorrhage. *Journal of Human Lactation, 11*(2), 123–128.

World Health Organization. (1981). *International code of marketing of breast milk substitutes.* Geneva: Author.

World Health Organization (1986). *Ottawa charter for health promotion.* Ottawa, ON: Author.

World Health Organization. (2004). *Promoting proper feeding for infants and young children.* Geneva: Author.

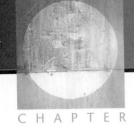

CHAPTER

# 7 Mental Health Nursing

**Directions:** Below are 200 multiple-choice questions and short answer questions totaling 250 points. These questions will test your knowledge of nursing with a mental health population. These questions offer a wide array of case-based and stand-alone questions representing the taxonomies of critical thinking, application, and knowledge/comprehension. Also reflected in these questions are the nursing competencies of health and wellness, alterations in health, professional practice, and nurse–person relationship. After completing these practice questions, check your work in the Answers and Rationales section located at the end of the chapter. Please note the topic areas and types of questions you found difficult and develop a plan to review study sources and increase your knowledge of these areas.

## ▶ Multiple-Choice Questions

1. Cross-tolerance to a drug is a situation in which:
   A. One drug can prevent withdrawal symptoms from another drug.
   B. One drug can increase the potency of another drug.
   C. The client has an allergic reaction to a classification of drugs.
   D. One drug can result in a lessened response to another drug.

2. The most important role of a nurse in caring for a client with a mental health disorder is to:
   A. Establish trust and rapport.
   B. Know how to solve the client's problems.
   C. Set limits with the client.
   D. Offer advice.

3. Contemporary mental health practice is highly collaborative and includes a number of

professional and paraprofessional workers. Which of the following tasks may be delegated to a nursing assistant in an acute mental health setting?
   A. Assessing mental status on admission.
   B. Doing a physical examination.
   C. Discussing the treatment plan.
   D. Checking for sharp objects.

4. When caring for a client diagnosed with body dysmorphic disorder, the client verbalizes disapproval of her physical features. In this situation, the nurse should:
   A. Compliment the client on her appearance.
   B. Encourage verbalizations about fears and stressful life situations.
   C. Agree with the client because that physical feature is awful.
   D. Ignore the comment and talk about less threatening issues.

5. A voluntary client in a facility decides to leave the unit against medical advice. In an effort to coerce the client to remain in the hospital, the nurse refuses to return the client's personal effects. This action is an example of which of the following?
   A. Limit setting.
   B. Violation of client rights.
   C. Slander.
   D. Violation of confidentiality.

6. Upon returning home from college, a young man discovers that his mother has been diagnosed with cancer. Initially, he responds to the news by stating: "No, I don't believe it. It can't be true." Which defence mechanism is he using?
   A. Suppression.
   B. Introjection.
   C. Denial.
   D. Repression.

7. A strong therapeutic nurse–person relationship is based on the nurse's:
   A. Sound knowledge of psychiatric nursing.
   B. Sincere desire to help others.
   C. Acceptance of others.
   D. Self-awareness and understanding.

8. The nurse documents that "the client describes her husband's abuse in an emotionless tone and with a flat facial expression." This assessment is document the client's:
   A. Mood.
   B. Affect.
   C. Feelings.
   D. Blocking.

9. Dina, a client in an outpatient mental health clinic, asks the nurse, "Do you think I should leave my husband?" The nurse responds to Dina by saying, "You aren't sure if you should leave your husband?" Which therapeutic technique is the nurse using in this situation?
   A. Offering a general lead.
   B. Reflecting.
   C. Reframing.
   D. Referencing.

10. Reading someone else's mail, using personal possessions without asking permission, and touching other people without their permission are all examples of:
    A. Manipulation.
    B. Antisocial behaviour.
    C. Poor boundaries.
    D. Passive–aggressive behaviour.

11. A client in an acute care setting tells the nurse, "I don't think I can face going home tomorrow." The nurse's response, "Do you want to talk more about it?" is an example of which of the following techniques?
    A. Restating.
    B. Exploring.
    C. Making observations.
    D. Presenting reality.

12. A woman reports to her family doctor that she has become increasingly afraid of riding in elevators. One day, she experiences palpitations, shortness of breath, dizziness, and trembling while in the elevator at her office building. Her physician can find no physiologic basis for these symptoms and refers her to a psychiatric clinical nurse specialist for outpatient counselling. Which of the following therapeutic approaches is most likely to help reduce the client's anxiety level?
    A. Systematic desensitization.
    B. Referral for evaluation for electroconvulsive therapy.
    C. Psychoanalytic-oriented psychotherapy.
    D. Group psychotherapy.

13. A client recently developed paralysis of the arms and was diagnosed with conversion disorder after tests failed to identify a physical cause for the paralysis. Which intervention should the nurse include in the plan of care?
    A. Teaching the client how to use nonpharmacologic pain control methods.
    B. Working with the client rather than the family.
    C. Insisting that the client eat without assistance.
    D. Exercising the client's arms regularly.

14. A client runs to the nursing station reporting breathing difficulty, chest pain, and palpitations related to a panic attack. The client is pale with his mouth held open and his eyebrows raised. What is the priority activity for the nurse to implement?
    A. Orient the client to person, place, and time.
    B. Assist the client to breathe deeply into a paper bag.
    C. Administer an IM anxiolytic agent.
    D. Set limits for acting-out, delusional behaviours.

15. A physical examination on an anxious client is being conducted. During the examination, the nurse would expect to find which of the following parasympathetic nervous system effects?
    A. Decreased urine output.
    B. Hyperactive bowel sounds.
    C. Muscle tension.
    D. Constipation.

16. While working with Walter, an anxious client, the nurse begins to feel tense and jittery herself and notices that she is having some difficulty concentrating on what Walter is telling her. The nurse is experiencing:
    A. Empathized anxiety.
    B. Secondary anxiety.
    C. Introjected anxiety.
    D. Maturational anxiety.

---

***Case Study:*** *Two staff nurses working in a psychiatric emergency department are being considered for a highly sought after promotion. The promotion is to* *be announced via a memo on the unit bulletin board. The psychiatric emergency nurses operate in a collaborative team environment. The two staff nurses vying for the promotion have worked together for 15 years and socialize outside of the work setting. Questions 17 to 23 relate to this scenario.*

17. After hearing from a colleague who read the notice on the bulletin board that she was not promoted, the nurse leaves the room in tears. This behaviour is an example of:

    A. Conversion.
    B. Regression.
    C. Introjection.
    D. Rationalization.

18. The nurse who was not promoted goes to the staff coffee room and slams several cupboard doors while looking for facial tissues. This behaviour exemplifies:

    A. Displacement.
    B. Sublimation.
    C. Conversion.
    D. Reaction formation.

19. When the nurse who was not promoted goes into the staff coffee room and slams several cupboard doors, a custodian goes into the staff room and remarked, "You seem pretty upset." The nurse replied that she is not the least bit upset. In this instance, the nurse is probably using:

    A. Reaction formation.
    B. Repression.
    C. Compensation.
    D. Denial.

20. Upon hearing she was not promoted, the nurse tells a friend, "Oh, well. I really didn't want the job anyway." This is an example of:

    A. Rationalization.
    B. Denial.
    C. Projection.
    D. Compensation.

21. Learning that she was not the successful candidate in the bid for promotion, the nurse tells another friend, "I knew I'd never get the job. The nurse manager hates me." If she actually believes this of the manager, who actually knows little of her, she is demonstrating:

    A. Compensation.
    B. Reaction formation.
    C. Projection.
    D. Denial.

22. The nurse who was not promoted meets the newly promoted nurse in the cafeteria and suddenly finds she has lost her voice and is unable to offer her congratulations. She is probably demonstrating:

    A. Denial.
    B. Conversion.
    C. Suppression.
    D. Repression.

23. The nurse who was not promoted initially experienced feelings of loss, but over time she goes out of her way to be supportive of the new head nurse and helps make the transition smooth. She offers to take on additional responsibilities to help out and is often heard encouraging others. She tells a friend, "I feel good about the way things are turning out. I have an investment in this psychiatric emergency department and want the best for our staff and clients." This development has its basis in:

    A. Altruism.
    B. Suppression.
    C. Displacement.
    D. Passive aggression.

24. A client diagnosed with depression is administered venlafaxine (Effexor) 75 mg/day PO. Venlafaxine is what type of agent?

    A. Lithium derivative.
    B. Monamine oxidase inhibitor.
    C. Tricyclic antidepressant.
    D. Selective serotonin reuptake inhibitor (SSRI).

25. A community mental health nurse is teaching her client about the initiation of lithium carbonate (Lithonate). The metabolism and excretion of the drug are important to consider for safe medication ingestion and symptom management. Reviewing the drug information, she can most accurately describe the metabolism and excretion of lithium as:

    A. Metabolised in the liver and excreted in the feces.
    B. Metabolised and excreted by the kidneys.
    C. Metabolised in the kidneys and excreted in urine.
    D. Not metabolised and excreted unchanged by the kidneys.

26. When planning the care for a client with Alzheimer's disease, the nurse should focus on:

    A. Assisting the client to reverse the disease.
    B. Provision of a safe and structured environment.

C. Support for the client to recognize his or her physical limitations.

D. Prevention of the loss of cognitive functions.

27. Don, a client with Alzheimer's disease, engages in a rambling conversation, mumbling incoherently and in a confused manner. The nurse can assist by redirecting the client's attention by encouraging him to:

A. Participate in dance therapy group.

B. Participate in reminiscence therapy group.

C. Fold towels and pillowcases.

D. Play cards with another client.

28. Stephanie, a new RN graduate, is providing care for inpatients with severe mood disorders. When evaluating a client for suicidal ideation, Stephanie must remember to assess for:

A. Deterioration of self-worth.

B. Vegetative shifts.

C. Hoarding of prized possessions.

D. Ideas and a plan to harm oneself.

---

**Case Study:** *Darlene is a 55-year-old client diagnosed with bipolar disorder. Her care is being followed by the community health nurse and a fly-in psychiatrist who she sees once a month. Weather has prohibited visits with her psychiatrist for the past 2 months, and her usual community health nurse has been recently been replaced. During this transition, Darlene discontinued her treatment with lithium. Currently in a manic state, she is being treated by generalist RN staff in an open ward of the rural hospital 1 hour outside of her community. Questions 29 to 31 relate to this scenario.*

29. The plan of care for Darlene in the general hospital during her manic state would include:

A. Setting limits, providing a low-stimulation environment, and maintaining a neutral attitude from the staff.

B. Offering high-calorie meals and insisting she finish all meals.

C. Allowing the client maximum opportunity for freedom and self-expression.

D. Insisting that the client remains active throughout the day so she will sleep through the night.

30. Darlene constantly belittles other clients on the general ward and is demanding special favours from the nurses. The most appropriate nursing intervention for Darlene is:

A. Ask other clients and staff members to ignore Darlene's behaviour.

B. Provide Darlene with an antianxiety agent whenever her belittling or demanding behaviour occurs.

C. Set limits with specific and consistent consequences for belittling or demanding behaviour.

D. Offer Darlene a variety of stimulating activities to distract her from other clients and from making demands on the nurses.

31. At shift change, the oncoming staff nurse is unable to locate Darlene. She is not in her room or the common area where clients gather. The nurse reports Darlene missing, and 2 hours later, she is returned to the hospital by the police, who found her swimming in the local creek in her hospital gown. Darlene states she was "being baptised by Mother Nature, who loves and worships me." Assessing her mental state, the nurse can describe Darlene's current alterations in mental status as:

A. Visual hallucinations.

B. Grandiose delusions.

C. Neologisms.

D. Dysphoria.

---

**Case Study:** *Evan is a 14-year-old boy who has been diagnosed with depression. His parents have reported that Evan has difficulty in school and have brought him to the community mental health centre for further assessment and treatment. Questions 32 to 34 relate to this scenario.*

32. Which additional problem would the nurse expect Evan to be experiencing?

A. Cognitive impairment.

B. Anxiety disorder.

C. Behavioural difficulties.

D. Labile moods.

33. The nurse at the mental health centre must remember that depression manifests differently in adolescents and adults. In Evan's case, signs and symptoms of his worsening depression are likely to include:

A. Obsession with body image.

B. Stealing from family members and truancy.

C. Hopelessness and helplessness.

D. Social withdrawal and oppositional behaviour.

34. Upon completion of assessment, the nurse determines that Evan's social withdrawal has left him isolated and lonely. An appropriate intervention is:

A. Implementation of regular ongoing family therapy.

B. Referral to an after-school social recreation program.

C. Referral to a residential program for youths with conduct disorders.

D. Supportive listening and goal setting.

---

***Case Study:*** *Joseph and Amina are new immigrants to an urban Canadian city. Amina has been experiencing increasing despair and depression because the recent death of their 7-month-old daughter from sudden infant death syndrome. She has been neglecting her housework and her husband. She has lost 9.1 kg over the past 8 weeks and has not left the house. Questions 35 to 37 relate to this scenario.*

**35.** Amina is admitted to an inpatient psychiatric unit with a diagnosis of depression. The nurse provides a unit orientation to Amina, and while observing her unpack, the nurse can expect her to exhibit:

A. A desire to initiate conversation with her roommates.

B. Expansive and dramatic movements.

C. Decelerated movements and flat affect.

D. Overly excited interest in her admission.

**36.** As Amina is treated and recovering, Joseph asks the nurse if Amina will experience future depressive episodes. The most appropriate response of the nurse would be:

A. "When an individual has depression, she will experience the problem all of her life."

B. "Depression is situational. The loss of your young child caused this, so it should never happen again."

C. "There are patterns with this illness. If a person has one depressive episode, she has a 60% chance of experiencing another."

D. "All people are at risk of depression. Nine out of 10 people will have depression in their lives."

**37.** Amina remains extremely depressed and expresses her increasing suicidal ideation to her primary nurse, Sheila. Sheila's priority nursing intervention should be:

A. Exploring the grief and loss issues concerning her baby's death.

B. Encouraging Amina to express her feelings of isolation and recent immigration.

C. Encouraging attendance at group cognitive behavioural therapy on the unit.

D. Ensuring that Amina is not permitted to use anything that would be potentially dangerous.

**38.** A therapy program nurse, Marc, is planning care for a client with dysthymia. Which of the following cognitive or behavioural nursing interventions should Marc include in the plan?

A. Teaching about the impact of negative beliefs and other assumptions.

B. Recommendations for an occupational therapy assessment.

C. Arranging for a comprehensive physical examination.

D. Administering phototherapy.

**39.** A nurse addressing a client in a manic state would best respond to the client's expansive mood with which statement?

A. "Don't worry; you'll come out of this soon."

B. "The best part of the illness is this state right now. How do you use your manic energy to your best advantage?"

C. "You are too elevated to discuss things rationally right now. After you stabilize, we can arrange to plan your treatment more collaboratively."

D. "I notice your energy level seems high right now. What has seemed to help you relax enough to manage your usual tasks in the past?"

**40.** Steve has been diagnosed with schizophrenia and is now preparing for discharge by reviewing relapse prevention with his family and the nurse at the early interventions clinic. The family and nurse are reassured that Steve has a good understanding of when to seek help in the future by which comment?

A. That he has a part-time job he will resume upon discharge.

B. That he understands the stressors and situations that precipitated his recent psychotic episode.

C. That he has the home phone numbers of all his therapists and his psychiatrist.

D. That he knows exactly when to take his prescribed medication.

**41.** Which comment by a client with a delusional disorder would indicate that he has made improvements?

A. "My spouse is having an affair."

B. "Dr. Davies is in love with me."

C. "I don't have any signs of cancer."

D. "The Hells Angels are casing my house and reporting on me to their leaders."

**42.** Despite antipsychotic medication treatment, a client experiences chronic auditory hallucinations. He is learning how to cope with them from his community mental health nurse. The best advice the nurse can give to the client for coping enhancement is:

A. "When you hear the voices, talk back to them."
B. "Focus on your internal feelings and sensations."
C. "Daydreaming and distracting yourself when you feel lonely are the most helpful."
D. "Maintaining a structured schedule and trusted supports can provide some means of coping."

**43.** Which of the following is the most likely rationale a client's family may share with the nurse as to why they believe the client's brief psychotic episode could be considered normal?

A. It is accepted within their religion or as part of a cultural belief, ceremony, or ritual.
B. The client has an infection.
C. It was only a brief episode and only happened once before.
D. The client is a drug addict.

**44.** As a nurse planning care for a client with paranoid delusions, which of the following will be your priority goal?

A. Eliminating all delusions.
B. Encouraging participation in all unit activities.
C. Enhancing independence.
D. Establishing trust.

**45.** A client who is experiencing auditory hallucinations tells the nurse, "I can hear the other clients talking about me and laughing." The best nursing response is:

A. "Those other clients aren't saying anything about you."
B. "I feel for you. That must be very painful."
C. "You *are* kidding, aren't you?"
D. "I don't hear anything, but tell me more about what you are hearing."

**46.** A nurse caring for a client with schizophrenia should monitor the client for signs of positive symptoms such as:

A. Hallucinations and delusions.
B. Weight gain and anhedonia.
C. Improved socialization and greater motivation.
D. Flat affect and low mood.

**47.** Jean is a nurse caring for a client with schizoaffective disorder who is currently experiencing auditory hallucinations. Which of the following nursing actions should Jean take as first priority?

A. Encouraging the client to engage in one-on-one therapeutic conversations.
B. Discussing with the client how to prevent relapse.
C. Engaging the client in reality-based conversations.
D. Acknowledging the client's strengths and accomplishments.

**48.** A nurse working with Virginia, a client with borderline personality disorder, could establish which of the following as outcome criteria for Virginia's treatment plan:

A. Display anger more frequently.
B. Act out her neediness.
C. Filter her concerns and insecurities through the nurse.
D. Experience troubling thoughts without self-mutilation.

**49.** The family of a client with Alzheimer's dementia who is admitted to a psychiatric unit awaiting placement to a long-term care facility indicates to the nurse and understanding of the prognosis when they state:

A. "We are investigating herbal and vitamin therapy."
B. "Does another hospital have a better treatment?"
C. "We are waiting for this medicine to kick in so he can go back to his lodge."
D. "What supports are available for the long term?"

**50.** A 70-year-old woman is brought into emergency department in a confused state, incoherent, and agitated after she reportedly spray painted her metal lawn furniture with metal paint earlier that day. She has no history of illness and is not on any medication. Which of the following assessment would be appropriate for the nurse to make in the psychiatric emergency assessment?

A. Dementia related to organic illness.
B. Distress related to a physical task in the heat of the day.
C. Delirium related to toxin exposure.
D. Depression related to aging.

**51.** A client with Alzheimer's disease has random violent outbursts, wanders, and is incontinent. She can no longer identify people who were once familiar and is unable to identify common objects. The nurse should give highest priority to which aspects during care planning?

A. Impaired communication skills.
B. Risk for injury.
C. Altered patterns of elimination.
D. Self-care deficits.

52. Matthew is a 4-year-old boy with severe autism. The nursing care in an outpatient mental health centre will most likely include:

A. Social skills training.
B. Cognitive behavioural therapy.
C. Play therapy.
D. Psychotropic medications.

53. Soha is from a cultural group that views emotional or mental illnesses as behaviour that is out of control and that brings shame upon the family. Which of the following responses to psychological distress would be mostly likely to occur for Soha given this cultural view?

A. Obsessive–compulsive behaviour.
B. Depression.
C. Somatising disorder.
D. Phobias.

*Case Study:* Mildred, age 70 years, has been hospitalized for a major depression after she was found to be almost nonfunctional at her home for more than 2 weeks. She had been seeing her psychiatrist in the community on an outpatient basis and taking antidepressant medication with no improvement in her symptoms. She has been admitted to have a medical workup for the initiation of a series of electroconvulsive therapy (ECT) treatments. Questions 54 to 57 relate to this scenario.

54. While the nurse is conducting pretreatment education with the family, Mildred's daughter asks, "Isn't this treatment dangerous?" The most appropriate nursing response would be:

A. "No, this treatment is absolutely safe."
B. "There are some side effects to the treatment, but they are not life threatening."
C. "There are risks involved, but with a depression as serious as your mother's, the benefits outweigh the risks because she will recover quicker with ECT."
D. "Although there are some risks, your mother will have a thorough examination in advance to ensure that she is a good candidate for the treatment."

55. Explaining to Mildred and her family about what to expect immediately after the ECT treatment,

which of the following statements would be appropriate?

A. "The client will have almost immediate positive results from the treatment and will feel much improved after the first ECT."
B. "The client will likely experience some confusion and disorientation after the treatment."
C. "The client may experience muscle soreness and tenderness after the treatment."
D. "The client will be heavily sedated after the treatment and may sleep for several hours."

56. Mildred's bilateral ECT is scheduled for tomorrow. The nurse caring for her should plan for which of the following activities?

A. Encourage the family to accompany Mildred to the treatment.
B. Encourage fluids 6 to 8 hours before the treatment.
C. Encourage caffeine intake the day before treatment to support seizure activity.
D. Provide frequent, supportive reorientation after the treatment.

57. After Mildred's ECT, which of the following would the nurse least expect to assess after the treatment?

A. Headache.
B. Disorientation.
C. Memory loss.
D. Paralytic ileus.

*Case Study:* Brittany is a 14-year-old ballet dancer who is underweight with recent hair loss, yellowish skin, facial lanugo, and peripheral edema. Her parents have brought Brittany to the community health centre with concerns that their daughter may have a liver problem. Questions 58 to 60 relate to this scenario.

58. The nurse can assess Brittany's symptoms as indicative of which of the following disorders?

A. Ulcerative colitis.
B. Bulimia nervosa.
C. Anorexia nervosa.
D. Acquired immunodeficiency syndrome.

59. Brittany is hospitalized to manage her eating disorder. Which of the following interventions should the nurse include for the plan of care?

A. Encourage Brittany to talk about food during mealtimes.
B. After Brittany returns from home visits, ask her if she has brought in any food, laxatives, or diuretics.

C. Discourage any discussion with nutritional counsellors or dieticians at the hospital.

D. Provide highly structured mealtimes with regular meals of sufficient caloric intake to promote weight gain.

60. Every time Brittany is weighed on the inpatient unit, she cries. Which of the following nursing interventions is most appropriate?

A. Instruct Brittany to close her eyes when being weighed.

B. Inform Brittany that she has to gain weight or she will die.

C. Remind Brittany that she is thin and looks fine.

D. Request that Brittany stand backward on the scale when being weighed.

---

*Case Study: Judy is a 46-year-old woman who is recently divorced and whose daughter, Rebecca, has left home to live with a religious community that restricts her contact with her mother. Judy has been experiencing non–medically founded pain at several sites over the past month and has now been admitted for inpatient psychiatric treatment after being diagnosed with somatoform disorder. Questions 61 to 63 relate to this scenario.*

61. When planning Judy's care on the inpatient unit, it will be important for the nurses to consider which aspect of treatment?

A. Ensuring the option for alternative medicines.

B. Providing instruction and assessment for stress management techniques.

C. Administering antipsychotic medications.

D. Providing behaviour modification for the family.

62. Early in her admission, Judy continues to complain of pain. It is essential that the nurse caring for her considers which of the following as assessment data?

A. Judy's performance of reality testing.

B. The duration and intensity of the pain.

C. The absence of laboratory findings to support clinical manifestation of the pain.

D. Judy's patterns of sleep, nutrition, and other vegetative shifts.

63. To optimize treatment goals for Judy, the nurse should pay attention to which priority area?

A. Avoiding focus on stressors.

B. Implementing medication treatment regimens.

C. Encouraging Judy to identify feelings and body sensations associated with stress.

D. Requesting a family meeting with Judy's ex-husband and daughter.

64. Jim has generalized anxiety disorder and is treated with buspirone hydrochloride (BuSpar). The nurse realises he needs additional medication teaching when he says:

A. "I won't drink any alcohol."

B. "I'll report any troubles with my heart or vision."

C. "I'll have my blood checked monthly."

D. "I take my medication as soon as I feel increased anxiety."

65. While teaching a client about her new antianxiety medication, alprazolam (Xanax), which of the following must the nurse include?

A. Cautionary teaching about ingesting foods with tyramine.

B. Instruction to take the medication with food.

C. Instruction to avoid drinking alcohol while on this medication.

D. Instruction to double up on the medication if she forgets a dose.

66. Suzanne is admitted to a psychiatric unit to initiate treatment for obsessive–compulsive disorder (OCD). Which of the following is an indication that the treatment with the medication sertraline (Zoloft) is having the desired effect?

A. Suzanne is able to sleep up to 4 hours per night.

B. The delusions Suzanne experiences are becoming less entrenched.

C. Suzanne is performing fewer rituals.

D. Suzanne experiences elevated mood and increased excitability.

67. A client's daughter complains that her mother's depression is not improving after 1 week on the chosen treatment, Elavil (amitriptyline), and that her mother is thinking about stopping her medication altogether. The nurse's best response to this concern is to:

A. Suggest that they consult the doctor about trying an alternative antidepressant.

B. Question the daughter about what sort of improvements she is expecting.

C. Let the daughter know that she will contact the physician.

D. Remind the daughter and the client that it may take 1 to 3 weeks for the medication to take effect.

68. Don, a client with schizophrenia, is taking trifluoperazine (Stelazine), and he begins to exhibit

restlessness, severe extrapyramidal symptoms, a high temperature, and diaphoresis. Caring for Don, you suspect neuroleptic malignant syndrome. Your best action given the above symptoms is to:

A. Have him stop taking the trifluoperazine immediately.
B. Administer antiparkinsonian medication.
C. Withhold foods with tyramine.
D. Administer antianxiety medications.

69. When providing medication teaching to a client who is taking clozapine (Clozaril), what must the nurse include?

A. Instruction that the IM injection must be taken every 4 weeks.
B. Discussion about the high incidence of extrapyramidal side effects and their treatment.
C. Caution that the medication can cause weight loss.
D. Instruction about the signs and symptoms of blood dyscrasias.

70. Randall is in an acute manic phase of bipolar disorder. He is pacing the halls and talking in a loud voice and with pressured speech. He is seen to be overly involved with co-clients and frequently threatens and disrupts others on the unit. Providing medication treatment for Randall, the nurse can expect the plan of care to include:

A. Monitoring Randall's phototherapy response.
B. Monitoring blood lithium levels.
C. Teaching Randall to avoid foods with tyramine.
D. Assessing for post–electroconvulsive therapy disorientation and confusion.

71. Evan's family is referred to family therapy after Evan was suspended from junior high school with behavioural problems. Which of Evan's father's statements indicates that he understands the purpose of family therapy?

A. "Evan will just have to realize that he has consequences for his behaviours and must try harder to behave at school."
B. "I suspect the therapist will notice how my wife babies our son. She has to make some changes, or Evan will never become a man."
C. "I hope we can all learn some new skills and begin to problem solve better with the help of the therapist."
D. "The therapist will tell us how to make our son behave better so he can go back to school."

72. A 6-year-old client being assessed at a children's mental health clinic can typically be expected to be in the process of developing what?

A. Understanding basic rules.
B. Imitating the actions of others.
C. Recognizing object permanence.
D. Understanding abstract concepts.

73. Joan has been admitted to an inpatient psychiatric unit and has hovered around the nursing station all day. When the nurse speaks with other clients during mealtimes, Joan tries to regain the nurse's attention by shouting at her, "You're just like my mother. You pay attention to everyone else but me!" The nurse can interpret this behaviour as:

A. A demonstration of resistance to therapy.
B. Evidence that the nurse is failing to meet the client's needs.
C. A demonstration of transference.
D. Evidence of family abuse.

74. You are beginning to establish a trusting rapport with a client who is coming to your community mental health centre for treatment of chronic and disabling anxiety. Just as you are initiating the working phase of therapy, this client begins to regularly arrive late for appointments and focuses her conversation on her busy schedule, difficulties in getting parking, and other reasons for being late. You can most likely interpret this behaviour as:

A. Transference.
B. Countertransference.
C. Identification.
D. Resistance.

75. A man who has never been admitted to a psychiatric unit is pacing the halls after his admission and orientation to the unit. To support the client's treatment and establish the nurse–client relationship, which actions should the nurse try first?

A. Apply restraints and have security watch over the client until he is calmer.
B. Explain the importance of his telling the truth to staff so that they can have an accurate assessment.
C. Invite him to sit down in a quiet place and reorient him to the nurse's name and the unit routines.
D. Call the psychiatrist for sedation.

76. Genevieve, who is unknown to the clinic staff, walks into the community mental health clinic in her small town stating, "I've had it. I can't go on

any longer. You've got to help me." The nurse asks Genevieve to be seated in a private interview room. What action should the nurse take next?

A. Reassure Genevieve that she will be helped.
B. Assess the client's situation, history, and mental status and inquire about contacting others for assessment information.
C. Call Genevieve's family and friends to get collateral information right away.
D. Call the police to initiate a committal under the mental health act.

77. As part of a task force on teenage suicide, you are considering the following steps in an effort to reduce teen suicide in your community. Which of the following represents primary prevention?

A. Advocate an increase in the number of adolescent psychiatric unit beds available in the community.
B. Educate teachers, parents, counsellors, and community health nurses about recognition and early intervention with suicidal teens.
C. Encourage emergency room staff to request psychiatric consultations for teen clients who are admitted with overdoses.
D. Support an increase in community programs, such as camp programs, music, sports, and other creative expressions, that increase self-esteem for children and teens.

78. While planning group strategies and approaches for group therapy, what ways can the facilitators promote group cohesiveness?

A. Make decisions in advance of the group meeting so that they can be announced and the group can move forward quickly.
B. Seat the most talkative members closest to the facilitators so they can be seen and heard more and take over as co-facilitators.
C. Help the group establish shared goals that are consistent with the individual goals of members.
D. Ensure that all group members know the ground rules established by the facilitators.

79. You are the leader of an outpatient group therapy program. Members of your current group relate superficially and test each other and the established group rules. Some members compete for your attention during group sessions. This behaviour is characteristic of which phase of group development?

A. Termination.
B. Feedback.

C. Working phase.
D. Orientation.

80. When communicating with a client experiencing paranoid thought distortions, the nurse should use which guiding principle?

A. Use a logical and persistent approach.
B. Encourage the ventilation of anger and frustration.
C. Express doubt and do not argue.
D. Agree with all delusions to create a calm environment.

81. The most appropriate activity to suggest for a client who is experiencing anxiety is:

A. Competitive sports.
B. Trivial pursuits.
C. Daily walks.
D. Bingo.

82. Physical exercise is an effective relaxation technique that nurses can recommend for clients with anxiety because it:

A. Stresses and strengthens the cardiovascular system.
B. Decreases the metabolic rate.
C. Decreases levels of norepinephrine in the brain.
D. Provides a natural outlet for the release of muscle tension.

83. A nurse is evaluating a family in which chronic child abuse has occurred and the parents have experienced chronic alcohol and drug abuse. The children have twice been removed for foster care within the past 2 years because they were required to be hyperresponsible in caring for their parents and their siblings at very young ages. Since that time, significant social supports have been instated by social services. The children are back home, and the parents have both received drug and alcohol treatment. What outcome would indicate progress for these parents?

A. The parents report continued use of spanking as discipline.
B. The parents report high expectations for the young children to manage the household tasks.
C. The parents report an understanding of normal growth and development.
D. The parents say they hope to attend parenting classes.

84. A 6-year-old girl is brought to the walk-in clinic in her neighbourhood for symptoms of a urinary

tract infection (UTI). The nurse's assessment reveals bruises in the child's genitals and rectal area. The mother reports that she left the little girl with her boyfriend the night before while she worked the night shift. The nurse's first priority with this client is to:

A. Obtain a urine sample to confirm the UTI.
B. Teach the mother about symptoms and treatment of UTIs.
C. Report the suspected child abuse to social services.
D. Assess the child for other health problems.

**85.** A nurse is assessing the family of a child brought into the emergency department with severe injuries. What behaviour by the parents might indicate child abuse?

A. Encouraging the child to explain his own injuries.
B. Providing a detailed description of the events before the injuries.
C. Having a panic-stricken and anxious attitude.
D. Having a delay in seeking treatment for the child's injuries.

**86.** A nurse is interviewing Julia, who has experienced both physical and psychological abuse by her common-law husband, Derrick. Which of the following statements indicates the greatest need for more teaching about abuse?

A. "Now that I have left Derrick, I don't need to worry."
B. "I have left him twice before, and I know there are many things that draw me back. Derrick can be so charming."
C. "I know it is not the case, but I feel like the abuse was my fault. That is what Derrick has repeatedly told me anyway."
D. "I worry about the children, that he will try to take them from me."

**87.** When working with adolescent clients, the nurse's general approach should be one of:

A. Asserting adult authority at all times.
B. Interacting with the client as a friend.
C. Being flexible and allowing occasional exceptions to the rules.
D. Being firm and not reacting to provocation.

**88.** A 14-year-old child with a history of conduct disorder is brought to the community mental health centre. When obtaining a history and mental health assessment, which of the following behaviours would suggest support for this diagnosis?

A. The parents have excessively high expectations of the child.

B. The parents are overly involved with the child.
C. The child has no siblings.
D. The parents use inconsistent limit setting oscillating with very harsh discipline.

**89.** A 6-year-old client has been diagnosed with attention deficit hyperactivity disorder (ADHD). Which medication is most likely to be prescribed?

A. Amitriptyline (Elavil).
B. Paroxetine (Paxil).
C. Methylphenidate (Ritalin).
D. Benztropine (Cogentin).

**90.** When planning the care for a young child with oppositional defiant disorder, you should include:

A. Emotive therapy.
B. Reminiscence therapy.
C. Behaviour modification.
D. Cognitive restructuring.

**91.** As a nurse working in a child and youth mental health clinic, you will likely assess for this most common anxiety disorder in young children.

A. Simple phobia.
B. Separation anxiety.
C. Posttraumatic stress disorder (PTSD).
D. Obsessive–compulsive disorder (OCD).

**92.** In speaking with a community group at a public health clinic, a mental health nurse evaluates her teaching as effective upon hearing the group state that the common behavioural signs of autism are:

A. Highly imaginative play.
B. Early language development.
C. Indifference to being held or hugged.
D. Overly affectionate behaviour toward parents.

**93.** Aside from treating depression, some antidepressants are also known to be effective in treating individuals with:

A. Autistic disorders.
B. Eating disorders.
C. Thought disorders.
D. Conduct disorders.

**94.** When caring for a client who has been unable to cope, is feeling confused, and is unable to make decisions after the sudden loss of a job, the nurse can understand this condition as:

A. Adventitious crisis.
B. Social crisis.
C. Maturational crisis.
D. Situational crisis.

**95.** A client who expressed suicidal ideations and was admitted to a psychiatric inpatient unit tells the nurse the next day that he feels fine, is at peace, and wants to go home now against medical advice. The nurse understands that this client:

A. Has had sufficient time to consider his situation and has a realistic appraisal of the serious nature of his suicidal ideations.

B. Is likely ready to be discharged home because his suicidal intent has been resolved.

C. Has resolved his feelings and is no longer at risk of self-harm.

D. Is possibly at more serious risk because he may have gained sufficient energy to act on his suicidal ideation; he requires further assessment.

**96.** Bernard is transferred to the psychiatric inpatient unit from the surgical intensive care unit after being treated for a self-inflicted gunshot wound. Meeting with Bernard one on one in an initial assessment and orientation to the unit, the nurse should maintain which of the following expectations of the intervention?

A. Bernard will spontaneously initiate contact with the nurse.

B. Bernard will identify past suicidal ideations and behaviour.

C. Bernard will explore the life events that led to the suicide attempt.

D. After he is able to ambulate, Bernard will begin group therapy and attend all programs on the unit and remain seated for 45 minutes.

**97.** A woman is admitted to the psychiatric inpatient unit after being found walking on a highway at night talking to herself. She is unkempt and appears thin and dirty. The best way to assess her immediate nutritional status and changes significant to her mental health status is to:

A. Compare her current weight with her usual weight.

B. Discuss her recent dietary intake.

C. Arrange for a medical consult.

D. Observe her at mealtimes.

**98.** A client with a diagnosis of paranoid schizophrenia tells the nurse that he hears a voice telling him, "Don't take those poisoned pills from that nurse!" The nurse can report which of the following objective assessments regarding this statement?

A. Impaired verbal communication related to disturbances in thought process as evidenced by use of symbolic references.

B. Disturbed thought processes related to anxiety as evidenced by delusions of persecution.

C. Disturbed perceptions related to anxiety as evidenced by auditory hallucinations.

D. Increased anxiety-related delusions of persecution evidenced by distorted thought content.

**99.** Julie is admitted to the emergency department with diaphoresis, chest pain, vertigo, and palpitations. On initial assessment, it appears there is no physiologic basis for these complaints. The client is seen by the psychiatric emergency room nurse who, on recognition that Julie has had four similar episodes in the past month, suspects that Julie has:

A. Panic disorder.

B. Schizoaffective disorder.

C. Obsessive–compulsive disorder.

D. Depression.

**100.** You are caring for a client with panic disorder who is experiencing difficulty sleeping and is up at the nurses' station late at night. What will best help the client achieve healthy sleeping patterns?

A. Suggest he stay up and play pool in the day area of the unit until he is tired.

B. Tell him to talk to the other client who is up and pacing the halls.

C. Encourage the use of relaxation exercises or techniques.

D. Administer sleeping medication.

**101.** Steve arrives to the psychiatric unit exhibiting extreme agitation, disorientation, and incoherence of speech with frantic and aimless physical activity and grandiose delusions. Which of the following concerns takes highest priority in planning your nursing interventions?

A. Hopelessness.

B. Ineffective individual coping.

C. Risk for injury.

D. Identity disturbance.

**102.** Charmaine, age 42 years, is admitted for a surgical biopsy of a suspicious lump in her right breast. At the time the nurse arrives to take her to surgery, Charmaine is finishing a letter to her to children. She tearfully tells the nurse, "I just want to leave this for my children in case anything goes wrong in the surgery." Which nursing response will be most therapeutic?

A. "This really is a minor procedure. You'll be back in your room before you know it."

B. "Try to take a few deep breaths and relax. I have some medications that will help."

C. "In case anything goes wrong? What are you concerned about right now?"

D. "I'm sure your children know how much you love them. You'll be out of surgery and able to talk with them in no time."

103. You are helping a client in your outpatient mental health practice who has a fear of public speaking that is preventing him from advancing in his career. He has conquered some of his other social phobias, such as using public bathrooms. During your interview to evaluate his progress, he makes all of the following statements. Which statement concerns you and is a priority for teaching?

A. "I try to take deep breaths when people talk to me."

B. "It helps me to have one or two drinks at lunch."

C. "I've met someone who I'd like to ask out on a date."

D. "One of my subordinates just got a promotion to a job I was interested in."

104. Sylvie is meeting with a client who has been prescribed alprazolam (Xanax). During a discussion about this medication, which instruction should Sylvie be certain to give to her client?

A. "Be sure to discontinue this medication immediately if you experience nausea."

B. "Apply sunscreen to prevent photosensitivity."

C. "Notify your physician if you experience urinary retention."

D. "Inform your physician immediately if you become pregnant or intend to do so."

105. A client experienced the loss of her home and beloved family dog in flood waters this past spring. Months later, she tells the nurse at the community mental health centre that even though she and her family are nicely settled into a new home, she finds it harder and harder to "feel anything." She says she can't concentrate on simple tasks, thinks about the flood incessantly, and fears losing control. She reports that she becomes extremely anxious whenever the flood is mentioned and must

leave the room if people talk about it. The admitting nurse suspects she has:

A. Conversion disorder.
B. Adjustment disorder.
C. Phobia (with depression).
D. Posttraumatic stress disorder (PTSD).

106. Trevor is a student nurse who is assessing a client with borderline personality disorder. He notes that this client has a tendency to view others and situations with extremes of "bad" or "good." Trevor documents this assessment finding as:

A. Manipulation.
B. Dissociation.
C. Dialectical behaviour.
D. Splitting.

107. A nurse is working Phil, a client with a dependant personality disorder. Phil reports numerous physical complaints. What is the best nursing response?

A. Avoid discussion of these complaints.
B. Disregard these complaints until the emotional issues are explored.
C. Encourage Phil to talk about his symptoms.
D. Explore the expressed symptoms in a matter-of-fact way.

108. Cheri is at her general practitioner's clinic, where the drug and alcohol nurse specialist in the shared care team meets with her on the request of her physician. Cheri admits to taking "meth." The nurse identifies this substance as belonging to the drug group:

A. Antidepressants.
B. Hallucinogens.
C. Stimulants.
D. Sedatives.

109. Josee is a drug and alcohol nurse specialist who is teaching an inservice about the signs and symptoms of severe alcohol withdrawal. During a learning check, Josee realizes that more teaching is needed when the group includes which symptom in the list they are compiling?

A. Dry heaves.
B. Elevated diastolic and systolic blood pressure.
C. Total wakefulness.
D. Drowsiness.

110. When a nurse is assessing a client with moderate alcohol withdrawal, which assessment finding could be expected?

A. Restlessness.
B. Marked disorientation and confusion.

C. Slight diaphoresis.

D. Vague, transient hallucinations.

111. Gemma is a young client in the early psychosis inpatient unit. Her psychosis has recently been clarified as a symptom of schizophrenia. When caring for Gemma on the unit, which nursing intervention will be *least* effective?

   A. Asking Gemma to clarify her expressed neologisms.

   B. Rewarding Gemma for positive behaviour.

   C. Performing all activities for Gemma so her needs are met.

   D. Exploring the content of Gemma's hallucinations with her.

112. A client with a thought disorder says, "Bud, dud, crud, mud. . . I'm a big stud." As a matter of correct mental health assessment terminology, the nurse documents this manner of speech as:

   A. Word salad.

   B. Neologism.

   C. Echolalia.

   D. Clang association.

113. Dave is a 28-year-old man with schizophrenia who is currently single, lives independently, and works in the automotive industry. His mental health has been stable with treatment for several years, and he is functioning well; however, he is very discouraged with his personal life. He presents to the nurse at the community mental health centre suggesting that he wants to stop taking his antipsychotic and antidepressant medication because of problems with his sexuality (low libido and erectile dysfunction). The nurse's best response is that the sexual problems are caused:

   A. Primarily by hallucinations and delusions.

   B. Exclusively by medication effects.

   C. Mostly by social stigma.

   D. By a combination of positive and negative symptoms and medication effects.

114. A client with schizophrenia began taking Haldol 1 week ago. She is now experiencing jerking movements of her neck and mouth. The primary nurse can interpret these symptoms as indicative of:

   A. Negative symptomatology.

   B. Akathisia.

   C. Tardive dyskinesia.

   D. Dystonia.

115. Amy is diagnosed with posttraumatic stress disorder (PTSD) at an outpatient mental health clinic after being raped while walking her dog in a public park. She receives counselling and support to address the trauma, but 3 months later, Amy returns to the clinic with concerns that she continues to experience fear, feelings of loss of control, and helplessness. Which nursing intervention is most appropriate for Amy at this time?

   A. Allow the client time to heal and reassure her that "it takes time."

   B. Explore the meaning of the traumatic event with Amy, asking, "What happened, and what has changed?"

   C. Suggest sleep medications, as prescribed, to restore a normal sleep–wake cycle, reminding Amy that "without proper sleep, recovery will be difficult."

   D. Recommend a high-protein, low-fat diet, suggesting to Amy that "without energy-boosting nutrition, recovery will take longer."

116. During treatment with the benzodiazepine alprazolam (Xanax), which dose-related adverse reaction must you monitor for?

   A. Blood dyscrasia.

   B. Hepatomegaly.

   C. Rash.

   D. Ataxia.

117. Dean is a 34-year-old client admitted to the psychiatric unit with obsessive–compulsive disorder. He is troubled and increasingly disabled by a ritual whereby he must brush the hair back from his forehead 15 times before carrying out any activity. The nurse caring for Dean notices that his hair is thinning and the skin on Dean's forehead is raw, bleeding, and inflamed (effects of the ritual). Planning for Dean's care, the nurse should assign the highest priority to:

   A. Setting consistent limits on this hair-brushing ritual because it is harmful to Dean.

   B. Helping Dean to identify how the ritual interferes with his daily activities.

   C. Exploring with Dean the purpose of the ritual behaviour.

   D. Using problem solving to help Dean to more effectively manage his anxiety.

118. A visibly anxious client is admitted to the psychiatric unit. The nurse assessing this client could expect to see which of the following cardiovascular effects produced by the sympathetic nervous system?

   A. Increased heart rate.

   B. Decreased blood pressure.

C. Syncope.
D. Decreased pulse rate.

119. The fear of having a heart attack or of losing one's mind is most likely to occur in individuals with:

   A. Dissociative identity disorder.
   B. Generalized anxiety disorder.
   C. Social phobia.
   D. Panic disorder.

120. Your client at a community mental health clinic describes a fear of being in places that are difficult or embarrassing to leave. He wants assistance to stop these troubling symptoms, which are beginning to disable him in social and occupational functioning. As the nurse, you are able to plan care after determining that these are symptoms of:

   A. Social phobia.
   B. Panic disorder.
   C. Agoraphobia.
   D. Generalized anxiety disorder.

121. Marg is a new client at an outpatient mental health service. At her intake appointment, she states, "When I have to face new people or situations—any situations in public, really—I start to perspire. My face gets so red I want to hide. I'm so afraid of embarrassing myself in public that I end up embarrassing myself. The words just can't come out. . . I'm a disaster!" The intake nurse can interpret these statements as indications of:

   A. Panic disorder.
   B. Generalized anxiety disorder.
   C. Agoraphobia.
   D. Social phobia.

122. Rebecca is a 43-year-old client with a panic disorder who describes a sensation of being "choked" or "trapped" after experiencing a panic attack. To assist Rebecca in understanding her situation, the nurse could anticipate exploring the meaning of which kind of loss?

   A. Youth.
   B. Control.
   C. Memory.
   D. Identity.

123. Ivan is a client on the adolescent psychiatric unit of an urban hospital. He was admitted with a diagnosis of body dysmorphic disorder. He has not been able to attend school or his part-time work, and he has not managed to maintain any friendships over the past year as a result of

certain body obsessions. Recently, he shaved the hair all over his body, claiming "it is all growing weird. . . . It is just too weird." As a treatment plan, the staff have Ivan pull on an elastic band around his wrist to produce a painful stimulus to modify his obsession with his body hair. This technique is a form of:

   A. Systematic desensitization.
   B. Thought stopping.
   C. Aversion therapy.
   D. Response prevention.

---

*Case Study:* Rosalind is a nurse leading an insight-oriented group therapy session in an outpatient mental health program for clients with mood and anxiety disorders. One client, Stuart, is continually sarcastic in group sessions. Question 124 relates to this scenario.

124. Stuart's sarcasm in group therapy sessions continues to challenge Rosalind. In one group session, he angrily responds to a peer, "You, buddy, are always whining. No wonder we're all pissed off with you in this group. Here's the world's smallest violin playing the world's saddest song for you!" Which role can Rosalind ascertain that Stuart is playing in the group?

   A. Aggressor.
   B. Monopoliser.
   C. Facilitator.
   D. Harmonizer.

---

*Case Study:* After taking 300 acetaminophen (Tylenol) tablets in an attempt to kill herself after a relationship breakup, Stephanie (age 16 years) is admitted to the adolescent psychiatric unit. She is refusing to talk with the nurse. Questions 125 to 127 relate to this scenario.

125. What is the most important nursing approach at this stage of the helping relationship?

   A. Appropriate self-disclosure to support a trusting relationship.
   B. Challenging Stephanie so that she begins to look not at her embarrassment for being admitted but at the realities of her feelings and actions.
   C. Allowing Stephanie time for self reflection and insight development.
   D. Supporting suicide precautions and safety measures for Stephanie on the unit.

126. During psychotherapy on the adolescent unit, it is clear that Stephanie rarely expresses her feelings and remains passive in her care and life

decisions. When in situations when she is **angry**, however, Stephanie's blood pressure increases to 175/100 mm Hg, her face becomes flushed, and she tends to leave the situation rather than seeing it through to some resolution. In family systems interviewing, it is established that her parents generally have a passive and easygoing style of communicating with Stephanie and others. Stephanie's primary nurse can help her understand her defence mechanisms, discussing her management of anger as which of the following?

A. Projection.
B. Assumptions.
C. Introjection.
D. Displacement.

**127.** Stephanie's nurse documents that "the patient describes the recent breakup of her dating relationship with an emotionless tone and a flat facial expression." The nurse will be able to document this quality as a descriptive statement of Stephanie's:

A. Blocking.
B. Feelings.
C. Affect.
D. Mood.

**128.** Six-year-old Matthew is diagnosed with enuresis after tests reveal there is no medical cause attributed to his bed wetting. Matthew's mother is upset and is blaming Matthew's father, from whom she has recently separated, for the problem. "It is all his father's fault!" Matthew's mother declares to the nurse. The nurse's best response would be:

A. "These things are generally no one's fault."
B. "You seem really upset by this situation."
C. "Why do you say that, exactly?"
D. "Why are you blaming Matthew's father?"

*Case Study: Jules has been working in psychiatric mental health nursing for several years. However, he has a scattered work history, often leaving to gain employment in a new province or territory. He has had several complaints about his professional practice but nothing that has led to any criminal charges or final revocation of his professional license. Concerns have been raised about his practice at the rural community mental health centre where he now works. Questions 129 and 130 relate to this scenario.*

**129.** Several former patients from another province have recently collected their stories to corroborate that Jules attempted to befriend them rather than engage in the community mental health therapy they required. Furthermore, they say that during their therapy, Jules encouraged them to invest in his food cooperative and seed business. Jules' behaviour with these former patients can best be described as:

A. Passive–aggressive.
B. Antisocial behaviour.
C. Having poor boundaries.
D. Dismissive.

**130.** Previously unaware of Jules' history of coercing clients into his business schemes, you have now been told that he has recently invited a group of mental health centre clients to join a multilevel marketing program for seeds and fertilizers. As a colleague of Jules in the rural community mental health centre, what is your best response?

A. Take over the care of Jules' clients because you notice a conflict of interest.
B. Report your concerns to Jules' manager with a request that the provincial nursing association investigate his practice.
C. Call the provincial representatives from Industry Canada to report the coercion of vulnerable clients into business deals.
D. Contact the media to file a "consumer report" on the multilevel marketing scam.

**131.** Which of the following is an appropriate strategy to reorient a confused client to where her room is?

A. Let all the other residents or co-patients know where her room is.
B. Remind the client frequently where her room is.
C. Have her wear a wristband with her name clearly labelled on it.
D. Place pictures of her family and other personal items on her bedside table to jog her memory.

**132.** Which statement best describes the guidelines for decision making and actions that are considered legal mental health nursing practice?

A. Providing only the care clients say they want.
B. Following the physician's orders and documenting care with appropriate terminology and in a timely manner.
C. Practicing as legislated by provincial and territorial scope of practice documents.
D. Reading clients their rights under the mental health act.

**133.** A client at an urgent mental health clinic presents after slashing her wrists with a large piece of glass. This client has a history of visits to the urgent clinic with crisis experiences, conflicts, and acting out as primary concerns. When the nurse is assisting in the management of the acute injury to the wrists, the client asks the nurse, "I did a good job, didn't I?" What is the best nursing response?

    A. "It seems to me you are getting attention in a negative way. How is that approach working for you?"

    B. "How many times have you done this in the past?"

    C. "You sure did. You are going to have one heck of a scar now."

    D. "What were you feeling and experiencing before you hurt yourself?"

**134.** Rita is a 48-year-old client at a community mental health centre. She experiences chronic generalized anxiety and expresses dependency traits. Rita asks the nurse, "Do you think I should leave my husband?" The nurse responds, "You have questions about whether you should leave your husband." What communication technique is the nurse using with Rita?

    A. Mirroring.

    B. Restating.

    C. Reframing.

    D. Reflecting.

**135.** Justin is a 23-year-old client admitted to the inpatient psychiatric unit with anxiety and adjustment disorder and demonstrating antisocial personality traits. He has off-unit passes to be accompanied by staff only. The designated smoking area is a gazebo at the back entrance of the unit. Justin is feeling particularly anxious and is asking for an additional smoke break off the unit. The nurse can best respond by saying:

    A. "I'd like to be able to take you, Justin, but I am busy right now."

    B. "Your breaks are designated at particular times that we all have to follow. Let's think about what can see you through to that time."

    C. "Smoking is harmful to your health, and I don't want to contribute to that bad habit."

    D. "Okay, Justin, if it seems like it will help, we can make an exception to the rule. I'll just need a minute to finish another matter."

**136.** An accepted criterion and characteristic expression of mental health is:

    A. Happiness.

    B. Self-acceptance.

    C. Freedom from anxieties.

    D. The ability to control others.

**137.** Daniel is a 38-year-old client who reports to his community mental health nurse a series of difficulties and feelings, including that he has recently lost his job, a situation that is will likely require him to move to more affordable accommodations. Consequently, he also feels intimidated about pursuing his current dating relationship, asking, "What do I have to offer my girlfriend now?" The nurse responds by stating, "Let's talk about your employment situation right now." What therapeutic technique is the nurse using with this statement?

    A. Exploring.

    B. Restating.

    C. Making observations.

    D. Focusing.

**138.** In a therapeutic interaction with a client, the nurse can use silence for various therapeutic purposes, including:

    A. An expression of intolerance and frustration.

    B. Allowing space for response and an expression of patience.

    C. Challenging the client to meet the intensity of the therapist.

    D. Ensuring that the client takes the lead in therapy.

**139.** Darren loses a major contract with his engineering firm and later gets a flat tire on the way home from work. That evening, he finds fault with his family at home. What defence mechanism is Darren expressing?

    A. Sublimation.

    B. Regression.

    C. Displacement.

    D. Projection.

**140.** During a mental status examination, a nurse asks a client to interpret the proverb "a rolling stone gathers no moss." The purpose of this assessment of mental status is to determine the client's:

    A. Judgement.

    B. Ability to rationalize.

    C. Ability to think abstractly.

    D. Ability to recall and remember.

**141.** Which of the following activities illustrates a psychiatric mental health nurse's role in primary prevention?

    A. Conducting a postdischarge goals group on an inpatient psychiatric unit.

B. Providing education about relationships in a high school's sexual health class.

C. Conducting medication monitoring and teaching in a home visit in the community.

D. Managing crisis intervention in a psychiatric emergency department.

142. Of the following, which clinical condition meets the requirement for involuntary admission?

A. A person who requests admission because he is scared by his suicidal thoughts and the seriousness of his plan.

B. A person who lives alone and has delusions and auditory hallucinations and is unable to follow through on employment opportunities.

C. A single parent who leaves her minor children at home all night while she goes out drinking.

D. A man who threatens to kill his wife.

143. During a mental health assessment interview, a client does not make eye contact with the nurse. The nurse suspects this behaviour is culturally based. What should the nurse do first in relation to this assumption?

A. Accept this behaviour because it is likely culturally based.

B. Observe how the client and the client's family interact with each other and with other staff members.

C. Read several articles about this cultural group and their behaviours.

D. Ask staff members of a similar cultural group about their habits and behaviours.

144. Which psychotropic medication is administered based on an individualized dosage according to blood levels of the drug?

A. Clozapine (Clozaril).

B. Alprazolam (Xanax).

C. Lithium carbonate (Lithane).

D. Thioridazine (Mellaril).

145. A 29-year-old woman is admitted to the psychiatric unit after her fiancé is killed in a helicopter crash at his work site. Several weeks after the accident, she is unable to sleep, eat, or work. Her response is considered:

A. A grief response.

B. A crisis of anticipated life transitions.

C. A generalized anxiety response.

D. A crisis caused by traumatic stress.

146. Working with a client with obsessive–compulsive disorder (OCD), a nurse notices that the client is attempting to resist his compulsion. While working with this client, the nurse should anticipate which concern with the client?

A. Increased depression.

B. Decreased sense of self-worth.

C. Increased anxiety.

D. Excessive fear.

147. Performing a physical examination on a client experiencing anxiety, the nurse can expect which of the following effects produced by the parasympathetic nervous system?

A. Decreased urine output.

B. Hyperactive bowel sounds.

C. Constipation.

D. Muscle tension.

---

*Case Study:* Monica is a client receiving treatment for acute anxiety at an outpatient mental health clinic. She has always considered herself "high strung," but over the past couple of weeks, she has been experiencing wakeful sleep, which is now disrupting her ability to concentrate at work and contributing to irritability. Questions 148 and 149 relate to this scenario.

148. Monica's condition would be considered chronic and generalized when symptoms of excessive worry and anxiety over two or more circumstances persists for at least:

A. 2 months.

B. 4 months.

C. 6 months.

D. 12 months.

149. Monica is diagnosed with generalized anxiety disorder and has been prescribed a new medication by her physician. During medication teaching at the clinic, which of the following questions or statements would be the most effective nursing response?

A. "We know another medication change worries people with anxiety, but in the long run, this medication should greatly reduce your anxiety, Monica."

B. "Your cooperation and compliance with this treatment is of the utmost importance if it is to be successful."

C. "What are you hoping will happen with this treatment, Monica? We need to know what your expectations are so you can be realistic and avoid disappointment."

D. "While you are starting this new treatment, what concerns or questions do you have, Monica?"

150. Shirley is a 41-year-old client with bipolar disorder who has been taken to the hospital by her husband in an extremely agitated state. Shirley has been admitted several times in the past, and over the past week, her condition has worsened in the community to the point that Shirley has spent $12,000 in a week buying two used vehicles and has also made a petition to legally change her name. She is admitted for treatment of her acute manic state. Which nursing approach would be the best therapeutic response to Shirley's condition at this time?

    A. Using reflection and open-ended questions to promote insight-oriented communications.
    B. Challenging Shirley about her inappropriate behaviours.
    C. Maintaining a firm but nonthreatening manner.
    D. Assisting Shirley in addressing the practical financial, legal, and personal repercussions of her actions.

151. A client with depression tells a nurse, "Life is not worth living. I just want to die." Which is the best nursing response to this client?

    A. "No one really wants to die. Maybe you just don't want to go on living in this depressed state."
    B. "Why you want to die, exactly?"
    C. "This must be a very difficult time for you."
    D. "Be patient. You'll feel better soon and will again appreciate life and all it has to offer you."

152. Which of the following traits is most common among suicidal clients?

    A. Remorse.
    B. Anger.
    C. Psychosis.
    D. Ambivalence.

153. When admitted to the psychiatric unit with major depression, Gurpreet reports to nursing staff that she doesn't want the hospital to release any information about her care or stay to anyone in her family because she has a family member who has been physically abusive. When the alleged abusive family member calls the unit demanding information about Gurpreet, the correct nursing response would be:

    A. "I'm sorry, I can't give any information. Goodbye."
    B. "To protect the confidentiality of our clients, we cannot give you information about whether your relative is receiving treatment here."
    C. "Gurpreet is not receiving any calls."
    D. "Your family member didn't sign a release so that information can be shared with you, so I am not at liberty to report."

154. Lynne recently attempted suicide and is admitted on the inpatient psychiatric unit of an urban hospital. She tells the nurse personal details that impacted her suicide attempt, including her husband's serious gambling addiction, which is destroying their family financially. Lynne asks the nurse not to share these details from their conversation. The best nursing response will be to say:

    A. "I will need to share information that is relevant and important to your treatment to the health care team."
    B. "I promise to keep what we say in our conversations in confidence."
    C. "Please don't tell me things that I can't share with the health care team."
    D. "Unless you give me permission, I will not share aspects of our conversations with anyone."

155. Katia is a 20-year-old client being treated for depression on the inpatient psychiatric unit. She discloses to the nurse that she was raped by her stepfather when she was 7 years old. Katia describes having nightmares about the experience and states that she continues to have a fear of men. The nurse suspects that Katia is experiencing:

    A. Borderline personality disorder.
    B. Posttraumatic stress disorder (PTSD).
    C. Delusional disorder.
    D. Anxiety disorder.

156. Pam is a nurse working with clients with personality disorders in a community rehabilitation program. David is a client with antisocial personality disorder who is set for an intake appointment. He has a history of violence, cruelty to animals, and stealing. During her assessment, what trait is Pam likely to uncover in David's assessment interview?

    A. Expressions of guilt and shame.
    B. Demonstrated ability to maintain stable relationships.
    C. Concern and dedication to an employer.
    D. A low tolerance for frustration.

157. A community health nurse is assessing a 7-year old girl for symptoms of sexual abuse. Which of

the following behavioural symptoms would support the possibility of sexual abuse?

A. Stuttering, rocking, and impulsivity.
B. Excessive fearfulness, thumb sucking, and withdrawal from peers in play settings.
C. Hyperactivity, rocking, and inattention.
D. Enuresis, impulsivity, and a decline in performance in schoolwork.

---

**Case Study:** *Ashleigh is a 19-year-old college student seen in the emergency department after an incident of date rape. She is undergoing a forensic examination and is being assessed by the psychiatric emergency response team, who are concerned by her response to the trauma. Questions 158 to 160 relate to this scenario.*

158. The nurse notices during her assessment that Ashleigh describes the series of events leading up to the rape with a blank facial expression, ending her description by saying, "I feel like it didn't happen at all." Which of the following statements most accurately describes Ashleigh's response?

A. Ashleigh is using denial as a defence mechanism to cope with the pain of the attack.
B. Ashleigh is experiencing the shock phase of a crisis event and is repressing her feelings associated with the attack.
C. Ashleigh is using reaction formation to manage the anger she feels toward her attacker.
D. Ashleigh is experiencing dissociation as a defence mechanism to cope with the attack.

159. The psychiatric nurse assessing Ashleigh in the emergency department should have which of the following as her primary concern?

A. Assist Ashleigh with crisis interventions.
B. Understand that Ashleigh will have a long recovery period.
C. Provide support and comfort.
D. Assist Ashleigh in developing prevention strategies for future dating situations.

160. The campus health nurse is caring for Ashleigh after she was sexually assaulted. Which of the following provides an indication to the nurse that Ashleigh is making a successful adjustment to the trauma?

A. Ashleigh takes courses in the martial arts.
B. She is silent about the assault, preferring to "just move on."
C. Ashleigh selects to move to another city to go to a different college to "get away from it all."
D. Ashleigh resumes her course work and campus activities.

161. Emily is a 13-year-old young woman who is brought to the emergency department by her aunt after a suicide attempt. During the interview, the nurse finds that Emily has been doing poorly in school, is engaging in high-risk sexual behaviour with older boys at school, and has a history of running away from home to stay with her aunt. The nurse should make it a point to assess for:

A. Pregnancy.
B. Sexual abuse.
C. Parental neglect.
D. Sexually transmitted diseases.

162. How should the nurse, Grant, respond if his client, Danielle, asks him not to share information about her with others?

A. "I will not share information with your family or friends without your permission. I will, however, need to share information that relates to your reason for being here with other staff who work with you."
B. "The nice thing about a therapeutic relationship is that it is just between the nurse and the client. You will have to tell the team exactly what you will want them to know about you and the problems that led to your hospitalization."
C. "It really depends on what you choose to tell me. I will be glad to disclose at the end of each session what I will report to other staff."
D. "I really cannot tell anyone about you. It will be as though I am talking about my own problems, and we can help each other by keeping it between us."

163. A nurse plans to teach a client, Dave, about his antipsychotic medication before his discharge. Dave is known to be severely and persistently mentally ill, and his history has revealed several hospitalizations during which he was treated with an antipsychotic medication. Because his pattern after discharge from the hospital to the community has involved a failure to keep aftercare appointments and unreliability in taking his medication, which long-acting antipsychotic medication is the most likely choice for Dave?

A. Chlorpromazine (Thorazine).
B. Thioridazine (Mellaril).
C. Fluphenazine decanoate (Prolixin decanoate).
D. Lithium carbonate.

**164.** Which statement made by a client who washes her hands compulsively identifies the thinking typical of a client with obsessive–compulsive disorder (OCD)?

    A. "I know I'll get my hands clean eventually; it just takes time."

    B. "I need a milder soap that won't damage my hands so much."

    C. "I feel so much better when my hands are clean. I can get on to do other things."

    D. "I feel driven to wash my hands, although I don't like doing it."

**165.** To assist a client with a somatoform disorder to increase her self-esteem, an appropriate nursing intervention would be to:

    A. Encourage the client to use avoidant interactional patterns rather than assertive patterns.

    B. Focus attention on the client as a person rather than on the symptom.

    C. Set large goals so the client can see positive gains.

    D. Discuss the client's childhood to link present behaviours with past traumas.

**166.** Annette is concerned that she may have serious heart disease. She seeks help at the mental health centre after a referral from an internist who has told her that she has no physical illness. Annette reports that she has experienced tightness in her chest and the sensation of her heart missing a beat. Because of her concerns over her symptoms, she has missed much time from work over the past 2 years, which is troubling to her and is creating financial worries. Her social life has also been severely restricted because she believes she must rest every evening, which is also distressing to her. Annette can be assessed as having symptoms consistent with:

    A. Conversion disorder.

    B. Dysthymic disorder.

    C. Antisocial disorder.

    D. Hypochondriasis.

**167.** To effectively assess clients, nurses must understand that an essential difference between somatoform disorders and dissociative disorders is that:

    A. Whereas symptoms of somatoform disorders are under the person's voluntary control, symptoms of dissociative disorders are unconscious and automatic.

    B. Symptoms of dissociative disorders are precipitated by psychological factors, and symptoms of somatoform disorders are related to stress.

    C. Whereas dissociative disorders involve stress-related disruptions of memory, consciousness, or identity. Somatoform disorders involve expression of psychological stress via somatic symptoms.

    D. Whereas symptoms of dissociative disorders are individually determined and related to childhood sexual abuse, symptoms of somatoform disorders are culture bound.

**168.** Shanda, age 18 years, and her mother begin to explore colleges for Shanda to go to next fall. When not traveling, Shanda spends the summer cooking gourmet meals for her family. Eventually, her mother notices that Shanda is eating only tiny portions of the food. Shanda says she isn't hungry because she samples the food while cooking. At summer's end, Shanda has a physical examination for the school sports program. Her weight has dropped from 130 to 95 lb, and she has amenorrhea. The physician refers Shanda to the mental health centre for treatment. The psychiatric nurse clinical specialist focuses on Shanda's feelings about assuming an autonomous adult role as she prepares for college. With which theory of etiology of eating disorders is this focus consistent?

    A. Psychological model.

    B. Family model.

    C. Sociocultural model.

    D. Biological model.

**169.** While performing an assessment of a client with the binge–purge type of bulimia, the nurse should be particularly alert for signs and symptoms of:

    A. Hypernatremia.

    B. Hypokalemia.

    C. Hypercalcemia.

    D. Fluid volume excess.

**170.** A student nurse caring for a depressed client reads in the client's medical record: "This client clearly shows the vegetative signs of depression." What can the student expect to observe?

    A. Suicidal ideation.

    B. Feelings of hopelessness, helplessness, and worthlessness.

    C. Constipation, anorexia, and sleep disturbance.

    D. Anxiety and psychomotor agitation.

**171.** It has been assessed that a severely depressed client shows vegetative signs of depression.

Which of the following interventions would **not** be appropriate to address these problems?

A. Providing frequent small meals and monitoring food and fluid intake.
B. Encouraging venting about sexual frustration.
C. Teaching encouraging relaxation techniques.
D. Doubling daily caffeine intake.

172. When the spouse of a client diagnosed with dysthymia asks what the major difference is between dysthymia and major depressive disorder, the nurse can point out that in major depressive disorder:

A. The symptoms persist for 2 or more years.
B. There is evidence of an earlier hypomania episode.
C. There is always evidence of suicidal ideation.
D. The client does not give a history of feeling depressed for years.

173. A depressed client is being seen in clinic and is being treated with selective serotonin reuptake inhibitors (SSRIs). She tells the nurse that she has some pills that she formerly took for depression and that they are called MAOIs. She tells the nurse she thinks she should start taking them right now in place of her current medication. The most important information the nurse should convey is:

A. She needs to have her blood pressure carefully monitored.
B. The SSRI antidepressant will be more effective as the weeks go by.
C. Dietary restrictions are required when taking MAOIs.
D. There is a risk of a serious reaction if she stops the SSRIs and begins the MAOIs.

---

*Case Study:* Three policemen bring Erica to the mental health unit for admission. She had been directing traffic on a busy city street. She shouted rhymes, such as "to work, you jerk, for perks," and made obscene gestures at cars that came too close to her. When her husband is contacted at work, he reports that Erica stopped taking her lithium 3 weeks ago and has not slept or eaten for 3 days, telling her husband she was "too busy." Questions 174 to 176 relate to this scenario.

174. During the initial assessment, which two features characteristic of the manic phase of bipolar disorder can be identified?

A. Increased muscle tension and anxiety.
B. Disinhibition, affective lability, and elevated mood.

C. Poor judgement and hyperactivity.
D. Vegetative signs and poor grooming.

175. On admission to the psychiatric unit, Erica is dressed in a red leotard and an exercise bra and has an assortment of chains and brightly coloured scarves on her head, waist, wrists, and ankles. Her first words to the nurse are, "I'll punch you, munch you, crunch you," as she dances into the room, shadow boxing. Then she shakes the nurse's hand and says cheerfully, "We need to become better acquainted. I have the world's greatest intellect, and you are probably an intellectual midget." Erica's mood can be documented as:

A. Belligerent and blunted.
B. Expansive and grandiose.
C. Anxious and unpredictable.
D. Suspicious and paranoid.

176. Which behaviours listed below will be of priority concern as the nurse begins a care plan for Erica?

A. Bizarre, colourful, inappropriate dress.
B. Grandiose thinking and poor concentration.
C. Insulting, provocative behaviour directed at staff.
D. Hyperactivity and ignoring eating and sleeping.

177. Adrienne is a manic client who became hyperactive after discontinuing her lithium. She has not eaten or slept for 3 days. Which of the following behaviours would be appropriate to focus on during Adrienne's care?

A. Powerlessness.
B. Risk for injury.
C. Fatigue.
D. Activity intolerance.

178. Rudy, a client experiencing mania, is an executive in an urban accounting firm. He tells the nurse that his job is only his cover, that he's really the "right-hand man to the prime minister of Canada" and that he has been sent to this city to reorganize the RCMP. A goal for nursing care related to Rudy would be to:

A. Assist Rudy to maintain contact with reality.
B. Explain to Rudy that his illusions are irrational.
C. Ignore Rudy's delusions.
D. Encourage Rudy to suppress verbal expression of his delusions.

179. Bryan, a salesman, has had difficulty holding a job because he accuses coworkers of conspiring

to take his sales. Today he argued with several officemates and threatened to kill one of them. The police were called, and he was brought to the urgent care health centre for evaluation. Bryan has had previous admissions to the inpatient psychiatric unit for stabilization of symptoms of paranoid schizophrenia. When the nurse meets him, he points at staff in the nursing station and shouts loudly, "They're all plotting to destroy me! Isn't that true?" An appropriate response for the nurse would be:

- A. "No, that's not true. People here are trying to help you, if you'll let them."
- B. "Everyone is trying to help you. No one wants to harm you."
- C. "Thinking that people want to destroy you must be very frightening."
- D. "That's absurd, Bryan. The staff here are health care workers, not members of the mob."

180. Denis, a newly admitted client with paranoid schizophrenia, is hypervigilant and constantly scans the environment. He states that he saw two doctors talking in the hall and knows they were plotting a way to kill him. The nurse may correctly assess Denis' behaviour as:

- A. An idea of reference.
- B. A delusion of infidelity.
- C. An auditory hallucination.
- D. Echolalia.

181. Corbin is a newly admitted client who has paranoid schizophrenia. Corbin's family mentions that they don't understand what caused his illness. The nurse should answer in terms of the:

- A. Neurobiologic–genetic model.
- B. Stress model.
- C. Family theory model.
- D. Developmental model.

182. Terry's plan of care includes the nursing intervention "assess for auditory hallucinations." What behaviours suggest that the client may be hallucinating?

- A. Aloofness, haughtiness, and suspicion.
- B. Elevated mood, hyperactivity, and distractibility.
- C. Performing rituals and avoiding open places.
- D. Darting the eyes, tilting the head, and mumbling to oneself.

183. Katia is newly diagnosed with paranoid schizophrenia. She is withdrawn, suspicious, and aloof. What activity would be most appropriate to plan for her?

- A. A basketball game.
- B. Ping-pong.
- C. Paint-by-number.
- D. Euchre (card game).

*Case Study: Jenn is in the withdrawn phase of catatonic schizophrenia. This is her first admission to an early psychosis program at an urban hospital. At present, she is completely stuporous. Questions 184 and 185 relate to this scenario.*

184. While giving care to Jenn during this phase of her symptoms, the nurse must:

- A. Explain all physical care activities in simple, explicit terms as though expecting a response.
- B. Maintain a quiet atmosphere, speaking as little as possible to Jenn.
- C. Provide as much sensory stimulation as possible using conversation, radio, television, and so on.
- D. Ask the client to do exactly the opposite of what is desired.

185. Which behaviour listed below is of highest priority for nursing care of a stuporous catatonic client?

- A. Noncompliance.
- B. Impaired verbal communication.
- C. Ineffective coping.
- D. Refusal to eat and drink.

*Case Study: Michelle, a client with borderline personality disorder, has had 21 admissions to the mental health unit. Every admission was precipitated by a suicide attempt, usually resulting in superficial cuts on her arm. On this admission, Michelle has developed a relationship with the nurse, Jessie, who has been highly supportive. Michelle has progressed to having a pass to spend an afternoon in a nearby shopping mall. Jessie is shocked when the emergency room nurse calls to say that Michelle has just been brought in with multiple self-inflicted lacerations. Jessie asks another more experienced nurse, "Why? Everything was going well. How could she do this to me?" Questions 186 and 187 relate to this scenario.*

186. What response by the emergency room nurse to Jessie reflects an understanding of Michelle's borderline disorder?

- A. "I know what you mean. You put a lot of energy into working with Michelle. It must be disappointing to have her do something like this."

B. "I could have told you this would happen. A client like Michelle always gets you in the end. I hope this will teach you not to get so involved."

C. "I know Michelle's behaviour seems personal, but it's really not. Clients with borderline disorder act out to relieve anxiety, and I suspect having the pass provoked a great deal of anxiety."

D. "I wonder if all this could have been avoided if I'd clued you in on Michelle. This is a usual pattern for her. She burned me once, too, when I first worked here."

187. For future planning, it is important for the staff to consider the reason for the self-mutilation. Michelle's self-mutilation may be explained as:

A. The result of an inherited disorder that manifests itself as an incapacity to tolerate stress.

B. Related to fear of abandonment brought on by movement toward autonomy and independence (i.e., earning a pass).

C. Use of projective identification to reduce anxiety.

D. A constitutional inability to regulate affect that predisposes her to psychic disorganization.

188. George tells the nurse that he is planning to hire a private detective to follow his wife, who he believes is having an extramarital affair. The nurse assesses him to be suspicious based on his looking behind the door to be sure no one is eavesdropping and his asking the nurse what she did with his medical record after he left. The behaviours manifested by George can be assessed as being most consistent with the clinical picture of:

A. Antisocial personality disorder.

B. Obsessive–compulsive personality disorder.

C. Paranoid personality disorder.

D. Schizoid personality disorder.

189. When assessing situational support, an appropriate question for the nurse to ask would be:

A. "Has anything upsetting occurred in the past few days?"

B. "What led you to seek help at this time?"

C. "How does this problem affect your life?"

D. "Who can be helpful to you during this time?"

190. The unit milieu most likely to have a low incidence of violent behaviour is one that has:

A. A rigid and authoritarian structure.

B. Little structure and haphazard routines.

C. Unpredictable routines and permits directing ventilation of anger at staff.

D. Predictable routines and high client autonomy.

191. Which understanding is vital for nurses to apply when planning care for severely and persistently mentally ill clients?

A. Cognitive impairment and medication side effects make compliance with the medication regimen difficult for many clients.

B. Referrals to multiple agencies are ideal in a community in which many resources are available.

C. Health teaching should focus primarily on medication action and side effects.

D. Deinstitutionalization resulted in greater access to health care than was available in state mental hospitals.

192. What is the reciprocal relationship between the family and the mentally ill member that nurses must be aware of to plan care for severely and persistently mentally ill clients?

A. The greater the number of mentally ill clients in a family, the greater burden the family places on community resources.

B. Families with a mentally ill member tend to bear increased financial, physical, and emotional stress, which affects family dynamics and often limits the resources available to the client.

C. Community resources available for severely and persistently mentally ill individuals usually meet all the needs of this population, thus requiring little additional support from families.

D. Mental health services need to be adjusted to the specific problems of each severely and persistently mentally ill individual.

193. Florie, age 15 years, has been referred to the adolescent mental health clinic by a juvenile court after being arrested for prostitution. She has run away from home several times and has lived in homeless shelters. Her parents have told the court they cannot manage her because she has been physically abusive to her mother and defiant and hostile to her father. From Florie's history, the nurse might anticipate that the psychiatrist will consider the diagnosis of:

A. Attention deficit hyperactivity disorder (ADHD).

B. Autistic disorder.

C. Conduct disorder.

D. Childhood depression.

**194.** Which of the following pieces of data obtained during nursing assessment would cause the nurse to consider a child at risk for the development of a psychiatric disorder?

    A. Being raised by a depressed mother.
    B. Regular prenatal care for the mother.
    C. Developmental milestones achieved on schedule.
    D. Harmonious parental relationships in the household.

**195.** John, age 84 years, is stopped for going through a red light in a small town where he has lived all his life. He tells the officer, "It wasn't there yesterday." He is unable to tell the officer his address and demonstrates labile mood, seeming pleasant one minute and angry the next. The officer knows that John is a nice old man, and instead of ticketing him, he takes him home to discuss his condition with the family. John lives with his wife, who is legally blind. She mentions, "John's my eyes, and I'm his mind." She also relates that John wanders around the neighbourhood occasionally, taking tools from people's garages, saying they belong to him. She reluctantly agrees that John should be admitted to the psychogeriatric inpatient unit for evaluation. His admitting diagnosis is Alzheimer's disease. Which early symptoms of Alzheimer's disease is John demonstrating?

    A. Aphasia.
    B. Apraxia.
    C. Agnosia.
    D. Memory disturbance.

**196.** A nursing intervention based on a behaviour modification approach is used in the treatment of a 15-year-old girl with anorexia nervosa. A model of such treatment might be:

    A. Restricting the client's privileges until she gains 3 lb.
    B. Providing a high-calorie, high-protein diet with between-meal snacks.
    C. Encouraging the client to have an outlet for her feelings and aggression through vigorous exercise.
    D. Role playing the client's interactions with her parents.

**197.** Wilfred, age 79 years, tells the home visiting nurse, "I've been feeling down for the last few days. I don't have much to live for. My family and friends are all dead. My money's running out, and my health is failing." The nurse should assess this as:

    A. Normal pessimism of the elderly.
    B. A cry for sympathy.
    C. Normal grieving.
    D. Evidence of high suicide potential.

**198.** Frank is an elderly depressed client who is being treated with a tricyclic antidepressant (TCA). He should be observed carefully for:

    A. Orthostatic hypotension and urinary retention.
    B. Photosensitivity and skin rashes.
    C. Pseudoparkinsonism and tardive dyskinesia.
    D. Diarrhea and electrolyte imbalance.

**199.** Phillip, an elderly, confused client, is going to be treated with donepezil (Aricept). This drug is often chosen for some elderly clients because it is effective in treating clients:

    A. Who are confused because of depression.
    B. With age-related neurologic changes.
    C. With early-stage Alzheimer's disease.
    D. With delirium.

**200.** An inpatient group is meeting in the solarium. The group is discussing aftercare. Zane tells the group about the activities of a psychosocial club for former inpatients. He explains the club's purpose, the referral process, and the club's location. In this interaction, Zane has taken the role of:

    A. Harmonizer.
    B. Evaluator.
    C. Information giver.
    D. Procedural technician.

## ▶ Short Answer Questions

**201.** During a mental health assessment at a walk-in mental health centre, a client complains of "not feeling human." This symptom is characteristic of what clinical disorder? (1 point)

**202.** A client is brought to the psychiatric emergency department after experiencing a seizure on the morning of her performance appraisal meeting with the bank where she works part time. The medical workup and electroencephalogram have negative results. This client seems indifferent to the condition. What disorder would the nurse consider as primary to this condition? (1 point)

**203.** When a client assessed at the psychiatric emergency room is considered to be malingering, what behaviour would characteristically be observed in this client? (1 point).

**Case Study:** *Henri, an 83-year-old man, is brought into the emergency department (ED) by his daughter, Chantal. He has a history of major depression and recently lost his wife of 55 years, moved into an assisted living residence, and had to give up the family pet to make the move. Henri was unresponsive when found by Chantal and his son-in-law, Marc, after ingesting an unknown quantity of antidepressant medication and sleeping pills. Stabilized in the ED, Henri is now admitted to a geriatric psychiatric unit for hospitalization. Question 204 relates to this scenario.*

**204.** What four intervention outcomes can the nurse anticipate in Henri's case? (4 points)

**205.** Lucille is a client at a community mental health and addictions centre in her rural community. She is starting treatment with disulfiram, and the mental health nurse is instructing her about expectations and contraindications. List three possible symptoms of ingesting alcohol while taking disulfiram. (3 points)

**206.** A male client is admitted to the inpatient psychiatric unit with acute anxiety related to a severe situational crisis. During a period of extreme anxiety, the client becomes agitated

and bangs his head against the wall in his hospital room. The physician orders a stat dose of diazepam 2.5 mg IM for agitation with acute anxiety. The ward stock vial label reads "diazepam 5 mg/mL." How many millilitres should the nurse administer in the IM injection? (1 point)

**Case Study:** *The terms "judgement" and "insight" are often confused in professional documentation, yet they refer to distinct aspects of the mental status examination. Questions 207 and 208 relate to this scenario.*

**207.** Complete the following statements to demonstrate a clear distinction of the terms. (2 points)

a. Insight is the ability to _____.

b. Judgement is the ability to _____.

**208.** A nurse is conducting a psychiatric mental health assessment on a client newly admitted to an inpatient psychiatric unit. What question can the nurse ask to assess the client's judgement? (2 points)

**Case Study:** *John is working on the psychiatric short-stay assessment unit. He arrives to work dishevelled and unkempt in appearance and smells of alcohol. John is loud even though it is the night shift and the patients are settled. One of John's colleagues asks him about his ability to provide care this night shift, but he denies that he has a problem. Questions 209 and 210 relate to this scenario.*

**209.** What is the best approach for John's colleague on the night shift to manage this situation? (2 points)

**210.** Which of the Canadian Nurses Association values from the Code of Ethics for Registered Nurses applies to John's practice concerns at this time? (1 point)

**211.** What are three hallmark signs of autism? (3 points)

**212.** What are three types of behaviour therapy? (3 points)

**213.** Describe three key nursing interventions for a client in the manic phase of bipolar illness. (3 points)

**214.** Describe what is significant about vegetative signs or symptoms of depression and list three such signs. (4 points)

before moving onto the next topic and sentence. What symptom is Steve experiencing? (1 point)

**216.** To assess Steve's orientation, what are five questions the nurse might ask Steve? (5 points)

**217.** Steve resolves from his medication-induced brief psychotic episode and begins group therapy to manage his stress and generalized anxiety. What are three techniques for easing anxiety that would be appropriate for clients with generalized anxiety? (3 points)

**218.** List four key elements of the mental status examination. (4 points)

**219.** Name three positive and three negative symptoms of schizophrenia. (6 points)

___

**Case Study:** *The psychiatric emergency room nurse is assessing Steve, a 27-year-old man experiencing a psychotic episode. He has no history of mental health problems but recently started a demanding, high-stress job. His girlfriend reports that Steve has been anxious and has had difficulties sleeping, for which he has been taking an over-the-counter sleeping remedy. His girlfriend is concerned because Steve is now mumbling incoherently and has not been able to attend to any goal-directed activity for the past 2 days. Questions 215 to 217 relate to this scenario.*

**215.** While the nurse is assessing Steve, she notices he is having difficulties completing a sentence

## ▶ Answers and Rationales

**1. D.** One drug can result in a lessened response to another drug.

*Rationale*
Cross-tolerance occurs when a drug with a similar action causes a decreased response to another drug. A drug that can prevent withdrawal symptoms from another drug describes cross-dependence. Cross-tolerance is not an allergic reaction to a classification of drugs. A drug that can increase the potency of another drug describes potentiating effects.

*Classification*
Competency Category: Nursing Practice: Alterations in Health
Taxonomic Level: Knowledge/Comprehension

**2. A.** Establish trust and rapport.

*Rationale*
It is extremely important that the nurse establishes trust and rapport. The nurse should not offer advice; rather, he or she should help the client develop the coping mechanisms necessary to solve his or her own problems. Setting limits is important but can only be developed after trust and rapport have been established.

*Classification*
Competency Category: Nurse–Person Relationship
Taxonomic Level: Application

**3. D.** Checking for sharp objects.

*Rationale*
A nursing assistant may be assigned to search a client's luggage or room for potentially harmful objects such as glass or sharp metal. A mental status assessment should be conducted by the nurse upon the client's admission. The physical examination should be completed by a licensed physician. A nurse or physician is responsible for discussing the treatment plan with the client.

*Classification*
Competency Category: Professional Practice
Taxonomic Level: Application

**4. B.** Encourage verbalizations about fears and stressful life situations.

*Rationale*
Encouraging the client to discuss stressful life situations helps keep the focus on the underlying issues. The client's preoccupation with a specific physical feature is a means of not coping with life. Ignoring the client or complimenting the client would not help this ineffective coping mechanism. The client would not be able to accept the compliment, and agreeing with her would only strengthen her problem.

*Classification*
Competency Category: Nursing Practice: Alterations in Health
Taxonomic Level: Critical Thinking

**5. B.** Violation of client rights.

*Rationale*
Confining a voluntary client against his or her will is considered a violation of rights. Slander is oral defamation of character. The nurse has not given out any information about the client, so confidentiality has not been violated.

*Classification*
Competency Category: Professional Practice
Taxonomic Level: Application

**6. C.** Denial.

*Rationale*
Denial is the avoidance of reality by ignoring or refusing to acknowledge unpleasant incidents. This defence mechanism is used to allay anxiety immediately after a stressful event. Introjection is an intense form of identification in which a person has incorporated the values or qualities of another person or group into his or her own ego structure. Suppression is the conscious analogue of repression; a person intentionally uses suppression to consciously exclude material from awareness. Repression is the unconscious exclusion of painful episodes from awareness.

*Classification*
Competency Category: Nursing Practice: Alterations in Health
Taxonomic Level: Knowledge/Comprehension

**7. D.** Self-awareness and understanding.

*Rationale*
Although all of the options are desirable, knowledge of oneself is the basis for building a strong therapeutic nurse–person relationship. Being aware of and understanding one's personal feelings and behaviours are prerequisites for understanding and helping clients.

*Classification*
Competency Category: Nurse–Person Relationship
Taxonomic Level: Application

**8. B.** Affect.

*Rationale*
Affect refers to a person's emotional expression (in this case, the manner in which the client talks about her experiences). Feelings are emotional states or perceptions. Blocking is the interruption of thoughts. Moods are prolonged emotional states expressed by the affect.

*Classification*
Competency Category: Nursing Practice: Alterations in Health
Taxonomic Level: Application

**9. B.** Reflecting.

*Rationale*
Reflection is correct because the nurse is referring feelings back to the client to explore. Reframing is offering a new way to look at a situation. The nurse's response is specific and is not offering a general lead.

*Classification*
Competency Category: Nurse–Person Relationship
Taxonomic Level: Critical Thinking

**10. C.** Poor boundaries.

*Rationale*
The described behaviours indicate poor personal boundaries, which is the inability to differentiate between oneself and others. Poor boundaries are symptoms of antisocial and passive–aggressive behaviour. Manipulation is an attempt to control another person.

*Classification*
Competency Category: Nursing Practice: Alterations in Health
Taxonomic Level: Application

**11. B.** Exploring.

*Rationale*
The nurse is using the technique of exploring because she is willing to delve further into the client's concern. She is not presenting reality, making observations, or simply restating. Rather, the nurse is encouraging the client to explore his or her feelings.

*Classification*
Competency Category: Nurse–Person Relationship
Taxonomic Level: Application

**12. A.** Systematic desensitization.

*Rationale*
Phobias are considered a learned response to anxiety that can be unlearned with interventions such as behaviour modification. One form of behaviour modification, systematic desensitization, helps a client relearn a sense of calm by reducing anxiety and potentially eradicating the phobia through gradual exposure to anxiety-producing stimuli. Psychoanalytic-oriented therapy and group therapy may also be effective in the reduction of anxiety, but they are long-term approaches that may require years of therapy. Electroconvulsive therapy is indicated for clients with severe depression or psychosis who respond poorly to other treatments.

*Classification*
Competency Category: Nursing Practice: Alterations in Health
Taxonomic Level: Knowledge/Comprehension

**13. D.** Exercising the client's arms regularly.

*Rationale*
Regular passive range of motion exercises with the client's arms serve to maintain muscle tone and mobility and prevent contractures. Because the client cannot consciously control his symptoms and move his arms, it is not advisable that the nurse insist that the client use his arms such as in eating without assistance. Furthermore, such insistence may anger the client and disrupt the therapeutic relationship. Including family members is important because they may be a part of the client's stress or conflict and are important in helping the client learn about these triggers and in regaining function of the arms. Education regarding pain management is not required because the client is not experiencing pain.

*Classification*
Competency Category: Nursing Practice: Alterations in Health
Taxonomic Level: Application

**14. B.** Assist the client to breathe deeply into a paper bag.

*Rationale*
When a client is experiencing a panic attack, his or her physiologic needs are of primary importance. Deep breathing into a paper bag corrects hyperventilation and restores a normal breathing pattern, which should relieve the client's other symptoms. The symptoms presented do not indicate a lack of orientation, so reorientation would not be a first priority. Furthermore, acting out and delusion have not been demonstrated, and during a panic attack, clients are not likely to act out, although they may strike out if they feel threatened or is gasping for air. In this case, an anxiolytic agent may be effective but is not the first priority, and IM administration may not be necessary. (Treatment should be done from least invasive to most depending on the priority.)

*Classification*
Competency Category: Nursing Practice: Alterations in Health
Taxonomic Level: Application

**15. B.** Hyperactive bowel sounds.

*Rationale*
Increased gastrointestinal motility, resulting in hyperactive bowel sounds and possibly leading to diarrhea

is an effect of the parasympathetic nervous system. Decreased urine output, muscle tension, and constipation would result from effects of the sympathetic nervous system stimulation.

*Classification*
Competency Category: Nursing Practice: Alterations in Health
Taxonomic Level: Knowledge/Comprehension

**16. A.** Empathized anxiety.

*Rationale*
Feelings of empathy enable anxiety to be transmissible from one person to another. A physical disorder must be present for secondary anxiety to materialize. A situation in which there is a threat to achievement of a developmental task results in maturational anxiety. Last, introjection is a defence mechanism, so introjected anxiety is an incorrect answer.

*Classification*
Competency Category: Nurse–Person Relationship
Taxonomic Level: Critical Thinking

**17. B.** Regression.

*Rationale*
Regressive behaviour is exhibited when the ego returns to an earlier, comforting, and less mature way of behaving in the face of disappointment. Crying is an example of a regressive behaviour. The unconscious transformation of anxiety into a physical symptom is an example of conversion. Intense unconscious identification with another person is referred to as introjection. Rationalization is the process of developing acceptable explanations to justify unacceptable ideas, actions, or feelings.

*Classification*
Competency Category: Nursing Practice: Alterations in Health
Taxonomic Level: Knowledge/Comprehension

**18. A.** Displacement

*Rationale*
Unconsciously transferring emotions associated with a person, object, or situation to another less threatening person, object, or situation is called displacement. The unconscious process of substituting constructive activity for unacceptable impulses is called sublimation; slamming of cupboard doors cannot be considered a constructive activity. Conversion involves unconsciously transforming anxiety into a physical symptom. Reaction formation occurs when a person keeps unacceptable feelings or behaviours

out of awareness by using the opposite feeling or behavior.

*Classification*
Competency Category: Nursing Practice: Alterations in Health
Taxonomic Level: Knowledge/Comprehension

**19. D.** Denial.

*Rationale*
Denial is an unconscious process of escaping an unpleasant reality by ignoring its existence such as this case in which the nurse is unable to acknowledge her true feelings. Reaction formation is an unconscious process that occurs when a person displays a feeling that is the opposite of anger. Repression happens when a person attempts to exclude an event from his or her awareness. Compensation is a mechanism in which a person unconsciously tries to make up for perceived deficits by excelling in another area to maintain self-esteem.

*Classification*
Competency Category: Nursing Practice: Alterations in Health
Taxonomic Level: Knowledge/Comprehension

**20. A.** Rationalization.

*Rationale*
Rationalization is an unconscious form of self-deception whereby a person makes excuses. The unconscious process that would call for the nurse to ignore the existence of the situation is denial. Projection on to others (e.g., blaming others) operates unconsciously. Compensation is an unconscious attempt to make up for a perceived weakness by emphasizing a strong point.

*Classification*
Competency Category: Nursing Practice: Alterations in Health
Taxonomic Level: Knowledge/Comprehension

**21. C.** Projection.

*Rationale*
Unconsciously adopting blaming behaviour is called projections, and it allows people to attribute unacceptable attributes to other people. A nurse who is unconsciously attempting to emphasize a strong point in an attempt to make up for a perceived weakness is engaging in compensation. Unconsciously adopting behaviour that is the opposite of one's actual feelings is called reaction formation. Unconsciously ignoring the existence of an unpleasant reality is called denial.

*Classification*
Competency Category: Nursing Practice: Alterations in Health
Taxonomic Level: Knowledge/Comprehension

**22. B.** Conversion.

*Rationale*
Conversion, a form of somatization, unconsciously transforms anxiety into a physical symptom that has no organic basis (e.g., the nurse losing her voice). Unconsciously determining to ignore the existence of an unpleasant reality is called denial. Suppression occurs when an event, idea, or feeling is placed out of awareness. This is distinct form repression, which occurs when a person unconsciously puts an event, idea, or feeling out of awareness.

*Classification*
Competency Category: Nursing Practice: Alterations in Health
Taxonomic Level: Knowledge/Comprehension

**23. A.** Altruism.

*Rationale*
When a person deals with emotional conflict by meeting the needs of others and receiving gratification through meeting others' needs, it is referred to as altruism.

*Classification*
Competency Category: Nursing Practice: Alterations in Health
Taxonomic Level: Application

**24. D.** Selective serotonin reuptake inhibitor (SSRI).

*Rationale*
Venlafaxine is an SSRI that is prescribed to treat depressive disorders.

*Classification*
Competency Category: Nursing Practice: Alterations in Health
Taxonomic Level: Knowledge/Comprehension

**25. D.** Not metabolised and excreted unchanged by the kidneys.

*Rationale*
Lithium is not metabolised and is excreted unchanged by the kidneys.

*Classification*
Competency Category: Nursing Practice: Alterations in Health
Taxonomic Level: Critical Thinking

**26. B.** Provision of a safe and structured environment.

*Rationale*
Injury prevention is a primary goal of care for clients with Alzheimer's disease. The nurse can help achieve this through provision of a safe and structured environment. Other care goals include management of effective communication with the client and family to help in the adjustment to the client's altered cognitive abilities. Cognitive losses themselves cannot be prevented, and because Alzheimer's disease is a degenerative dementia, it cannot be reversed.

*Classification*
Competency Category: Nursing Practice: Health and Wellness
Taxonomic Level: Application

**27. C.** Fold towels and pillowcases.

*Rationale*
Intervention activities, such as folding towels and pillowcases, are simple tasks that can be used to redirect a client's attention. Typically, this sort of activity is familiar, and the client is likely to perform it successfully. Dance therapy is excessively stimulating and complicated. Cards and reminiscence group therapies require cognitive abilities that are too complicated for a confused client.

*Classification*
Competency Category: Nursing Practice: Alterations in Health
Taxonomic Level: Critical Thinking

**28. D.** Ideas and a plan to harm oneself.

*Rationale*
Suicidal ideation refers to thoughts or plans of suicide. To assess for these, the nurse must ask directly if the client is thinking about or planning suicide. A lifting of depression and giving away of prized possessions can be common indicators of increased risk of suicide rather than a further deterioration of self-worth. Vegetative shifts are indicative of depression, not necessarily of suicidal ideation.

*Classification*
Competency Category: Nursing Practice: Alterations in Health
Taxonomic Level: Application

**29. A.** Setting limits, providing a low-stimulation environment, and maintaining a neutral attitude from the staff.

*Rationale*

Nurses in a generalist setting should be aware of attending to the special needs of the mental health clients on the general unit. Management of the health care environment will benefit Darlene as well as other clients on the unit. The nurse should set limits and create a low-stimulation, neutral environment to facilitate de-escalation of Darlene's manic state. High-calorie finger foods can be offered to supplement a client's diet if he or she cannot remain seated long enough to complete a meal.

*Classification*

Competency Category: Nursing Practice: Alterations in Health
Taxonomic Level: Application

**30. C.** Set limits with specific and consistent consequences for belittling or demanding behaviour.

*Rationale*

The nurse will need to set limits and consequences for behaviour such as belittling and being demanding of others because this is inappropriate behaviour. Requiring that others ignore the client is likely to increase those behaviours. Offering Darlene stimulating activities would be counterproductive, and providing her with antianxiety medication would provide no motivation for her to adjust her behaviours.

*Classification*

Competency Category: Nursing Practice: Alterations in Health
Taxonomic Level: Critical Thinking

**31. B.** Grandiose delusions.

*Rationale*

Disturbed thinking marked by expanded sense of self with false beliefs, such as religious connections or physical powers, can be described as grandiose delusions. Visual hallucinations are perceptual disturbances, which Darlene did not describe. Neologisms are made-up words, which are also not present in this description of Darlene's mental state. Also, Darlene is not experiencing dysphoria (chronic low mood) at this time.

*Classification*

Competency Category: Nursing Practice: Alterations in Health
Taxonomic Level: Application

**32. C.** Behavioural difficulties.

*Rationale*

Adolescents with depression typically demonstrate irritability and behavioural problems. Anxiety disor-ders are most commonly associated with younger children. Cognitive impairments are typically comorbid with delirium, dementia, and learning difficulties. Labile mood would be more characteristic of a client with bipolar disorder.

*Classification*

Competency Category: Nursing Practice: Alterations in Health
Taxonomic Level: Application

**33. D.** Social withdrawal and oppositional behaviour.

*Rationale*

For adolescents, depression typically manifests as social withdrawal and oppositional behaviour. For adults, it usually produces hopelessness and helplessness. Drug use may lead to stealing and truancy. Adolescents quite commonly display obsession with body image.

*Classification*

Competency Category: Nursing Practice: Alterations in Health
Taxonomic Level: Application

**34. B.** Referral to an after-school social recreation program.

*Rationale*

When social isolation has been identified, it is most appropriate to refer the client to an age-appropriate social and recreational program. More intensive family therapy is not indicated at this time. Evan is not displaying conduct disorder, so he does not require a residential program. Supportive listening and goal setting would further isolate Evan from his peer group.

*Classification*

Competency Category: Nursing Practice: Alterations in Health
Taxonomic Level: Application

**35. C.** Decelerated movements and flat affect.

*Rationale*

Slow movements, fatigue, and flat affect typically present in individuals with depression. The other responses indicate an elevated mood.

*Classification*

Competency Category: Nursing Practice: Alterations in Health
Taxonomic Level: Application

**36. C.** "There are patterns with this illness. If a person has one depressive episode, she has a 60% chance of experiencing another."

*Rationale*
If a person has a depressive episode, there is a 60% chance of a second episode. The other statements are false.

*Classification*
Competency Category: Nursing Practice: Health and Wellness
Taxonomic Level: Knowledge/Comprehension

**37. D.** Ensuring that Amina is not permitted to use anything that would be potentially dangerous.

*Rationale*
Although grief and loss as well as isolation are impacting her depressed state, the priority intervention is to prevent Amina from self-harm. All of the interventions listed are appropriate, but ensuring safety from potential danger is the priority.

*Classification*
Competency Category: Nursing Practice: Health and Wellness
Taxonomic Level: Application

**38. A.** Teaching about the impact of negative beliefs and other assumptions.

*Rationale*
Cognitive and behavioural therapy assists the client in becoming more aware of his or her thoughts and feelings and behavioural responses to upsetting situations. Only the teaching about beliefs is indicative of a cognitive behavioural intervention. The others are specific treatments or assessments.

*Classification*
Competency Category: Nursing Practice: Health and Wellness
Taxonomic Level: Application

**39. D.** "I notice your energy level seems high right now. What has seemed to help you relax enough to manage your usual tasks in the past?"

*Rationale*
Acknowledging the client's manic state and then asking about things that have helped in the past is the most therapeutic response to a client in a manic state. It would not be therapeutic to tell the client not to worry, to describe mania as the best part of the illness, or to postpone discussing treatment options.

*Classification*
Competency Category: Nursing Practice: Health and Wellness
Taxonomic Level: Critical Thinking

**40. B.** That he understands the stressors and situations that precipitated his recent psychotic episode.

*Rationale*
A client who can verbalize an understanding of the stressors and events that have preceded past psychotic episodes recognizes the information that can be applied to different situations. Although having a job and knowing when to take medications support wellness, they do not necessarily indicate that he knows when to seek help in the future. Having the home phone numbers of therapists indicates bad boundaries.

*Classification*
Competency Category: Nursing Practice: Health and Wellness
Taxonomic Level: Application

**41. C.** "I don't have any signs of cancer."

*Rationale*
The comment indicating that the client has no signs of cancer would indicate that a client is free of somatic delusions. The client saying that his doctor is in love with him is expressing an erotomanic delusion. The client who believes his spouse is having an affair is expressing jealous delusions, and the client who states the Hells Angels are following or reporting on him has a persecutory delusion.

*Classification*
Competency Category: Nursing Practice: Alterations in Health
Taxonomic Level: Critical Thinking

**42. D.** "Maintaining a structured schedule and trusted supports can provide some means of coping."

*Rationale*
Suggesting to a client who is experiencing hallucinations to talk back to voices, focus on internal feelings, or daydream would all be counterproductive. Offering the suggestion of maintaining a structured schedule is most helpful because this approach will provide the client the chance to remain functional even while experiencing a perceptual disturbance.

*Classification*
Competency Category: Nursing Practice: Health and Wellness
Taxonomic Level: Application

**43. A.** It is accepted within their religion or as part of a cultural belief, ceremony, or ritual.

*Rationale*

Some religions and cultures may accept particular experiences, including seeing visions and hearing voices, as completely normal even though these manifestations may meet the criteria for a psychotic episode.

*Classification*

Competency Category: Nurse–Person Relationship
Taxonomic Level: Application

**44. D.** Establishing trust.

*Rationale*

Establishing a trusting relationship is the priority goal when working with clients with delusions. Only after trust is established can other assessment and goal setting or interventions take place. Being free of delusions, participating in unit activities, and performing tasks independently are important but are not initial priorities.

*Classification*

Competency Category: Nurse–Person Relationship
Taxonomic Level: Application

**45. D.** "I don't hear anything, but tell me more about what you are hearing."

*Rationale*

This response provides a reality orientation without refuting the experience of the client. It also seeks to find out more because it is important to assess if commands are part of the hallucination. Refuting the experience is not helpful and does not provide any support. Oversympathizing is not the best response because it does not reorient the client, and sarcasm is not productive, either.

*Classification*

Competency Category: Nursing Practice: Alterations in Health
Taxonomic Level: Critical Thinking

**46. A.** Hallucinations and delusions.

*Rationale*

Only the hallucinations and delusions are considered positive symptoms. The other responses are not considered "positive" symptoms, or symptoms that are clinical manifestations that appear odd and unusual additions to the client's character. Negative symptoms include flat affect, avolition, and anhedonia with withdrawal.

*Classification*

Competency Category: Nursing Practice: Alterations in Health
Taxonomic Level: Knowledge/Comprehension

**47. C.** Engaging the client in reality-based conversations.

*Rationale*

Although encouraging therapeutic conversations, discussing relapse prevention, and acknowledging the client's strengths are all important with a client experiencing hallucinations, engaging in reality orientation is the first priority for the nursing care.

*Classification*

Competency Category: Nursing Practice: Alterations in Health
Taxonomic Level: Application

**48. D.** Experience troubling thoughts without self-mutilation.

*Rationale*

Clients with borderline personality disorder frequently engage in impulsive acts, particularly self-mutilation. The behaviour described in answer D indicates a positive outcome for a client who has such maladaptive behaviours as the typical impulsivity of self-mutilation.

*Classification*

Competency Category: Nursing Practice: Alterations in Health
Taxonomic Level: Critical Thinking

**49. D.** "What supports are available for the long term?"

*Rationale*

This response indicates that the family members are aware that support will be required and that this is a long-standing, deteriorating condition. It is unlikely that a return to the client's previous condition and living situation will evolve because Alzheimer's dementia is a progressive and deteriorating condition. Vitamin and herbal therapies are not a solution, and another care facility will not offer any miracle solutions.

*Classification*

Competency Category: Nursing Practice: Alterations in Health
Taxonomic Level: Application

**50. C.** Delirium related to toxin exposure.

*Rationale*

Delirium is a state of mental confusion and excitation. Symptoms include mind wandering, incoherent speech, and often continued aimless physical activity. The onset is usually rapid (i.e., within hours). Metal paint is a toxin that is known to cause delirium.

*Classification*
Competency Category: Nursing Practice: Health and Wellness
Taxonomic Level: Critical Thinking

**51. B.** Risk for injury.

*Rationale*
Risk for injury to self and others should maintain the highest priority in care planning. In this case, the client's wandering, memory loss, and aggression pose hazards for accidents, falls, and injuries.

*Classification*
Competency Category: Nursing Practice: Alterations in Health
Taxonomic Level: Application

**52. C.** Play therapy.

*Rationale*
Given the developmental stage of the client, play therapy is the only intervention of the list that would be indicated. A 4-year-old boy with autism would not be a candidate for social skills, cognitive behavioural therapy, or psychotropic medications.

*Classification*
Competency Category: Nursing Practice: Alterations in Health
Taxonomic Level: Knowledge/Comprehension

**53. C.** Somatising disorder.

*Rationale*
For a cultural group in which expressions of emotional or mental illness are shameful, the anxiety or a distressing circumstance is likely to manifest as a somatic disorder, which is an adaptive sort of expression of the anxiety.

*Classification*
Competency Category: Nursing Practice: Alterations in Health
Taxonomic Level: Critical Thinking

**54. D.** "Although there are some risks, your mother will have a thorough examination in advance to ensure that she is a good candidate for the treatment."

*Rationale*
Supportive and informative teaching requires a description of the risk and the measures of that risk through the assessment and examination process.

Explaining that the treatment is absolutely safe would be false, and suggesting that there are side effects but that they are not life threatening is vague and not reassuring to the family. Explaining that she will recover quicker is giving a false sense of hope.

*Classification*
Competency Category: Nursing Practice: Alterations in Health
Taxonomic Level: Application

**55. B.** "The client will likely experience some confusion and disorientation after the treatment."

*Rationale*
Clients typically experience some confusion and disorientation after treatment; this generally recovers quite quickly. Clients are not heavily sedated after treatment. Muscle soreness is rare. Clients do not have immediate benefits after treatment; the typical course of treatment is six to 10 treatments.

*Classification*
Competency Category: Nursing Practice: Alterations in Health
Taxonomic Level: Application

**56. D.** Provide frequent, supportive reorientation after the treatment.

*Rationale*
Common side effects of bilateral ECT treatments are confusion, disorientation, and short-term memory loss. The nurse should plan frequent, brief, and succinct reorientation statements.

*Classification*
Competency Category: Nursing Practice: Alterations in Health
Taxonomic Level: Application

**57. D.** Paralytic ileus.

*Rationale*
Although ECT is an operative procedure, the intestinal obstruction and failure of peristalsis known as paralytic ileus that can accompany some surgical procedures or bowel disturbances is least expected after ECT. Headache, disorientation, and memory loss are common short-term side effects.

*Classification*
Competency Category: Nursing Practice: Alterations in Health
Taxonomic Level: Knowledge/Comprehension

**58. C.** Anorexia nervosa.

*Rationale*
The assessment data support a diagnosis of anorexia nervosa.

*Classification*
Competency Category: Nursing Practice: Alterations in Health
Taxonomic Level: Knowledge/Comprehension

**59. D.** Provide highly structured mealtimes with regular meals of sufficient caloric intake to promote weight gain.

*Rationale*
Structured mealtimes should be encouraged. During mealtimes, non–food-related social conversation is the encouraged treatment. Nutritional counselling is also encouraged. Sneaking food, laxatives, and diuretics is a much greater concern in clients with bulimia nervosa than in those with anorexia nervosa.

*Classification*
Competency Category: Nursing Practice: Health and Wellness
Taxonomic Level: Critical Thinking

**60. D.** Request that Brittany stand backward on the scale when being weighed.

*Rationale*
The most appropriate intervention is to have Brittany stand backward on the scale. Instructing Brittany to close her eyes may not be sufficient because the impulse to check the weight and concern with gaining weight may be so great that she will open her eyes and experience further distress.

*Classification*
Competency Category: Nursing Practice: Alterations in Health
Taxonomic Level: Application

**61. B.** Providing instruction and assessment for stress management techniques.

*Rationale*
Conditions of stress (e.g., Judy's isolation, her marital breakup, and isolation from her daughter) exacerbate somatoform disorders. Alternative medicines are not proven to benefit people with somatoform disorders. Psychotic symptoms are not common or present in this case, so antipsychotic medications are not indicated. Behaviour modification would be appropriate for the client and is not indicated for the family.

*Classification*
Competency Category: Nursing Practice: Health and Wellness
Taxonomic Level: Application

**62. C.** The absence of laboratory findings to support clinical manifestation of the pain.

*Rationale*
One of the key criteria for the diagnosis of somatoform disorder is the absence of clinical or laboratory findings to support any physical manifestations of the described pain. Reality testing is not a factor because Judy is not delusional. The cause of somatoform disorder is psychological and out of the client's awareness. Patterns of vegetative shift are notable in people with depression.

*Classification*
Competency Category: Nursing Practice: Alterations in Health
Taxonomic Level: Critical Thinking

**63. C.** Encouraging Judy to identify feelings and body sensations associated with stress.

*Rationale*
By encouraging identification of feelings and body sensations, the client can gain awareness and some recognition of somatising patterns. Avoiding stressors and learning about stressors would be counterproductive. Medication is generally not indicated and creates dependency and further somatisation of the psychological condition as well. Although addressing family concerns can be important to assist in support and stress management, these family members are currently not part of Judy's support system.

*Classification*
Competency Category: Nursing Practice: Health and Wellness
Taxonomic Level: Application

**64. D.** "I take my medication as soon as I feel increased anxiety."

*Rationale*
BuSpar is taken as a maintenance drug rather than as a prn response to acute symptoms. Improvements with this treatment are noted in 7 to 10 days, but full effects may take 3 to 4 weeks. Other shorter acting anxiolytics are prescribed for short-term anxiety.

*Classification*
Competency Category: Nursing Practice: Alterations in Health
Taxonomic Level: Critical Thinking

**65. C.** Instruction to avoid drinking alcohol while on this medication.

*Rationale*
Alcohol will potentiate the depressant effects of alprazolam, causing harmful sedation.

*Classification*
Competency Category: Nursing Practice: Health and Wellness
Taxonomic Level: Critical Thinking

**66. C.** Suzanne is performing fewer rituals.

*Rationale*
Zoloft is a selective serotonin reuptake inhibitor that is effective in treating people with OCD, specifically with the ritualistic behaviours associated with sensations of anxiety. A decrease in ritualistic behaviours indicates that the treatment is having the desired effect.

*Classification*
Competency Category: Nursing Practice: Alterations in Health
Taxonomic Level: Critical Thinking

**67. D.** Remind the daughter and the client that it may take 1 to 3 weeks for the medication to take effect.

*Rationale*
The client may need to take the Elavil for 1 to 3 weeks before the desired effect is seen. Suggesting a medication change would only complicate matters. Questioning the daughter's expectations will not assist in informing her about the facts about this effect of the medication. Deferring to the physician is not necessary because the nurse should be well aware of the course of action of this medication, and it is her role to teach the family.

*Classification*
Competency Category: Nursing Practice: Health and Wellness
Taxonomic Level: Application

**68. A.** Have him stop taking the trifluoperazine immediately.

*Rationale*
The neuroleptic agent should be immediately discontinued. Because this is a potentially fatal condition, medical treatment and assessment should be initiated.

*Classification*
Competency Category: Nursing Practice: Alterations in Health
Taxonomic Level: Knowledge/Application

**69. D.** Instruction about the signs and symptoms of blood dyscrasias.

*Rationale*
A dangerous side effect of clozapine is blood dyscrasia. Symptoms of blood dyscrasias, including sore throat, fever, general malaise, and unusual bleeding, need to be taught to the client. Weekly white blood cell counts are often ordered when a client is started on clozapine.

*Classification*
Competency Category: Nursing Practice: Health and Wellness
Taxonomic Level: Application

**70. B.** Monitoring blood lithium levels.

*Rationale*
Lithium is the drug of choice for clients with bipolar illness and has an antimanic effectiveness in 78% of people. Lithium decreases the intensity, frequency, and duration of manic and depressive episodes. Blood levels need to be monitored for therapeutic levels during the acute phase (1.0–1.5 mEq/L) and during longer term maintenance. Other treatments that could be expected for patients during mania include sedatives or antipsychotics. Electroconvulsive therapy, phototherapy, and monoamine oxidase inhibitors are not typically indicated during manic phases.

*Classification*
Competency Category: Nursing Practice: Health and Wellness
Taxonomic Level: Critical Thinking

**71. C.** "I hope we can all learn some new skills and begin to problem solve better with the help of the therapist."

*Rationale*
Family therapy is aimed at improving communication and problem solving within the family group. The focus is on the family as a group, not on correcting the behaviour of any one family member.

*Classification*
Competency Category: Nurse–Person Relationship
Taxonomic Level: Critical Thinking

**72. D.** Understanding abstract concepts.

*Rationale*
Children who are 5 to 7 years old are learning to integrate abstract concepts based on relationships.

Children this age typically have long been able to understand basic rules and instructions, imitate others, and recognize object permanence.

*Classification*
Competency Category: Nursing Practice: Health and Wellness
Taxonomic Level: Knowledge/Comprehension

**73. C.** A demonstration of transference.

*Rationale*
The unconscious transfer of qualities originally associated with another relationship to a nurse or therapist is referred to as transference. Quite often these qualities are those of a parent, family member, or authority figure and may provoke responses that are not appropriate to the new situation to which they are ascribed.

*Classification*
Competency Category: Nurse–Person Relationship
Taxonomic Level: Critical Thinking

**74. D.** Resistance.

*Rationale*
The conscious or unconscious introduction of actions that sabotage the helping relationship, thus helping the client avoid confronting actual issues of therapy, are considered resistance.

*Classification*
Competency Category: Nurse–Person Relationship
Taxonomic Level: Critical Thinking

**75. C.** Invite him to sit down in a quiet place and reorient him to the nurse's name and the unit routines.

*Rationale*
Many clients are anxious at the time of admission and are often reassured by repetition of orientation information along with a calming professional approach. This should always be tried first before any more invasive discussions or medical or physical measures.

*Classification*
Competency Category: Nurse–Person Relationship
Taxonomic Level: Application

**76. B.** Assess the client's situation, history, and mental status and inquire about contacting others for assessment information.

*Rationale*
Before any interventions are planned with a client without any history at the mental health centre, the nurse must thoroughly assess the client's mental status and current situation.

*Classification*
Competency Category: Nursing Practice: Alterations in Health
Taxonomic Level: Critical Thinking

**77. D.** Support an increase in community programs, such as camp programs, music, sports, and other creative expressions, that increase self-esteem for children and teens.

*Rationale*
Primary prevention strategies must involve changes that will be made in the community that promote health and prevent disease.

*Classification*
Competency Category: Nursing Practice: Health and Wellness
Taxonomic Level: Critical Thinking

**78. C.** Help the group establish shared goals that are consistent with the individual goals of members.

*Rationale*
When goals are established by the group that fit their individual needs and meet a great group need, group cohesiveness is easier to establish.

*Classification*
Competency Category: Nursing Practice: Nurse–Client Relationship
Taxonomic Level: Application

**79. D.** Orientation.

*Rationale*
During the orientation phase, group members often test the boundaries of the group to establish their roles, discover norms, and explore their ability to trust within the group.

*Classification*
Competency Category: Nurse–Person Relationship
Taxonomic Level: Knowledge/Comprehension

**80. C.** Express doubt and do not argue.

*Rationale*
Paranoid clients develop a delusional system to defend against anxiety. It is best to insert doubt but not argue with the client because refuting and

arguing with the delusion would just add to the anxiety of the client. Encouraging venting of frustration would not address the thought distortion, and a logical, persistent approach would not be a match with the distorted thinking.

*Classification*
Competency Category: Nursing Practice: Alterations in Health
Taxonomic Level: Application

**81. C.** Daily walks.

*Rationale*
Taking daily walks allows the client to expend energy and establish a trusting, neutral relationship with the nurse. The other suggestions are higher stimulation activities that insert competition and added anxiety to the situation.

*Classification*
Competency Category: Nursing Practice: Health and Wellness
Taxonomic Level: Application

**82. D.** Provides a natural outlet for the release of muscle tension.

*Rationale*
Clients experiencing anxiety often experience the stress response, which creates considerable muscle tension. Physical exercise allows for a release of this tension, which decreases the experience of stress for anxious clients.

*Classification*
Competency Category: Nursing Practice: Health and Wellness
Taxonomic Level: Knowledge/Comprehension

**83. C.** The parents report an understanding of normal growth and development.

*Rationale*
Understanding normal growth and development helps the parents have more reasonable expectations of their children. Spanking indicates the parents have not learned other forms of discipline. Expecting hyperresponsible behaviour is not healthy, and merely hoping to attend parenting classes does not indicate an understanding of the concepts.

*Classification*
Competency Category: Nursing Practice: Health and Wellness
Taxonomic Level: Critical Thinking

**84. C.** Report the suspected child abuse to social services.

*Rationale*
The child's initial examination shows signs of sexual abuse that must be reported. The other responses of gathering further data and teaching will be later priorities.

*Classification*
Competency Category: Nursing Practice: Professional Practice
Taxonomic Level: Critical Thinking

**85. D.** Having a delay in seeking treatment for the child's injuries.

*Rationale*
A delay in seeking treatment for a child's serious injuries is a sign of abuse. Anxiety is expected and is a normal response. Vague descriptions of the injuries are more common in abuse cases than detailed ones, and abusers often prevent a child from explaining the nature of his or her injuries rather than encouraging it.

*Classification*
Competency Category: Nursing Practice: Alterations in Health
Taxonomic Level: Critical Thinking

**86. A.** "Now that I have left Derrick, I don't need to worry."

*Rationale*
The period of time after a victim leaves a relationship is the most dangerous time; having left, the victim is in greater danger in many ways. It often takes several times before a person leaves an abuser for good; the honeymoon phase can cloud the better judgement of the victim involved in the cycle of violence. Often victims are afraid that their abusers will attempt to sabotage custody of their children and often feel guilty. These other issues are later priorities to address than the immediate danger one must realize when first leaving an abuser.

*Classification*
Competency Category: Nursing Practice: Health and Wellness
Taxonomic Level: Critical Thinking

**87. D.** Being firm and not reacting to provocation.

*Rationale*
Adolescent clients often challenge authority to clarify their boundaries. Remaining firm, neutral, and not reactive is the best approach. Asserting authority would likely be counterproductive, and although it is helpful to be supportive and friendly, the nurse should maintain professional boundaries and should

not approach the client as a friend. Creating exceptions to rules would create confusion for the client.

*Classification*
Competency Category: Nurse–Person Relationship
Taxonomic Level: Application

**88. D.** The parents use inconsistent limit setting oscillating with very harsh discipline.

*Rationale*
Issues of inconsistent limit setting and very harsh discipline are often typical of families with children who have conduct disorder. High expectations and parental overinvolvement are more characteristic of anxiety disorders. Being an only child is not correlated in any way with conduct disorder.

*Classification*
Competency Category: Nursing Practice: Alterations in Health
Taxonomic Level: Knowledge/Comprehension

**89. C.** Methylphenidate (Ritalin).

*Rationale*
Ritalin (a central nervous system stimulant) is commonly prescribed for the management of ADHD in children and adolescents. Ritalin increases the ability to focus attention by blocking other irrelevant thoughts and impulses. Elavil and Paxil are antidepressant medications that are occasionally used in the treatment of clients with ADHD but not commonly so. Cogentin is an antiparkinsonian agent that is not indicated at all in this case.

*Classification*
Competency Category: Nursing Practice: Alterations in Health
Taxonomic Level: Knowledge/Comprehension

**90. C.** Behaviour modification.

*Rationale*
Behaviour modification is quite effective for children and adolescents with defiance and oppositional behaviours. Emotive therapies and cognitive restructuring are more effective in older adults and for anxiety and depression therapy. Reminiscence therapy is used more for elderly individuals and older adults with memory impairment.

*Classification*
Competency Category: Nursing Practice: Alterations in Health
Taxonomic Level: Application

**91. B.** Separation anxiety.

*Rationale*
Although separation anxiety can occur at any age, it is the most common anxiety problem of children. The peak onset is between ages 7 and 9 years. OCD, simple phobia, and PTSD are less common in young children.

*Classification*
Competency Category: Nursing Practice: Alterations in Health
Taxonomic Level: Knowledge/Comprehension

**92. C.** Indifference to being held or hugged.

*Rationale*
Children with autistic disorders are highly indifferent to the show of affection of others. These children often have repetitive and unimaginative play, have delayed language development, and tend not to be affectionate.

*Classification*
Competency Category: Nursing Practice: Health and Wellness
Taxonomic Level: Application

**93. B.** Eating disorders.

*Rationale*
Antidepressants have been effective in treating some clients with eating disorders. Antidepressants have not been found to be effective in treating individuals with thought disorders, conduct disorders, or autism.

*Classification*
Competency Category: Nursing Practice: Alterations in Health
Taxonomic Level: Knowledge/Comprehension

**94. D.** Situational crisis.

*Rationale*
Situational crisis occurs when a client experiences stress that he or she is unable to cope with that occurs with a life change, transition, or crisis event.

*Classification*
Competency Category: Nursing Practice: Alterations in Health
Taxonomic Level: Knowledge/Comprehension

**95. D.** Is possibly at more serious risk because he may have gained sufficient energy to act on his suicidal ideation; he requires further assessment.

*Rationale*
This is a classic sign that a person is at high risk for suicide.

*Classification*
Competency Category: Nursing Practice: Alterations in Health
Taxonomic Level: Critical Thinking

**96. B.** Bernard will identify past suicidal ideations and behaviour.

*Rationale*
It is important for the nurse to accurately assess the client's suicide ideation and past behaviour.

*Classification*
Competency Category: Nurse–Person Relationship
Taxonomic Level: Critical Thinking

**97. A.** Compare her current weight with her usual weight.

*Rationale*
When a client is unable to be specific about her recent activities or eating habits, comparing her current weight as it relates to her usual weight is the best determinant of her nutritional status and weight change.

*Classification*
Competency Category: Nursing Practice: Alterations in Health
Taxonomic Level: Application

**98. C.** Disturbed perceptions related to anxiety as evidenced by auditory hallucinations.

*Rationale*
Hallucinations are sensory experiences of perception without corresponding stimuli in the environment. This client objectively reports to the nurse the fearfulness and experience of this hallucination. The other responses are not founded in objective information based on the client's statement.

*Classification*
Competency Category: Nursing Practice: Alterations in Health
Taxonomic Level: Application

**99. A.** Panic disorder.

*Rationale*
Julie displays classic symptoms of panic disorder resulting from acute anxiety. Panic disorder may cause a variety of physiologic symptoms, including those listed in Julie's case as well as dyspnea, choking, feelings of unreality, shaking or trembling, and hot or cold flashes. The disorder is marked by a history of three or more panic attacks within 3 weeks that are unrelated to extreme physical exertion or life-threatening situations. Symptoms of schizoaffective disorder are mood and thought focused, depression symptoms are mood focused, and OCD symptoms are ritual and compulsions focused.

*Classification*
Competency Category: Nursing Practice: Alterations in Health
Taxonomic Level: Critical Thinking

**100. C.** Encourage the use of relaxation exercises or techniques.

*Rationale*
Relaxation exercises or techniques, such as deep breathing, progressive muscle relaxation, and imagery or relaxing visualization, can all help the client gain control over anxiety in a way that promotes sleep. These exercises help produce a physiologic response opposite to that produced by stress (i.e., the relaxation response). Providing sleeping pills would provide short-term relief from the sleeplessness but would not promote healthy sleeping patterns. Suggesting the client stay up and talk or play pool would not help him develop longer term sleep habits or control stress or anxiety. In fact, playing games and engaging in talk late into the evening may produce *more* of a stress response.

*Classification*
Competency Category: Nursing Practice: Health and Wellness
Taxonomic Level: Application

**101. C.** Risk for injury.

*Rationale*
Steve is at increased risk for injury because of his hyperactivity, agitation, and disorientation. Although the other concerns are important for Steve's care, the client's safety always takes highest priority. The nurse should plan first and foremost to prevent injury and harm for which Steve is at risk given his current condition.

*Classification*
Competency Category: Nursing Practice: Health and Wellness
Taxonomic Level: Critical Thinking

**102. C.** "In case anything goes wrong? What are you concerned about right now?"

*Rationale*
The most therapeutic response is one in which the nurse reflects back to the client what she has said and

asks the client to reflect further. All of the other responses do not adequately invite reflection or demonstrate listening and concern for the client's situation and feelings.

*Classification*
Competency Category: Nurse–Person Relationship
Taxonomic Level: Critical Thinking

**103. B.** "It helps me to have one or two drinks at lunch."

*Rationale*
Alcohol and drug abuse in an attempt to reduce anxiety is a common response to phobic disorders. The statement indicating potential alcohol abuse should be the priority concern for the nurse's teaching. Telling the nurse about strategies for managing anxiety, such as deep breathing and expressing desire to ask someone out on a date, demonstrate small steps that the client is overcoming his fears. Expressing to the nurse that someone else got a job the client was interested in shows insight into the impact of his disorder and demonstrates trust in the nurse.

*Classification*
Competency Category: Nursing Practice: Health and Wellness
Taxonomic Level: Application

**104. D.** "Inform your physician immediately if you become pregnant or intend to do so."

*Rationale*
Xanax is contraindicated during pregnancy, and the medication should not be taken if the client is or intends to become pregnant imminently. Nausea, photosensitivity, and urinary retention are all side effects but are not contraindications.

*Classification*
Competency Category: Nursing Practice: Health and Wellness
Taxonomic Level: Knowledge/Application

**105. D.** Posttraumatic stress disorder (PTSD).

*Rationale*
Survivors of trauma, disasters, and events outside of the usual ranges of human experiences may experience PTSD. People who have PTSD usually relive the event mentally and experience emotional numbness and the difficulty concentrating that this client displays. Inability to function in daily life because of memory, sleep, and concentration impairments can be disabling. In phobic disorders,

clients fear objects that do not pose particular danger. The primary features of depressive illness are mood changes. With adjustment disorders, the stressor is usually less severe and more within usual range of experience than with PTSD. Conversion disorders are an expression of anxiety that suggests a physical disorder (without physiologic findings).

*Classification*
Competency Category: Nursing Practice: Alterations in Health
Taxonomic Level: Critical Thinking

**106. D.** Splitting.

*Rationale*
The defence mechanism of splitting is identified when a client views others as all good or all bad. Manipulation occurs when a client attempts to use and reform situations and people for his or her own gain regardless of the distortion or validity. Dialectical behavioural approaches are psychosocial approaches to the treatment of people with bipolar disorder. Dissociation refers to the separation of objects from their emotional significance. Trevor's correct documentation of this symptom is important to the client's overall care and treatment planning.

*Classification*
Competency Category: Nursing Practice: Professional Practice
Taxonomic Level: Knowledge/Comprehension

**107. D.** Explore the expressed symptoms in a matter-of-fact way.

*Rationale*
The nurse should address Phil's symptoms promptly and in a matter-of-fact way. The nurse should avoid a lengthy discussion about the symptoms to avoid anchoring dependency but should not avoid the discussion or disregard the described symptoms altogether, which would be counterproductive.

*Classification*
Competency Category: Nurse–Person Relationship
Taxonomic Level: Application

**108. C.** Stimulants.

*Rationale*
"Meth" is a common street name of methamphetamine, a stimulant.

*Classification*
Competency Category: Nursing Practice: Alterations in Health
Taxonomic Level: Knowledge/Comprehension

**109. D.** Drowsiness.

*Rationale*
Clients experiencing severe alcohol withdrawal are likely to be hyperwakeful, so drowsiness is not a symptom that would be expected. The other listed symptoms are indeed characteristic of severe alcohol withdrawal.

*Classification*
Competency Category: Nursing Practice: Health and Wellness
Taxonomic Level: Critical Thinking

**110. D.** Vague, transient hallucinations.

*Rationale*
With moderate alcohol withdrawal, the nurse can expect the client to experience vague transient hallucinations (visual or auditory). Restlessness and slight diaphoresis are usually present in individuals with mild withdrawal. Marked disorientation and confusion are expected in those with more severe withdrawal.

*Classification*
Competency Category: Nursing Practice: Alterations in Health
Taxonomic Level: Application

**111. C.** Performing all activities for Gemma so her needs are met.

*Rationale*
Gemma's nurse should not perform all activities for her; rather, the nurse should encourage Gemma to attend to her daily living needs to avoid dependence. Rewarding positive behaviour is part of a behavioural management approach that helps promote productive behaviour. Exploring neologisms and hallucination content is not done in depth but must be attended to in order to make note of command hallucinations and to help promote reality checks.

*Classification*
Competency Category: Nursing Practice: Health and Wellness
Taxonomic Level: Application

**112. D.** Clang association.

*Rationale*
Documenting assessment findings accurately is paramount in building a sense of the clinical picture and ascertaining accurate diagnosis and treatment for the client. In this case, the expressed thought process is assessed as a clang association because of the rhyming, rhythmic associations of words.

*Classification*
Competency Category: Professional Practice
Taxonomic Level: Knowledge/Comprehension

**113. D.** By a combination of positive and negative symptoms and medication effects.

*Rationale*
Although antipsychotic and antidepressant medications may have sexual side effects (including low libido and erectile dysfunction) for some patients, the effects of the positive and negative symptoms of schizophrenia also impact sexuality and sexual functioning. The nurse should emphasize that the treatment is not the only factor to begin to look at problem solving. Encouraging a balanced understanding of the situation is important for promotion of mental and sexual health. Hallucinations and delusions may impact libido and functioning but are not the primary problem in Dave's case. Social stigma does impact social relations but is also not the key problem in this case.

*Classification*
Competency Category: Nursing Practice: Health and Wellness
Taxonomic Level: Application

**114. D.** Dystonia.

*Rationale*
Dystonia is an extrapyramidal side effect of high-potency typical antipsychotics. It is marked by muscle contractions and twisting or jerking movements, especially of the neck, mouth, and tongue. Dystonia typically occurs early in drug therapy. Tardive dyskinesia is marked by repetitive, involuntary movements and is caused by prolonged use of typical antipsychotic medications. Akathisia involves pacing and restless movements, and negative symptoms are characterized by apathy, withdrawal, and poverty of expression.

*Classification*
Competency Category: Nursing Practice: Alterations in Health
Taxonomic Level: Knowledge/Comprehension

**115. B.** Explore the meaning of the traumatic event with Amy, asking, "What happened, and what has changed?"

*Rationale*
A client who has experienced trauma needs encouragement to examine and understand the meaning of the traumatic event and consequent losses. Without this critical examination, symptoms may worsen, and

the client may become depressed or anxious or engage in self-destructive behaviours such as substance abuse. Without this exploration of meaning, the client will not heal, no matter how much time passes. Behavioural techniques, such as sleep and nutrition management, may be helpful, and a physician may even prescribe sleeping medication. However, the most immediate intervention for the nurse is to assess the client's understanding of the event and encourage this dialogue. Specific diet and sleep medications would only be indicated if sleep and diet were problematic for the client and her recovery.

*Classification*
Competency Category: Nurse–Person Relationship
Taxonomic Level: Knowledge/Application

**116. D.** Ataxia.

*Rationale*
Benzodiazepines have dose-related adverse reactions, including ataxia, dysrhythmia, headache, weakness, dizziness, drowsiness, tremor, nystagmus, a glassy-eyed appearance, vertigo, and syncope. As therapy continues, these dose-related reactions diminish, which is why nurses should instruct their clients to avoid driving or using heavy equipment when clients are first prescribed these medications or the medications are increased in dose.

Although hepatomegaly may occur with benzodiazepine use, it is a rare adverse reaction rather than a dose-related reaction. Idiosyncratic reactions (e.g., rash) to benzodiazepine use may also occur, but they are not typically dose related. Blood dyscrasia is an adverse reaction of some novel antipsychotics.

*Classification*
Competency Category: Nursing Practice: Alterations in Health
Taxonomic Level: Cognitive/Knowledge

**117. A.** Setting consistent limits on this hair-brushing ritual because it is harmful to Dean.

*Rationale*
As with all interventions, client safety is the paramount concern and must be maintained. Setting consistent limits on any potentially harmful ritualistic behaviour must take highest priority. Although the other options are important, they are not the highest priority. When a client like Dean has ritualistic behaviours that interfere with daily activities, the condition will have an impact on his motivation for addressing his coping behaviours. Exploring the purpose of the ritualistic behaviour helps the client see this behaviour as an attempt to control anxiety. As Dean learns new ways to manage anxiety over the longer term, the ritualistic behaviour is likely to decrease.

*Classification*
Competency Category: Nursing Practice: Health and Wellness
Taxonomic Level: Critical Thinking

**118. A.** Increased heart rate.

*Rationale*
Responses to stress that are produced by the sympathetic nervous system impacting the cardiovascular system include increased heart rate, cardiac output, and blood pressure as well as peripheral vasoconstriction. Syncope is a response to parasympathetic stimulation.

*Classification*
Competency Category: Nursing Practice: Alterations in Health
Taxonomic Level: Application

**119. D.** Panic disorder.

*Rationale*
When people feel so anxious that they fear having a heart attack or losing their mind, they are most likely having a panic attack associated with panic disorder. People with social phobia, generalized anxiety disorder, and dissociative disorders are all likely to have anxiety symptoms associated with those conditions but are less likely to experience panic symptoms.

*Classification*
Competency Category: Nursing Practice: Alterations in Health
Taxonomic Level: Critical Thinking

**120. C.** Agoraphobia.

*Rationale*
The fear of being in places that are difficult and embarrassing to leave is known as agoraphobia. Social phobia is a fear of social performance. Generalized anxiety disorder is marked by anxiety symptoms that are persistent and out of proportion to the stimulus. Panic disorder involves recurrent, unexpected, and severe symptoms of panic.

*Classification*
Competency Category: Nursing Practice: Health and Wellness
Taxonomic Level: Critical Thinking

**121. D.** Social phobia.

*Rationale*
The dread of social situations and overwhelming fear of being scrutinized and embarrassed in public is known as social phobia. Generalized anxiety disorder involves anxiety that is persistent and out of proportion to the stimulus. Panic disorder involves the acute and severe experience of anxiety in the form of panic attacks. Agoraphobia is a specific phobia related to being unable to leave a space.

*Classification*
Competency Category: Nursing Practice: Alterations in Health
Taxonomic Level: Critical Thinking

**122. B.** Control.

*Rationale*
During panic attacks, clients often fear a loss of control, that they are losing control of their minds and bodies so that they feel sensations of being trapped or extremely frightened about their situations. Forgetfulness and confusion and the fears surrounding those experiences are more often experienced by people who are concerned with a loss of memory. People who fear a loss of youth often experience narcissism or self-consciousness about their appearance. People who experience depersonalization or nihilistic beliefs may experience a loss of identity.

*Classification*
Competency Category: Nurse–Person Relationship
Taxonomic Level: Application

**123. C.** Aversion therapy.

*Rationale*
This is an example of aversion therapy, in which a painful stimulus is applied to create an aversion to an obsession (in this case, Ivan's obsession with his body hair). Systematic desensitization is a systematic, slow process of exposing a client to the object of his or her unwarranted fear. Thought stopping is a technique of having an intense distraction stimulus to assist a client in stopping a repeated and disturbing thought. Response prevention is a technique of using distraction or redirection to prevent a compulsive behaviour.

*Classification*
Competency Category: Nursing Practice: Alterations in Health
Taxonomic Level: Application

**124. A.** Aggressor.

*Rationale*
Stuart is taking the role of the aggressor in the group, challenging co-patients (often to distract from his own concerns) or challenging the facilitator. The role as aggressor takes that challenging role into the aggressive realm without regard for the sensitivities of the group or needs of the facilitator's pacing. A monopoliser in a group takes over the conversation with his or her own concerns and needs. A facilitator facilitates the group's progress. A harmonizer seeks balance and harmony (at all costs) in a group.

*Classification*
Competency Category: Nurse–Person Relationship
Taxonomic Level: Knowledge/Comprehension

**125. D.** Supporting suicide precautions and safety measures for Stephanie on the unit.

*Rationale*
Although all the other aspects of forming a helping relationship and successful therapy on the unit are important, the priority nursing approach is supporting safety and suicide precautions. Supporting Stephanie's involvement in group therapy will be more important later on in the treatment, as will challenging and appropriate self-disclosure.

*Classification*
Competency Category: Nurse–Person Relationship
Taxonomic Level: Knowledge/Application

**126. C.** Introjection.

*Rationale*
It is most likely that Stephanie has adopted the defence mechanism of introjection because of her parents' belief that anger should not be expressed outwardly. She may also be somatising, as evidenced by the increase in blood pressure in emotionally charged scenarios and her fight-or-flight response. Projection is the attribution of one's own thoughts onto another person, and displacement is the discharge of negative feelings onto the other person. Assumptions are not a defence mechanism but rather a pattern of cognition.

*Classification*
Competency Category: Nurse–Person Relationship
Taxonomic Level: Critical Thinking

**127. C.** Affect.

*Rationale*
Affect is the term for a person's emotional expression and the manner in which a person talks about his or

her experiences. Blocking is the interruption of thoughts. Feelings are a person's emotional states or perceptions, and moods are prolonged emotional states expressed by affect. Knowledge of correct terminology for documentation is imperative for professional mental health practice.

*Classification*
Competency Category: Professional Practice
Taxonomic Level: Knowledge/Application

**128. B.** "You seem really upset by this situation."

*Rationale*
Hearing her son's diagnosis has led Matthew's mother to express her emotions and project blame. Acknowledging her feelings would build further trust and encourage her to discuss her thoughts and feelings. Asking her to pinpoint blame or denying her feelings will not build the helping relationship during this time of perceived distress.

*Classification*
Competency Category: Nurse–Person Relationship
Taxonomic Level: Application

**129. C.** Having poor boundaries.

*Rationale*
Although Jules has dismissed the actual needs of these clients when they were in his care, his behaviour is an example of poor boundaries or the failure to differentiate between the needs of oneself and others in his professional role. Poor boundaries are often a symptom of passive–aggressive and antisocial traits, but these behaviours are indicative of Jules' failure to distinguish between himself and his clients in order to stand by his professional obligations and the needs of his clients.

*Classification*
Competency Category: Nursing Practice: Professional Practice
Taxonomic Level: Application

**130. B.** Report your concerns to Jules' manager with a request that the provincial nursing association investigate his practice.

*Rationale*
The correct lines of communication must be followed in addressing professional practice concerns. The first line of communication is to directly communicate your concerns to the person. If this has been attempted or is not possible, then the manager or direct supervisor should be called upon for problem solving and decision making. In this case, because patient safety is of paramount concern, the professional association must be notified to review Jules' professional practice in a larger investigation.

*Classification*
Competency Category: Professional Practice
Taxonomic Level: Critical Thinking

**131. B.** Remind the client frequently where her room is.

*Rationale*
It is the nurse's role to assess the client's confusion and to reorient her to her room. Asking co-patients to reorient the client would not be appropriate. A wristband would not necessarily build the helping relationship or assist in orientation. Placing personal items at the bedside may not assist the client in finding her way.

*Classification*
Competency Category: Nursing Practice: Health and Wellness
Taxonomic Level: Knowledge/Application

**132. C.** Practicing as legislated by provincial and territorial scope of practice documents.

*Rationale*
The Health Professions Acts at the provincial and territorial level outline the scope of practice for mental health and other nursing decisions and actions. These are the legal frameworks for practice and must be followed. The nursing Code of Ethics also describes the requirement to follow the competencies and scope outlined by the provincial and territorial governments and within the employment site.

*Classification*
Competency Category: Professional Practice
Taxonomic Level: Knowledge/Comprehension

**133. D.** "What were you feeling and experiencing before you hurt yourself?"

*Rationale*
When clients are unable to express their feelings related to experiences, they may engage in self-destructive behaviours such as self-mutilation. The best nursing responses to self-mutilating behaviours are ones that encourage clients to express themselves in a more adaptive and functional manner. All the other responses are judgemental and fail to acknowledge the client's problem communicating her feelings.

*Classification*
Competency Category: Nurse–Person Relationship
Taxonomic Level: Application

**134. D.** Reflecting.

*Rationale*
Reflecting is the correct response because the nurse's response is referring back feelings for the client to explore at more depth. Mirroring is when the nurse mirrors behaviour for the client to see as feedback. Restating is simply stating back what the client said, and reframing is feeding back to the client an alternative way of looking at the client's statement.

*Classification*
Competency Category: Nurse–Person Relationship
Taxonomic Level: Application

**135. B.** "Your breaks are designated at particular times that we all have to follow. Let's think about what can see you through to that time."

*Rationale*
Consistency of approach is essential when working with clients with personality disorder traits. "Special exceptions" reinforce their antisocial traits and manipulation. It is best to be specific and look to alternatives rather than dismiss the request altogether or provide judgemental responses such as in answer C.

*Classification*
Competency Category: Nursing Practice: Health and Wellness
Taxonomic Level: Critical Thinking

**136. B.** Self-acceptance.

*Rationale*
Self-acceptance is a generally accepted criterion for mental health and is the foundation for healthy relationships with others. Freedom from anxiety is not necessarily an indicator of mental health because anxiety serves as a motivator and influences personal growth and learning. Self-control and direction, rather than the control of others, is an indicator of mental health. Happiness, although desirable, is not an indication of mental health because at times of loss and crisis, unhappiness is a mentally healthy response.

*Classification*
Competency Category: Nursing Practice: Health and Wellness
Taxonomic Level: Cognitive/Knowledge

**137. D.** Focusing.

*Rationale*
By focusing, the nurse can take a series of concerns and help the client begin to discuss a specific issue rather than becoming overwhelmed by all the interconnected difficulties. In this statement, the nurse did not seek to explore the situation further, make any observations, or restate the client's concerns.

*Classification*
Competency Category: Nurse–Person Relationship
Taxonomic Level: Application

**138. B.** Allowing space for response and an expression of patience.

*Rationale*
Silence is an expression of patience and acceptance of the client's process. It is not an expression of intolerance, an effort to challenge the client, or a request that the client take the lead. It is one of the most challenging but important therapeutic techniques for nurses to learn.

*Classification*
Competency Category: Nurse–Person Relationship
Taxonomic Level: Application

**139. C.** Displacement.

*Rationale*
Darren is demonstrating displacement, the discharge of feelings from one area into another area that is considered safe (i.e., anger about work and his car toward others at home). Projection is an act of attributing one's emotions to or blaming them on others. Regression is the mechanism of acting and behaving in a manner previously used and acceptable in another time and developmental stage.

*Classification*
Competency Category: Nursing Practice: Alterations in Health
Taxonomic Level: Critical Thinking

**140. C.** Ability to think abstractly.

*Rationale*
Abstract thinking is the ability to interpret meaning. Asking a client to interpret a proverb is one technique for inquiring about abstract thinking. Abstract thought is a higher level of thought than concrete thinking. Rational thinking involves logic, sequence, and making judgements. Memory and judgement are not assessed through proverbs but through questions about past activities (memory) and ethical decisions (judgement).

*Classification*
Competency Category: Nursing Practice: Alterations in Health
Taxonomic Level: Knowledge/Application

**141. B.** Providing education about relationships in a high school's sexual health class.

*Rationale*
Preventing psychiatric and mental health problems is an example of primary prevention. Education on relationship and sexual health is primary prevention. The others are examples of secondary and tertiary prevention.

*Classification*
Competency Category: Nursing Practice: Health and Wellness
Taxonomic Level: Critical Thinking

**142. D.** A man who threatens to kill his wife.

*Rationale*
The criteria for involuntary admission include dangerousness to oneself or others, unwillingness to seek treatment, and serious and acute mental illness. The man threatening to kill is wife meets these criteria, but the person who has suicidal thoughts and is seeking admission does not. A patient with delusions who is unable to work may live a safe and productive life without hospitalization. A neglectful parent should seek social services support and be reported but does not meet the criteria for an involuntary admission.

*Classification*
Competency Category: Professional Practice
Taxonomic Level: Cognitive/Knowledge

**143. B.** Observe how the client and the client's family interact with each other and with other staff members.

*Rationale*
Assessing a client's interactions with others is a helpful way to determine the client's usual behavioural patterns. This may also help a nurse determine what a behaviour means to a client. Reading and consulting others about a cultural behavioural pattern is only useful in assisting an understanding of an individual client after a nurse has had an opportunity to assess and observe the client directly. The nurse has to be able to assess and care for the client as an individual as well as a member of a cultural community.

*Classification*
Competency Category: Nurse–Person Relationship
Taxonomic Level: Application

**144. C.** Lithium carbonate (Lithane).

*Rationale*
The doses of lithium (an antimania drug) are individualized based on a standardized safe level of 0.6 to 1.2 mEq/L.

*Classification*
Competency Category: Nursing Practice: Alterations in Health
Taxonomic Level: Cognitive/Knowledge

**145. D.** A crisis caused by traumatic stress.

*Rationale*
Traumatic stress can create symptoms such as an inability to sleep, eat, or work. People experiencing extreme and traumatic events may experience nonpathologic psychological pain that can be disabling. The event illustrates a person in crisis and is not the cause of usual life transitions, a usual grief response, or an anxiety episode.

*Classification*
Competency Category: Nursing Practice: Alterations in Health
Taxonomic Level: Critical Thinking

**146. C.** Increased anxiety.

*Rationale*
A compulsion is a ritualized behaviour that serves to neutralize or minimise the experience of anxiety in response to a certain obsession. When a client attempts to resist those rituals, he or she client can be expected to experience increased anxiety. A client with OCD may feel increased depression and fear and a decreased sense of self-worth; however, these are not necessarily responses to resisting the compulsions.

*Classification*
Competency Category: Nursing Practice: Alterations in Health
Taxonomic Level: Critical Thinking

**147. B.** Hyperactive bowel sounds.

*Rationale*
The parasympathetic nervous system would produce increased gastrointestinal motility, leading to hyperactive bowel sounds and possibly diarrhea. All of the other symptoms result from sympathetic nervous system stimulation.

*Classification*
Competency Category: Nursing Practice: Alterations in Health
Taxonomic Level: Cognitive/Knowledge

**148. C.** 6 months.

*Rationale*
The diagnostic criteria from the *Diagnostic and Statistical Manual of Mental Disorders* for generalized anxiety

disorder include excessive worry and anxiety over two or more circumstances for at least 6 months.

*Classification*
Competency Category: Nursing Practice: Alterations in Health
Taxonomic Level: Cognitive/Knowledge

**149. D.** "While you are starting this new treatment, what concerns or questions do you have, Monica?"

*Rationale*
Asking a question opening the therapeutic conversation to dialogue and the concerns of the patient is the best response in this case. Monica has anxiety, and placating her or dismissing the potential anxiety over starting a new treatment would be counterproductive and would cause more worry for her.

*Classification*
Competency Category: Nurse–Person Relationship
Taxonomic Level: Application

**150. C.** Maintaining a firm but nonthreatening manner.

*Rationale*
Maintaining a firm but nonthreatening approach is important when working with a client in a manic and agitated state. Because Shirley cannot control her extreme behaviour at this time, confronting and challenging her or asking her to address the practical matters would not be productive. Asking open-ended and insight-oriented questions is also not productive when clients are in a manic state; rather, managing a calm environment, providing short and direct questions, and providing feedback is the approach a nurse should take with the client at this time.

*Classification*
Competency Category: Nurse–Person Relationship
Taxonomic Level: Application

**151. C.** "This must be a very difficult time for you."

*Rationale*
Allowing the client to express his feelings without judgement is important. This response allows the client to have that expression and acknowledges the difficulties of his current state of mind. The other comments either make judgements or may make the client defensive or intellectualize the feeling state.

*Classification*
Competency Category: Nurse–Person Relationship
Taxonomic Level: Affective/Knowledge

**152. D.** Ambivalence.

*Rationale*
The struggle between self-survival and self-destruction sets up an inherent ambivalence in clients who are suicidal. Often these doubts are expressed by clients who attempt suicide and later attempt to get rescued or saved. Anger and remorse may be present in people who experience depression but are not universally present in those with suicidal ideation. Similarly, individuals with psychosis may or may not experience suicidal ideation.

*Classification*
Competency Category: Nursing Practice: Alterations in Health
Taxonomic Level: Affective/Knowledge

**153. B.** "To protect the confidentiality of our clients, we cannot give you information about whether your relative is receiving treatment here."

*Rationale*
Clients have the right to have their confidentiality respected. Both answers A and B do not breech confidentiality, but answer B is more respectful and diplomatic about the place of confidentiality in the hospital.

*Classification*
Competency Category: Professional Practice
Taxonomic Level: Critical Thinking

**154. A.** "I will need to share information that is relevant and important to your treatment to the health care team."

*Rationale*
Anything that impacts the care and treatment of the client must be shared with the team, and the client should be made aware of this practice. The nurse should not promise to hold information in confidence because this signifies a blurred professional boundary. The nurse should also not discourage the client from sharing information or working with the team approach to her recovery.

*Classification*
Competency Category: Nurse–Person Relationship
Taxonomic Level: Knowledge/Application

**155. B.** Posttraumatic stress disorder (PTSD).

*Rationale*
Katia's memories of the traumatic incident, current nightmares, and fears are all hallmark signs of PTSD. She does not demonstrate the impulsivity and

extreme behaviours indicative of borderline personality disorder or the delusional thinking associated with delusional disorder. Although she does describe fears, they are associated with a trauma, which indicates a diagnosis of PTSD rather than generalized anxiety disorder.

*Classification*
Competency Category: Nursing Practice: Alterations in Health
Taxonomic Level: Critical Thinking

**156. D.** A low tolerance for frustration.

*Rationale*
Emotional immaturity, a low tolerance for frustration, and impulsivity are traits common to clients with antisocial personality disorder. Clients with antisocial personality disorder typically have difficulties maintaining personal and work relationships and have little expression of guilt, shame, or remorse for behaviours, believing that others are to blame for the consequences of their maladaptive behaviours.

*Classification*
Competency Category: Nursing Practice: Alterations in Health
Taxonomic Level: Cognitive/Knowledge

**157. B.** Excessive fearfulness, thumb sucking, and withdrawal from peers in play settings.

*Rationale*
Regression is a common symptom of 6- to 8-year-old children who are victims of sexual abuse. Some symptoms of regression in children this age include thumb sucking, shyness with peers, fears, clinging to adults, sexual acting out, and possibly running away.

*Classification*
Competency Category: Nursing Practice: Alterations in Health
Taxonomic Level: Critical Thinking

**158. D.** Ashleigh is experiencing dissociation as a defence mechanism to cope with the attack.

*Rationale*
When a client strips an event of its emotional significant, the client is using dissociation as a defence mechanism to cope with the intensity of the event and feelings. Dissociation is common in victims of violent events such as rape.

*Classification*
Competency Category: Nursing Practice: Alterations in Health
Taxonomic Level: Critical Thinking

**159. A.** Assist Ashleigh with crisis interventions.

*Rationale*
A rape or assault of any kind is a crisis situation, and the primary nursing focus should be crisis intervention. Providing support and comfort and appreciating the recovery period are important, but the priority should be crisis management. Prevention strategies and teaching would not be appropriate at this time because they would impart to Ashleigh that she should have prevented this situation. At this time, she needs to recover from the crisis response.

*Classification*
Competency Category: Nursing Practice: Health and Wellness
Taxonomic Level: Critical Thinking

**160. D.** Ashleigh resumes her course work and campus activities.

*Rationale*
The goal of crisis intervention is to support clients to resume pre-crisis levels of functioning. Resuming activities and schoolwork in time would indicate Ashleigh's successful adjustment after her crisis experience.

*Classification*
Competency Category: Nursing Practice: Health and Wellness
Taxonomic Level: Critical Thinking

**161. B.** Sexual abuse.

*Rationale*
The assessment findings of sexual behaviour, suicide attempt, and running away from home are indicators of possible sexual abuse. Assessment of neglect, sexually transmitted diseases, and pregnancy are all important but are secondary to the urgent assessment of possible sexual abuse.

*Classification*
Competency Category: Nursing Practice: Health and Wellness
Taxonomic Level: Application

**162. A.** "I will not share information with your family or friends without your permission. I will, however, need to share information that relates to your reason for being here with other staff who work with you."

*Rationale*
It is a professional responsibility for Grant to work collaboratively with the mental health team in caring

for his clients. It is important to the therapeutic responsibility that Grant informs Danielle about the professional boundaries and ways her care is planned collaboratively while maintaining confidentiality.

*Classification*
Competency Category: Professional Practice
Taxonomic Level: Knowledge/Application

**163. C.** Fluphenazine decanoate (Prolixin decanoate).

*Rationale*
A long-acting injectable depot medication will be a likely choice because it can be administered every 1 to 4 weeks, which may assist in concerns about Dave not taking his medication while in the community. It is considered a relapse prevention strategy for such clients.

*Classification*
Competency Category: Nursing Practice: Health and Wellness
Taxonomic Level: Critical Thinking

**164. D.** "I feel driven to wash my hands, although I don't like doing it."

*Rationale*
When caring for clients with OCD, it is important to understand that their compulsive behaviours are not wilful or enjoyable. In most cases, the compulsions and behaviours are a ritualized outlet for the inordinate anxiety and obsessive thoughts they experience. The drive is overwhelming, and the behaviours are necessary to relieve anxiety. Planning for care and interventions needs to take into account this anxiety relieving and the disdain the client experiences as important aspects of the ritual behaviours.

*Classification*
Competency Category: Nursing Practice: Alterations in Health
Taxonomic Level: Critical Thinking

**165. B.** Focus attention on the client as a person rather than on the symptom.

*Rationale*
Through focusing on themselves rather than on their symptoms, clients with somatoform disorder may gain abilities to directly understand and act on their emotions. Assertiveness and small goal attainment are important techniques in developing great self-awareness and self-esteem. Linking to past traumas is rarely helpful. Emphasis on here-and-now functioning is paramount in gaining self-esteem and mastery and managing somatoform illness.

*Classification*
Competency Category: Nursing Practice: Alterations in Health
Taxonomic Level: Application

**166. D.** Hypochondriasis.

*Rationale*
Annette is experiencing a persistent conviction that she has a serious disease despite medical evidence to the contrary. Her persistence is based on bodily sensations and symptoms that are misinterpreted. The pattern whereby she has no secondary gain and is distressed by the situation is consistent with hypochondriasis. Conversion disorder includes neurologic symptoms and impacts a certain body part or sensation. Dysthymia is a consistent low mood with some symptoms of depression lasting more than 2 years. Antisocial personality disorder is characterized by a long-standing pattern of disregard for the needs and rights of others, lack of remorse and empathy, and impulsivity.

*Classification*
Competency Category: Alterations in Health
Taxonomic Level: Knowledge/Comprehension

**167. C.** Dissociative disorders involve stress-related disruptions of memory, consciousness, or identity. Somatoform disorders involve expression of psychological stress via somatic symptoms.

*Rationale*
Precipitating factors in each can be stress, anxiety, and traumatic events. Symptoms are very different in each disorder. Dissociative disorders symptoms include; loss of memory, loss or altered conciousness and an altered sense of identity. Somatoform illness symptoms are physical illness symptoms that have a psychological rather than physiologic base.

*Classification*
Competency Category: Nursing Practice: Alterations in Health
Taxonomic Level: Cognitive/Knowledge

**168. A.** Psychological model.

*Rationale*
Psychological models or factors of eating disorders consider the impact of self-esteem, identity, role development, and fears concerning adulthood and sexuality development. Family models emphasize the mother–daughter and parental relationships, family boundaries, and concerns about control and release within families. Biological theories emphasise that eating disorders tend to run in families and that

neurochemical factors have been linked to eating disorders. Social models are concerned with the societal expectations of appearance.

*Classification*
Competency Category: Nursing Practice: Alterations in Health
Taxonomic Level: Critical Thinking

**169. B.** Hypokalemia.

*Rationale*
Dehydration and electrolyte imbalances (including hypokalemia, metabolic alkalosis, and hypochloremia) are symptoms and signs of a bulimia in which clients consume abnormally large quantities of food and have compensatory measures to prevent weight gain (e.g., self-induced vomiting, diuretic or laxative use).

*Classification*
Competency Category: Nursing Practice: Alterations in Health
Taxonomic Level: Cognitive/Knowledge

**170. C.** Constipation, anorexia, and sleep disturbance.

*Rationale*
Vegetative signs of depression include signs and symptoms of changes to life-sustaining functioning, including loss of appetite and decreased nutritional intake, disturbances in sleep, loss of sex drive, gross alterations in bowel functioning and urination, and disturbances in memory and concentration.

*Classification*
Competency Category: Nursing Practice: Alterations in Health
Taxonomic Level: Knowledge/Comprehension

**171. A.** Providing frequent small meals and monitoring food and fluid intake.

*Rationale*
When a client is experiencing vegetative signs of depression, sleep and nutrition are altered. Although encouraging and teaching relaxation techniques to promote sleep would be useful, when someone is experiencing vegetative signs, he or she is often not able to get involved in teaching or learning as usual. The best intervention is to provide frequent small meals and to monitor the client's food and fluid intake.

*Classification*
Competency Category: Nursing Practice: Health and Wellness
Taxonomic Level: Application

**172. D.** The client does not give a history of feeling depressed for years.

*Rationale*
Teaching about the distinction between dysthymia and major depression requires that the nurse focus on the duration and intensity of symptoms. With major depression, the duration of symptoms is shorter (at least 2 weeks), and the intensity of symptoms is more severe than in dysthymia (which is diagnosed only when symptoms are present for 2 or more years).

*Classification*
Competency Category: Nursing Practice: Alterations in Health
Taxonomic Level: Application

**173. D.** There is a risk of a serious reaction if she stops the SSRIs and begins the MAOIs.

*Rationale*
Severe interactions and contraindications occur when clients taking SSRIs begin MAOI intervention. There is a 5-week "washout" period required for clients switching from SSRIs to MAOIs. For clients switching from an MAOI to an SSRI, the "washout" period is 2 weeks. This must be the first point of teaching. The client was formerly taking MAOIs, so although there would need to be teaching about the dietary restrictions (tyramine) and the potential for hypertensive crisis, the first point of teaching should be about the risk of a drug reaction if she immediately switches from the SSRI to the MAOI.

*Classification*
Competency Category: Nursing Practice: Health and Wellness
Taxonomic Level: Knowledge/Application

**174. C.** Poor judgement and hyperactivity.

*Rationale*
Symptoms of poor judgement (i.e., directing traffic, making obscene gestures at cars) and hyperactivity (i.e., not sleeping and reporting to being "too busy") are assessment findings in this scenario that relate to the characteristics of mania. Increased muscle tension and anxiety are symptoms of anxiety-type disorders, and vegetative signs and poor grooming would be notable in major depressive episodes. Although affective lability, disinhibition, and elevated mood can be assessed in the manic phase of bipolar disorder, these symptoms are not described in this scenario.

*Classification*
Competency Category: Nursing Practice: Alterations in Health
Taxonomic Level: Cognitive/Knowledge

**175. B.** Expansive and grandiose.

*Rationale*
Erica is demonstrating an expansive and grandiose mood state. Although she also exhibits aspects of belligerence, she does not have a blunted affect. She is not demonstrating anxious or unpredictable behaviour that would be consistent with a crisis or anxiety situation, nor suspiciousness or paranoia, which would be more consistent with a major thought disorder. Accurate documentation of Erica's mood state is imperative at the time of admission.

*Classification*
Competency Category: Professional Practice
Taxonomic Level: Application

**176. D.** Hyperactivity and ignoring eating and sleeping.

*Rationale*
Safety needs are always the first priority in care planning. A client such as Erica who has not eaten or slept for several days and has been extremely hyperactive may be at risk of exhaustion and malnutrition and the implications of those states. Although thought disorder, expansive mood, and dress are important assessment information, priority interventions must centre on the basic needs listed in answer D.

*Classification*
Competency Category: Nursing Practice: Health and Wellness
Taxonomic Level: Application

**177. B.** Risk for injury.

*Rationale*
Safety needs are always the first priority in care planning. A client who has not eaten or slept for several days and has been extremely hyperactive may be at risk for injury from exhaustion and malnutrition and the implications of those states. A client who is hyperactive is not experiencing fatigue and has an expanded tolerance for activity. A client in this state of mania may feel a heightened sense of power, although hospitalization may create a sense of powerlessness for the client. The priority focus should be on the risk of injury to the client.

*Classification*
Competency Category: Nursing Practice: Health and Wellness
Taxonomic Level: Critical Thinking

**178. A.** Assist Rudy to maintain contact with reality.

*Rationale*
Assisting a client who is experiencing delusions to maintain contact with reality and decelerate a speeded thought process is the priority goal. The longer a client experiences delusions, the more impairment and harm that can result from them (including professional harm or social embarrassment). A priority goal is to orient Rudy to reality. Explaining the irrationality of delusion is not usually productive when someone is in a manic state. In Rudy's case, there are no illusions described. Ignoring or suppressing the symptom is not productive in reestablishing stability.

*Classification*
Competency Category: Nurse–Person Relationship
Taxonomic Level: Application

**179. C.** "Thinking that people want to destroy you must be very frightening."

*Rationale*
It is important to validate the feelings and experience of a person in a delusional state without reinforcing the delusion. Providing this support and acknowledgement assists in building a trusting relationship even when the client is feeling suspicious. Denying the experience or ignoring the feelings would be countertherapeutic and would not assist in establishing trust.

*Classification*
Competency Category: Nurse–Person Relationship
Taxonomic Level: Application

**180. A.** An idea of reference.

*Rationale*
An idea of reference is a false impression that outside events have special meaning for oneself. In Denis' case, the doctors' conversation is assumed by Denis to be about a plot to kill him. A delusion of infidelity is a jealous delusion. An auditory hallucination is a perceptual disturbance (i.e., hearing voices that are not there). Echolalia is the pattern of repeating speech. Correct documentation and terminology are imperative for professional practice and planning safe and effective patient care.

*Classification*
Competency Category: Professional Practice
Taxonomic Level: Knowledge/Comprehension

**181. A.** Neurobiologic–genetic model.

*Rationale*
Although the precise cause of schizophrenia is unknown, it is best explained as an interplay of genetic, biochemical, anatomic, and other factors. The presence of abnormalities that affect neurotransmitters is an important factor. Social support and family problems may occur when there is a lack of information about the disease and the way stress impacts the disease. However, stress and family and developmental situations are not the causes of the illness, and family members who can understand this are much more supportive.

*Classification*
Competency Category: Nursing Practice: Health and Wellness
Taxonomic Level: Critical Thinking

**182. D.** Darting the eyes, tilting the head, and mumbling to oneself.

*Rationale*
Clients who are hallucinating may dart their eyes, present with a blunted affect, move their heads, grimace, or mumble to themselves. Performing rituals and avoiding open spaces would be present in people with some anxiety disorders. Elevated mood, hyperactivity, and distractibility are present in people with mania, and aloofness, haughtiness, and suspicion can be seen in people with paranoid personality disorder. Accurate clinical assessment is essential to care planning for accountable, responsible professional practice.

*Classification*
Competency Category: Professional Practice
Taxonomic Level: Application

**183. C.** Paint-by-number.

*Rationale*
A client who is suspicious will have difficulties and likely become agitated from activities that involve cooperation with other clients (e.g., playing basketball, ping-pong, or cards). A solitary activity with a defined outcome and the potential for the client to come and go to the activity (e.g., a paint-by-number) is most appropriate in this instance.

*Classification*
Competency Category: Nursing Practice: Alterations in Health
Taxonomic Level: Application

**184. A.** Explain all physical care activities in simple, explicit terms as though expecting a response.

*Rationale*
A client in a stuporous state is not in a position to negotiate, discuss, or gather insight. At this stage of a psychotic experience, a client requires clear and simple explanations of all activities. Not speaking much would be confusing and increasing anxiety, but excessive information and stimuli would also not benefit goal-directed activities.

*Classification*
Competency Category: Nurse–Person Relationship
Taxonomic Level: Application

**185. D.** Refusal to eat and drink.

*Rationale*
A client in a stuporous state may refuse to eat or drink, which can interfere with life functioning. Although noncompliance (e.g., with medication), impaired communication, and coping are all important concerns, the priority for nursing care is to assess and intervene if the client refuses to eat and drink. Higher levels of care may be required, and it is a priority for the nurse to assess this state.

*Classification*
Competency Category: Nursing Practice: Health and Wellness
Taxonomic Level: Critical Thinking

**186. C.** "I know Michelle's behaviour seems personal, but it's really not. Clients with borderline disorder act out to relieve anxiety, and I suspect having the pass provoked a great deal of anxiety."

*Rationale*
It will be instructive for the more experienced nurse to share with Jessie the rationale behind Michelle's self-inflicted injuries as a feature of her borderline personality disorder. Understanding professional boundaries is a vital nursing role. Reinforcing an overhelping relationship or boundary blurring would not be professional or instructive, and berating the client and her behaviours would not be professional.

*Classification*
Competency Category: Professional Practice
Taxonomic Level: Application

**187. B.** Related to fear of abandonment brought on by movement toward autonomy and independence (i.e., earning a pass).

*Rationale*
The best explanation is that Michelle is experiencing anxiety and fear related to obtaining the pass and the

independent actions required while she is out of the unit. She does not have an inherited disorder manifesting as an inability to manage stress, and she does not exhibit projective identification. Borderline personality pathology is not a constitutional inability to regulate affect; rather, it consists of maladaptive behaviour patterns that usually present at times of stress or perceived threat (e.g., regarding fears of rejection, abandonment, and failure).

*Classification*
Competency Category: Nursing Practice: Alterations in Health
Taxonomic Level: Knowledge/Comprehension

**188. C.** Paranoid personality disorder.

*Rationale*
A characteristic that fits the clinical picture of paranoid personality disorder is being suspicious and distrustful of others' motives. The corresponding behaviours may include the signs noted in this case study. Clients with schizoid personality disorders tend toward emotional detachment and withdrawal and have little concern for the feelings of others. Clients with obsessive–compulsive personality disorder display a desire for perfection at the expense of others with little flexibility and an overwhelming concern for controlling situations. Clients with antisocial personality disorder display no regard, concern, or empathy for others' rights and needs.

*Classification*
Competency Category: Nursing Practice: Alterations in Health
Taxonomic Level: Knowledge/Comprehension

**189. D.** "Who can be helpful to you during this time?"

*Rationale*
An appropriate question to ask regarding situational support is who can be helpful at this time. Finding out about a client's means of coping with a crisis or situation is key in any interview for planning care and assessing the balancing factors regarding a situation.

*Classification*
Competency Category: Nurse–Person Relationship
Taxonomic Level: Application

**190. D.** Predictable routines and high client autonomy.

*Rationale*
Managing the milieu of an inpatient psychiatric unit is the responsibility of the nursing staff. Clear limits with latitude for individual autonomy is the most supportive atmosphere for managing the mix of clients and the potential for aggression and violence. Rigid structure often creates a venue for resistance among clients, and little structure with minimal routine is confusing and can create anxiety and the potential for violence. Unpredictability and ventilation of anger to staff members are also not productive in managing a calm and supportive milieu free of violence.

*Classification*
Competency Category: Nursing Practice: Health and Wellness
Taxonomic Level: Critical Thinking

**191. A.** Cognitive impairment and medication side effects make compliance with the medication regimen difficult for many clients.

*Rationale*
One important aspect of care planning with clients who have severe and persistent mental illness is that compliance with medication regimens can be very challenging because of many social determinants. The plan of care should work to ameliorate these problems and continually seek to assess and make treatment in the community work. Referral to multiple agencies does not tend to support this nor does solely providing teaching on medications and side effects. Clients and families need to know more about their own signs and symptoms and ways to support each other (i.e., through psychoeducation). Deinstitutionalization has not resulted in greater access to health care in many communities.

*Classification*
Competency Category: Nursing Practice: Health and Wellness
Taxonomic Level: Critical Thinking

**192. B.** Families with a mentally ill member tend to bear increased financial, physical, and emotional stress, which affects family dynamics and often limits the resources available to the client.

*Rationale*
Families with a member who has a severe and persistent mental illness tend to experience great stressors, which often creates less-than-optimal supports to clients who greatly need support. The supportive community mental health system can step in and assist the whole family in this matter. Addressing the individual client's needs is important, but supporting the whole family can better the situation for everyone.

*Classification*
Competency Category: Nurse–Person Relationship
Taxonomic Level: Critical Thinking

**193. C.** Conduct disorder.

*Rationale*
Key signs and symptoms of conduct disorder in children are aggressive behaviour, destruction of property, deceitfulness, theft, and disregard for socially appropriate behaviour and rules. ADHD is characterized by inattention, hyperactivity, and impulsivity, and autism is characterized by social withdrawal and an inability to focus on more than one object.

*Classification*
Competency Category: Nursing Practice: Alterations in Health
Taxonomic Level: Critical Thinking

**194. A.** Being raised by a depressed mother.

*Rationale*
Having a mother with a depressive illness has an impact on the child's health. Regular prenatal care would not place the child at risk. Similarly, harmony in the home and reaching developmental milestones would not place the child at increased risk for developmental or psychiatric disorders.

*Classification*
Competency Category: Nursing Practice: Health and Wellness
Taxonomic Level: Knowledge/Comprehension

**195. D.** Memory disturbance.

*Rationale*
In the case study, John is demonstrating memory disturbance, which is foremost among stage 1 characteristics of Alzheimer's-type dementia. Aphasia, apraxia, and agnosia are particular to people with vascular-type dementia and stroke.

*Classification*
Competency Category: Nursing Practice: Alterations in Health
Taxonomic Level: Cognitive/Knowledge

**196. A.** Restricting the client's privileges until she gains 3 lb.

*Rationale*
Behaviour modification approaches involve creating positive and negative consequences for desirable and undesirable behaviour. The benefit of gaining weight in this case will mean the adding of privileges.

*Classification*
Competency Category: Nursing Practice: Health and Wellness
Taxonomic Level: Application

**197. D.** Evidence of high suicide potential.

*Rationale*
This elderly man has many of the characteristic risk factors for suicide, including older age, male gender, losses, chronic health problems, financial worries, and mentioning of his suicidal thoughts. The nurse must use appropriate screening tools in clients with depression and a suicide risk.

*Classification*
Competency Category: Nursing Practice: Health and Wellness
Taxonomic Level: Critical Thinking

**198. A.** Orthostatic hypotension and urinary retention.

*Rationale*
Orthostatic hypotension and urinary retention are common side effects of TCAs. Photosensitivity, skin rashes, and pseudoparkinsonism and tardive dyskinesia are common side effects of older antipsychotics, and diarrhea and electrolyte imbalances are side effects of lithium.

*Classification*
Competency Category: Nursing Practice: Health and Wellness
Taxonomic Level: Knowledge/Comprehension

**199. C.** With early-stage Alzheimer's disease

*Rationale*
Aricept is used to manage some of the early symptoms of Alzheimer's disease. It is not a cure; rather, it is a treatment that is known to slow the progress of the disease and manage some symptoms.

*Classification*
Competency Category: Nursing Practice: Alterations in Health
Taxonomic Level: Knowledge/Comprehension

**200. C.** Information giver.

*Rationale*
In this case, Zane is giving information freely to co-patients. A harmonizer seeks harmony in group conflict. An evaluator sums up the findings and discussion. A procedural technician keeps the activities on task, manages time, and so on.

*Classification*
Competency Category: Nurse–Person Relationship
Taxonomic Level: Critical Thinking

**201. Answer:** Dissociative identity disorder.

*Rationale*
The sense of not feeling human is a classic symptom in cases of dissociative identity disorder.

*Classification*
Competency Category: Nursing Practice: Alterations in Health
Taxonomic Level: Knowledge/Comprehension

**202. Answer:** Conversion disorder.

*Rationale*
In conversion disorder, the individual has one or more clinical manifestations that suggest a neurologic or medical disorder. Psychological stressors (in this case, the performance appraisal) contribute to the clinical manifestation, and indifference to the condition is characteristically exhibited.

*Classification*
Competency Category: Nursing Practice: Alterations in Health
Taxonomic Level: Critical Thinking

**203. Answer:** Attention-seeking behaviour and secondary gain.

*Rationale*
Attention-seeking behaviour and secondary gain are key diagnostic criteria for malingering.

*Classification*
Competency Category: Nursing Practice: Alterations in Health
Taxonomic Level: Application

**204. Answers:**

- Henri will experience no physical harm to himself.
- Henri will set realistic goals for himself and the future.
- Henri will express optimism and hope for the future.
- Henri will openly discuss his concerns and experiences with the nurse.
- Henri will develop insight into his illness.
- Henri will understand strategies to help him manage his symptoms.

*Rationale*
These are the priority outcomes for a client who is depressed and experiencing suicidal ideation.

*Classification*
Competency Category: Nursing Practice: Health and Wellness
Taxonomic Level: Critical Thinking

**205. Answer:** Within 2 weeks of taking disulfiram, a client who ingests alcohol may experience any of the following: headache, chest pain, diaphoresis or sweating, tachycardia, vomiting, facial flushing, red eyes, shortness of breath, hypotension, and fainting.

*Rationale*
These are the key symptoms of alcohol intake while taking disulfiram.

*Classification*
Competency Category: Nursing Practice: Health and Wellness
Taxonomic Level: Application

**206. Answer:** 0.5 mL.

*Rationale*
0.5 mL should be administered per the formula 2.5 mL/5 mL × 1 mL.

*Classification*
Competency Category: Nursing Practice: Professional Practice
Taxonomic Level: Critical Thinking

**207. Answers:**

a. explain the nature of one's problems or situation.
b. make appropriate choices and behave in an appropriate manner.

*Rationale*
Insight is the ability to explain the nature of one's problems or situation. It is more than knowing one's diagnosis because a client may know his diagnosis but not have an understanding of its impact on his situation and current problems. Judgement is the ability to make appropriate choices and behave in an appropriate manner.

*Classification*
Competency Category: Nursing Practice: Professional Practice
Taxonomic Level: Knowledge/Comprehension

**208. Answers:**

- What would you do if you were in a movie theatre and someone yelled "Fire!"?

- What would you do if you found an addressed and stamped letter lying on the ground?
- What would you do if you found a wallet with $100 in it while you were on the bus?

*Rationale*
Any hypothetical ethical situation posed as a question can invite assessment of judgment.

*Classification*
Competency Category: Nurse–Person Relationship
Taxonomic Level: Application

**209. Answer:** The best approach would be to report the incident to the nurse supervisor and ensure that John is not assigned any clients. He cannot work the shift.

*Rationale*
It is important that the nurse immediately reports unsafe practice of nursing colleagues to the appropriate authority. It is important that John is not allowed to work the shift.

*Classification*
Competency Category: Professional Practice
Taxonomic Level: Critical Thinking

**210. Answers:** Safe, competent, and ethical care

*Rationale*
This situation fits within the ethical value of safe, competent, and ethical care.

*Classification*
Competency Category: Professional Practice
Taxonomic Level: Critical Thinking

**211. Answers:**

- Inappropriate responses to environmental stimuli.
- Disordered thinking.
- Indifference toward others.
- Lack of intonation and expression in speech.
- Repetitive rocking motions.
- Hand flapping.
- A dislike of changes in routine and daily activities.
- An unusual fascination with inanimate objects.
- A dislike of touching or cuddling.
- No fear of danger.
- Appearance of hearing failure during infancy.

- Regression at age 2 years after seemingly normal development.
- Impaired language development appearance of hearing failure during infancy.

*Rationale*
Autism is typically diagnosed by age 3 years and occurs in 10 to 12 of every 10,000 children. Its hallmark signs are listed above.

*Classification*
Competency Category: Nursing Practice: Alterations in Health
Taxonomic Level: Application

**212. Answers:**

- Assertiveness training.
- Aversion therapy.
- Flooding.
- Desensitization.
- Positive conditioning.
- Response prevention.
- Thought stopping.
- Thought switching.
- Token economy.

*Rationale*
Many types of behaviour therapy exist. Any of the above therapies may be used when a behavioural therapy approach is required. Behaviour therapies are often used to assist individuals in changing behaviours that do not support good mental health and coping skills.

*Classification*
Competency Category: Nursing Practice: Health and Wellness
Taxonomic Level: Application

**213. Answers:**

- Provide emotional support and assist the client in setting realistic goals.
- Provide for the client's dietary needs.
- Assist the client in reestablishing sleep habits.
- Establish clear limits for the client.
- Maintain a calm, clear, and self-confident manner.
- Support the client in managing personal hygiene.
- Involve the client in activities that require gross motor movement.

- Maintain a consistent team approach, seeking assistance when necessary for the client's acting-out behaviours.

*Rationale*
Clients in the manic phase of bipolar illness may not focus adequately to maintain adequate nutrition, elimination, sleep, and hygiene to sustain life. These clients may be disruptive to other clients or engage in acting-out behaviours that pose a danger to the client.

*Classification*
Competency Category: Nursing Practice: Health and Wellness
Taxonomic Level: Critical Thinking

**214. Answers:**

These are symptoms of a major depressive episode or clinical depression and include:

- Changes in appetite and eating (weight loss).
- Alterations in sleep.
- Decreased sex drive or libido.
- Decreased concentration.
- Decreased memory.

*Rationale*
Vegetative signs are symptoms of depression that interrupt life-sustaining functioning.

*Classification*
Competency Category: Nursing Practice: Health and Wellness
Taxonomic Level: Critical Thinking

**215. Answer:** Flight of ideas.

*Rationale*
Flight of ideas is a rapid succession of speech in which the client jumps from one topic to another.

*Classification*
Competency Category: Nursing Practice: Alterations in Health
Taxonomic Level: Application

**216. Answers:**

- Can you tell me what time of the day it is?
- What day of the week is it?
- What is the month?
- Can you tell me what year it is?
- Can you tell me who you are and who I am?
- Can you tell me where we are right now?

*Rationale*
Testing orientation involves asking the client the time, date, day, year, month, and location (city, street, hospital, unit).

*Classification*
Competency Category: Nursing Practice: Alterations in Health
Taxonomic Level: Application

**217. Answers:**

- Progressive muscle relaxation and other relaxation therapies.
- Guided imagery.
- Deep breathing.
- Time management skills.
- List making.
- Realistic goal setting.
- Cognitive restructuring.

*Rationale*
Various techniques can help ease anxiety. These approaches help reduce hyperventilation, help the client gain awareness of his or her body sensations, assist the client in focusing on something besides his or her anxiety, and interrupt the flow of negative thoughts.

*Classification*
Competency Category: Nursing Practice: Health and Wellness
Taxonomic Level: Application

**218. Answers:** Level of consciousness, general appearance, behaviours, speech, mood and affect, perceptions, intellectual performance, judgement, insight, thought process, and content are all assessed in the mental status examination. Aspects of the patient interview, such as patient history, medical history, presenting problem, family and social history, and medication and substance use, are also important but are not considered mental status data.

*Rationale*
All of these areas assess the person's overall mental status. All of these areas should be assessed to fully be aware of the client's mental status.

*Classification*
Competency Category: Nursing Practice: Professional Practice
Taxonomic Level: Application

**219. Answers:** Positive symptoms include hallucinations, delusions, illusions, agitation, hostility, bizarre behaviours, and association disturbances (e.g., echolalia, echopraxia, clang associations, illogical or disorganized thinking, neologisms, word salad).

Negative symptoms include avolition, amotivation, anergia, anhedonia, social withdrawal, alogia, ambivalence, affective flattening, restricted emotions, lack of ego boundaries, lack of self care, dependency, and sleep disturbances.

*Rationale*

Positive symptoms indicate a distortion or excess of normal functioning. Negative symptoms indicate a loss or lack of normal functioning; these develop over time and hinder the client's ability to endure life tasks.

*Classification*

Competency Category: Nursing Practice: Alterations in Health

Taxonomic Level: Knowledge/Comprehension

---

## ▶ Self-Analysis for Chapter 7

200 Multiple choice questions × 1 point each = /200 points

+

19 Short answer questions for a total of 50 points = /50 points

*Total Mental Health Nursing review questions = /250 points*

## SUPPLEMENTAL RESOURCES

Boyd, M.A. (2006). *Psychiatric nursing: Contemporary practice* (3rd ed.). Philadelphia: Lippincott Williams & Wilkins.

Canadian Nurses Association. (2002). *Code of ethics for registered nurses*. Ottawa, ON: Author.

Canadian Nurses Association. (2005). *The Canadian registered nurse exam prep guide* (4th ed.). Ottawa, ON: Author.

Hogan, M.A., & Smith, G.B. (2003). *Mental health nursing reviews and rationales*. Upper Saddle River, NJ: Prentice Hall.

Ren Kneisl, C., Skodal Wilson, H., & Trigoboff, E. (2003). *Contemporary psychiatric-mental health nursing*. Upper Saddle River, NJ: Prentice Hall.

Schilling McCann, J.A. (2006). *Straight A's in psychiatric and mental health nursing: A review series*. Philadelphia: Lippincott Williams & Wilkins.

Stein, A.M. (2007). *Nursing review series: Psychiatric nursing*. New York: Thomson Delmar Learning.

Townsend, M.C. (2003). *Instructors guide to accompany psychiatric/mental health nursing: Concepts of care* (4th ed.). Philadelphia: F.A. Davis Company.

Varacrolis, E.M., Benner Carson, V., & Shoemaker, N.C. (2006). *Foundations of psychiatric mental health nursing: A clinical approach* (5th ed.). St. Louis: Saunders Elsevier.

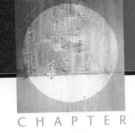

# 8 Comprehensive Practice Exams I & II

**Directions:** The following are two comprehensive practice exams similar in format to the Canadian Registered Nursing Exam (CRNE). These practice exams offer a wide variety of both multiple-choice and short answer questions and are representative of professional practice, adult health, child health, maternal–child health, and mental health nursing. Complete these practice exams as if you were preparing to write the actual CRNE. Schedule approximately 3 hours per practice exam and plan to write these exams in a quiet place where you will not experience interruptions. Focus on using the study tips provided in Chapters 1 and 2 of the this book when completing the practice exam questions. After you have completed these practice exams, compare your answers with the correct ones provided at the end of the chapter.

## COMPREHENSIVE PRACTICE EXAM I

### ▶ Professional Practice Multiple-Choice Questions

1. Carol is an RN working an evening shift on an intake unit of a long-term care facility. She must ask one of the unregulated health care workers (UHCWs) to perform a treatment on a resident. What must the RN ensure before delegating a task to an UHCW?

   A. The worker has practiced the task.
   B. The worker has the appropriate knowledge and skills.
   C. The worker is supervised during the performance of the task.
   D. The worker will be guided through the task by another nurse.

2. Angela, a RN, overhears another RN, John, making plans to meet a hospitalized client "for a drink" the next time the client is released from the unit on evening pass. What should Angela do?

   A. Tell the client that she should not meet the nurse socially.
   B. Report the conversation to the nurse manager of your unit.
   C. Discuss the overheard conversation directly with John.
   D. Encourage the interaction with the client after discharge.

3. Professional regulations and laws that govern nursing practice are in place for which of the following reasons?

   A. To limit the number of nurses in practice.
   B. To ensure that nurses are of good moral standing.
   C. To protect the safety of the public.
   D. To ensure that enough new nurses are available.

*Case Study: Jessica Smith is 20-years-old and has a diagnosis of depression. She is admitted to the mental health unit, where she is encouraged to participate in group sessions and to eat her meals in the common room with other patients. Questions 4 to 6 relate to this scenario.*

4. John Stewart, RN, is assigned to work with Jessica. Jessica asks John if he is married or has a girlfriend. John responds by saying, "I am curious about why you asked this question. However, what is important is how you are feeling today." John's response would be considered which of the following?

   A. Inappropriate; Jessica was just interested in John's personal situation.

B. Inappropriate; John should have answered her to establish a therapeutic relationship.

C. Appropriate because John is neither married nor has a girlfriend.

D. Appropriate because the focus of a therapeutic relationship is on the client.

5. During the night shift, Jessica tells a nurse that she is going to kill herself and is placed on constant observation. When she asks to use the toilet, the nurse follows her into the bathroom. Jessica says, "I don't need you to follow me into the bathroom. Give me some space." Which of the following statements by the nurse would be considered the most appropriate?

A. "You are right; I don't need to come into the bathroom with you. I will wait outside the door."

B. "I must stay with you until we are sure you are not going to hurt yourself."

C. "If you think you are going to be alright, I will check on you in 5 minutes."

D. "I can't imagine that there is anything dangerous in the bathroom, so go ahead, and I will wait for you in the hallway."

6. Jessica is ready to be discharged and states to the nurse: "It would be really good for me if we could meet for coffee if I am feeling depressed again." Which of the following statements indicates that the nurse understands the boundaries of the therapeutic relationship?

A. "That would be okay as long as we go to a public place. Where would you like to meet?"

B. "Before you leave the hospital, I will make sure you have the information about the crisis centre."

C. "We could go to the gym together. Exercise can be very therapeutic for patients experiencing depression."

D. "I often meet with people after they are discharged because it is sometimes difficult to deal with situations after they leave the hospital".

7. Andrew, an RN, is employed by a community nursing service and is scheduled for a daily visit to Mr. H. for a blood pressure check. Andrew is very busy and is running late, so he decides to skip the visit to Mr. H. today. He bases this decision on the rationale that his blood pressure was normal yesterday. This decision would be:

A. Inappropriate; it would be considered neglect of duty.

B. Appropriate; it would be considered a knowledgeable assessment of the client's situation.

C. Inappropriate; it would be considered client abuse.

D. Appropriate; it would be considered an effective way to prioritize his workload for the day.

8. An RN is working night shift with another nurse and notices that the other nurse is charting vital signs that she did not actually take on her patients. What should the nurse observing this situation do first?

A. Discuss the observations with the other nurse.

B. Nothing; it is not the nurse's place to report this behaviour.

C. Notify the union steward representing the nursing employees.

D. Do the vital signs on the patients for the other nurse.

---

***Case Study:*** *Mr. Edwards lives in a long-term care facility and has signed a form to state that he does not want to be resuscitated. During the winter, he develops an upper respiratory infection that progresses to pneumonia. His health has rapidly deteriorated, and he is no longer competent. His family states they want everything possible done for Mr. Edwards. Questions 9 and 10 relate to this scenario.*

9. Which of the following should the nurse anticipate?

A. He should be treated with antibiotics for his pneumonia.

B. He should be resuscitated if he has a respiratory arrest.

C. The wishes of his family will be followed.

D. Pharmacologic intervention should not be initiated.

10. On morning rounds, the nurse finds Mr. Edwards without vital signs. What should the nurse do?

A. Notify the physician that the patient has no vital signs.

B. Begin CPR and call for an ambulance.

C. Call the supervisor for further directions.

D. Go to the desk and review the chart to determine the resuscitation status.

11. Mr. Ralph has been prescribed a narcotic analgesic to be given around the clock for his cancer-related pain. He is competent and has actively been involved in decisions regarding his

care. What should the nurse do when Mr. Ralph refuses his next dose?

A. Try to persuade him to take the medication as ordered by the doctor.

B. Ensure that he understands the rationale for taking the medication as ordered.

C. Ask his wife to hold his hands while you put the pill under his tongue.

D. Document his choice and reassess his pain in 1 hour.

12. A 70-year-old man is admitted to the emergency department unconscious with a ruptured abdominal aortic aneurysm. No family members are present, and the surgeon instructs the staff to take the client directly to the operating room for lifesaving surgery. Which of the following actions should the nurse take regarding informed consent?

A. Take the client to the operating room for surgery without informed consent.

B. Keep the patient in the emergency department until the family has been contacted.

C. Ask the nursing supervisor to contact the hospital lawyer.

D. Contact the hospital chaplain so he can sign the consent on the client's behalf.

13. Linda is a staff nurse who suspects that one of her coworkers is self-administering illegal drugs during work hours. Which of the following is Linda's first priority?

A. Notify the nurse manager and document the situation.

B. Determine if this is a breach of any hospital policy.

C. Report the nurse to the provincial or territorial governing body.

D. Discuss her concerns with one of the doctors.

14. A nurse is caring for a client with a fresh postoperative wound after a femoral–popliteal revascularization procedure. The nurse fails to routinely assess the pedal pulses on the affected leg, and the blood vessel becomes occluded. The nurse is at risk for being accused of which of the following?

A. Malpractice.

B. Negligence.

C. Refusal of treatment.

D. Forgetfulness.

15. A patient on a surgical unit asks a nurse her opinion of her surgeon. The nurse replies, "He is a rude man, and his patients always end up with infections." The nurse is at risk of being accused of which of the following?

A. Libel.

B. Slander.

C. Negligence.

D. Assault.

16. A nurse on a medical unit charts in the patient's medical records: "The doctor was tardy and negligent in his follow-up care." The nurse is at risk of being accused of which of the following?

A. Negligence.

B. Slander.

C. Libel.

D. Ignorance.

17. A nurse reports to a physician that a client receiving a blood transfusion has an increased temperature of 1°C greater than his baseline and is complaining of a headache. The doctor tells the nurse to continue the blood infusion. By following the order, the nurse is at risk of being accused of which of the following?

A. Negligence.

B. Malpractice.

C. Assault.

D. Unethical conduct.

18. Mr. Brown uses a wheelchair. On one occasion, he is unable to call the nurse to assist him to the toilet. He urinates in his wheelchair. His nurse scolds him in front of other residents for his "accident." The nurse has demonstrated which of the following?

A. Verbal abuse.

B. Incompetence.

C. Reinforcement.

D. Negligence.

19. Maureen, a nurse working on a medical unit, is caring for Sally, a client with anemia. Maureen has a part-time business selling vitamins and supplements and approaches Sally, offering to sell her vitamins to help "improve her blood." When another nurse overhears this conversation, he should discuss which of the following with Maureen?

A. How he can also start selling the vitamins and supplements.

B. That Maureen is in a conflict of interest.

C. How impressed he is with the initiative Maureen has taken.

D. The cost of the supplements she is selling.

20. After surgery, the surgeon writes "resume pre-op meds" as an order on a patient's chart. What should the nurse do with this order?

    A. Contact the surgeon for clarification because this is not a complete order.
    B. Transcribe the preoperative medication orders as the surgeon has ordered.
    C. Ask the pharmacist for a list of preoperative medications for the client.
    D. Ask the anaesthetist to clarify the order.

## Professional Practice Short Answer Questions

21. A physician writes an order for insulin on a sliding scale. Which part of the physician's order will lead to a medication error if the order is carried out as written? (1 point)

    Blood glucose 0–8 mmol/L: Give 3 units of regular insulin subcutaneous.

    Blood glucose 9–12 mmol/L: Give 5 units of regular insulin subcutaneous.

    Blood glucose 13–15 mmol/L: Give 8 units of regular insulin subcutaneous.

22. A 50-year-old man is admitted to the emergency department with a suspected forearm fracture. He has multiple tattoos and scars on his forearms, indicating that he could be an IV drug user. The physician orders an HIV test as part of the routine admission blood work. Give three reasons why giving an HIV test based on these observations is inappropriate. (3 points)

23. A nurse is sending laboratory results by fax machine to a physicians' office. The fax ends up going to the wrong address. What should the nurse do in this situation? (1 point)

## Care of Adults and Older Adults Multiple-Choice Questions

24. A 62-year-old male client had drainage of a pelvic abscess secondary to diverticulitis 6 days ago. While drinking water, he begins to cough violently. His daughter runs to the nurse's station, screaming that her father has "exploded." Upon entering the room, the nurse observes that the client's wound has dehisced and a small segment of bowel is protruding. What should the nurse's priority action be?

    A. Ask the client what has occurred, call the physician, have the daughter stay with her father, and cover the area with the bed sheet soaked in water.
    B. Have a nursing assistant hold the incision together while you obtain the vital signs, call the physician, and flex the client's knees.
    C. Obtain vital signs, call the physician, obtain emergency orders, and explain to the daughter exactly what has occurred.
    D. Have the nursing assistant call the physician while you remain with the client, flex the client's knees, and cover the incision with sterile gauze.

25. When monitoring a patient who is at risk for hemorrhage, which assessment data is significant?

    A. Warm, dry skin; hypotension; and bounding pulse.
    B. Hypertension; bounding pulse; and cold, clammy skin.
    C. Weak, thready pulse; hypertension, and warm, dry skin.
    D. Hypotension; cold, clammy skin; and weak, thready pulse.

**Case Study:** *Mrs. Jacob, age 78 years, is admitted to the rehabilitation unit after a cardiovascular accident (CVA). She is bedridden and aphasic. The next morning, the physician orders an indwelling catheter because the client has been incontinent during the night. Questions 26 to 28 relate to this scenario.*

26. Mrs. Jacob's emotional responses to her illness would be most influenced by:

    A. Her past experiences and coping abilities.
    B. Her urinary incontinence.
    C. Her relationship with the health care staff.
    D. Her ability to understand her illness.

27. When supporting Mrs. Jacob to develop independence, the nurse should:

    A. Demonstrate ways she can regain independence in activities.
    B. Reinforce success in tasks accomplished.
    C. Establish long-term goals for the client.
    D. Point out her errors in performance.

28. To ensure optimum nutrition, the nurse may find that Mrs. Jacob needs assistance with eating. To accomplish this, what action should the nurse take?

    A. Encourage her to participate in the feeding process.
    B. Feed Mrs. Jacob to conserve her energy.
    C. Request that her food be pureed.
    D. Have her niece feed her her meals.

29. A nurse is developing care plan for Mrs. Williams, age 54 years, who is experiencing anxiety after the loss of her job. Mrs. Williams is verbalizing her concerns regarding her ability to meet her role expectations and financial obligations. Which nursing diagnosis would be most appropriate for Mrs. Williams?

    A. Altered family process.
    B. Altered thought process.
    C. Potential for improved health.
    D. Ineffective individual coping.

---

**Case Study:** *Mr. Kenn, a 39-year-old man, arrives at the hospital to undergo a total laryngectomy and radical neck dissection. Questions 30 to 33 relate to this scenario.*

30. Mr. Kenn enters the operating room and appears relaxed. Then Mr. Kenn begins talking rapidly, commenting, "I'm really nervous and scared about the operation." What action should the nurse take next?

    A. The client is experiencing anxiety; the nurse should listen attentively and provide realistic verbal reassurance.
    B. The client is experiencing an adverse effect of Meperidine; the nurse should report it to the physician.
    C. The client is typically anxious; the nurse should proceed with the assessment and preparation for surgery.
    D. The client needs additional sedation; the nurse should request an order from the anaesthesiologist.

31. It is Mr. Kenn's first postoperative day. Which of the following is a priority goal?

    A. Communicate by use of esophageal speech.
    B. Improve body image and self-esteem.
    C. Prevent aspiration.
    D. Maintain a patent airway.

32. When preparing to suction Mr. Kenn's tracheostomy, the nurse should be aware that the maximum time frame recommended for intermittent suction is:

    A. 1 to 5 seconds.
    B. 5 to 10 seconds.
    C. 10 to 15 seconds.
    D. 16 to 20 seconds.

33. When performing deep tracheal suctioning for Mr. Kenn, the nurse should:

    A. Be sure the cuff of the tracheostomy is inflated during suctioning.
    B. Instil acetylcysteine (Mucomyst) into the tracheotomy before suctioning to loosen secretions.
    C. Apply negative pressure as the catheter is being inserted.
    D. Preoxygenate the client before suctioning.

34. A client has been immobilized in traction for 3 weeks. Why should the nurse assess for the development of renal calculi?

    A. Urinating in a supine position predisposes a client to urinary retention.
    B. Decreased fluid intake because immobilization impairs osteoblastic activity.
    C. Lack of muscle action and normal tension cause calcium withdrawal from the bone.
    D. Fracture healing requires more calcium and thus increases total calcium metabolism.

35. What is an appropriate nursing action to detect early signs of metabolic complications of total parental nutrition (TPN)?

    A. Assess lung sounds.
    B. Weigh the patient daily.
    C. Monitor urine output.
    D. Monitor vital signs.

36. The nurse should be aware that the patient's serum blood glucose should be maintained below

which level when receiving total parental nutrition?

A. 3 mmol/L.
B. 4.2 mmol/L.
C. 5.5 mmol/L.
D. 8.3 mmol/L.

37. After a laminectomy, a male client has a palpable bladder and complains of lower abdominal discomfort. He is voiding 60 to 80 mL of urine every 4 hours. What is the best nursing intervention?

A. Observe for worsening discomfort.
B. Administer the prescribed analgesic.
C. Obtain an order for urinary catheterization.
D. Reassure the client that this is a normal voiding pattern.

38. A physician orders a low-residue diet for a client with an acute exacerbation of colitis. The nurse would know that the dietary teaching is understood when the client reports that he can eat:

A. Cream soup and crackers, omelettes, mashed potatoes, peas, orange juice, and coffee.
B. Stewed chicken, baked potatoes with butter, strained peas, white bread, plain cake, and milk.
C. Baked fish, macaroni with cheese, strained carrots, fruit gelatine, and milk.
D. Lean roast beef, buttered white rice with egg slices, white bread with butter and jelly, and tea with sugar.

---

**Case Study:** *Mrs. Hillster has a diagnosis of a bowel obstruction. She complains of nausea, is vomiting dark bile material, and has severe cramping and intermittent abdominal pain. This condition is caused by intussusceptions, and surgery is scheduled. Questions 39 to 41 relate to this scenario.*

39. Four days after surgery, Mrs. Hillster has not passed any flatus, and there are no bowel sounds. Even though her abdomen has become more distended, she feels little discomfort. Paralytic ileus is suspected. What causes this condition?

A. Impaired blood supply.
B. Impaired neural functioning.
C. Perforation of the bowel wall.
D. Obstruction of the bowel wall.

40. Mrs. Hillster requires additional surgery, and an ileostomy is performed. What knowledge should

guide the nurse in the care of Mrs. Hillster's ostomy?

A. Expect the stoma to start draining 72 hours after surgery.
B. Explain that the drainage can be controlled with daily irrigations.
C. Anticipate that emotional stress can increase intestinal peristalsis.
D. Be aware that bleeding from the stoma is a medical emergency.

41. Why is Mrs. Hillster at risk for developing anemia?

A. The hemopoietic factor is absorbed only in the terminal ileum.
B. Folic acid is absorbed only in the terminal ileum.
C. Iron absorption is dependent on simultaneous bile salt absorption in the terminal ileum.
D. Trace elements required for hemoglobin synthesis are present only in the ileum.

42. When caring for a client within the first 24 hours after a cardiac catheterization, the nurse should:

A. Keep the patient NPO for 2 to 4 hours after catheterization.
B. Check the pulse distal to the catheter insertion site.
C. Ensure that the patient is kept flat in bed for 8 hours after the procedure.
D. Ensure that the doctor has ordered antiarrhythmic medications for the patient.

43. What is the purpose of water in a closed chest drainage chamber?

A. It facilitates emptying of bloody drainage from the chest.
B. It fosters the removal of chest secretions by capillarity.
C. It prevents the entrance of air into the pleural cavity.
D. It decreases the danger of a sudden change in pressure in the tubing.

44. A doctor orders a nurse to assess the amount of chest tube drainage. The normal amount of drainage in 24 hours is approximately:

A. 300 mL.
B. 750 mL.
C. 1200 mL.
D. 1500 mL.

45. While delivering a tube feeding by gravity, an observation that indicates that the client is

unable to tolerate continuation of the feeding would be:

A. Passage of flatus.
B. The rapid flow of the feeding.
C. Epigastric tenderness.
D. A rise of formula in the tube.

46. A client's cardiac monitor shows ventricular fibrillation. The nurse from the coronary care unit should prepare for:

A. An IM injection of digoxin (Lanoxin).
B. An IV line for emergency medications.
C. Immediate defibrillation.
D. Elective cardioversion.

47. Diabetic coma results from an excess accumulation of which of the following in the blood?

A. Nitrogen from protein catabolism, causing ammonia intoxication.
B. Ketones from rapid fat breakdown, causing acidosis.
C. Glucose from rapid carbohydrate metabolism, causing drowsiness.
D. Sodium bicarbonate, causing alkalosis.

48. A client with diabetes mellitus has had declining renal function over the past several years. He is placed on hemodialysis because of persistently elevated creatinine levels. Which diet regimen would be best for the client on days between dialysis?

A. High-protein with a prescribed amount of water.
B. Low-protein diet with a prescribed amount of water.
C. Low-protein diet with an unlimited amount of water.
D. No protein in the diet and use of a salt substitute.

49. A 28-year-old woman has had type I diabetes mellitus for 10 years. She is doing home blood glucose monitoring and checking her urinary dipsticks for acetone. She asks the nurse why she has to dipstick her urine, too. Upon which of the following rationales would the nurse base her answer?

A. A positive test reaction indicates too much glucose.
B. A positive test reaction indicates too much insulin.
C. A positive test reaction indicates ketoacidosis.
D. The test measures protein in the urine.

---

**Case Study:** *Mr. Mulji, age 28 years, is found in a coma in his hospital room. There is a strong odour of acetone on his breath. He is married, climbs mountains, and is a triathlete. Previous health records do not reveal that Mr. Mulji has diabetes mellitus. Emergency measures are instituted immediately. Questions 50 and 51 relate to this scenario.*

50. A nursing action that should be included in the plan of care for Mr. Mulji is:

A. Regulating insulin dosage according to the amount of ketones found in the urine.
B. Withholding glucose in any form until the ketoacidosis is corrected.
C. Observing for signs of hypoglycemia as a result of treatment.
D. Giving fruit juices, broth, and milk as soon as he is able to take fluids orally.

51. Important to both Mr. Mulji and his wife, Ryann, is an understanding that a diabetic diet:

A. Is based on nutritional requirements that are the same for all clients.
B. Can be planned around a wide variety of commonly available foods.
C. Should be rigidly controlled to avoid similar diabetic emergencies.
D. Must not include processed foods because they have too many variable seasonings.

52. A 78-year-old woman has been discharged recently from the hospital after experiencing heart failure related to long-standing hypertension and coronary artery disease. A community health nurse is evaluating her compliance with medication therapy. Which of the following factors best indicates that the client is complying with digoxin (Lanoxin) therapy?

A. Her ability to count her radial pulse correctly.
B. Her weight gain of 2 lb in less than a week.
C. An apical heart rate of 101 bpm.
D. Absence of a pericardial friction rub.

53. A client with chronic obstructive pulmonary disease (COPD) is being discharged after treatment for an acute exacerbation. Which statement by the client indicates proper understanding of the discharge instructions?

A. "I should take my bronchodilator at bedtime to prevent insomnia."
B. "I should do my most difficult activities when I first get up in the morning."
C. "I should try to eat several small meals during the day."
D. "I should plan to do my exercises after I eat."

54. A 48-year-old foreman at a local electric company comes to the emergency department complaining of severe substernal chest pain radiating down his left arm. He is admitted to the coronary care unit with a diagnosis of myocardial infarction (MI). Which of the following should the nurse do first when the patient is admitted to the coronary care unit?

    A. Begin EGG monitoring.
    B. Obtain a family health history.
    C. Auscultate the lung fields bilaterally.
    D. Determine the quality of the client's pain.

55. When performing external cardiac compressions, the nurse should exert downward vertical pressure on the lower sternum by placing:

    A. The heels of each hand side by side, extending the fingers over the chest.
    B. The heel of one hand on the sternum and the heel of the other on top of it with the fingers interlocking.
    C. The fingers of one hand on the sternum and the fingers of the other hand on top of them.
    D. The heel of one hand on the sternum and the fleshy part of a clenched fist on the lower sternum.

*Case Study:* The nurse manager on a surgical unit is holding a meeting with the nursing team to discuss management's decision to reduce staffing on the nursing unit. During the discussion, one of the staff nurses stands up and yells at the nurse manager, using profanity and threatening "to take this decision further." Questions 56 to 58 relate to this scenario.

56. To defuse this situation, which of the following would be the best step for the nurse manager to take?

    A. Tell the nurse who is acting out that she is suspended for her behaviour.
    B. Call a break in the meeting and talk to the nurse in a private place or in his or her office.
    C. Ask the rest of the staff if they also feel the same way.
    D. Tell the nurse who is acting out settle down and to act professionally.

57. The nurse manager speaks to the nurse in her office or in a private place. The acting-out nurse is still speaking to the manager with a raised voice. The manager realizes she must set some limits on the nurse's behaviour. Which of the following statements would indicate that the manager effectively sets limits?

    A. "Settle down, or I will call someone for help."
    B. "Get ahold of yourself, or things will be worse for you."
    C. "Please lower your voice, or you will not be able to return to the meeting."
    D. "That is enough, or I will have you escorted out."

58. The nurse manager knows that setting limits on unacceptable behaviour should include consequences that are appropriate, enforceable, and which of the following?

    A. Consistent.
    B. Courteous.
    C. Concurrent.
    D. Consensual.

59. Andrew has been admitted to the intensive care unit after decompression of a cervical fracture. The nurses are concerned that after Andrew begins to wake up, he may try to pull out his endotracheal tube. The nurses decide to apply wrist restraints to Andrew's hands until he is alert and the tube is removed. What must the nurses do before applying the wrist restraints?

    A. Obtain consent from Andrew's next of kin.
    B. Nothing; this is a nursing decision.
    C. Try using ankle restraints because they are more effective.
    D. Discuss the decision with the physiotherapist.

60. Roger is a nurse working on a surgical unit and is stuck with a used hypodermic needle while walking to the sharps container located in the medicine room. This unit has a higher incidence of needlestick injuries compared with other units within the agency. Which of the following actions by the nursing manager would demonstrate advocacy for a quality practice environment?

    A. Have a meeting with staff to see how they can improve on methods to decrease needlestick injuries.
    B. Demonstrate how to use retractable needles.
    C. Track and verbally reprimand the nurses with needlestick injuries.
    D. Institute a "zero tolerance" policy regarding needlestick injuries.

61. A nurse is assisting an anaesthetist during the intubation of a patient. The anaesthetist visualizes the vocal cords with the laryngoscope and says to the nurse, "This is an easy one. Why don't you give it a try?" indicating that the nurse

should put in the endotracheal tube. What would be the most appropriate response by the nurse?

A. "As long as you watch, I will do it."
B. "It would be a good experience for me in case I need to do it in an emergency."
C. "I have done it before, so it would be good for me to do it again."
D. "No, it is not within my scope of practice."

62. During emergency surgery, a client is given a unit of blood. After the surgery, it is learned that the patient is a Jehovah's Witness. Which of the following would be an appropriate action after the transfusion and surgery?

A. Nothing; the patient will never know about the transfusion.
B. Disclose to the patient that she was given a blood transfusion.
C. Ask if the patient would accept blood, and if she says yes, tell her about the transfusion.
D. Tell her while she is still sleepy in the recovery room so she may not remember.

63. A client is complaining that he is having difficulty sleeping. The nurse notes that the client has dimenhydrinate (Gravol) ordered PRN for nausea. The nurse is aware that this medication often produces sedation and gives the client the medication. Which of the following is an accurate statement regarding the nurse's action?

A. The nurse used appropriate judgment in giving the medication.
B. The nurse demonstrated a client-focused intervention.
C. The nurse must only give the medication for the appropriate indication.
D. This action is within scope of practice of a registered nurse.

64. An individual has been advised to stop smoking. Which of the following statements by the nurse is considered therapeutic?

A. "I know how you feel. I had to stop smoking when I was pregnant."
B. "Stopping 'cold turkey' will give you the best chance for success."
C. "I can offer you some information outlining a variety of ways to stop smoking."
D. "The most effective way to stop smoking is to use the nicotine patch. Let me ask the doctor to order it for you."

65. A previously healthy male client, age 78 years, has been newly diagnosed with hypothyroidism. He lives in his own apartment in a community development designed for elderly individuals. He

asks the nurse assigned to his building complex for advice about his condition. What would be the best advice the nurse could give this client?

A. "Stop taking your self-prescribed daily aspirin."
B. "Don't become overtired by attending too many activities."
C. "Keep the temperature in your apartment cooler than usual."
D. "Increase the amount of fibre and fluids in your diet."

## ▶ Care of Adults and Older Adults Short Answer Questions

66. A nurse is working on a medical unit. Three hours into her shift, she needs to leave the workplace because of a family emergency. The nurse assuming care for the first nurse's patients reviews the medication sheets and notes that the nurse has signed for the medications for the entire shift. List three priority actions the nurse should take. (3 points)

67. Describe one characteristic of a healthy stoma. (1 point)

68. A man is admitted to the intensive care unit after a cerebrovascular accident (CVA) caused by a blood clot. The client's same-sex partner is present when the doctor arrives to obtain consent for the administration of tissue plasminogen activator (TPA), the "clot-busting" drug. The partner insists that he knows what his partner's wishes would be. The client is still legally married to his wife even though they stopped living together 1 year ago. Who has the right to provide consent in this situation? (1 point)

69. Mrs. Jules is a 77-year-old woman who has had problems with urinary urgency for the past

3 years. She is trying to deal with the problem herself by using an absorbent pad, but she feels that everyone notices it. She states that the bulk and odour are embarrassing and that she does not like to go out as a result. Provide two recommendations that can help Mrs. Jules regain control of her urinary elimination. (2 points)

**70.** Identify two precautions taken to prevent dislodgement or disconnection of a central line. (2 points)

**71.** Explain the purpose of antiembolism stockings. (1 point)

# ▶ Child Health
## Multiple-Choice Questions

**72.** A 10-month old child has been presented in the emergency department with respiratory compromise. Which of the following indicates respiratory compromise?

A. Nasal flaring.
B. Cyanosis.
C. Dyspnea.
D. Tachypnea.

*Case Study:* An 8-year-old child with a long-standing diagnosis of bronchial asthma arrives in the emergency department (ED). The child has an audible expiratory wheeze and intercostal retractions and is quite anxious. This is the second related visit to the ED this month, and the parents are in attendance; both are smokers. Questions 73 and 74 relate to this scenario.

**73.** The parents of this 8-year-old child with bronchial asthma have stated they require health teaching to address their concerns that their child has had two visits to the ED in the past month. The nurse should explain which of the following?

A. The cause of asthma is often allergens and infection.
B. Pediatric patients outgrow asthma.
C. Pediatric patients readily tolerate asthmatic episodes.
D. The environment has little impact on the child's asthma.

**74.** The child's mother reports that the child experiences symptoms daily with nighttime symptoms more than once a week. This child's asthma would be classified as which of the following?

A. Severe persistent asthma.
B. Moderate persistent asthma.
C. Moderate intermittent asthma.
D. Mild intermittent asthma.

**75.** Which of the following is a classic clinical manifestation of cystic fibrosis?

A. Steatorrhea.
B. Hyponatremia.
C. Urinary tract infections.
D. Integumentary compromise.

*Case Study:* A nurse is assessing a 17-year-old adolescent with a previous head injury. The parents inform the nurse of drastic personality changes with aggressive behaviour since the injury. Questions 76 and 77 relate to this scenario.

**76.** The nurse can determine that the injury was in which lobe of the brain?

A. Frontal.
B. Occipital.
C. Temporal.
D. Parietal.

**77.** On further assessment of this teen 1 hour later, the nurse identifies apnea, bradycardia, and a widening pulse pressure. What is occurring at this time?

A. The patient's condition is stabilizing.
B. Intracranial pressure is increasing.
C. The patient likely has a bladder infection.
D. The patient has received too much pain medication.

**78.** A nurse is providing an inservice to the community focusing on preventing the incidence of hepatitis in children. Which type of hepatitis could a child contract from a contaminated diaper changing table?

A. Hepatitis A.
B. Hepatitis B.
C. Hepatitis C.
D. Hepatitis D.

79. A young infant presents with a notched vermilion border, dental anomalies, and variably sized clefts. These signs are indicative of which of the following?

A. Cleft lip.
B. Cleft palate.
C. Cleft lip and palate.
D. Esophageal atresia.

80. During initial health teaching, identify the correct information that the nurse would provide to the parents of a child newly diagnosed with cleft lip or palate.

A. "Your child will not be able to breastfeed."
B. "A glass bottle is the best choice for your child."
C. "Feed your child in an upright position."
D. "Burp your child after the entire feed is finished."

81. If a child requires a repair of a cleft lip, what is the ideal age category that the parents can anticipate for this corrective surgery?

A. 1 to 2 months.
B. 3 to 6 months.
C. 9 to 11 months.
D. 12 to 18 months.

82. A 12-year-old patient is scheduled for surgery in 1 hour to repair a fractured tibia. The child's preoperative vital signs show him to be febrile. What is the best course of action to take at this point?

A. Inform the surgeon.
B. Record the temperature only.
C. Administer oral antipyretics.
D. Place cool compresses on the child.

83. A nurse is assessing a fresh postoperative 7-year-old for pain and finds him playing in bed with his toys. The nurse should determine which of the following?

A. Some children distract themselves with play while in pain.
B. A child who resumes his or her usual play activity is not experiencing pain.
C. Nurses can accurately estimate children's pain from physical appearance or activity.

D. Narcotic analgesics are too dangerous for young children.

84. The parents of a pregnant adolescent are outraged that they are being refused medical information about their daughter's condition from the nursing team. What is the best response to address their anger?

A. "Your daughter's medical information is considered confidential, and you aren't entitled to it just because you're her parents."
B. "I'm not supposed to tell you, but she's pregnant and will need your support."
C. "I can appreciate your concerns. If we obtain permission from your daughter, we can include you in our discussions."
D. Your daughter will now have to be responsible for her own health.

85. You are caring for a 5-year-old girl who has a history of multiple admissions for fractures and cuts. Her mother explains that the child fractured her femur by falling but does not give any further details. The child indicates that the mother's boyfriend was with her when the injury occurred, and her recollection of the event is in conflict with the information her mother has provided. The nurse's immediate responsibility is to:

A. Keep the child safe and assess for abuse.
B. Collect forensic specimens for laboratory analysis.
C. Call the police department and report abuse.
D. Restrict family visiting the child.

86. Of the following four medical diagnoses, which would be the priority when providing nursing care?

A. Epiglottitis.
B. Appendectomy.
C. Pneumonia.
D. Sickle cell disease.

87. A nurse is caring for a 14-year-old boy with type I diabetes mellitus. Health teaching has been focused on reviewing the signs and symptoms of hypoglycemia. The nurse determines that the adolescent needs further teaching when he says:

A. "If my blood sugar is low, I will be able to deal with it."
B. "If my blood sugar is low, I will feel sweaty and anxious."
C. "If my blood sugar is low, my heart rate will speed up."
D. "If my blood sugar is low, my blood pressure will increase."

88. A 13-year-old patient is being taught to self-administer insulin. Which of the following would a nurse emphasize in the health teaching?

    A. Activity levels rarely determine insulin requirements.
    B. Meal sizes are not usually considered when determining insulin needs.
    C. The need for insulin always decreases when strenuous sports are played.
    D. Insulin is always administered subcutaneously.

89. Identify the stage of development of a pediatric patient who would be frightened of intrusive procedures such as assessing temperature and blood pressure.

    A. Toddler.
    B. Preschool.
    C. School-aged.
    D. Adolescent.

90. Identify the stage of development of a pediatric patient who is most receptive to the use of puppets and dolls for explanation of illness or surgery.

    A. Toddler.
    B. Preschool.
    C. School-aged.
    D. Adolescent.

91. Sharon is a nurse caring for the child with a urinary tract infection and is 1 hour late administering the child's prescribed antibiotic therapy and pain medication despite the child's mother repeatedly asking for it. Liz, the charge nurse, challenges Sharon about the lateness of the medications. Sharon responds, "It's no big deal. At least he got the medication." What is the best course of action for Liz to take?

    A. No course of action because the nurse is working on a busy floor.
    B. Reassign responsibility of this patient to another nurse.
    C. Speak to the unit manager so he or she can handle the situation.
    D. Speak to the unit manager and fill out a medication error form.

92. You are assessing the health of a 6-month-old patient who is sitting in her mother's lap. Suddenly, a loud noise is heard from the hall, but the child does not startle. What should the nurse suspect?

    A. The child is well adjusted and happy.
    B. The child may have a hearing impairment.

    C. The child is accustomed to loud noises.
    D. The child was distracted at the time.

## ▶ Child Health Short Answer Questions

93. Identify two potential causes of increased intracranial pressure in children. (2 points)

94. Identify three factors that influence a child's response to pain. (3 points)

## ▶ Maternal–Child Health Multiple-Choice Questions

95. Shirley, age 25 years, is 2.5 months pregnant. She asks the nurse if feeling like she has to "go to the bathroom every 5 minutes" is normal. Which of the following is the best response to Shirley?

    A. "You probably have a bladder infection and should contact your primary care provider."
    B. "Women in early pregnancy are naturally preoccupied with their bodily functions."
    C. "Bladder capacity normally increases throughout the pregnancy."
    D. "The growing uterus puts pressure on the bladder, so urinary frequency is normal."

96. Jessica is in her second trimester of pregnancy. Thomas, her husband, accompanies her to her prenatal visits. He tells the nurse that he is worried about being a good father to their new baby. Which of the following nurse's response would be appropriate for Thomas?

    A. "Develop a fathering role similar to that of an admired close friend."
    B. "Can you help me understand what aspect of being a father concerns you?"
    C. "Begin by following the basic pattern that your father used with you."
    D. "Preparation for fatherhood is not necessary because your role will come naturally."

97. Sandy and Timothy arrive at the hospital with their birth plan. Their birth plan states that they wish to birth a healthy infant without the use of analgesics or anaesthetic agents. Which of the following nursing actions would be most beneficial to Sandy and her husband while she is in labour?

    A. Act as an advocate for the couple and verbalize their wishes to nurses and primary care providers.
    B. Provide privacy for the couple and respect their wishes for being left alone during labour.
    C. Provide information about the nature and availability of drugs for Sandy.
    D. Encourage the use of drugs if Sandy has difficulty maintaining control during labour.

98. Debra is seeking information from the nurse about having a home birth with registered midwives. The nurse discusses Debra's questions and provides her with information. Which of the following statements lets the nurse know Debra has considered the risks and benefits of using a midwife?

    A. "I will look for an obstetrician because it's hard to find a general practitioner who provides maternity services."
    B. "I am safer having a home birth with a physician."
    C. "I will develop a list of questions to use in interviewing primary care providers."
    D. "I understand the complications that could occur in a home birth setting."

99. Stacey, age 15 years, gravida 1, para 0, is admitted to the antenatal unit with a history of nausea and vomiting for the past week. Stacey tells the nurse she is from another province and is staying with friends. When the nurse asks Stacey if the father of the baby is supportive of the pregnancy, Stacey begins to cry and states, "He left 3 weeks ago, and I haven't heard from him." What is the nurse's most appropriate response?

    A "Will your parents be able to support you?"
    B. "It appears that you are concerned about where the baby's father is living right now."
    C. "Tell me more about how you are feeling."
    D. "Would you like to speak to the hospital social worker?"

100. Margaret is attending her first prenatal appointment. She states that she drank beer throughout her last pregnancy to "build iron" in her blood. Margaret asks the nurse if it is okay to have a few drinks during this current pregnancy. Which of the following responses by the nurse would be most appropriate?

    A. "It is not safe to consume alcohol during pregnancy."
    B. "It is safe to consume one or two drinks per week in the first trimester."
    C. "It is safe to consume wine and beer in moderation during pregnancy."
    D. "It is safe to consume one or two drinks per week in the third semester."

101. A nurse completes the initial assessment of a newborn. According to the due date (EDC) on the antenatal record, the baby is 12 days postmature. Which of the following physical findings does not confirm that this newborn is 12 days postmature?

    A. Meconium aspiration.
    B. Absence of lanugo.
    C. Hypoglycemia.
    D. Increased amounts of vernix.

---

*Case Study:* Riley is 34-years-old, gravida 4, para 3. She delivered a 3850 g baby. Her estimated blood loss was 400 mL. Her immediate vital signs after delivery were blood pressure, 110/70 mm Hg; temperature, 37°C; pulse, 68 bpm; and respirations, 20 breaths/min. She delivered 2 hours ago and is now on the postpartum unit. The nurse begins her postpartum assessment. Questions 102 to 105 relate to this scenario.

102. The nurse assesses Riley's fundus. Where would the nurse expect the fundus to be located at this time?

    A. At the umbilicus.
    B. Above the umbilicus.
    C. 1 cm below the umbilicus.
    D. 2 cm below the umbilicus.

103. The nurse palpates Riley's fundus, and it is 1 to 2 cm above the umbilicus and displaced to the right. Which of the following nurse's actions would be appropriate?

    A. Start a pad count.
    B. Notify the charge nurse.
    C. Massage the fundus and express clots.
    D. Have Riley void and reassess the fundus.

104. One hour later, the nurse notes that Riley is trickling blood from the vagina and has soaked a pad in about 30 to 40 minutes. Her vital signs are blood pressure, 90/68 mm Hg; pulse, 100 bpm; and respirations, 24 breaths/min. She

appears restless. Which of the following immediate actions would be appropriate by the nurse?

A. Notify the physician or midwife.
B. Have Riley turn on her left side.
C. Palpate and massage her fundus to assess firmness.
D. Do nothing because this is a normal finding.

105. Riley's husband enters the room and becomes very agitated with the fact that the nurse is taking so long to assess his wife. He starts pacing within the small room and raises his voice. Which of the following is the best nurse's response?

A. Tell the husband to calm down.
B. Ask the husband to leave the room and come back later.
C. Hurry with her assessment so as not to agitate him further.
D. Succinctly explain the need to do a proper assessment.

___

***Case Study:*** *Baby Wong was born 1 hour ago at 3575 g with Apgar scores of 8 at 1 minute and 9 at 5 minutes and has just been transferred to the newborn nursery. He was breastfed in the delivery room. The nurse begins the newborn assessment. Questions 106 to 110 relate to this scenario.*

106. Baby Wong is asleep. The nurse counts his apical pulse at 100 bpm. Which of the following statements is accurate about his pulse?

A. This finding is dangerously low.
B. This finding is abnormally high.
C. This finding is on the high end of the normal range.
D. This finding is at the low end of the normal range.

107. What is the primary reason for administration of vitamin K to babies after birth?

A. To stimulate growth of intestinal flora.
B. To promote absorption of fat-soluble nutrients.
C. To speed conjugation of bilirubin.
D. To prevent synthesis of clotting factors from the liver.

108. During Baby Wong's assessment, his temperature drops. Which of the following does the nurse recognize as a cause of temperature instability?

A. Excessive heat loss.
B. Impaired thermogenesis.

C. Immature central control by the hypothalamus.
D. Lack of glycogen stores.

109. What nursing action will best improve Baby Wong's body temperature?

A. Uncover him and place him on the radiant warmer.
B. Bundle him and return him to his bassinet.
C. Do nothing because his temperature will increase naturally within the next hour.
D. Feed him a small amount of formula.

110. The nurse assesses Baby Wong's neurologic system. Which of the following behaviours would the nurse interpret as a normal reflex response?

A. Draws his hand away when palm of hand is stimulated.
B. Turns his head away when his cheek is stroked.
C. Flexes his toes slightly when the sole of his foot is stroked.
D. Makes a walking movement when he is held upright with one foot touching the table.

111. Tamara, age 29 years, has a history of cardiac disease and is expecting her third baby. Tamara will most likely experience signs of cardiac decompensation in which of the following times during her pregnancy?

A. 8 to 12 weeks gestational age.
B. 16 to 20 weeks gestational age.
C. 22 to 26 weeks gestational age.
D. 28 to 32 weeks gestational age.

112. A nurse observes decreased fetal heart rate variability on the fetal heart tracing of a labouring woman. Which of the following is not an indication for decreased fetal heart rate variability?

A. Prolapsed cord.
B. Fetal sleep.
C. Prematurity of birth.
D. Fetal hypoxia.

113. Which of the following is an accurate statement about the impact of hemodynamic changes occurring during pregnancy?

A. Hematocrit decreases.
B. There is an increased risk of transient tachycardia.
C. Circulatory blood volume decreases.
D. Cardiac output decreases.

114. Which of the following is true regarding partner abuse in pregnancy in Canada?

A. It occurs most frequently in new immigrant families.

B. Partner abuse in pregnancy is rare.

C. Partner abuse may increase during pregnancy.

D. It occurs in approximately 3% to 5% of pregnant women.

## ▶ Maternal–Child Health
## Short Answer Questions

***Case Study:*** *Sunita, gravida 3, para 2, is a married woman whose pregnancy is at 39 weeks gestational age. Her pregnancy has been unremarkable. Sunita has been experiencing irregular contractions all day. She tells the nurse at the hospital that her contractions are coming "sooner and stronger now." Sunita is focused and breathing well through the uterine contractions. Question 115 relates to this scenario.*

115. The nurse finds that Sunita's contractions occur every 2 minutes, are strong, and last 90 seconds each. Her cervix is 5 cm dilated and 80% effaced. The presenting part is at 0 station. Sunita continues to cope well. She is focused on her contractions and does not want to be touched. What six factors may contribute and influence how Sunita is responding to labour? (3 points)

116. List four areas of self-care and precautions about which you need to instruct a newly delivered hepatitis B carrier mother. (2 points)

## ▶ Mental Health
## Multiple-Choice Questions

117. When caring for a client taking central nervous system (CNS) stimulants, the nurse must monitor the client for which of the following conditions?

A. Hypotension, listlessness, and weight gain.

B. Arrhythmias, slowing of sensorium, and increased appetite.

C. Mood swings, tachycardia, and weight loss.

D. Slow pulse, hyperpyrexia, and weight gain.

118. During a mental status assessment, the nurse must assess the client's judgment. To accomplish this, the nurse should ask the client to:

A. Discuss hypothetical ethical situations.

B. Spell words backwards.

C. Interpret proverbs.

D. Count by serial sevens.

119. In a crisis intervention situation, the main goal is to:

A. Provide a rapid means for admission to an acute care facility.

B. Solve the client's problems for him or her.

C. Resolve the immediate crisis.

D. Establish a means for long-term therapy.

120. During the working phase of a nurse-led group therapy, what is the nurse's main task?

A. Encourage group cohesiveness.

B. Explain the purpose and goals of the group.

C. Offer advice to help resolve conflicts.

D. Encourage a discussion of feelings of loss regarding termination.

121. The primary indication for electroconvulsive therapy (ECT) is:

A. Noncompliance with treatment.

B. Major depression with psychotic features.

C. Antisocial behaviour.

D. Severe agitation.

122. A client reports to the emergency department complaining of suicidal ideation and feelings of worthlessness. He has a family history of suicide. In assessing the client to determine treatment recommendations, the most important factor for the nurse to consider is:

A. The client's religion and social status.

B. An active suicide plan and the means to carry it out.

C. A previous suicide attempt.

D. Social support and marital status.

123. A client who was brought to the hospital in an agitated state is admitted to a psychiatric unit for observation and treatment. On admission, he is found to be talking rapidly, folding and unfolding garments several times while putting his personal effects away. The client can't seem to settle down. Which nursing assessment would be of top priority at this time?

A. Self-care deficit.

B. Anxiety.

C. Impaired verbal communication.

D. Powerlessness.

124. When using the technique of self-disclosure during a nurse–client interaction, the nurse should:
    A. Discuss the nurse's experience in detail.
    B. Have the client explain his or her perception of what the nurse has revealed.
    C. Ensure relevance to the client's experiences and quickly refocus on them.
    D. Allow the client time to ask questions about the nurse's experience.

125. Although smoking is prohibited on hospital property, a client with antisocial personality disorder smokes in the client lounge and refuses to follow other unit and hospital rules. The client gets others to do his laundry and other personal chores, and refuses to work with nurses he does not like. The plan of care for this client should focus primarily on:
    A. Engaging in power struggles to minimize manipulate behaviour.
    B. Using behaviour modification to decrease negative behaviour by using negative reinforcement.
    C. Isolating the client to decrease contact with easily manipulated clients.
    D. Consistently enforcing unit rules and facility policy.

126. You are working in a community mental health clinic. Your client who has been diagnosed with schizophrenia is taking clozapine (Clozaril) and complains of a sore throat. This symptom may be an indication of which of the following adverse reactions?
    A. Tardive dyskinesia.
    B. Reye's syndrome.
    C. Agranulocytosis.
    D. Extrapyramidal reaction.

---

*Case Study:* Enrique, a 33-year-old new Mexican immigrant, meets with a community health nurse. His concerns centre on his professional and social life. He states that his job as an engineer provides a lot of stress, and he has been working 60 to 70 hours a week because he cannot say no to his boss. Enrique feels vulnerable in his job because his immigrant status depends on this employment. Enrique has never been married and has no time to date. He has very little social time available for family or friends. Questions 127 to 130 relate to this scenario.

127. Enrique has identified to the community health nurse that his lack of assertive behaviour with his boss has contributed to long work hours. To assist Enrique, which question would be most appropriate for his nurse to ask?
    A. "When is the best time of day to approach your boss?"
    B. "What other ways could you approach your boss?"
    C. "What have you done so far to try to solve this problem?"
    D. "Which alternative seems like the best decision at this time?"

128. In assessing Enrique's social supports, which would be the most important question for the nurse to ask?
    A. "In what ways are you able to be a positive support system to others?"
    B. "With how many family members do you maintain close contact?"
    C. "What do you do for fun in your free time?"
    D. "What kind of emotional or material support do you receive from others?"

129. In addition to assessing social support, which intervention would be most helpful in assisting Enrique in implementing change in his work situation?
    A. Teach him about the effects of long-term stress on the body.
    B. Encourage him to vent about his feelings about his boss.
    C. Role play with the nurse assuming the role of the boss.
    D. Explore alternative work settings with Enrique.

130. Enrique has identified isolation and loneliness as part of his current stress. He recognizes that he has become withdrawn but does not know how to change the situation. The most appropriate step for the nurse to take next is:
    A. Refer him to special interest clubs for newcomers to the city.
    B. Model culturally appropriate interactional skills.
    C. Support him in developing attainable goals to enhance his socialization.
    D. Have him plan a social activity with his boss for the upcoming weekend.

131. A 49-year-old painter recently fractured his tibia while skiing. Now unable to work, he is worried about his finances. His physician prescribes buspirone (BuSpar), 5 mg by mouth three times per day, to treat his anxiety. During buspirone

therapy, the client is advised to avoid which of the following drugs?

A. Monoamine oxidase inhibitors (MAOIs).
B. Antiparkinsonian drugs.
C. Antineoplastic drugs.
D. Beta-adrenergic blockers.

132. A psychiatric inpatient unit nurse is caring for a client with obsessive–compulsive disorder. The psychiatrist orders lorazepam (Ativan), 1 mg by mouth 3 times a day, as part of the client's treatment plan. During client teaching about this new medication, the nurse should remind the client to:

A. Stay out of the sun.
B. Maintain an adequate salt intake.
C. Avoid caffeine.
D. Avoid aged cheeses.

---

*Case Study:* Eloise is a 50-year-old recently divorced woman experiencing symptoms of generalized anxiety, particularly excessive worry. She has no siblings; her parents died last year; and she has contact with her ex–in-laws who, she feels, subtly blame her for the divorce. Eloise is seeking assistance with her anxiety concerns at the local community mental health clinic. Questions 133 to 135 relate to this scenario.

133. When the nurse asks Eloise to describe her social supports, she says that she is divorced, has no siblings, her parents died last year, and she has contact with her once-supportive ex–in-laws. However, since the divorce, her ex–in-laws constantly complain about her behaviour. Regarding the relationship with her ex–in-laws, the nurse can base plans of care on the knowledge that:

A. The ex–in-laws offer the only opportunity for the client to obtain social support.
B. Low-quality support relationships often negatively affect coping in a crisis.
C. The relationship with the ex–in-laws can enhance the client's sense of control and competence.
D. Strong social support is of relatively little importance as a mediating factor.

134. Eloise is experiencing considerable stress in this change of role from being married to being divorced. She says that her in-laws believe that her excessive drinking was the cause of the divorce. She states, "These days, a couple of glasses of wine in the evenings helps calm my

nerves." A coping strategy the nurse might suggest for Eloise is:

A. Ceasing all contact with her ex–in-laws to decrease her anxiety.
B. Using previously learned deep breathing and muscle relaxation techniques.
C. Relying on the support of her work colleagues.
D. Using assertiveness techniques in talking with her ex–in-laws.

135. Eloise remains in the hospital, and her sensorium clears after 3 days. A few days later, while the nurse is caring for her, she tells the nurse that drinking helps her cope with her anxiety related to her recent divorce. Which response by the nurse would help Eloise view her drinking more objectively?

A. "Sooner or later, your drinking will kill you."
B. "I hear a lot of defensiveness in your voice. You don't really believe what you're saying, do you?"
C. "If you were coping so well, what are you doing here?"
D. "Tell me what happened the last time you felt you were under a lot of stress and were drinking to cope."

136. A client with borderline personality disorder tells the nurse that she wants to "fire" her psychiatrist, who has refused to give her a pass because she returned intoxicated after having engaged in impulsive and unprotected sexual behaviour during her last pass. The best nursing response is to:

A. Suggest that the client bring up the concerns in the community meeting.
B. Ignore the client's attention seeking and tell her to discuss the issue with her psychiatrist.
C. Ask the client to explore why she feels so angry.
D. Set limits and reinforce that the psychiatrist's refusal of the pass was a consequence and response to the behaviours on her last pass.

## ▶ Mental Health Short Answer Questions

---

*Case Study:* Henri, an 83-year-old man, is brought into the emergency department (ED) by his daughter, Chantal. He has a history of major depression and recently lost his wife of 55 years, moved into an assisted living residence, and had to give up the

family pet to make the move. Henri was unresponsive when found by Chantal and his son-in-law,
Marc, after having ingested an unknown quantity of
antidepressant medication and sleeping pills. Stabilized in the ED, Henri is now admitted to a geriatric
psychiatric unit for hospitalization. Questions 137
and 138 relate to this scenario.

**137.** What are three risk factors for suicide that
should be considered in Henri's case? (3 points)

**138.** What are two priority nursing interventions the
nurse should consider in planning Henri's care?
(2 points)

# COMPREHENSIVE PRACTICE EXAM II

## ▶ Professional Practice Multiple-Choice Questions

**1.** Michelle is a public health nurse responsible for
contact tracing of individuals identified in
confirmed cases of sexually transmitted
infections. Michelle telephones an individual
named by an infected client. The individual on
the telephone demands to be told the name of
the person who identified him as a contact.
Which of the following is the appropriate
response from Michelle?

A. "Just as I will protect your privacy, I must
protect the privacy of the other people
involved."
B. "If you tell me the name of the person you
have had sex with, I will tell you if it is the
same person who identified you."
C. "I can only disclose the name if you consent
to having treatment for your infection."
D. "The individual who named you asked for
anonymity or confidentiality regarding this
situation."

**2.** An individual returns to the nursing unit after
being discharged demanding Tylenol #3's. He is
advised that he is no longer a patient on the unit

and this medication cannot be administered.
He states that everyone is incompetent and says,
"I know where you park your cars, and you'd
better watch out when you leave here tonight."
What is the next appropriate step that the nurse
should take?

A. Bring the client to the emergency room
immediately.
B. Call the police.
C. Administer two Tylenol #3's immediately.
D. Nothing; the client is just expressing his frus-
tration.

**3.** During morning rounds, an RN assesses that her
elderly patient's IV line has gone interstitial. She
obtains the necessary equipment to restart the IV
and attempts venipuncture in the opposite arm.
Hospital policy states that each nurse may
attempt the initiation of an IV twice, and if
unsuccessful, he or she must ask a more experienced nurse to take over. The RN attempts four
times, and the client becomes distressed. What
action should the nurse manager take in this situation?

A. Document this incident and discuss with the
nurse that she did not follow agency policy
and distressed the client.
B. Nothing; the nurse needed to get the IV
restarted, and two attempts are not enough
for an elderly client.
C. Ask the other nurses if this is a reasonable
policy and follow their comments.
D. Ask the patient not to say anything to
the physician because it is not a significant
injury.

**4.** A physician writes an order for a nurse to
administer an IV medication STAT, which,
according to the hospital policy, can only be
given by a physician. The nurse informs the
physician that she cannot administer the
medication, and the physician tells her, "Give it,
and I will cover you." What should the nurse do
in this situation?

A. Administer the medication as ordered.
B. Refuse to administer the medication.
C. Call another nurse to see if he or she would
give it.
D. Give the medication but have the physician
sign for it.

**5.** Hilary is a new RN on a mental health unit.
During the assessment of a client, she has noticed
that periods of silence occur. Which of the
following actions would indicate that Hilary

understands what should occur during these periods of silence?

- A. She leaves the client because the conversation is obviously finished.
- B. She changes the subject by introducing a new topic of interest.
- C. She tells the client that she is too busy to sit there in silence.
- D. She sits quietly and allows the client to process his or her thoughts.

6. Angela is a nurse on a surgical unit where the physician has ordered methadone for a client. When the medication arrives on the unit, Angela is unable to find a policy regarding the storage of this medication. She knows that methadone belongs to the opioid family of drugs and places it in the narcotic cupboard. Angela is demonstrating which of the following?

- A. Appropriate professional judgment in the absence of a policy.
- B. Inappropriate storage of medication that should be at the bedside.
- C. Practicing outside of her scope; the pharmacist should be involved.
- D. Lack of knowledge of how opioids should be stored.

7. During a surgical dressing change, the nurse touches the sterile gauze on the outside of the dressing tray, resulting in the contamination of the swab. What would be the most appropriate action of the nurse?

- A. Discard the swab and use another piece of sterile gauze.
- B. Nothing; the dressing change is almost finished.
- C. Use the gauze anyway because the wound already has some redness.
- D. Nothing; the outside of the tray is considered sterile

8. A nurse observes a consent form signed by a male client indicating his permission for the insertion of a feeding tube before the beginning of chemotherapy. One hour before the procedure, the client states that he has changed his mind and now does not want the feeding tube. What would be the most appropriate response by the nurse?

- A. "You have a right to withdraw consent. Let's discuss your decision."
- B "You must have the feeding tube inserted before the chemotherapy."
- C. "After you have given consent in writing, you cannot change your mind."

- D. "Changing your mind now would be really inconvenient for the surgeon."

9. A nurse is examining the Foley catheter of a client who is in a four-bed ward of the surgical unit. The nurse does not pull the curtains and does not cover the client while performing this assessment. Which of the following qualities of ethical care is the nurse violating?

- A. Dignity.
- B. Confidentiality.
- C. Justice.
- D. Choice.

---

***Case Study:*** *A student nurse has been asked to develop an education activity for a grade 8 class regarding nutrition. She realizes that she needs to include information on the importance of fibre in the diet. Questions 10 to 12 relate to this scenario.*

10. Which of the following food choices would she encourage this age group to consume to increase their dietary fibre content?

- A. Baked French fries with ketchup.
- B. Sandwiches on whole wheat bread.
- C. Grape-flavoured juice boxes.
- D. Chicken legs with gravy.

11. One of the students attending the session states, "I hate fibre, and this is a stupid idea." Which of the following is the best response by the student nurse?

- A. "A lot of people don't like fibre. Why don't we talk about ways you can add fibre to your diet that you may not have thought about?"
- B. "It is not about whether you like fibre or not. It is about what's good for you. Let's talk more about fibre."
- C. "You are only thinking of yourself. I am going to speak to the entire class. Who does like to eat fibre?"
- D. "Do you think you are the only one who hates fibre? Sometimes we need to eat things we hate. What are other sources of fibre?"

12. The student nurse will know that her educational activity has been effective if the students do which of the following at the end of the session?

- A. Thank her for coming, give her a card, and clap when she leaves.
- B. List five sources of fibre they would include in their food choices.

C. Get a 50% on the quiz at the end of the workshop.

D. Ask the teacher if the nursing student can talk to them about sexuality.

13. Reggie, an RN, is caring for a client who is learning to use a walker after a total knee replacement. The client states, "I hate this stupid thing. Everything is going wrong. I wish you would leave me alone." Reggie responds by saying, "You sound frustrated. This surgery has impacted your ability to be active, and that must be difficult for you." Reggie is demonstrating which therapeutic communication technique?

A. Empathy.

B. Sharing of feelings.

C. Asking relevant questions.

D. Paraphrasing.

14. Elizabeth is an RN who is to administer 5000 U of heparin subcutaneously to her patient. She obtains a vial of heparin and draws up the dose. Elizabeth is aware that the hospital policy for administering heparin requires that she have the dose verified with another RN. To comply, she approaches another nurse. The second nurse should do which of the following?

A. Read the medication administration record, read the label on the vial, calculate the dosage, and look at the amount drawn up in the syringe.

B. Look at Elizabeth's calculation sheet and verify her math. Then look at the syringe and the amount drawn up.

C. Look at the medication administration record and the syringe because the only strength of heparin on this unit is 10,000 U/mL.

D. Tell Elizabeth that "independent double check" is only for IV heparin.

15. A nurse applies to work in a weight loss clinic and is required to promote a 940-calorie-per-day diet for rapid weight loss. Clients are required to attend the clinic on a daily basis to discuss their progress with the nurse. Which of the following statements is accurate regarding this scenario?

A. It is good that the clients are monitored by an RN.

B. This would be an appropriate job for an RPN or LPN.

C. This would not be an appropriate job for an RN.

D. This would be an ideal job for a new graduate in nursing.

*Case Study:* *A nurse on an orthopaedic unit assesses her client's right foot after the application of a knee-to-toe circular cast. The client sustained a fractured tibia in a motor vehicle accident and was admitted through the emergency department to the orthopedic unit with an elevated blood alcohol level. Questions 16 to 18 relate to this scenario.*

16. The client complains of pain in her right heel. In addition to assessing for circulation, the nurse would also assess for which of the following to ensure that a complete, focused assessment has been done?

A. Assess for drainage at the heel site.

B. Assess if the client has voided.

C. Assess for symptoms of a hangover.

D. Assess the client's recollection of the accident.

17. The nurse concludes that there is no compromise of circulation in the client's right foot and administers an analgesic. The client experiences no pain relief and states that her heel pain is worse. What intervention should the nurse do?

A. Repeat the dose of analgesia every hour.

B. Call the physician to report the finding.

C. Massage the client's foot in a circular motion.

D. Apply warm, moist heat to the right ankle area.

18. The physician tells the nurse that he does not want to be bothered with phone calls regarding this client, saying, "She was drunk when she came in and has an addictive personality." He also tells the nurse that she is incompetent and should "figure these things out for herself." Which of the following would be the best action by the nurse?

A. Inform the client of the conversation and let her know that she is receiving inferior care from the physician.

B. Document the assessment and the conversation with the physician only.

C. Reassess the client, document both the conversation and the assessment, and notify the nursing supervisor.

D. Suggest to the client that if she has her own narcotics with her, she should take some until the next dose is due.

19. Jane and Ashley work on a medical unit of a hospital. Jane overhears Ashley tell a peer that she forgot to pay her annual dues to the provincial or territorial governing body, which means she is technically working without a current license. She states, "No one ever checks anyway,

and if they do, I will just play dumb." What action, if any, should Jane take?

A. No action because Jane is not responsible for ensuring that nurses have current registration.

B. Remind the nurse manager of her responsibility to ensure that all nurses have current registration and to recommend a deadline for staff to show proof of registration.

C. Leave a note for Ashley to pay her registration because she does not want to see her get in trouble.

D. Jane should not pay either because no one checks these things anyway, or if she is caught, she will "play dumb" as well.

20. On a busy evening shift in a regional trauma unit, two motor vehicle accident victims are brought into the emergency department. One of the victims is a young mother who was hit by another vehicle. The second patient is the male driver of the vehicle that hit the young mother. It is obvious that this man is drunk. The nurse manager of the trauma unit is short staffed and has called for additional staff. Because of this, she elects to treat the young woman and have the drunk driver wait for the backup staff. Which of the following is an accurate reflection of this scenario?

A. The nurse has made the best decision based on the circumstances.

B. Drunk drivers who cause accidents should be treated last.

C. The nurse must treat each client equally without prejudice.

D. The woman was not drinking, so she should be treated first.

21. A woman who is visiting her husband on your nursing unit asks the nurse about another patient on the unit, who happens to be her friend. The visitor states that she saw this patient's name on the computer screen that another nurse was using at the desk. What should you do?

A. Discuss the matter with the other nurse, reminding him or her not to leave client information in view of visitors.

B. Tell the visitor that the friend is a patient on the unit but do not disclose any further information.

C. Tell the visitor that she should not be reading information that is confidential.

D. Ask the friend to come to the visit the client's room to meet with the wife.

22. The nurse enters information on the client's chart and then realizes a mistake has been made. The appropriate steps in correcting the entry error would be which of the following?

A. Use correction fluid to cover the mistake and write the correct information over top.

B. Erase the entry and write the correct information in the appropriate place.

C. Blacken out the entry with a marker and add the correct data after it.

D. Draw a line through the incorrect entry and date it and initial it followed by the correct data.

23. A client who was instructed not to get out of bed by himself repeatedly gets out at night anyway and is at an increased risk of falling because of his unsteady gait. The physician orders a bed alarm. The alarm goes off every time the client turns over, and the nurse turns the alarm off until it can be repaired. When the client gets out of bed and falls, which of the following statements is accurate?

A. The nurse is responsible for the injuries sustained by the client.

B. The maintenance department is responsible for the injuries sustained by the client because of the faulty alarm.

C. No one is responsible when the patient fell out of bed.

D. The family is responsible because they should have stayed with the client during the night.

## ▶ Professional Practice Short Answer Questions

24. The nurse caring for a postoperative client hangs an IV solution that contains potassium chloride ($K^+$) 40 mEq/L. The client has a urinary output of 20 mL/hr for each of the past 3 hours. Why would hanging this infusion be an unsafe act on behalf of the nurse? (1 point)

25. Mrs. Black is an 88-year-old patient who is receiving care in her home by a visiting nurse. The nurse shares with Mrs. Black that she is experiencing financial difficulty and has to work two jobs. Mrs. Black gives the nurse an envelope with a significant amount of money in it, stating, "It's a tip for the good care you give me." Identify

two actions a nurse should take after receiving this offer. (2 points)

**26.** A nurse administers meperidine (Demerol) as ordered for pain. The client experiences nausea and vomiting and a decrease in respiratory rate. Identify three actions the nurse should take when documenting the client's adverse reaction to this medication. (3 points)

## ▶ Care of Adults and Older Adults Multiple-Choice Questions

**27.** You make a home care visit to your client, 86-year-old Martha Marlin. She seems confused regarding the date and is not sure whether she took her medicines today. What assessments would be most important?

   A. Assess her cognitive status, how she is managing with activities of living, and what supports she has available.
   B. Assess her orientation to person, time, and place and her capacity to make decisions regarding her health status.
   C. Assess her respiratory and cardiovascular system to determine if chronic illness is presenting.
   D. Assess for stages of depression, sensory deprivation, and social isolation.

**28.** You have been assigned a patient with a diagnosis of autonomic dysreflexia. You are unfamiliar with this diagnosis. How would you prepare to competently care for this patient?

   A. Look up the term in the dictionary and consult with other nurses.
   B. Search the Internet for the definition and problems that present.
   C. Review the condition in a textbook and review the chart and nursing care plan.
   D. Assess the patient's knowledge about the condition and consult the physician.

*Case Study:* *You are the home care nurse assigned to a 65-year-old patient, John Grill, with chronic emphysema that has resulted in chronic obstructive*

*pulmonary disease (COPD). When you visit him, you see that he is using the accessory muscles for breathing and is in tripod position. Questions 29 to 35 relate to this scenario.*

**29.** Which of the following other physical assessment techniques would provide the most valuable information to assess his breathing?

   A. Inspection and vibration.
   B. Breath screening techniques and vital capacity measurements.
   C. Auscultation and percussion.
   D. Exertional effects on breathing and pursed-lip breathing.

**30.** Which of the following are signs of hypoxia?

   A. Decreased pulse rate, increased blood pressure, and capillary refill time of 4 seconds.
   B. Increased pulse rate, oxygen saturation of 88%, and circumoral cyanosis.
   C. Eupnea, oxygen saturation of 95%, and orthopnea.
   D. Pallor, hypotension, and bradypnea.

**31.** John has oxygen at 2 L/min ordered and is very short of breath when you come to administer his medications. He asks you, "Why has my doctor ordered such a low oxygen level because I obviously need more?" How would you respond?

   A. "I must follow the doctor's orders, so I will need to keep the oxygen at 2 L/min."
   B. "You need a low supplemental oxygen because oxygen is toxic to your condition."
   C. "Your body is stimulated to breathe by low oxygen levels, so you don't want to increase the level of oxygen."
   D. "Your body needs the extra carbon dioxide to stimulate respirations, so you should not increase the oxygen."

**32.** John's arterial blood gases (ABGs) are taken, and the results are $PO_2$ of 68 mm Hg, $PCO_2$ of 55 mm Hg, and pH of 7.3. What would these findings indicate?

   A. Hypoxemia, hypercapnia, and respiratory acidosis.
   B. High oxygen levels, increased carbon dioxide, and respiratory alkalosis.
   C. Anoxia, decreased carbon dioxide levels, and metabolic acidosis.
   D. Hypoxia, normal carbon dioxide levels, and normal acid–base balance.

33. What measures would assist with more effective breathing for John?

   A. Pursed-lip breathing exercises, coughing exercises, oxygen, and high Fowler's position.
   B. Deep apical breathing, low Fowler's position, and regular exercise and ambulation.
   C. Postural drainage, Trendelenburg position, incentive spirometer, and coughing.
   D. Maintaining a patent airway, stacked coughs, and supine position.

34. For the evaluation step of the nursing process, which charting notes would indicate nursing actions were effective in reducing breathing problems?

   A. Respirations at 26 breaths/min, circumoral cyanosis present, orthopneic.
   B. Anxiety decreased, oxygen saturation levels at 90%, nonproductive cough, respirations at 22 breaths/min.
   C. Disoriented; oxygen saturation levels at 85%; coughing large amount thick, white sputum; dyspnea on exertion.
   D. Edema of the extremities, laboured respirations, colour normal.

35. John develops signs of cor pulmonale. What observations would alert you to this condition?

   A. Irregular radial pulse and decreased pulse rate.
   B. Pulmonary edema.
   C. Edema of the extremities and distended neck veins.
   D. Decreased urine formation because of decreased arterial blood flow.

---

*Case Study: Jana, age 17 years, has developed glomerulonephritis 6 weeks after a strep sore throat. She has 400 cc/day of urine, headaches, and pitting edema. Her blood pressure is 146/90 mm Hg. She has been hospitalized to undergo diagnostic tests. Questions 36 to 38 relate to this scenario.*

36. Jana is unsure of function of the kidneys. How would you explain the function of the kidneys?

   A. The kidneys excrete wastes and maintain fluid and electrolyte balance.
   B. The kidneys are responsible for detoxifying foods and drugs and eliminating toxins.
   C. The kidneys strain urine and reabsorb waste products.
   D. The kidneys remove extra bicarbonate to help maintain the body in a slightly acid state.

37. Jana asks you about the role of the glomerulus. Which of the following is the most accurate description about the role of the glomerulus?

   A. The glomerulus filter allows a small amount of water through and then concentrates waste products of creatinine and urea and excretes them.
   B. The glomerulus filters out waste products, and the tubules reabsorb needed fluids, nutrients, and electrolytes.
   C. The glomerulus normally allows blood cells and protein to filter out then be reabsorbed.
   D. The primary purpose of the glomerulus is to reduce blood flow through the kidneys.

38. In addition to physical problems, which other psychosocial problems could likely affect Jana?

   A. Altered sexuality patterns related to surgical interventions.
   B. Impaired physical mobility related to bone reabsorption.
   C. Anxiety related to poorly functioning kidneys and body image disturbance.
   D. Altered breathing patterns related to dehydration.

39. You are asked to accurately assess urine output. Which of the following statements is true regarding urine output?

   A. Daily early morning weight helps to identify retention of fluids.
   B. If the patient perspires from a fever, there will be more urine output.
   C. The presence of pitting edema helps to determine dehydration.
   D. Urine output is decreased with glomerulonephritis.

---

*Case Study: Mr. James Maurice, age 46 years, is admitted with severe abdominal pain. He has a history of esophageal varices secondary to cirrhosis of the liver. Questions 40 to 46 relate to this scenario.*

40. When completing his physical assessment, what signs would alert you to an internal hemorrhage?

   A. Pulse, 110 bpm; temperature, 38.9°C; soft abdomen; sounds in all four quadrants.
   B. Pulse, 80 bpm; temperature, 37.3°C; pain in the right lower quadrant; constipation.
   C. Pulse, 108 bpm; temperature, 36.5°C; distended abdomen; nausea.
   D. Pulse, 60 bpm; temperature, 39°C; rebound tenderness in the right lower quadrant; diarrhea.

41. James has a gastrointestinal bleed and experiences hematemesis and cramping melena diarrhea. He is very anxious and afraid he will die. Laboratory reports are as follows: Hgb, 90 g/L; Hct, is 35%. What priorities are most important?

    A. Ensuring urine output is at least 1200 cc/24 hrs.
    B. Maintaining adequate tissue perfusion and oxygenation.
    C. Giving medications to reduce the cramps and diarrhea.
    D. Giving an antiemetic to lessen nausea and vomiting.

42. He asks you, "Will I make it?" How would you respond?

    A. "You'll be okay after the doctor has the bleeding under control."
    B. "That's a difficult question to answer. This must be very frightening for you."
    C. "Why? Do you think you're not going to make it?"
    D. "Chronic alcoholism has serious consequences."

43. James' blood is typed and cross-matched and for 3 U of packed cells. What are important precautions to take before initiating the packed cells?

    A. Initiate an IV with dextrose, take baseline vital signs, and check blood type.
    B. Initiate an IV with normal saline, take vital signs, and have two nurses check the blood type and identity.
    C. Warm the blood to room temperature, initiate an IV with dextrose, and take vital signs.
    D. Initiate an IV with normal saline, connect the packed cells, and take baseline vital signs.

44. When James' condition is stabilized, you ask him about his alcohol intake. What important aspects would you ask about?

    A. Amount of alcohol intake, physical symptoms indicating abuse, and whether he is in denial.
    B. Amount and pattern of alcohol intake, influence on employment, and influence on relationships.
    C. Whether he has had delirium tremens and how it has influenced his decision regarding alcohol intake.
    D. Whether he understands that his bleeding is a direct result of his alcoholism and that it means permanent damage has occurred.

45. When James' condition has been stabilized, you involve him in developing a plan of care. What would be important aspects to include in this plan?

    A. Identifying nursing goals and explaining the importance of following these goals.
    B. Discussing his goals and involving him in identifying and prioritizing important interventions.
    C. Informing him regarding the extent of damage to the liver and drawing up a contract to start his rehabilitative process.
    D. Identifying his potential and actual problems, informing him regarding his options, and arranging for him to attend Alcoholics Anonymous.

46. Twenty minutes after the packed cell transfusion is initiated, James complains of shivering, headache, and lower back pain. His vital signs show a normal temperature, increased pulse, and respiratory rate. What would you do?

    A. Stop the transfusion, continue with saline infusion, and notify the doctor regarding a suspected hemolytic reaction.
    B. Slow the transfusion, notify the doctor regarding a possible febrile reaction, and follow the doctor's orders.
    C. Slow the transfusion, give an antihistamine as ordered, and notify the doctor regarding a possible allergic reaction.
    D. Stop the transfusion, check the oxygen saturation levels, and check the urine volume.

47. A doctor in a clinic asks you to perform an IV insertion. You have not done an IV start for many years. What would you do?

    A. Quickly review the procedure and perform the IV insertion.
    B. Explain that you are unable to perform the IV start until you have completed an inservice and practice session on IV insertions.
    C. State that it is not within your scope of practice as a nurse working in a clinic.
    D. Explain that you do not have malpractice insurance to cover this skill.

48. You are working with a licensed practical nurse (LPN) and delegating the taking of vital signs for a preoperative patient. When you are reviewing the chart as the patient is leaving for the operating room, you note that the temperature is 38.4°C and the pulse 110 is bpm. What would you do?

    A. Have the LPN take the vital signs again, phone the operating room, and cancel the surgery.

B. Take the vital signs yourself and in the future do not delegate this preoperative responsibility.

C. Notify the surgeon and await his or her decision; reinforce with the LPN the importance of reporting abnormal preoperative vital signs.

D. Sign off the chart but flag that vital signs are abnormal; allow the patient to go down to the operating room.

49. You are on a surgical unit and have been assigned four patients. When you receive a report, you find out that you have a patient who had a transurethral resection of the prostate (TURP) today. A postoperative patient from yesterday is requesting pain medication. A patient with a postoperative infection needs to have an IV antibiotic given in 30 minutes. Another patient is to be discharged shortly when his family arrives. Which patient would be your first priority to complete an initial assessment?

A. The patient who had the TURP.

B. The patient requesting pain medication.

C. The patient with the postoperative infection to get IV medication ready.

D. The patient being discharged.

50. Mr. Jones, 78 years old, has Parkinson's disease. He slept very poorly last night, was nauseated when he got up this morning, and feels weak and tired. He eats a small portion of his breakfast. He is scheduled to go down to physiotherapy in 1 hour. What action should the nurse take?

A. Give him an antiemetic to reduce the nausea and get him up and dressed to go to physiotherapy.

B. Assess his nausea and sleep interferences; call the physiotherapy department to cancel or reschedule his appointment.

C. Notify the dietician to change his diet to clear fluids; cancel physiotherapy until his strength resumes.

D. Ask the dietician to visit with him regarding food preferences and recommend that the doctor order sleeping pills for him.

51. A nurse has been newly hired in an acute care hospital. What important guidelines should be used to ensure accountability for communications?

A. Knowing the organizational structure and the lines of communication for the new position.

B. Developing informal lines of communication with peer staff members.

C. Delegating responsibilities to allied health workers without knowing their scope of practice.

D. Relying on previous experience to determine the lines of communication.

52. There have been concerns that the patient assignment (workload allocation) on the unit has not been done fairly. You believe that this has made it very difficult to provide high-quality nursing care. The nursing unit manager calls a meeting to discuss concerns. Which of the following is the least appropriate professional response?

A. Giving your opinion and identifying the nurses who have the reduced workload.

B. Gathering information and examining the level of care required by different patients over a few weeks.

C. Participating in brainstorming what factors need to be considered when patient workload is determined.

D. Suggesting new ways for patient assignment allocation and taking responsibility for evaluating the results.

53. Which of the following is an example of social interaction rather than a therapeutic professional nursing interaction?

A. Considering the verbal and nonverbal messages and meaning expressed by a client.

B. Equal sharing of time for discussion of problems so there is mutuality in the relationship.

C. An interaction that involves facilitative qualities of caregivers, including empathy, respect, and empowerment.

D. An interaction used to assess the coping abilities of the person and views regarding health.

54. Mrs. Piazza, age 32 years, had a breast biopsy that was positive for adenocarcinoma, and she is scheduled for a mastectomy. She has two young children and is very concerned with her prognosis. She states that she feels at an "all time low in my life" and wants to know ways to help her adjust to this news. Which question or statement would best assess her coping abilities?

A. "Why are you so worried? Wait until the surgery is done, and then you will have a better idea of the extent of the cancer."

B. "What ways have you used to help reduce stress and help you cope with significant events in your life?"

C. "Could you get some spiritual help from your church or pastor?"

D. "You've managed well in your life so far. For the sake of your children, I know you will handle this situation capably."

55. Mrs. Lemongrass, a 42-year-old First Nations resident from the local reserve, has been admitted with non–insulin-dependent diabetes mellitus. She asks to have her local medicine man come and help her decide what traditional aboriginal medicines could help her. What would you do?

A. Tell her that traditional healing methods are not likely to work for control of diabetes.

B. Suggest that she inform and discuss with her doctor how traditional therapies could be integrated into her plan of care.

C. Let her know she has a choice and needs to make a decision as to whether she uses traditional or medical means to control her diabetes.

D. Recommend that she wait until her diabetes is under control and she is discharged before she starts using traditional medicines.

56. What important considerations would you make when teaching and caring for a newly diagnosed 13-year-old young woman with diabetes mellitus?

A. Involving her in the development of the teaching plan and encouraging her to question and actively participate.

B. Informing her regarding all the complications that could occur if she is noncompliant.

C. Allowing her to develop the teaching plan and assess her own readiness to learn about different aspects about the disease.

D. Having her work closely with another teenager who has diabetes to learn about the condition and control.

57. Mr. Arndt, age 67 years, has recently been prescribed a diuretic to help control his blood pressure. He was up four times during the night to go to the bathroom. He says that he didn't sleep all night long. He is refusing to take his 40-mg dose of furosemide the next morning. What actions would you take?

A. Reinforce the reason he is taking the medication. Respect his decision if he still refuses the medication and chart his refusal.

B. Take his blood pressure and warn him about the dangers of an increased blood pressure.

C. Tell him that the extra fluid will be gone and he won't be going to the bathroom as much now.

D. Reinforce how much his edema has decreased and how effective the medication has been and encourage him to take the medication.

58. You are caring for a patient who has returned from the operating room after an exploratory laparotomy. He has had 150 cc/hr of IV solution. He has not voided for 8 hours. Postoperative orders read: "Catheterize prn. Conservative measures to stimulate voiding have not been successful." What assessments and actions should you take?

A. Palpate all four abdominal quadrants and assess his intake and output record.

B. Inspect and palpate the lower abdomen; if it is distended and uncomfortable, insert a straight catheter.

C. Give him pain medication and catheterize him as soon as possible to lessen the possibility of a bladder and kidney infection.

D. Wait until the patient experiences considerable discomfort in the bladder region and then catheterize him.

---

***Case Study:*** *Carla Jenna, a single 24-year-old mother of a 3-month-old baby, has been admitted with deep vein thrombosis in her left leg. Her left leg is edematized and cold. She has a heparin drip running. She becomes very agitated and states that she is nursing her baby and needs to leave the hospital to help her mother take care of her baby. Questions 59 to 61 relate to this scenario.*

59. How would you respond to this patient?

A. Inform her that she needs to make a choice in resolving her health problems or taking care of her baby.

B. Explain the importance of the Heparin in resolving the thrombosis and examine ways that her baby could room in with assistance from her mother.

C. Call the doctor to help resolve the situation in the best interests of the patient.

D. Call the social worker to arrange child care alternatives.

60. Which of the following would not be an appropriate response to Carla's needs?

A. Involving her in a plan of care and working with her to identify her priority needs.

B. Working with her to establish target dates for resolution of her problems and realistic discharge goals.

C. Letting her decide which nursing measures are most important and implementing these measures.

D. Explaining the rationale for nursing measures and involving her in the timing of these measures.

61. After care measures have been implemented, important follow-up would include:

A. Document the list of problems that have been identified.

B. Individualize the care plan according to your evaluation and document care measures and the patient's response.

C. Document the evaluation of the effectiveness of care given and identify the strengths and challenges experienced as well as your plan for revisions.

D. Reassess the client and redevelop the care plan based on the reassessment.

---

**Case Study:** *Mrs. Snow, age 74 years, has recently had a cerebrovascular accident (CVA) and is on an acute care medical unit. She has left-sided hemiparesis, is hoping to regain the strength in her left side, and is anxious to be able to go home. Questions 62 to 67 relate to this scenario.*

62. What would be important nursing measures after the CVA?

A. Perform passive range of motion on both sides and turn the patient from the supine position to the left lateral and then right lateral position every 4 hours.

B. Perform active range of motion on both sides and reposition the patient from the supine to the prone position every 2 hours.

C. Perform passive range of motion exercises on the left side and turn the patient from the supine to the right lateral position every 2 hours.

D. Perform isometric exercises on the affected side, reposition the patient from the right lateral to left lateral position and then to the supine position, ensuring that you support the affected leg in external rotation.

63. Mrs. Snow states that she has an aching pain in her back and finds it difficult to get comfortable when she is lying on her back. She refuses to take any medications for pain. What actions would you take to alleviate her back pain?

A. Suggest that she only alternate sidelying positions to lessen the back pain and give her back a rest.

B. Provide lumbar support when in the supine position, offer her a back rub, and check regarding the possibility of heat treatments to relieve the pain.

C. Reinforce the importance of changing positions and the possibility of pressure ulcer formation.

D. Encourage her to take the medications so she can get optimal rest.

64. Which health team members could assist in achieving her goals?

A. Social worker and respiratory technologist.

B. Nursing aid and Meals on Wheels.

C. Physiotherapist and occupational therapist.

D. Home care nurse attendant and radiology technician.

65. What are important nursing responsibilities when a referral to other health team members has been made?

A. Ensuring that the physician reports the level of functioning of the patient.

B. Recommending that each health team member independently completes his or her own assessment and determination of problems and then consult with each other.

C. Recommend that each member read the history and nurse's notes to understand the patient's progress.

D. Sharing assessment information and information on the patient's capability and level of participation in meeting activities of daily living.

66. Mrs. Snow is anxious to know when the rehabilitation process can begin. You would reinforce that:

A. "Rehabilitation will start as soon as your discharge date has been confirmed."

B. "We will begin exercises and turning now and start getting you up walking after your condition has stabilized."

C. "You will be responsible for exercising your weak side after your condition has stabilized."

D. "Rehabilitation is a long process, and it's most important that you rest and recuperate at this time."

67. The home care coordinator is planning a home visit in preparation for Mrs. Snow's discharge to her home. Mrs. Snow has been performing the following activities with minimal assistance: dressing, bathing at the sink, basic cooking, ambulation with a walker, and toileting. What

would be important environmental assessments for the home care coordinator to include?

A. Checking the cleanliness of the home, ensuring removal of clutter, and organizing all essentials on one level of the house.

B. Reinforcing the importance of having renovations done before discharge to enable wheelchair access and accessibility to all needs for daily living.

C. Checking access to the home with a walker, access and safety measures in the bathroom, and access to food preparation in the kitchen and ensuring safety in her sleeping environment.

D. Ordering a wheelchair, special utensils, and .a raised toilet seat and rearranging the furniture in her home.

## ) Care of Adults and Older Adults Short Answer Questions

**Case Study:** *Olga Proznik, age 60 years, has been admitted to the unit. Upon admission, she tells you that she had a mini stroke, and the doctor's history indicates the differential diagnosis of transient ischemic attack (TIA). She had right-sided paresis and was unable to speak for 1 hour. Questions 68 to 71 relate to this scenario.*

68. Identify two possible causes of TIA. (2 points)

69. Mrs. Proznik's daughter states that she is relieved that her prayers have been answered and that her mother's problems have been resolved. How would you respond to her and inform her of the possible risk factors? (1 point)

70. The mother and daughter want to know what they can change in their lifestyle. Identify two

modifiable risk factors that contribute to CVAs. (2 points)

71. The doctor has ordered ticlopidine (Ticlid). State the reason this medication is administered. (1 point)

**Case Study:** *Mrs. Marge Evenrude, age 88 years, is admitted to the unit from the emergency department after having a cerebrovascular accident (CVA) affecting the right side of her body. She is aphasic and chokes when taking fluids. Her daughter was at her home and witnessed the CVA 2 hours ago. The doctor has ordered IV tissue plasminogen activator (TPA) to be given. Questions 72 and 73 relate to this scenario.*

72. Identify the reason for TPA and why accuracy of timing is important with this medication. (2 points)

a) Reason:

b) Accuracy of timing:

73. Identify three priority nursing assessments to complete after a client initially presents with a CVA. (3 points)

## ) Child Health Multiple-Choice Questions

74. The nurse is aware that the parents of a child newly diagnosed with juvenile arthritis require more health teaching when the mother states:

A. "I help my child perform daily range of motion exercises."

B. "I give my child NSAIDs only when she is having pain."

C. "I apply heat pads to the joints when my child is having pain."

D. "I encourage my child to attend school regularly."

75. A public health nurse is providing an information session focusing on injury prevention for young children diagnosed with juvenile arthritis. Of the information offered below, what should be included in this session?

    A. Parents should promote rest by doing most of the child's activities for them.
    B. Children should not attend school but be homeschooled instead.
    C. Children should be encouraged to run and play at will to expend energy.
    D. Daily range of motion exercises are required to support joint mobility.

76. Identify a common method of evaluating the urine output for newborns, infants, and toddlers who are not potty trained.

    A. Weighing the child before and after feeds.
    B. Weighing the diaper before and after micturition.
    C. Weighing the child before and after micturition.
    D. Measuring the formula before the child ingests it.

77. Which of the following describes the cause of cystic fibrosis?

    A. It is inherited as an autosomal dominant trait.
    B. It is inherited as an autosomal recessive trait.
    C. Its inheritance is based on the gestational age of the newborn.
    D. Its inheritance is affected by the child's gender.

78. A 16-year-old teen has been diagnosed with a basal skull fracture following a motor vehicle accident. The teen presents with increasing drowsiness and is febrile. Which is the teen most at risk for developing?

    A. Meningitis.
    B. Pneumonia.
    C. Renal failure.
    D. Paralytic ileus.

79. Which cranial nerve is being assessed when the nurse asks the child to repeat a whispered word?

    A. I.
    B. IV.

C. VIII.

D. X.

*Case Study:* A 12-year-old girl presents complaining of severe right lower quadrant pain. Her pulse and respirations are elevated, and she has localized tenderness and sluggish bowel sounds. Questions 80 to 82 relate to this scenario.

80. After being attended to in the emergency department for a short time, the child states that the pain has suddenly resolved and she feels better. Which of the following would the nurse suspect?

    A. Ruptured appendix.
    B. Gastroenteritis.
    C. Celiac disease.
    D. Food allergies.

81. What would be the priority treatment at this point?

    A. Preparation for emergency surgery.
    B. Initiation of antibiotic therapy.
    C. Referral for dietary revision.
    D. Modification of pain management strategies.

82. The child has been prescribed a 3-day course of treatment of gentamicin sulfate while recuperating. Which of the following manifestations would indicate that the child is developing gentamicin toxicity?

    A. Decreased renal output.
    B. Electrolyte disturbances.
    C. Joint discomfort.
    D. Visual disturbances.

83. You are taking the health history of an 8-year-old boy. His mother states that he continually has a cold all winter with a runny nose. He is not doing well in school and is itching all the time. The nurse suspects the child has

    A. Allergies.
    B. Sinusitis.
    C. Ringworm.
    D. Fifth disease.

*Case Study:* You have just admitted a 9-year-old child pulled from a house fire with a full-thickness burn involving the epidermis, dermis, and underlying subcutaneous tissue. Questions 84 to 86 relate to this scenario.

84. The child is not in pain. Identify the category of burn the child has:

    A. First degree.
    B. Second degree.
    C. Third degree.
    D. Fourth degree.

85. Based on the above information, identify the priority nursing diagnosis for this client.

    A. Body image disturbance.
    B. Risk for altered nutrition.
    C. Impaired social interaction.
    D. Impaired skin integrity.

86. The child's face, neck, and chest area are involved in the burns. Identify the priority potential health concern in this situation.

    A. Facial abnormalities.
    B. Airway obstruction.
    C. Localized pain.
    D. Ulceration.

87. A child who fell through ice and was submerged for longer than 1 minute is admitted to the emergency department with hypothermia near drowning. At which point will you best be able to determine the child's outcome status?

    A. Three days after the incident.
    B. As soon as CPR is successfully initiated.
    C. As soon as the patient is warmed.
    D. After the parents' initial visit.

88. Despite continuous health teaching, a 13-year-old boy will only use his left thigh for insulin administration. The nurse is aware this is happening because:

    A. The child is exerting control over the situation.
    B. This is attention-seeking behaviour.
    C. Repeatedly using the same site is less painful.
    D. The child is afraid of scarring.

89. Which age group would most likely identify their pain as punishment for past behaviour?

    A. Infant (age 9–12 months).
    B. Preschool or toddler (age 2–5 years).
    C. Children (age 6 –11 years).
    D. Adolescents (age 12–17 years).

*Case Study:* A nurse has admitted a 1-year-old patient to the unit with a diagnosis of influenza. Questions 90 and 91 relate to this scenario.

90. The nurse can anticipate which type of precautions will be required while caring for this child?

    A. Standard precautions.
    B. Airborne precautions.
    C. Droplet precautions.
    D. Contact precautions.

91. While hospitalized, this child develops a *Clostridium difficile* infection. The nurse can anticipate adding which of the following types of precautions?

    A. Standard precautions.
    B. Airborne precautions.
    C. Droplet precautions.
    D. Contact precautions.

92. You are caring for a 9-year-old hospitalized child who has a poor appetite, and your nursing interventions are focused on increasing the child's fluid intake. Identify the choice below that is least likely to be successful in meeting your patient's goal.

    A. Offering small glasses of fluid.
    B. Offering frequent ice chips.
    C. Offering popsicles and gelatine.
    D. Offering milkshakes and cream soups.

93. Methylphenidate hydrochloride (Ritalin) has been prescribed for a 6-year-old child with attention deficit hyperactivity disorder. Health teaching for the child' parents will include which of the following statements?

    A. "You will see a positive response to Ritalin in approximately 8 weeks."
    B. "You should give the dose to your child right before his evening bedtime."
    C. "Extended-release tablets may be crushed or chewed."
    D. "If discontinued, Ritalin must be tapered off slowly."

94. A 3-year-old African Canadian child presents to the physician's office with a protruding abdomen and icteric sclera and is febrile. The nurse suspects which of the following?

    A. Iron deficiency anemia.
    B. Sickle cell anemia.
    C. Pernicious anemia.
    D. Aplastic anemia.

95. Identify the situation that would potentially be most upsetting to a 5-year-old autistic child.

    A. Separation from his parents.
    B. The sound of a fire truck on the street.

C. Moving his toy box across the room.

D. The sound of music playing.

96. A 14-year-old young woman is brought to the emergency department with a lacerated finger. During her assessment, the nurse notices bruises of varying stages of healing on various areas of the teen's trunk and arms. The teen tells the nurse that, on occasion, her father hits her. She asks that the nurse not tell anyone. Which of the following statements is the most appropriate response from the nurse?

A. "I understand you want me to keep this a secret, but there is a legal obligation for health care providers to report suspected or real abuse."

B. "I understand you want me to keep this a secret. I will honour that."

C. "I will keep this a secret from your father, but I must tell your mother."

D. "I will tell the doctor about the bruises to see if she wants an x-ray ordered."

97. A 16-year-old young woman comes into the sexual health clinic and asks an RN for condoms. She asks that the nurse not tell her mother that she was there. What is the appropriate response by the nurse?

A. "I am bound by confidentiality not to tell anyone about your visit."

B. "If you were my daughter, I would want to know."

C. "Are you embarrassed that you are sexually active?"

D. "The doctor will need to speak to your mother before you get this prescription."

## ▶ Child Health
## Short Answer Questions

98. Identify the most common pathogen causing urinary tract infections in the pediatric population. (1 point)

99. A nurse is waiting in the checkout line of the grocery store and overhears an individual in front of her speaking about a pediatric client she is caring for in the home care setting. She mentions the client and the client's family by name and discusses the client's diagnosis. List two things the nurse in the line should do. (2 points)

100. Identify three nursing interventions directed at providing chronically ill school-age children with a sense of autonomy. (3 points)

## ▶ Maternal–Child Health
## Multiple-Choice Questions

101. Krista is 33 weeks pregnant. She tells the nurse that she was exposed to environmental toxins a few weeks ago and is concerned that it may cause abnormal fetal development. Which of the following is the nurse's correct response to Krista about when the embryo or fetus is most susceptible to teratogenic agents?

A. In the first 2 weeks after the first day of the last menstrual period (LMP).

B. At 15 to 60 days after conception.

C. At 16 to 20 weeks of the pregnancy.

D. At 32 to 36 weeks gestation.

102. Barbara's first child was born with spina bifida (a neural tube defect). Which of the following nurse's recommendations is appropriate as a supplement to Barbara's diet?

A. Iron.

B. Calcium.

C. Folic acid.

D. Vitamin K.

103. Norma is concerned about nutrition during pregnancy because she does not have much of an appetite. Which of the following is the nurse's best response to Norma?

A. "Pregnant women should increase their daily intake of all vitamins and minerals."

B. "Current research has shown that the amount of weight gained is not important."

C. "The placenta of underweight women will ensure adequate nutrition for the fetus."

D. "Supplements may be necessary to meet recommended amounts of vitamins and minerals."

104. Paula asks the nurse, "I smoke one pack of cigarettes a day. Will smoking hurt my baby?" Which of the following is the nurse's best explanation for why smoking is harmful to the fetus?
    A. "Yes. Carbon monoxide binds with the red blood cells, reducing the amount of oxygen they can carry to the baby."
    B. "Yes. Nicotine produces a variety of toxins in the mother's body, which can be harmful to the fetus."
    C. "Yes. Smoke will disrupt normal renal function in the pregnant woman and impede waste disposal for the fetus."
    D. "Yes. Nicotine damages the alveolar tissues of the fetus and will contribute to respiratory difficulties in the newborn."

105. Jill is 10 weeks pregnant with her first baby. Which of the following presumptive signs of pregnancy would the nurse expect to find when performing this assessment?
    A. Amenorrhea.
    B. Bluish discoloration of the vagina and the cervix.
    C. Fetal heart sounds.
    D. Positive pregnancy test.

106. Barbara is experiencing Braxton Hicks contractions in her third trimester of pregnancy. She asks the nurse the reason for having these contractions. Which of the following nurse's responses is correct about Braxton Hicks contractions?
    A. "They provide practice for true uterine contractions during labour."
    B. "They serve no practical purpose."
    C. "They generate increased muscle mass and enhance myometrial tone."
    D. "They enhance movement of blood through intervillous spaces."

107. Amira is a woman in the home-based, high-risk antenatal community care program with a diagnosis of hypertension in pregnancy. At the first home visit, the nurse discovers several warning signs of pregnancy that must be immediately investigated. Which of the following factors does not require immediate investigation?
    A. Vaginal bleeding.
    B. Nausea.
    C. Blurred vision.
    D. Severe headache.

108. Which of the following responses by the nurse would be most effective in helping a pregnant woman who is experiencing nausea and vomiting?
    A. "Drink fluids when feeling nauseated."
    B. "Increase intake of foods high in fat."
    C. "Eat your largest meal in the evening."
    D. "Eat dry, starchy foods upon awakening."

109. Angelina, age 29 years and in the third trimester of her first pregnancy, asks the nurse for advice about upper respiratory discomforts. Angelina complains of nasal stuffiness, nosebleeds, and shortness of breath. Which response by the nurse is correctly related to the cause of the symptoms?
    A. "It sounds like you are coming down with a cold. I'll ask the care physician to prescribe a safe medication for relief of symptoms"
    B. "A good vaporizer will help; avoid the hot steam kind. Also, try spending less time lying on your left side"
    C. "You are experiencing the results of increased blood supply; one of the pregnancy hormones, estrogen, causes them."
    D. "This is most unusual. I'm sure your obstetrician will want you to see an ear, nose, and throat specialist."

110. Lauren, whose pregnancy is at 41 weeks gestation, tells the nurse she has felt eight fetal movements in the past 24 hours. The number of fetal movements is:
    A. Normal and not concerning.
    B. Serious and requires intervention.
    C. Not a reliable indicator of fetal well-being.
    D. Only accurate when used in conjunction with a stress test.

111. A triage nurse is completing an initial assessment of the women in the waiting room. Which of the following statements helps the nurse to correctly recognize that a woman is in true labour?
    A. "I passed some thick, red-tinged mucus when I urinated this morning."
    B. "My baby dropped, and I have to urinate more frequently now."
    C. "The contractions in my uterus are 3 minutes apart and last 2 minutes each."
    D. "My bag of waters just broke."

112. For which of the following women is it appropriate for a nurse to perform a vaginal examination?
    A. A multiparous woman presenting at 32 weeks gestation in early labour with ruptured membranes.

B. A primigravida at 38 weeks gestation who has leaking membranes and is not in labour.

C. A multiparous woman with ruptured membranes presenting at 39 weeks gestation who is not in labour with a cervix dilated to approximately 3 cm.

D. A primigravida at 38 weeks gestation with ruptured membranes, 90-second contractions every 2 minutes, and a pronounced "bloody show."

113. Mrs. Willson tells the nurse that her last menstrual period (LMP) was February 1, 2008. Using Nägele's rule, what is Mrs. Willson's due date or estimated date of confinement (EDC)?

A. November 1, 2008.
B. November 8, 2008.
C. December 1, 2008.
D. December 8, 2008.

114. A married couple lives in a single-family house with their newborn daughter and the husband's daughter from a previous marriage. Based on the information given, which of the following family forms best describes this family?

A. Blended family.
B. Extended family.
C. Nuclear family.
D. Same-sex family.

115. Which of the following pregnancy situations does the nurse recognize as having the greatest risk for the fetus?

A. A fundal height of 27 cm at 32 weeks gestation.
B. A fetal heart rate of 170 bpm with fetal movements.
C. A breech lie.
D. A gestational birth age of 37 weeks.

---

*Case Study:* Mrs. Nyguen calls the labour and birth unit and tells the nurse that she is due in 4 weeks. She is concerned that despite a healthy pregnancy, the baby is not moving very much today. Questions 116 and 117 relate to this scenario.

116. Upon further questioning, the nurse learns that Mrs. Nyguen has just completed 1 hour of fetal kick counting, and only four movements were experienced. Which of the following is the nurse's most appropriate response?

A. Instruct the mother to contact her primary care provider in the morning.
B. Instruct the mother to come in immediately for evaluation.

C. Advise her that this is normal and she doesn't need to count anymore.
D. Instruct her to continue counting for 1 more hour and call back with the results.

117. Mrs. Nyguen arrives at the hospital later that evening. The nurse obtains a fundal height measurement of 30 cm. The nurse is alerted to which of the following possibilities?

A. Transverse lie.
B. IUGR.
C. Stillbirth.
D. Placenta previa.

---

*Case Study:* Marie-Claire is a single mother, age 22 years, gravid 3, para 2, and 8 weeks pregnant. She tells the emergency room nurse that she was attacked and raped a few hours ago. Questions 118 and 119 relate to this scenario.

118. Marie-Claire is exhibiting behaviours associated with fear, denial, and anger. Which of the following actions should the nurse perform immediately?

A. Contact the client's family members.
B. Assure her that everything will be fine.
C. Create a safe and secure atmosphere.
D. Explain the process of collecting legal evidence.

119. Marie-Claire tells the nurse that she works as an "escort" to support her two young children. Based on this information, the nurse recognizes that a gonorrhea culture should be obtained. What is the nurse's rationale for why a gonorrhea culture should be obtained?

A. Gonorrhea testing is required by federal law.
B. Increased number of partners increases the risk of gonorrhea.
C. Infection is usually associated with HIV infection.
D. All women with gonorrhea are initially asymptomatic.

120. When asked by the student nurse why the nurse included the parents in the initial newborn assessment, which of the following nurse's responses would be most accurate?

A. To teach the parents the importance of newborn assessment.
B. To foster prenatal independence in the baby's care.
C. To increase maternal and paternal role attainment.

D. To support collaborative relationships with family members.

## ▶ Maternal–Child Health
## Short Answer Questions

*Case Study:* Trista is 34 years old, gravida 3, para 2, and had a 28-hour labour and delivery. She has been transferred to the postpartum unit. Questions 121 and 122 relate to this scenario.

121. The nurse has begun Trista's postpartum assessment. Identify three nursing interventions that the nurse will implement when assessing Trista for postpartum hemorrhage. (3 points)

122. Postpartum hemorrhage may be classified as being of early or late onset. Describe the time of onset of early postpartum hemorrhage and list four factors that may cause an early postpartum hemorrhage. (4 points)

## ▶ Mental Health
## Multiple-Choice Questions

*Case Study:* Rosalind is a nurse leading an insight-oriented group therapy session in an outpatient mental health program for clients with mood and anxiety disorders. Questions 123 to 125 relate to this scenario.

123. During the group session, a client, Stuart, is restless and is starting to make sarcastic remarks to others in the therapy session. Rosalind responds by saying, "Stuart, you look angry." Rosalind is using which of the following communication techniques:

A. Reaffirming.
B. Clarification.
C. Mirroring.
D. Making observations.

124. During this insight group, another member, Shannon, demands a lot of attention, interrupts

others, and talks most of the time. Rosalind's best response to Shannon would be:

A. Ignore the behaviour, allowing Shannon to vent her feelings.
B. "Shannon, I imagine I speak for the group when I say I am frustrated with your behaviour."
C. "I invite you to briefly summarize your point, Shannon, so that we can hear from others."
D. "I find that your behaviour drains the group, Shannon."

125. Rosalind's insight-oriented group therapy is proceeding well, but certain members of the group are starting to ignore the group agreements to remain neutral and not socialize with each other in their off-therapy time. For instance, Shannon and Stuart have been having coffee after group sessions and gossip about other group participants. Unhealthy personal boundaries can be a result of unhealthy role modeling and dysfunctional family arrangements, and boundary problems can also occur where there has been a pattern of:

A. Consistent limit setting.
B. Abuse and neglect.
C. Attention and direction.
D. Supportive environments.

*Case Study:* Marcie and her boyfriend, Ryan, are in a single vehicle motorcycle accident, and the ambulance brings them to the emergency department (ED). Ryan is unconscious on arrival to the hospital and very badly hurt, but Marcie, who was driving, has only minor cuts and bruises. After being treated for her minor injuries, Marcie begins to exhibit symptoms of acute anxiety in the ED. Questions 126 to 128 relate to this scenario.

126. After being treated for minor cuts, Marcie appears confused and has trouble focusing on what the nurse is saying. She complains of nausea and dizziness, has tachycardia, and is hyperventilating as the nurse interviews her. She tells the nurse that she feels as though something awful is going to happen. The nurse should assess Marcie's level of anxiety as:

A. Mild.
B. Moderate.
C. Severe.
D. Panic.

127. Marcie appears confused and has trouble focusing on what the nurse is saying. She complains

of nausea and dizziness, has tachycardia, and is hyperventilating as the nurse interviews her. She tells the nurse that she feels as though she is having a heart attack. What anxiety relief behaviour is Marcie using?

A. Acting out.
B. Somatisation.
C. Withdrawal.
D. Problem solving.

128. Marcie is displaying considerable anxiety, including scattering of attention, dizziness, nausea, tachycardia, and hyperventilation. What statement would indicate that the nurse is reacting to Marcie's relief behaviour rather than her needs?

A. "It must have been a frightening experience to be in an accident."
B. "Accidents can result in all kinds of feelings. It must have been scary."
C. "I'll stay with you in case you would like to share your feelings with me."
D. "There is nothing physically wrong with you. You need to stop breathing so rapidly."

---

*Case Study:* Randy is a former soldier who served in Rwanda. Since being discharged from military service, Randy has been chronically unemployed and has a history of explosive anger and depression. Questions 129 to 131 relate to this scenario.

129. In a mental health interview, Randy reports feeling ashamed of being "weak" and of letting past experiences control his thoughts and actions in the present. What is the nurse's best response?

A. "It isn't too late for you to make changes in your life."
B. "Weak people don't want to make changes in their lives."
C. "No one can predict how he or she will react in a traumatic situation"
D. "Many people who have been in your situation experience similar emotions and behaviours."

130. Randy has been diagnosed with posttraumatic stress disorder (PTSD). Which of the following characteristics best describe the hallmark symptoms associated with PTSD?

A. Anger, guilt, and humiliation.
B. Flashbacks, recurring dreams, and numbness.
C. Fatigue and self-blame.
D. Denial of the event.

131. Three months after receiving his diagnosis of PTSD, Randy returns to the mental health clinic complaining of fear, loss of control, and feelings of helplessness. Which nursing intervention is most appropriate for Randy?

A. Allowing Randy time to heal.
B. Exploring the meaning of the traumatic event with Randy.
C. Giving sleep medication as prescribed to restore a normal sleep–wake cycle.
D. Recommending a high-protein, low-fat diet.

---

*Case Study:* Isabella is a 43-year-old married woman who has called in sick to work for the past 3 days. When she returns to work, her makeup cannot conceal the bruises on her face. A coworker who is a good friend to Isabella mentions the bruises and tells her that they look like the kind of bruises she used to get herself when her ex-husband used to beat her. Isabella claims the bruises were a result of "an accident. My husband just had a terrible day at his work. He's being so kind and gentle now. Yesterday he brought me flowers. He says he is going to get a new job, so it will never happen again." Questions 132 and 133 relate to this scenario.

132. Which phase of the cycle of violence does Isabella's response represent:

A. Phase 1, the tension-building phase.
B. Phase 2, the acute battering incident.
C. Phase 3, the honeymoon phase.
D. Phase 4, the resolution phase.

133. Isabella's coworker suggests that she seek assistance from their employee assistance program. Isabella refuses because she believes her husband has reformed. What is the *best* alternative suggestion her coworker can make at this point?

A. File for divorce.
B. Get a restraining order against her husband.
C. Carry the number of the distress centre and have the address of the nearest safe house for women.
D. Carry a weapon for protection.

134. What sort of role does the milieu plays in therapy initiated with clients admitted to an inpatient unit?

A. The milieu provides example of the consequences of one's behaviours so that rewards and punishments may aid the client's learning in a realistic manner.

B. The milieu is one of comfort and caregiving such that staff attend to the basic needs of inpatient clients.

C. The environment is irrelevant; the quality of psychotherapy is the foundation of the inpatient treatment program.

D. The therapeutic environment is structured so that stressors are used as opportunities for assessment and learning.

135. Howard, an elderly male client, is admitted to the hospital for dehydration. Although he lives in his son's basement, he was not accompanied by any family to the hospital, and a neighbour called for the ambulance when Howard fell in the front yard bringing in the mail. On admission, Howard is poorly dressed, has body odour, appears unkempt, and has unexplained bruises. The nurse's priority action will be to:

A. Inquire about medications.

B. Assess the history of the present illness.

C. Determine if Howard is experiencing abuse or neglect.

D. Ensure that Howard is given a bath.

136. In assessing an adolescent client at your clinic, you are able to recognize that depression in adolescents is often:

A. Similar in symptomatology to that of adult clients.

B. Often masked by aggressive behaviours.

C. Situational and not as serious as that of adult clients.

D. A sign that the teenager needs to be admitted to the hospital.

137. When working with clients in crisis, the nurse must be aware that crisis intervention differs from other forms of therapeutic intervention in that crisis intervention focuses on:

A. Determining the pathology that is the underlying reason for ineffective coping.

B. Exploring past experiences with a goal of self-actualization.

C. Immediate problems, as perceived by the client, with the short-term goal of problem solving.

D. Interpreting unconscious processes with the goal of personality integration.

138. Julie is a nurse working with clients at an urgent response mental health clinic. When working with clients in crisis, which of the following is *most* important in her initial assessment?

A. Determining the client's role in the emergence of the crisis.

B. Obtaining a complete assessment of the client's history.

C. Remaining focused on the immediate problem.

D. Assisting the client in identifying and gaining insight around how this crisis is similar to others in the client's life.

139. Carlynn, a 19-year-old female client, unknown to the psychiatric inpatient unit staff, is placed on one-on-one observations after a suicide attempt. As the nurse follows Carlynn into the bathroom, she objects strongly, yelling, "Leave me alone! I'm tired of being followed around and being watched like a child who can't be trusted." The nurse's best response would be:

A. "Yelling at me won't change the rules, and if you talk about suicide, then this is the rule."

B. "I understand that you are angry, but I must be able to see you at all times to make sure you are safe."

C. "Things would improve if you would concentrate on the positive things rather than the things that are getting you down."

D. "Because you are doing better, I will just wait outside the bathroom, and you can close the door until you are finished."

140. Bill comes to the walk-in mental health clinic in his neighbourhood health centre for assistance after being involved in clean-up efforts after a shooting at a local high school. Bill says he has been feeling anxious since his involvement in these efforts and is having some difficulty sleeping. The nurse working with Bill should choose which of the following to help him cope with the experience?

A. Advise him to avoid going back to work or anywhere near the school for at least 60 days.

B. Create an opportunity for Bill to talk about his experience, ask how he has coped thus far, and explore enhanced coping skills.

C. Arrange for spiritual counselling from his priest.

D. Send him to the emergency department for further evaluation because he is experiencing a crisis situation, which is an emergency.

## ▶ Mental Health Short Answer Questions

141. A nurse is discussing the use of monoamine oxidase inhibitors (MAOIs) with a client in the acute care setting. The nurse must emphasize

that the biggest complication with this class of drug is _____. (1 point)

142. What foods must someone taking MAOIs be advised to avoid? (2 points)

143. What are two hallmark symptoms of attention deficit hyperactivity disorder (ADHD)? (2 points)

## ▶ Answers and Rationales

## COMPREHENSIVE PRACTICE EXAM I

**1. B.** The worker has the appropriate knowledge and skills.

*Rationale*
The RN is accountable for his or her actions and for the delegation of tasks to UHCWs. The RN delegates tasks to UHCWs consistent with their level of expertise and education, the job description, agency policy, legislation, and personal need. Based on the choices offered, if the RN is confident that the UHCW has the appropriate knowledge regarding the task, the task can be delegated.

*Classification*
Competency Category: Professional Practice
Taxonomic Level: Knowledge/Comprehension

**2. C.** Discuss the overheard conversation directly with John.

*Rationale*
Planning to meet a client for a social event while she is still a patient could blur the boundaries of the therapeutic relationship, which may result in an unhealthy outcome for the client. Angela should take John aside and point out that this behaviour is inappropriate and not in the client's best interest.

*Classification*
Competency Category: Professional Practice
Taxonomic Level: Application

**3. C.** To protect the safety of the public.

*Rationale*
Provincial and territorial governing bodies, professional regulations, and laws are in place to protect the public by ensuring that nurses are accountable for safe, competent, and ethical nursing practice.

*Classification*
Competency Category: Professional Practice
Taxonomic Level: Knowledge/Comprehension

**4. D.** Appropriate because the focus of a therapeutic relationship is on the client.

*Rationale*
Every nurse has the responsibility to practice in a manner that is consistent with providing safe, competent, and ethical care. If John had shared his personal information with Jessica, he would have crossed the boundary of a therapeutic relationship and changed the focus of the discussion from a client focus to a social focus. It is very important in all areas of care, but especially in the mental health setting, that the relationship between the nurse and the patient has very clear boundaries and is client focused.

*Classification*
Competency Category: Nurse–Person Relationship
Taxonomic Level: Application

**5. B.** "I must stay with you until we are sure you are not going to hurt yourself."

*Rationale*
Jessica is depressed and has expressed suicidal thoughts. She has been placed on constant supervision as required by unit policy. Staying with Jessica, even when she is in the bathroom, demonstrates an understanding of constant observation and exercises professional judgment regarding the policy and the situation.

*Classification*
Competency Category: Nurse–Person Relationship
Taxonomic Level: Application

**6. B.** "Before you leave the hospital, I will make sure you have the information about the crisis centre."

*Rationale*
The nurse realizes that in addition to crossing boundaries within the therapeutic relationship if they met for coffee, it would not be consistent with promoting

health and wellness. Providing the number for the crisis worker at the crisis centre is an example of promoting a healthy strategy if Jessica feels she is becoming depressed again.

*Classification*
Competency Category: Professional Practice
Taxonomic Level: Application

**7. A.** Inappropriate; it would be considered neglect of duty.

*Rationale*
Andrew was scheduled to visit the client, and the client expected the visit, as did the agency he works for. Not attending to the client would be inappropriate and would constitute neglect.

*Classification*
Competency Category: Professional Practice
Taxonomic Level: Application

**8. A.** Discuss the observations with the other nurse.

*Rationale*
The first action one should take is to discuss what was witnessed with the other nurse and express concern that this behaviour is unethical, unprofessional, and illegal. The nurse manager should be notified so he or she can follow up with the nurse. Documenting vital signs that were not actually taken on a legal document is illegal and would result in professional misconduct. Additionally, the clients' health status and safety is a concern if their vital signs were not actually assessed during the shift.

*Classification*
Competency Category: Professional Practice
Taxonomic Level: Critical Thinking

**9. A.** He should be treated with antibiotics for his pneumonia.

*Rationale*
The patient has signed a document indicating his wish not to be resuscitated. Treating the pneumonia with antibiotics would not be considered resuscitation measures.

*Classification*
Competency Category: Professional Practice
Taxonomic Level: Critical Thinking

**10. A.** Notify the physician that the patient has no vital signs.

*Rationale*
The patient has signed a document indicating his wish not to be resuscitated. The nurse should be

aware of the client's "do not resuscitate" status and should not need to go to the desk to find out; this would delay the initiation of CPR if it were to be carried out. The nurse should notify the physician so he or she can pronounce the death and notify the family.

*Classification*
Competency Category: Alteration in Health
Taxonomic Level: Critical Thinking

**11. D.** Document his choice and reassess his pain in 1 hour.

*Rationale*
Mr. Ralph has the right to choose whether he wants to take the medication. The nurse should assess his pain on a regular basis and educate Mr. Ralph that taking the medication before the pain gets out of control would be a better pain management plan. Also, the nurse should try to determine the reason for not wanting the medication other than choice (e.g., side effects, fear of falling asleep and not waking).

*Classification*
Competency Category: Professional Practice
Taxonomic Level: Critical Thinking

**12. A.** Take the client to the operating room for surgery without informed consent.

*Rationale*
All attempts should be made to contact the family, but delaying life-saving surgery is not an option. The surgeon can perform surgery without consent if there is a risk of loss of life or limb if the surgery is not performed. The nurse should take the client to the operating room.

*Classification*
Competency Category: Professional Practice
Taxonomic Level: Critical Thinking

**13. A.** Notify the nurse manager and document the situation.

*Rationale*
The nurse has the responsibility to notify the manager of any behaviour that puts clients at risk or is against hospital, legal, or professional standards. Linda may want to confront the nurse at some point, but this was not one of the options provided.

*Classification*
Competency Category: Professional Practice
Taxonomic Level: Critical Thinking

**14. B.** Negligence.

*Rationale*
Negligence refers to careless acts on the part of an individual who is not exercising reasonable or prudent judgment. Negligence refers to the omission to do something that a reasonable person (another nurse) would do.

*Classification*
Competency Category: Professional Practice
Taxonomic Level: Knowledge/Comprehension

**15. B.** Slander.

*Rationale*
Slander is considered to be words that are communicated verbally to a third party and that harm or injure the personal or professional reputation of another person.

*Classification*
Competency Category: Professional Practice
Taxonomic Level: Knowledge/Comprehension

**16. C.** Libel.

*Rationale*
Libel is considered written words that harm or injure the person or professional reputation of another person.

*Classification*
Competency Category: Professional Practice
Taxonomic Level: Knowledge/Comprehension

**17. B.** Malpractice.

*Rationale*
Malpractice is a negligent act on the part of a professional; it relates to the conduct of a person who is acting in a professional capacity. Five elements must be in place for a nurse to be held liable for malpractice: presence of a nurse–person relationship, breach of duty, foreseen ability of harm, a failure to meet a standard of care with potential to injure the patient, and actual harm to the patient. The nurse is aware that a spike in temperature of 1°C or a headache is a significant symptom in a client receiving blood, and she should take further initiative to advocate for the client. She is aware that harm could come to the client.

*Classification*
Competency Category: Professional Practice
Taxonomic Level: Critical Thinking

**18. A.** Verbal abuse.

*Rationale*
Reprimanding a client for something that is beyond his control, especially in front of others, is considered abusive. It would also be considered a breach of confidentiality.

*Classification*
Competency Category: Professional Practice
Taxonomic Level: Critical Thinking

**19. B.** That Maureen is in a conflict of interest.

*Rationale*
Maureen is offering advice outside of the scope of practice for an RN. She could be accused of diagnosing and prescribing. Maureen is also working outside of the therapeutic relationship. The client may feel pressured to purchase the supplements to get nursing care or assistance from Maureen. This puts Maureen in a "power" position over the client.

*Classification*
Competency Category: Professional Practice
Taxonomic Level: Critical Thinking

**20. A.** Contact the surgeon for clarification because this is not a complete order.

*Rationale*
When a patient goes to the operating room, all orders become null and void. After surgery, all orders must be renewed as full orders, which requires complete orders, including the drug name, route, dose, and frequency. The nurse should not transcribe and follow this order as written.

*Classification*
Competency Category: Professional Practice
Taxonomic Level: Critical Thinking

**21. Answer:** The patient would receive insulin with a blood glucose level below 4 mmol/L, which is the lowest parameter of a normal glucose level. Giving insulin to someone with a blood glucose level below 4 mmol/L would be life threatening.

*Rationale*
The nurse is responsible for knowing if the medication is appropriate for the client as well as the appropriate dosing parameters. The nurse should recognize that this is a potential medication error and should intervene before it is implemented and the patient put at risk.

*Classification*
Competency Category: Professional Practice
Taxonomic Level: Knowledge/Comprehension

**22. Answers:**

- This test is being ordered based on a subjective observation of the client (i.e., tattoos and needle scars).
- The client's HIV status would not impact the cause or outcome of the injury for which he has been admitted.
- The client did not give informed consent for the test to be done.
- Universal precautions should be taken with all clients.

*Rationale*
The client's HIV status will not impact the cause of his forearm fracture or the treatment choices or outcomes. If the client had been admitted with a condition that would warrant investigation of HIV as a cause, then the physician should discuss the test with the client. The potential outcomes of a positive test result should also be explained to the client. Consent to testing must be given by the client before testing.

*Classification*
Competency Category: Professional Practice
Taxonomic Level: Critical Thinking

**23. Answer:** The nurse should contact the location where it was sent and ensure that the document is destroyed and the information kept confidential. The nurse should also notify the physician and complete an incident report.

*Rationale*
Sending medical information to the wrong fax number would be a breach in confidentiality. As a follow up, the generator of the information should be notified and an incident report completed.

*Classification*
Competency Category: Professional Practice
Taxonomic Level: Application

**24. D.** Have the nursing assistant call the physician while you remain with the client, flex the client's knees, and cover the incision with sterile gauze.

*Rationale*
This is an emergency situation. The physician must be notified, but further injury must be prevented by immediately flexing the client's knees and moistening the area with sterile towels and sterile saline. The moistening prevents dehydration of the intestines, which could lead to necrosis, and reduces the chance of infection.

*Classification*
Competency Category: Nursing Practice: Alterations in Health
Taxonomic Levels: Critical Thinking

**25. D.** Hypotension; cold, clammy skin; and weak, thready pulse.

*Rationale*
The decreased blood volume associated with hemorrhage reduces blood pressure and creates a weak, thready pulse. The skin becomes cold and clammy because of the constriction of peripheral blood vessels caused by the activation of the compensatory sympathetic nervous system.

*Classification*
Competency Category: Nursing Practice: Alterations in Health
Taxonomic Level: Application

**26. A.** Her past experiences and coping abilities.

*Rationale*
The major factors determining the reaction to illness are past experiences and coping mechanisms.

*Classification*
Competency Category: Nursing Practice: Health and Wellness
Taxonomic Level: Critical Thinking

**27. B.** Reinforce success in tasks accomplished.

*Rationale*
To increase or maintain motivation, the nurse should focus on the positive aspects of the client's progress.

*Classification*
Competency Category: Nurse–Person Relationship
Taxonomic Level: Application

**28. A.** Encourage her to participate in the feeding process.

*Rationale*
As a part of the rehabilitative process after a CVA, clients must be encouraged to participate in their own care to the extent that they are able and to extend their ability by establishing short-term goals.

*Classification*
Competency Category: Nursing Practice: Health and Wellness
Taxonomic Level: Knowledge/Comprehension

**29. D.** Ineffective individual coping.

*Rationale*
Ineffective individual coping may be evidenced by an inability to meet basic needs or role expectations and alterations in social participation.

*Classification*
Competency Category: Nursing Practice: Health and Wellness
Taxonomic Level: Critical Thinking

**30. A.** The client is experiencing anxiety; the nurse should listen attentively and provide realistic verbal reassurance.

*Rationale*
Clients routinely experience preoperative anxiety. Nurses should use basic therapeutic communication skills to reduce clients' apprehension.

*Classification*
Competency Category: Nurse–Person Relationship
Taxonomic Level: Application

**31. D.** Maintain a patent airway.

*Rationale*
Although all of the options are appropriate postoperative goals, maintaining a patent airway takes priority, especially on the first postoperative day. A laryngectomy tube is most likely to be in place, and suctioning is commonly needed to clear secretions. Edema and hematoma formation at the surgical site may increase the risk of a blocked airway.

*Classification*
Competency Category: Nursing Practice: Alterations in Health
Taxonomic Level: Application

**32. B.** 5 to 10 seconds.

*Rationale*
The total procedure time from catheter insertion to removal should not be longer than 15 seconds. Intermittent suctioning removes pharyngeal secretions and minimizes stress to the patient. Suctioning that lasts longer than 10 seconds can cause cardiopulmonary compromise, usually from hypoxemia or vagal overload.

*Classification*
Competency Category: Nursing Practice: Alterations in Health
Taxonomic Level: Knowledge/Comprehension

**33. D.** Preoxygenate the client before suctioning.

*Rationale*
Preoxygenation and deep breathing assist in reducing suction-induced hypoxemia. Preoxygenation decreases the risk of atelectasis caused by the negative pressure of suctioning.

*Classification*
Competency Category: Nursing Practice: Alterations in Health
Taxonomic Level: Application

**34. C.** Lack of muscle action and normal tension cause calcium withdrawal from the bone.

*Rationale*
All clients who are confined to bed for any considerable period risk losing calcium from their bones. This is precipitated in the urine and causes calculi.

*Classification*
Competency Category: Nursing Practice: Alterations in Health
Taxonomic Level: Critical Thinking

**35. C.** Monitor urine output.

*Rationale*
Hyperosmolar hyperglycemia is a metabolic complication of parenteral nutrition. Expansion of the blood volume combined with hyperglycemia can cause osmotic diuresis presenting as increased urine output. Intake and output should be recorded so that a fluid imbalance can be readily deterred. Urine can also be tested for hyperosmolar diuresis.

*Classification*
Competency Category: Nursing Practice: Alterations in Health
Taxonomic Level: Application

**36. D.** 8.3 mmol/L.

*Rationale*
Blood sugars should be maintained below a level of 8.3 mmol/L because hyperglycemia has been shown to be associated with decreased immune function and risk of complications.

*Classification*
Competency Category: Nursing Practice: Health and Wellness
Taxonomic Level: Knowledge/Comprehension

**37. C.** Obtain an order for urinary catheterization.

*Rationale*
The client has "overflow retention." A catheter relieves the discomfort by draining urine from the

bladder. Permitting further distension could injure the bladder. Although an analgesic may relieve the discomfort, it will not resolve the cause.

*Classification*
Competency Category: Nursing Practice: Health and Wellness
Taxonomic Level: Application

**38. D.** Lean roast beef, buttered white rice with egg slices, white bread with butter and jelly, and tea with sugar.

*Rationale*
A low-residue diet decreases the amount of fecal material in the lower intestinal tract. This is necessary in the acute phase of ulcerative colitis to prevent irritation of the colon. The juice contains cellulose, which is not absorbed and irritates the colon; cream soup contains lactose, which is irritating to the colon. Milk contains lactose, which is irritating to the colon and contraindicated in people with colitis.

*Classification*
Competency Category: Nursing Practice: Health and Wellness
Taxonomic Level: Critical Thinking

**39. B.** Impaired neural functioning.

*Rationale*
Paralytic ileus occurs when neurologic impulses are diminished, as from anaesthesia, infection, or surgery.

*Classification*
Competency Category: Nursing Practice: Alterations in Health
Taxonomic Level: Critical Thinking

**40. C.** Anticipate that emotional stress can increase intestinal peristalsis.

*Rationale*
Emotional stress of any kind can stimulate peristalsis and thereby increase the volume of drainage.

*Classification*
Competency Category: Nursing Practice: Health and Wellness
Taxonomic Level: Critical Thinking

**41. A.** The hemopoietic factor is absorbed only in the terminal ileum.

*Rationale*
Vitamin B12 (extrinsic factor) combines with intrinsic factor, a substance secreted by the parietal cells of

the gastric mucosa, forming hemopoietic factor. Hemopoietic factor is only absorbed in the ileum, from which it travels to bone marrow and stimulates erythropoiesis.

*Classification*
Competency Category: Nursing Practice: Alterations in Health
Taxonomic Level: Critical Thinking

**42. B.** Check the pulse distal to the catheter insertion site.

*Rationale*
The pulse should be assessed because trauma at the insertion site may interfere with blood flow distal to the site. There is also danger of bleeding or occlusion.

*Classification*
Competency Category: Nursing Practice: Alterations in Health
Taxonomic Level: Application

**43. C.** It prevents the entrance of air into the pleural cavity.

*Rationale*
Atmospheric pressure is greater than the pressure inside the pleural space. If a chest tube were not attached to underwater seal drainage, air would enter the pleural space and collapse the lung (pneumothorax). The water seal does not affect the amount of suction used.

*Classification*
Competency Category: Nursing Practice: Alterations in Health
Taxonomic Level: Knowledge/Comprehension

**44. B.** 750 mL.

*Rationale*
During the first 3 hours, 100 to 300 mL of fluid may drain from a chest tube in an adult after the first 3 hours. This rate decreases, and 500 to 1000 mL of drainage can be expected within the first 24 hours.

*Classification*
Competency Category: Nursing Practice: Alterations in Health
Taxonomic Level: Knowledge/Comprehension

**45. D.** A rise of formula in the tube.

*Rationale*
A rise in the level of formula within the tube indicates a full stomach. Passage of flatus reflects intestinal motility, which does not pose a potential problem.

*Classification*
Competency Category: Nursing Practice: Alterations in Health
Taxonomic Level: Critical Thinking

**46. C.** Immediate defibrillation.

*Rationale*
When ventricular fibrillation is verified, the first intervention is defibrillation. It is the only intervention that will terminate this lethal dysrhythmia.

*Classification*
Competency Category: Nursing Practice: Alterations in Health
Taxonomic Level: Application

**47. B.** Ketones from rapid fat breakdown, causing acidosis.

*Rationale*
Ketones are released when fat is broken down for energy.

*Classification*
Competency Category: Nursing Practice: Alterations in Health
Taxonomic Level: Knowledge/Comprehension

**48. B.** Low-protein diet with a prescribed amount of water.

*Rationale*
Although dialysis removes water, creatinine, and urea from the blood, the client's diet must still be maintained and monitored.

*Classification*
Competency Category: Nursing Practice: Health and Wellness
Taxonomic Level: Critical Thinking

**49. C.** A positive test reaction indicates ketoacidosis.

*Rationale*
Urinary acetone indicates the development of ketoacidosis. Ketoacidosis is a side effect of the breakdown of bodily fat stores.

*Classification*
Competency Category: Nursing Practice: Health and Wellness
Taxonomic Level: Knowledge/Comprehension

**50. C.** Observing for signs of hypoglycemia as a result of treatment.

*Rationale*
During treatment for acidosis, the client may develop hypoglycemia; careful observation for this complication should be made by the nurse.

*Classification*
Competency Category: Nursing Practice: Alterations in Health
Taxonomic Level: Application

**51. B.** Can be planned around a wide variety of commonly available foods.

*Rationale*
Each client should be given an individually devised diet selecting commonly used foods from the Canadian Diabetic Association's exchange diet. Family members should be included in the diet teaching.

*Classification*
Competency Category: Nursing Practice: Health and Wellness
Taxonomic Level: Knowledge/Comprehension

**52. A.** Her ability to count her radial pulse correctly.

*Rationale*
A client who complies with drug therapy is less likely to have a recurrence of cardiac failure. Client knowledge of how to check a radial pulse and actions to take if it is not within normal limits can prevent a toxic digoxin reaction.

*Classification*
Competency Category: Nursing Practice: Health and Wellness
Taxonomic Level: Critical Thinking

**53. C.** "I should try to eat several small meals during the day."

*Rationale*
Because digestion takes energy they need to devote to breathing instead, clients with COPD may feel full after only a small meal. They tolerate smaller, more frequent high-calorie meals better than larger meals.

*Classification*
Competency Category: Nursing Practice: Health and Wellness
Taxonomic Level: Application

**54. A.** Begin EGG monitoring.

*Rationale*
EGG monitoring should be started as soon as possible; life-threatening arrhythmias are the leading cause of death in the first hours after MI.

*Classification*
Competency Category: Nursing Practice: Alterations in Health
Taxonomic Level: Application

**55. B.** The heel of one hand on the sternum and the heel of the other on top of it with the fingers interlocking.

*Rationale*
This provides the best leverage for depressing the sternum. Thus, the heart is adequately compressed, and blood is forced into the arteries. Grasping the fingers keeps them off the chest and concentrates the energy expended in the heel of the hand while minimizing the possibility of fracturing ribs.

*Classification*
Competency Category: Nursing Practice: Alterations in Health
Taxonomic Level: Knowledge/Comprehension

**56. B.** Call a break in the meeting and talk to the nurse in a private place or in his or her office.

*Rationale*
When an individual is verbally acting out and others are present, it is advisable to isolate the individual by either removing him or her from the audience or removing the audience. By doing this, it gives the person an opportunity to regain control of rational thinking without embarrassment in front of his or her peers. It also avoids the audience from encouraging or coaching the acting-out individual and further escalating the situation.

*Classification*
Competency Category: Professional Practice
Taxonomic Level: Application

**57. C.** "Please lower your voice, or you will not be able to return to the meeting."

*Rationale*
When setting limits on behaviour, it is important to be clear as to which behaviour you are addressing. It is important to tell the acting-out person what the consequences of not changing the behaviour will be. The consequences need to be reasonable, enforceable, and consistent.

*Classification*
Competency Category: Professional Practice
Taxonomic Level: Application

**58. A.** Consistent.

*Rationale*
To be effective, limits must be set on unacceptable behaviour.

*Classification*
Competency Category: Professional Practice
Taxonomic Level: Application

**59. A.** Obtain consent from Andrew's next of kin.

*Rationale*
Before applying restraints, the nurse must obtain consent from the next of kin until the client is able to give consent himself.

*Classification*
Competency Category: Professional Practice
Taxonomic Level: Critical Thinking

**60. A.** Have a meeting with staff to see how they can improve on methods to decrease needlestick injuries.

*Rationale*
Based on research and occupational health and safety standards, employers must provide safety equipment for employees. When an accident is investigated and a plan is developed to prevent further accidents from occurring, the solution should be based on preventing the accident at the source. Therefore, meeting with staff to determine the best way to prevent needlestick injuries on the unit would be an appropriate intervention.

*Classification*
Competency Category: Professional Practice
Taxonomic Level: Critical Thinking

**61. D.** "No, it is not within my scope of practice."

*Rationale*
Intubating a patient is not within the scope of practice for a nurse, even with the anaesthetist directing the procedure. This is not an emergency situation, and the nurse should refuse to place the tube into the patient. If the nurse does insert the tube and the client is injured during the procedure, the nurse could be charged with malpractice.

*Classification*
Competency Category: Professional Practice
Taxonomic Level: Critical Thinking

**62. B.** Disclose to the patient that she was given a blood transfusion.

*Rationale*
The nurse is a patient advocate and should encourage the disclosure of the administration of blood. The

nurse should be honest with the client if she specifically asks if blood was administered.

*Classification*
Competency Category: Professional Practice
Taxonomic Level: Critical Thinking

**63. C.** The nurse must only give the medication for the appropriate indication.

*Rationale*
The nurse must only give a medication for which it is ordered or indicated.

*Classification*
Competency Category: Professional Practice
Taxonomic Level: Critical Thinking

**64. C.** "I can offer you some information outlining a variety of ways to stop smoking."

*Rationale*
Every nurse has the responsibility to practice in a manner that promotes the patient's right to choose.

*Classification*
Competency Category: Nurse–Person Relationship
Taxonomic Level: Application

**65. D.** "Increase the amount of fibre and fluids in your diet."

*Rationale*
Clients with hypothyroidism typically have constipation. A diet high in fibre and fluids can help prevent this.

*Classification*
Competency Category: Nursing Practice: Nurse–Client Relationship
Taxonomic Level: Application

**66. Answers:**

- Notify the supervisor.
- Call the previous nurse to establish which medications were actually given and when. Also notify the nurse that this is an inappropriate action.
- Complete an incident report.
- Ensure that the patients receive the medications that are ordered at the appropriate time.

*Rationale*
The nursing supervisor needs to be notified and an incident report completed to track this behaviour. This will allow the manager to follow up on previous occurrences. If this behaviour occurs frequently on this unit, it needs to be addressed in an educational session. The previous nurse should be aware of the inappropriate behaviour and should clarify with the oncoming nurse which medications have been given. The patients still require medication as prescribed.

*Classification*
Competency Category: Professional Practice
Taxonomic Level: Critical Thinking

**67. Answers:**

- Red (highly vascular).
- Moist with smooth surfaces (like the inside of the mouth).
- It may take up to 6 weeks for swelling to recede and for the stoma to achieve its normal size.
- The stoma should not be recessed below the level of the skin.

*Rationale*
All of the answers provided above are characteristic of a healthy stoma.

*Classification*
Competency Category: Nursing Practice: Health and Wellness
Taxonomic Level: Knowledge/Comprehension

**68. Answer:** The wife.

*Rationale*
Because the client is still legally married, his wife is considered next of kin and has the right to provide consent on his behalf.

*Classification*
Competency Category: Professional Practice
Taxonomic Level: Critical Thinking

**69. Answers:**

- Suggest a scheduled voiding time.
- Suggest bladder training techniques.
- Suggest the client keep a daily log of activities or lifestyle factors that are associated with urinary incontinence.
- Suggest and teach Kegel exercises.
- Advise her to use small pads in her pants when going out or exercising.
- Instruct her to avoid lifting heavy objects.
- Have her limit her fluid intake when going out and before bed.

*Rationale*

All of the above answers are practical recommendations aimed at helping Mrs. Jules regain control of urinary elimination. Gaining a thorough understanding of the activities or lifestyle factors associated with urinary incontinence is significant when developing care plans to support clients in regaining control of urinary continence.

*Classification*

Competency Category: Nursing Practice: Health and Wellness
Taxonomic Level: Application

70. **Answers:**

* Secure the central line to the chest wall with sutures or Steri-Strips.
* Coil and tape the extension tubing to the patient's chest.
* Place a tab of tape on the tubing and pin it to the patient's hospital's gown.
* Luer-lock all connections and tape them with clear tape.

*Rationale*

To prevent dislodgement or disconnection of a central line, all connections need to be Luer-locked and taped with clear tape.

*Classification*

Competency Category: Nursing Practice: Alterations in Health
Taxonomic Level: Knowledge/Comprehension

71. **Answer:**

Antiembolism stockings help prevent thrombus formation by facilitating the return of venous blood to the heart. They help to maintain external pressure on the muscles and vessels of the lower extremities and thus promote venous return and reduce the formation of emboli.

*Rationale*

Antiembolism stockings help to prevent thrombus formation by facilitating the return of venous blood to the heart.

*Classification*

Competency Category: Nursing Practice: Alterations in Health
Taxonomic Level: Knowledge/Comprehension

72. **A.** Nasal flaring.

*Rationale*

Nasal flaring refers to enlargement of the opening of the nostrils during breathing. Nasal flaring is seen mostly in infants and younger children and is often an indication that increased effort is required for breathing. Any condition that causes the infant to work harder to obtain enough air can cause nasal flaring. Although many causes of nasal flaring are not serious, some can be life threatening. In young infants, nasal flaring can be a very important sign of respiratory distress. All of the other choices would be seen in both the adult and pediatric populations.

*Classification*

Competency Category: Nursing Practice: Alterations in Health
Taxonomic Level: Knowledge/Comprehension

73. **A.** The cause of asthma is often allergens and infection.

*Rationale*

Respiratory tract infections cause epithelial damage and stimulate the production of IgE antibodies directed toward the viral antigens. They also increase airway responsiveness to other asthma triggers that may persist for weeks beyond the original infection; smoking is a main allergen. Triggers of bronchial asthma in children are usually allergies that initiate the inflammatory response. Because the child has long-standing asthma, the nurse should assess the parents' level of understanding about the disease before offering information. Given that both parents are smokers, allergen-triggered asthma is a probable cause. If it did not cause the asthma, it would aggravate it. Asthmatic episodes may be life threatening in all age groups.

*Classification*

Competency Category: Nurse–Person Relationship
Taxonomic Level: Critical Thinking

74. **B.** Moderate persistent asthma.

*Rationale*

Severe persistent asthma is continual symptoms with frequent nighttime symptoms. Moderate persistent asthma is daily symptoms with nighttime symptoms more than 1 night per week. Mild persistent asthma includes symptoms more than two times a week but not more than one time per day with night time symptoms more than two times per month. Mild intermittent asthma includes symptoms less than two times a week with nighttime symptoms less than two times per month.

*Classification*

Competency Category: Nursing Practice: Alterations in Health
Taxonomic Level: Knowledge/Comprehension

**75. A.** Steatorrhea.

*Rationale*
Steatorrhea are stools that are large, foul smelling, bulky, and greasy because of the lack of pancreatic enzymes in the duodenum, which means the child is unable to digest fats, proteins, and some sugars.

*Classification*
Competency Category: Nursing Practice: Alterations in Health
Taxonomic Level: Knowledge/Comprehension

**76. A.** Frontal.

*Rationale*
The frontal lobe regulates personality and judgment. The occipital lobe regulates vision. The temporal lobe regulates hearing. The parietal lobe regulates sensation.

*Classification*
Competency Category: Nursing Practice: Alterations in Health
Taxonomic Level: Application

**77. B.** Intracranial pressure is increasing.

*Rationale*
Apnea, bradycardia, and widening pulse pressure, collectively referred to as Cushing's triad, are hallmarks of increasing intracranial pressure, which indicates that the patient's condition is deteriorating.

*Classification*
Competency Category: Nursing Practice: Alterations in Health
Taxonomic Level: Critical Thinking

**78. A.** Hepatitis A.

*Rationale*
Modes of transmission of Hepatitis A in children include exposure to contaminated changing tables and ingestion of water or shellfish contaminated with feces.

*Classification*
Competency Category: Nursing Practice: Health and Wellness
Taxonomic Level: Critical Thinking

**79. A.** Cleft lip.

*Rationale*
A cleft lip involves a notched vermilion border, variably sized clefts, and dental anomalies.

*Classification*
Competency Category: Nursing Practice: Alterations in Health
Taxonomic Level: Knowledge/Comprehension

**80. C.** "Feed your child in an upright position."

*Rationale*
Feeding the child in an upright position allows gravity to assist in the feeding and decreases the chance of choking. Children with mild cleft lip or palate may be able to breastfeed. A plastic compressible bottle is best used to help squeeze the formula into the child's mouth; however, these children require frequent burping.

*Classification*
Competency Category: Nursing Practice: Health and Wellness
Taxonomic Level: Application

**81. B.** 3 to 6 months.

*Rationale*
Cleft lip repair is usually scheduled when the child is 3 to 6 months of age to facilitate bonding with the parents and the management of nutritional concerns. Additional surgery may need to be scheduled as the child grows.

*Classification*
Competency Category: Nursing Practice: Health and Wellness
Taxonomic Level: Knowledge

**82. A.** Inform the surgeon.

*Rationale*
The surgeon must be informed immediately so he or she can decide whether to proceed with the surgery. A child scheduled for surgery in 1 hour would be NPO, so oral antipyretics would not be an option. Although cool compresses might relieve some discomfort, the priority is to notify the physician.

*Classification*
Competency Category: Professional Practice
Taxonomic Level: Critical Thinking

**83. A.** Some children distract themselves with play while in pain.

*Rationale*
Some children distract themselves with play or music while in pain and may sleep because of exhaustion. Nurses commonly underestimate children's pain

when they do not rely on the child's self-report. Narcotics can be administered safely to children.

*Classification*
Competency Category: Nursing Practice: Alterations in Health
Taxonomic Level: Application

**84. C.** "I can appreciate your concerns. If we obtain permission from your daughter, we can include you in our discussions."

*Rationale*
The reality of the situation is that the parents may be included in the exchange of medical information but only with the daughter's consent. Sharing that fact with the parents clearly identifies that the decision is the daughter's to make and that she is entitled to make it. The nurse should support the client's right to privacy and confidentiality.

*Classification*
Competency Category: Professional Practice
Taxonomic Level: Critical Thinking

**85. A.** Keep the child safe and assess for abuse.

*Rationale*
The assessment for risk is the priority. This would include verbalizing your concerns to the most immediate supervisor and involving hospital social workers and the medical team. These initial steps need to be implemented and then the appropriate authorities need to be alerted.

*Classification*
Competency Category: Professional Practice
Taxonomic Level: Application

**86. A.** Epiglottitis.

*Rationale*
Epiglottitis would be the priority for care because there is potential for airway obstruction.

*Classification*
Competency Category: Nursing Practice: Health and Wellness
Taxonomic Level: Critical Thinking

**87. A.** "If my blood sugar is low, I will be able to deal with it."

*Rationale*
Hypoglycemia causes confusion and hallucinations. Patients may not always be able to respond appropriately to remedy the situation.

*Classification*
Competency Category: Nurse–Person Relationship
Taxonomic Level: Critical Thinking

**88. D.** Insulin is always administered subcutaneously.

*Rationale*
The goal of the session is "self-administration," so the information related to administering insulin is prioritized. A priority teaching point is that insulin is always self-administered through a subcutaneous route. Too much information during one session will confuse the child. A separate session should be dedicated to the actual insulin concerns.

*Classification*
Competency Category: Nursing Practice: Health and Wellness
Taxonomic Level: Critical Thinking

**89. B.** Preschool.

*Rationale*
Preschool children learn only one characteristic of an object, and they fear being hurt.

*Classification*
Competency Category: Nurse–Person Relationship
Taxonomic Level: Application

**90. B.** Preschool.

*Rationale*
Preschoolers believe that the puppets and dolls are actually talking to them, so this is a common method of teaching in many children hospitals.

*Classification*
Competency Category: Nursing Practice: Health and Wellness
Taxonomic Level: Application

**91. D.** Speak to the unit manager and fill out a medication error form.

*Rationale*
Nurses are expected to demonstrate professional conduct, including the safe administration of medication. Administering scheduled medications 1 hour late is a medication error and should be identified to the unit manager. The unit manager should speak directly with the nurse as per her or his job responsibilities.

*Classification*
Competency Category: Professional Practice
Taxonomic Level: Critical Thinking

**92. B.** The child may have a hearing impairment.

*Rationale*
Children of this age have a hyperreflexive reaction to loud noises. A lack of response might suggest that further testing is necessary to explore possible hearing loss.

*Classification*
Competency Category: Nursing Practice: Health and Wellness
Taxonomic Level: Critical Thinking

**93. Answers:**

- Persistent, frequent coughing.
- Chronic constipation and straining to pass stool.
- Moderate to severe levels of pain.
- Prolonged agitation.

*Rationale*
Chronic constipation and straining to pass stool, persistent and frequent coughing, pain, and being agitated are all potential causes of increased intracranial pressure in children.

*Classification*
Competency Category: Nursing Practice: Alterations in Health
Taxonomic Level: Application

**94. Answers:**

- Personality traits.
- Parental presence.
- Meaning of pain.
- Developmental level.
- Culture.
- Past experiences.

*Rationale*
Personality traits, the presence of the child's parents, the developmental level of the child, personal meanings of pain, culture, and past experiences all influence a child's response to pain.

*Classification*
Competency Category: Nursing Practice: Alterations in Health
Taxonomic Level: Application

**95. D.** "The growing uterus puts pressure on the bladder, so urinary frequency is normal."

*Rationale*
Shirley is not exhibiting any signs or symptoms of bladder infection other than urinary frequency.

Urinary frequency initially most likely results from increased bladder sensitivity and compression of the bladder from the enlarging uterus.

*Classification*
Competency Category: Nursing Practice: Health and Wellness
Taxonomic Level: Application

**96. B.** "Can you help me understand what aspect of being a father concerns you?"

*Rationale*
While listening to Thomas' concerns, the nurse determines that the developmental task at this stage in pregnancy is for him to negotiate with his partner concerning the role he will play in labour and to prepare for parenthood. He concentrates on his experience of the pregnancy and begins to think of himself as a father. Each man brings to pregnancy attitudes that affect the way that he adjusts, including experiences he has had with his own father and child care and the perceptions of the men in his life.

*Classification*
Competency Category: Nursing Practice: Health and Wellness
Taxonomic Level: Affective

**97. A.** Act as an advocate for the couple and verbalize their wishes to nurses and primary care providers.

*Rationale*
According to the Canadian Nurses Association Code of Ethics (2006), nurses are ethically responsible for giving childbearing families the autonomy to make informed choices about the care they receive. This also fosters a collaborative relationship with the family.

*Classification*
Competency Category: Nurse–Person Relationship
Taxonomic Level: Critical Thinking

**98. C.** "I will develop a list of questions to use in interviewing primary care providers."

*Rationale*
As consumers of health care, expectant families have the right to find a caregiver and place of birth that shares their philosophy of birth. This statement clearly reflects the understanding of "informed choice."

*Classification*
Competency Category: Nursing Practice: Health and Wellness
Taxonomic Level: Critical Thinking

**99. C.** "Tell me more about how you are feeling."

*Rationale*
This response further explores Stacey's feelings in order to assist her.

*Classification*
Competency Category: Nurse–Person Relationship
Taxonomic Level: Application

**100. A.** "It is not safe to consume alcohol during pregnancy."

*Rationale*
Complete abstinence from alcohol use during pregnancy is recommended. A safe level of alcohol consumption during pregnancy has not yet been established.

*Classification*
Competency Category: Nursing Practice: Health and Wellness
Taxonomic Level: Knowledge

**101. D.** Increased amounts of vernix.

*Rationale*
Vernix caseosa is a whitish substance that serves as a protective covering over the fetal body throughout pregnancy. Vernix usually disappears by term gestation. It is highly unusual for a 12-day postmature baby to have increased amounts of vernix. Discrepancies between the EDC and gestational age by physical examination may occur.

*Classification*
Competency Category: Nursing Practice: Alterations in Health
Taxonomic Level: Critical Thinking

**102. B.** Above the umbilicus.

*Rationale*
The fundus of the uterus may be palpated through the abdominal wall halfway between the umbilicus and the symphysis pubis within a few minutes after birth. One hour later, it has risen to the level of the umbilicus, where it will remain for the next 24 hours. After 24 hours after birth, the fundus will decrease one fingerbreadth (1 cm) per day in size.

*Classification*
Competency Category: Nursing Practice: Alterations in Health
Taxonomic Level: Knowledge/Comprehension

**103. D.** Have Riley void and reassess the fundus.

*Rationale*
A full bladder can cause uterine atony, increase the amount of lochia, and displace the position of the uterus for assessment of the involution of the uterus.

*Classification*
Competency Category: Nursing Practice: Alterations in Health
Taxonomic Level: Critical Thinking

**104. C.** Palpate and massage her fundus to assess firmness.

*Rationale*
Riley is displaying signs of a postpartum hemorrhage with the amount of blood loss in 30 minutes and a change in her vital signs. The most appropriate immediate response is to palpate and massage her uterus to determine if it is "boggy."

*Classification*
Competency Category: Nursing Practice: Alterations in Health
Taxonomic Level: Critical Thinking

**105. D.** Succinctly explain the need to do a proper assessment.

*Rationale*
This response informs the father of the need to do the assessment and empowers the nurse to do his or her work properly.

*Classification*
Competency Category: Nurse–Person Relationship
Taxonomic Level: Critical Thinking

**106. D.** This finding is at the low end of the normal range.

*Rationale*
During sleep, a newborn's pulse can be as low as 100 bpm.

*Classification*
Competency Category: Nursing Practice: Health and Wellness
Taxonomic Level: Application

**107. A.** To stimulate growth of intestinal flora.

*Rationale*
Newborns do not have the intestinal flora to produce vitamin K in the first week after birth. Administering

vitamin K promotes the formation of clotting factors in the liver and prevents hemorrhagic disease.

*Classification*
Competency Category: Nursing Practice: Health and Wellness
Taxonomic Level: Knowledge/Comprehension

**108. A.** Excessive heat loss.

*Rationale*
Newborns are at a distinct disadvantage in maintaining normal temperature. With a large body surface in relation to mass and a limited amount of insulating subcutaneous fat, newborns are susceptible to excessive heat loss.

*Classification*
Competency Category: Nursing Practice: Alterations in Health
Taxonomic Level: Application

**109. A.** Uncover him and place him on the radiant warmer.

*Rationale*
Placing newborns under a radiant heat source is an excellent mechanical measure to help conserve heat.

*Classification*
Competency Category: Nursing Practice: Alterations in Health
Taxonomic Level: Critical Thinking

**110. D.** Makes a walking movement when he is held upright with one foot touching the table.

*Rationale*
Newborns who are held in a vertical position with their feet touching a hard surface will take a few quick, alternating steps.

*Classification*
Competency Category: Nursing Practice: Health and Wellness
Taxonomic Level: Application

**111. D.** 28 to 32 weeks gestational age.

*Rationale*
During a normal pregnancy, the maternal cardiovascular system undergoes many changes that put a physiologic strain on the heart. The normal maternal heart is able to compensate for the increased workload to maintain the pregnancy, labour, and birth. The diseased heart is already hemodynamically challenged, with a 30% to 50% increase in cardiac output occurring at 22 to 26 weeks gestation during

pregnancy. A woman with a history of heart disease becomes symptomatic at 7 to 8 months gestation.

*Classification*
Competency Category: Nursing Practice: Alterations in Health
Taxonomic Level: Critical Thinking

**112. A.** Prolapsed cord.

*Rationale*
Fetal heart variability reflects the normal changes and fluctuations in the fetal heart rate over a period of time. A prolapsed cord would cause severe fetal heart decelerations rather than subtle changes in long- or short-term variability.

*Classification*
Competency Category: Nursing Practice: Alterations in Health
Taxonomic Level: Critical Thinking

**113. A.** Hematocrit decreases.

*Rationale*
The hematocrit measures the portion of whole blood that is composed of erythrocytes. The plasma volume during pregnancy has a greater increase than the erythrocyte increase. The hematocrit decreases during pregnancy.

*Classification*
Competency Category: Nursing Practice: Health and Wellness
Taxonomic Level: Critical Thinking

**114. C.** Partner abuse may increase during pregnancy.

*Rationale*
Pregnancy and birth are trigger points for intimate partner abuse because the abuser experiences a sense of loss of control. This is especially true if abuse occurred before the pregnancy. During pregnancy, the mother and baby take priority during the pregnancy, and the abuser attempts to maintain or regain control by abusing the woman.

*Classification*
Competency Category: Nursing Practice: Alterations in Health
Taxonomic Level: Knowledge/Comprehension

**115. Answers:**

- Culture.
- Acceptance of the pregnancy.
- Level of health and wellness.
- Support system.
- Previous childbirth experience.

- Childbirth education.
- Developmental level.
- Nursing care in labour.
- Pain of labour.
- History of abuse or violence.
- Previous experience with pain.

*Rationale*
Behaviours of labouring women vary from individual to individual. In practicing woman-centred care, health care professionals must have a clear understanding of the contributing factors that may affect women's behaviours and responses to labour and birth.

*Classification*
Competency Category: Nurse–Person Relationship
Taxonomic Level: Critical Thinking

**116. Answers:**

- Tell her to wash her hands before handling the baby.
- Provide precautions for blood spills, lochia, and perineal pads.
- Tell her why it is important to delay breast-feeding for 48 hours after administration of HBIG to the baby.
- Tell her how to inspect her breasts and nipples for infection or breaks in skin if breastfeeding. If infection or breaks are present, breastfeeding is not recommended.

*Rationale*
Hepatitis B carrier women should be taught how to prevent contamination and transmission of the infection to their newborn and others. It is important for women to wash their hands before handling the baby; be aware of precautions for blood spills, perineal pads, and lochia; and keep the baby away from soiled linens. Education is a critical component of the mother's care and should include why it is important to delay breastfeeding for 48 hours after HBIG administration and how to inspect the breasts for breaks or cracks in the skin.

*Classification*
Competency Category: Alterations in Health
Taxonomic Level: Critical Thinking

**117. C.** Mood swings, tachycardia, and weight loss.

*Rationale*
Stimulants produce mood swings, anorexia, weight loss, and tachycardia. The other symptoms listed indicate CNS depression.

*Classification*
Competency Category: Nursing Practice: Alterations in Health
Taxonomic Level: Knowledge/Comprehension

**118. A.** Discuss hypothetical ethical situations.

*Rationale*
The best way to assess a client's judgment is to discuss hypothetical ethical situations such as: "What would you do if you found on the ground a letter in an envelope that was addressed and stamped?"

*Classification*
Competency Category: Alterations in Health
Taxonomic Level: Application

**119. C.** Resolve the immediate crisis.

*Rationale*
The goal of crisis intervention is to resolve the immediate problem. The client must learn to solve his or her own issues. Although some clients do enter long-term therapy or are admitted to an acute care facility, these are not the goals of crisis intervention.

*Classification*
Competency Category: Alterations in Health
Taxonomic Level: Knowledge/Comprehension

**120. A.** Encourage group cohesiveness.

*Rationale*
During the working phase of a group, the nurse continues to encourage cohesiveness among its members. During the orientation (or initial) phase, the nurse leading the group should explain the purpose and goals of the group. During the termination (or final) phase, the leader should encourage a discussion of feelings associated with termination. When leading a group, the nurse should act as facilitator; offering advice is not appropriate. The group members should work together to resolve conflicts.

*Classification*
Competency Category: Nurse–Person Relationship
Taxonomic Level: Application

**121. B.** Major depression with psychotic features.

*Rationale*
ECT is indicated for depression. ECT is not indicated for severe agitation, antisocial behaviour, or treatment noncompliance.

*Classification*
Competency Category: Nursing Practice: Alterations in Health
Taxonomic Level: Knowledge/Comprehension

**122. B.** An active suicide plan and the means to carry it out.

*Rationale*
The presence of an actual plan would require a restrictive environment for the client. Although a previous suicide attempt, marital status, and social support can affect the rate of suicide, a serious plan is of primary concern for the nurse.

*Classification*
Competency Category: Nursing Practice: Health and Wellness
Taxonomic Level: Critical Thinking

**123. B.** Anxiety.

*Rationale*
Anxiety is the top priority at this time because the client's behaviour mimics some of the objective signs of anxiety, which include restlessness, irritability, rapid speech, inability to complete tasks, and verbal expressions of tension. The other aspects of the nursing assessment are significant but are not the priority because the nurse has not had the opportunity to determine the presence of these conditions.

*Classification*
Competency Category: Health and Wellness
Taxonomic Level: Critical Thinking

**124. C.** Ensure relevance to the client's experiences and quickly refocus on them.

*Rationale*
The nurse's self-disclosure should be brief and to the point so that the interaction can be refocused on the client's experiences. Because the client is the focus of the nurse–person relationship, the discussion should not dwell on the nurse's own experience.

*Classification*
Competency Category: Nurse–Person Relationship
Taxonomic Level: Application

**125. D.** Consistently enforcing unit rules and facility policy.

*Rationale*
Firmness and consistency regarding rules are the hallmarks of a plan of care for a client with personality disorder. Isolation is inappropriate and violates the client's rights. Power struggles should be avoided because the client may try to manipulate people through them. Behaviour modification usually fails because of staff inconsistency and client manipulation.

*Classification*
Competency Category: Nursing Practice: Alterations in Health
Taxonomic Level: Application

**126. C.** Agranulocytosis.

*Rationale*
The complaint of a sore throat may indicate an infection caused by agranulocytosis, a depletion in white blood cells. Although an extrapyramidal reaction or tardive dyskinesia may occur, a sore throat is not an indication of these conditions. Reye's syndrome is caused by a virus and is unrelated to clozapine.

*Classification*
Competency Category: Nursing Practice: Alterations in Health
Taxonomic Level: Critical Thinking

**127. C.** "What have you done so far to try to solve this problem?"

*Rationale*
To assist the client in resolving this situation, the nurse assists the client in understanding his situation by determining what has worked in the past. This general understanding helps the client to see the bigger picture and begin the problem-solving process. Immediately seeking an alternative is not advised. At this early stage of assessment, it is important to focus on helping the client identify his strengths to manage his work situation rather than providing quick solutions.

*Classification*
Competency Category: Nursing Practice: Alterations in Health
Taxonomic Level: Critical Thinking

**128. D.** "What kind of emotional or material support do you receive from others?"

*Rationale*
To assess social support, the nurse must first determine what kind of support the client currently receives. It is not significant at the early stage of assessment to know how the client supports others. The specific details of the client's family contact would be more appropriate at a later stage of assessment. The client has already stated that he has very little social life and is working overtime, so questions about free-time activities would not add to the initial assessment.

*Classification*
Competency Category: Nursing Practice: Alterations in Health
Taxonomic Level: Application

**129. C.** Role play with the nurse assuming the role of the boss.

*Rationale*
Practical role playing activities are effective in implementing change because they offer an opportunity to practice behaviour change. Encouraging ventilation of feeling offers Enrique an opportunity to express feelings however does not promote the implementation of change. Teaching about stress, while important as information, may not necessarily provide support for practical change; and exploring new work settings serves as a strategy to avoid the current problem at hand.

*Classification*
Competency Category: Nursing Practice: Health and Wellness
Taxonomic Level: Application

**130. C.** Support him in developing attainable goals to enhance his socialization.

*Rationale*
Supporting Enrique to set goals around social interaction is the first step in promoting change for wellness. Merely referring a client to a social activity is only a short-term solution and may not be desired by the client. Modeling is important, but interactional skills are an individual approach that must be authentic to the client in whatever culture they may be from. Suggesting solutions such as planning a specific activity with anyone (let alone the employer) is not appropriate to social wellness.

*Classification*
Competency Category: Nursing Practice: Health and Wellness
Taxonomic Level: Critical Thinking

**131. A.** Monoamine oxidase inhibitors (MAOIs).

*Rationale*
Buspirone interacts with MAOIs. The interaction produces a hypertensive reaction. Beta-adrenergic blockers, antineoplastic drugs, and antiparkinsonian drugs would not cause an interaction with buspirone and therefore can be administered simultaneously.

*Classification*
Competency Category: Nursing Practice: Alterations in Health
Taxonomic Level: Knowledge

**132. C.** Avoid caffeine.

*Rationale*
Consuming 500 mg or more of caffeine will significantly alter the effects of lorazepam, and other dietary restrictions are not necessary (e.g., aged cheeses, which are to be avoided with MAOIs). Staying out of the sun or using sunscreens is required during phenothiazine treatment, and adequate salt intake is indicated for clients taking lithium.

*Classification*
Competency Category: Health and Wellness
Taxonomic Level: Knowledge

**133. B.** Low-quality support relationships often negatively affect coping in a crisis.

*Rationale*
Strong social support enhances mental and physical health, providing a significant buffer against distress. Relationships of low-quality support are known to negatively impact a person's coping effectiveness.

*Classification*
Competency Category: Nursing Practice: Health and Wellness
Taxonomic Level: Critical Thinking

**134. B.** Using previously learned deep breathing and muscle relaxation techniques.

*Rationale*
Eloise is experiencing stress because of a recent role change subsequent to her recent divorce. Using previously learned relaxation techniques would be an appropriate way of decreasing her stress without using alcohol as a temporary solution. Ceasing contact with significant others in her life is extreme and in this case should not be recommended by the nurse.

*Classification*
Competency Category: Nursing Practice: Health and Wellness
Taxonomic Level: Critical Thinking

**135. D.** "Tell me what happened the last time you felt you were under a lot of stress and were drinking to cope."

*Rationale*
Helping Eloise see alcohol as a cause, not a solution, to her life problems is an objective and productive response. This response will assist Eloise to become receptive to the possibility of change. The other responses directly confront and attack defences against anxiety that Eloise still needs and may reflect the nurse's frustration with the client.

*Classification*
Competency Category: Nursing Practice: Alterations in Health
Taxonomic Level: Application

**136. D.** Set limits and reinforce that the psychiatrist's refusal of the pass was a consequence and response to the behaviours on her last pass.

*Rationale*
Setting limits and providing clear and consistent boundaries are important in the care of clients with borderline personality disorder. With a client who is impulsive and has a difficult time setting limits for herself, the team's consistent work in naming the limits is key to therapy. Suggesting that the client bring up the issue in the community meeting would not be productive. Ignoring the client's pursuit of limits and boundaries would likely lead to further attention seeking and impulsivity. Exploring the anger does not adequately address the behavioural aspect of her problems.

*Classification*
Competency Category: Nurse–Person Relationship
Taxonomic Level: Critical Thinking

**137. Answers:**

For 3 points, list any three of the following. For 2 points, list any two of the following.

- Age over 50 years.
- Male gender (at higher risk than females).
- Recently widowed.
- Mental or chronic illness (i.e., major depression).
- Recent losses (i.e., moving from home and loss of family pet).

*Rationale*
All of the answers provided are risk factors associated with suicide and should be considered when caring for Henri.

*Classification*
Competency Category: Alterations in Health
Taxonomic Level: Critical Thinking

**138. Answers:**

For 2 points, list any two of the following.

- Establish a therapeutic relationship.
- Ensure safety by assessing suicide assessment for the client.
- Ensure safety by observing and assessing the client's safety on the unit (e.g., checking belongings, providing observations on the unit).
- Place the client on close observation.
- Make a contract with Henri not to harm himself.

For 1 point, list any one of the following.

- Stay with the client.
- Listen to the client.
- Support the client's sense of hope.

*Rationale*
All of the answers provided are priority nursing interventions that could be implemented when planning care for Henri. Based on Henri's presenting symptoms, ensuring safety and regular assessment for suicidal ideation is significant. Also significant is establishing a therapeutic nurse–person relationship.

*Classification*
Competency Category: Alterations in Health:
Nurse–Person Relationship
Taxonomic Level: Critical Thinking

## ▶ Answers and Rationales

# COMPREHENSIVE PRACTICE EXAM II

**1. A.** "Just as I will protect your privacy, I must protect the privacy of the other people involved."

*Rationale*
The nurse must maintain client confidentiality at all times. If people thought that their names were going to be shared with people who they have identified as sexual partners, they would not likely disclose the names and would not want their names revealed, either. The nurse must assure all parties that no identifying information will be revealed.

*Classification*
Competency Category: Professional Practice
Taxonomic Level: Critical Thinking

**2. B.** Call the police.

*Rationale*
The nurse should call the police because the individual has threatened the staff, which is a chargeable offence under the Criminal Code of Canada. The individual's behaviour is unpredictable, and he could be a risk to himself and others.

*Classification*
Competency Category: Professional Practice
Taxonomic Level: Critical Thinking

**3. A.** Document this incident and discuss with the nurse that she did not follow agency policy and distressed the client.

*Rationale*

The manager should discuss with the nurse that she did not follow agency policy. The fact that the client became distressed could lead to the nurse's being accused of unprofessional conduct or battery. This should be documented, and if this incident is repeated, remediation or progressive discipline measures may be required.

*Classification*

Competency Category: Professional Practice
Taxonomic Level: Application

**4. B.** Refuse to administer the medication.

*Rationale*

The nurse should refuse to give the medication because hospital policy would not support her giving it. Giving a medication and having someone else sign for it would be unethical and illegal. Asking another nurse would not be appropriate because the first nurse is aware that the drug should be given by a physician.

*Classification*

Competency Category: Professional Practice
Taxonomic Level: Knowledge/Comprehension

**5. D.** She sits quietly and allows the client to process his or her thoughts.

*Rationale*

Silence should be respected as an integral quality of therapeutic communication. Clients often need brief periods of time to process their thoughts and develop answers to questions. The nurse should allow brief periods of silence to occur.

*Classification*

Competency Category: Professional Practice
Taxonomic Level: Application

**6. A.** Appropriate professional judgment in the absence of a policy.

*Rationale*

Option A is appropriate because it demonstrates that Angela exercises professional judgment in the absence of an agency procedure, protocol, or position statement. Opioids must be locked in the narcotic cupboard. She is practicing within her scope of practice and has demonstrated that she has knowledge of the medication.

*Classification*

Competency Category: Professional Practice
Taxonomic Level: Critical Thinking

**7. A.** Discard the swab and use another piece of sterile gauze.

*Rationale*

Answer A is the correct answer because it demonstrates that the nurse is aware that she contaminated the gauze, which should not be used on the client and should be thrown away. This demonstrates that the nurse is providing safe, competent, and ethical care. Using the contaminated gauze, especially when the nurse is aware of the risk of transferring bacteria to the client's wound, would not be demonstrating safe and competent care.

*Classification*

Competency Category: Professional Practice
Taxonomic Level: Knowledge/Comprehension

**8. A.** "You have a right to withdraw consent. Let's discuss your decision."

*Rationale*

Answer A is correct because it demonstrates that the nurse understands that a client must give consent for a procedure and may withdraw that consent if he or she chooses. This answer also demonstrates the nurse's understanding that the client's change of mind is worth exploring.

*Classification*

Competency Category: Professional Practice
Taxonomic Level: Application

**9. A.** Dignity.

*Rationale*

Dignity includes the provision of privacy. Nurses must respect the physical privacy of persons when care is given. They must provide care in a discreet manner and limit the number of interruptions and intrusions during care.

*Classification*

Competency Category: Professional Practice
Taxonomic Level: Application

**10. B.** Sandwiches on whole wheat bread.

*Rationale*

The nurse would know that, of the choices provided, the sandwiches on whole wheat bread is the best source of fibre.

*Classification*

Competency Category: Professional Practice
Taxonomic Level: Application

**11. A.** "A lot of people don't like fibre. Why don't we talk about ways you can add fibre to your diet that you may not have thought about?"

*Rationale*
Answer A is the most appropriate response because it acknowledges the student's opinion but also opens the discussion for further health education and some options that the student may not have considered. The other options are not reflective of a therapeutic response and may cause the audience to disengage.

*Classification*
Competency Category: Professional Practice
Taxonomic Level: Application

**12. B.** List five sources of fibre they would include in their food choices.

*Rationale*
Of the options provided, answer B is the most appropriate because it reflects the students' willingness to apply what they have learned. Answers A and D indicate that the students liked the student nurse but does not reflect the amount of learning. Answer C evaluates the learning of the students but does not measure the impact of the session on the students' ability to make food choices that include fibre.

*Classification*
Competency Category: Professional Practice
Taxonomic Level: Application

**13. A.** Empathy.

*Rationale*
Reggie is demonstrating empathy by stating that this is difficult for the client. He has also acknowledged that the client is frustrated. The other options are therapeutic techniques, but they are not reflected in Reggie's statement.

*Classification*
Competency Category: Professional Practice
Taxonomic Level: Critical Thinking

**14. A.** Read the medication administration record, read the label on the vial, calculate the dosage, and look at the amount drawn up in the syringe.

*Rationale*
Independent double checking can be used for any medication, including blood products, and should be carried out from the beginning of the process by each nurse independently. This means each nurse does the three checks and does his or her own math calculations.

*Classification*
Competency Category: Professional Practice
Taxonomic Level: Knowledge/Comprehension

**15. C.** This would not be an appropriate job for an RN.

*Rationale*
This job would put the nurse in a conflict with the ethical standards of nursing. Promoting a 940-calorie-per-day diet to all clients would be inappropriate. For most adults, 940 calories per day would be considered a starvation diet and would not promote a healthy lifestyle choice.

*Classification*
Competency Category: Professional Practice
Taxonomic Level: Critical Thinking

**16. A.** Assess for drainage at the heel site.

*Rationale*
A complete, focused assessment of the heel pain would include the assessment of pain, assessment of circulation in the foot and toes, and assessment for drainage at the heel site. The nurse is responsible for making a focused assessment. The other assessments are important but are not focused on the complaint of heel pain.

*Classification*
Competency Category: Professional Practice
Taxonomic Level: Knowledge/Comprehension

**17. B.** Call the physician to report the finding.

*Rationale*
The best response would be to notify the physician. The nurse cannot repeat the dose of analgesia without an order. Massaging the ankle and applying moist heat would be inappropriate for a number of reasons, namely, if the client is developing a deep vein thrombosis, it may dislodge an embolus. Unrelieved pain indicates that an adverse event is developing, and the physician should be made aware of the situation.

*Classification*
Competency Category: Professional Practice
Taxonomic Level: Critical Thinking

**18. C.** Reassess the client, document both the conversation and the assessment, and notify the nursing supervisor.

*Rationale*
The nurse should reassess the client and document the assessment findings. The conversation with the

physician, including the time of the phone call, should be documented as well. The nursing supervisor should be notified so that the nurse will be supported if further conflict occurs with the physician. The other answers do not have the client's best interests as a priority. The client should not be encouraged to take her own medications.

*Classification*
Competency Category: Professional Practice
Taxonomic Level: Critical Thinking

**19. B.** Remind the nurse manager of her responsibility to ensure that all nurses have current registration and to recommend a deadline for staff to show proof of registration.

*Rationale*
The employer is responsible, along with the registrant, to ensure that a current copy of a registration document is on file. Of the answers provided, answer B is the best because there may be other nurses who have not maintained their registration, and the manager needs to be aware of this. In some Canadian provinces, nurses are penalized financially for every day in which they practice without a license.

*Classification*
Competency Category: Professional Practice
Taxonomic Level: Application

**20. C.** The nurse must treat each client equally without prejudice.

*Rationale*
The nurse must make a decision based on the needs of each client, not on personal values and opinions that are based on personal judgment of the client or actions of the client.

*Classification*
Competency Category: Professional Practice
Taxonomic Level: Critical Thinking

**21. A.** Discuss the matter with the other nurse, reminding him or her not to leave client information in view of visitors.

*Rationale*
Leaving personal information in view of other people is a breach of confidentiality. The nurse should approach the nurse at the computer and inform him or her of the incident.

*Classification*
Competency Category: Professional Practice
Taxonomic Level: Critical Thinking

**22. D.** Draw a line through the incorrect entry and date and initial it followed by the correct data.

*Rationale*
Patient records are legal documents, so entries must not be erased, obliterated, or distorted in any way. Incorrect entries should have a single line placed through them and be then dated, timed, and initialled. The correct entry should be placed in the next available space. By following these steps, the nurse maintains clear, concise, accurate, and timely documentation.

*Classification*
Competency Category: Professional Practice
Taxonomic Level: Knowledge/Comprehension

**23. A.** The nurse is responsible for the injuries sustained by the client.

*Rationale*
The nurse would be responsible for the injuries because she did not take appropriate measures to have the alarm fixed and provide a safe environment for the client. The nurse was aware that the client was at risk of falling. By turning off the alarm, there was no alert that the client had gotten out of bed.

*Classification*
Competency Category: Professional Practice
Taxonomic Level: Critical Thinking

**24. Answer:** The client does not have sufficient urinary output to eliminate excess $K^+$. The client will be predisposed to becoming hyperkalemic.

*Rationale*
The nurse who hangs the IV with $K^+$ knowing the urinary output is less than sufficient (30 mL/hr) does not recognize the client's kidneys are not eliminating $K^+$ at an appropriate rate. This would lead to hyperkalemia, which would be a negative outcome for the client. The nurse would be acting in a negligent and unsafe manner.

*Classification*
Competency Category: Professional Practice
Taxonomic Level: Critical Thinking

**25. Answers:**

    a. Refuse to take the money.

    b. Advise the nursing supervisor.

    c. Document the conversation and her actions.

*Rationale*
The nurse should not accept the gift from the client. The nursing supervisor should be notified and the

conversation documented to ensure that it is clear that the nurse did not accept the gift. Gifts appropriate in value for the care given, such as chocolates or a donation that is made to a nursing unit for all the staff to access, would be appropriate. Accepting a significant amount of money from a client would be considered abuse and crosses the boundaries of the nurse–person relationship.

*Classification*
Competency Category: Professional Practice
Taxonomic Level: Application

26. **Answers:**

   - Document the event and assessment in the nurse's notes.
   - Document the notification of the event to the physician.
   - Document the nursing interventions.
   - Document the client's response to the nursing intervention.

*Rationale*
Documenting all of these steps will establish a record of events and will demonstrate that the nurse met the standards of patient care during the administration of this medication.

*Classification*
Competency Category: Professional Practice
Taxonomic Level: Knowledge/Comprehension

27. **A.** Assess her cognitive status, how she is managing with activities of living, and what supports she has available.

*Rationale*
This the most complete statement of the essential assessment necessary to complete for a client who is confused and with a questionable mental health status.

*Classification*
Competency Category: Professional Practice
Taxonomic Level: Critical Thinking

28. **C.** Review the condition in a textbook and review the chart and nursing care plan.

*Rationale*
Nurses need to have the knowledge and understand important considerations regarding assessment, setting of priorities, and important care measures before taking care of a patient with an unfamiliar diagnosis.

*Classification*
Competency Category: Nursing Practice: Alterations in Health
Taxonomic Level: Critical Thinking

29. **C.** Auscultation and percussion.

*Rationale*
These are important assessment tools to identify whether the client has respiratory problems. Inspection has already provided other vital information.

*Classification*
Competency Category: Nursing Practice: Alterations in Health
Taxonomic Level: Application

30. **B.** Increased pulse rate, oxygen saturation of 88%, and circumoral cyanosis.

*Rationale*
This combination of symptoms indicates hypoxia.

*Classification*
Competency Category: Nursing Practice: Alterations in Health
Taxonomic Level: Knowledge

31. **C.** "Your body is stimulated to breathe by low oxygen levels, so you don't want to increase the level of oxygen."

*Rationale*
This provides an explanation of the importance of low oxygen levels at a time when the client feels short of breath. This will also alert him not to increase the oxygen on his own.

*Classification*
Competency Category: Nursing Practice: Health and Wellness
Taxonomic Level: Application

32. **A.** Hypoxemia, hypercapnia, and respiratory acidosis.

*Rationale*
Accurate interpretation of laboratory test results indicates low oxygen, increased carbon dioxide, and respiratory acidosis.

*Classification*
Competency Category: Nursing Practice: Alterations in Health
Taxonomic Level: Critical Thinking

**33. A.** Pursed-lip breathing exercises, coughing exercises, oxygen, and high Fowler's position.

*Rationale*
These are the measures that support more efficient, effective breathing.

*Classification*
Competency Category: Nursing Practice: Alterations in Health
Taxonomic Level: Application

**34. B.** Anxiety decreased, oxygen saturation levels at 90%, nonproductive cough, respirations at 22 breaths/min.

*Rationale*
These show results of effective measures and reduction of breathing problems.

*Classification*
Competency Category: Professional Practice
Taxonomic Level: Critical Thinking

**35. C.** Edema of the extremities and distended neck veins.

*Rationale*
Cor pulmonale is right-sided heart failure caused by lung problems, so the symptoms outlined indicate edema and venous congestion, which are backup signs from right-sided failure.

*Classification*
Competency Category: Nursing Practice: Alterations in Health
Taxonomic Level: Application

**36. A.** The kidneys excrete wastes and maintain fluid and electrolyte balance.

*Rationale*
Health teaching regarding the normal role and function of the kidneys would focus on these functions. The other answers are inaccurate.

*Classification*
Competency Category: Nursing Practice: Health and Wellness
Taxonomic Level: Application

**37. B.** The glomerulus filters out waste products, and the tubules reabsorb needed fluids, nutrients, and electrolytes.

*Rationale*
This response accurately informs the patient regarding the role of the glomerulus.

*Classification*
Competency Category: Nursing Practice: Alterations in Health
Taxonomic Level: Knowledge/Comprehension

**38. C.** Anxiety related to poorly functioning kidneys and body image disturbance.

*Rationale*
This is the most plausible psychosocial problem for this client.

*Classification*
Competency Category: Nursing Practice: Alterations in Health
Taxonomic Level: Knowledge/Comprehension

**39. A.** Daily early morning weight helps to identify retention of fluids.

*Rationale*
Weight is the most accurate measure of output and fluid balance. The other statements are inaccurate.

*Classification*
Competency Category: Nursing Practice: Alterations in Health
Taxonomic Level: Knowledge/Comprehension

**40. C.** Pulse, 108 bpm; temperature, 36.5°C; distended abdomen; nausea.

*Rationale*
Increased pulse rate, a distended abdomen, and nausea signify the possibility of hemorrhage.

*Classification*
Competency Category: Nursing Practice: Alterations in Health
Taxonomic Level: Critical Thinking

**41. B.** Maintaining adequate tissue perfusion and oxygenation.

*Rationale*
The first priority is to ensure adequate nutrients to the tissues and return of waste products.

*Classification*
Competency Category: Nursing Practice: Alterations in Health
Taxonomic Level: Critical Thinking

**42. B.** "That's a difficult question to answer. This must be very frightening for you."

*Rationale*
This is an honest response that acknowledges the client's fears and concerns yet does not give false reassurance.

*Classification*
Competency Category: Nurse–Person Relationship
Taxonomic Level: Critical Thinking

**43. B.** Initiate an IV with normal saline, take vital signs, and have two nurses check the blood type and identity.

*Rationale*
Important actions before starting the packed cell transfusion include initiating a normal saline IV, obtaining baseline vital signs, and double checking to ensure proper cross-match of packed cells for the patient.

*Classification*
Competency Category: Nursing Practice: Health and Wellness
Taxonomic Level: Knowledge/Comprehension

**44. B.** Amount and pattern of alcohol intake, influence on employment, and influence on relationships.

*Rationale*
Honest, open questioning regarding alcohol intake patterns and effects in the client's life helps address the presenting problem. This could be an important turning point in his life.

*Classification*
Competency Category: Nursing Practice: Health and Wellness
Taxonomic Level: Application

**45. B.** Discussing his goals and involving him in identifying and prioritizing important interventions.

*Rationale*
Involvement of the patient in determining the goals and interventions is very important to enhance the client's compliance with the care measures.

*Classification*
Competency Category: Nursing Practice: Health and Wellness
Taxonomic Level: Critical Thinking

**46. A.** Stop the transfusion, continue with saline infusion, and notify the doctor for a suspected hemolytic reaction.

*Rationale*
Hemolytic reaction is one of the most severe blood reactions, so prompt action of stopping of the transfusion is very important, followed by ensuring the IV access is preserved.

*Classification*
Competency Category: Nursing Practice: Alterations in Health
Taxonomic Level: Critical Thinking

**47. B.** Explain that you are unable to perform the IV start until you have completed an inservice and practice session on IV insertions.

*Classification*
Competency Category: Professional Practice
Taxonomic Level: Critical Thinking

*Rationale*
This is a skill that requires knowledge and supervised practice, especially because of the invasive nature of the procedure. Honest acknowledgement of your lack of competency in a skill is an important professional responsibility, followed by actions to ensure you acquire the skill.

**48. C.** Notify the surgeon and await his or her decision; reinforce with the LPN the importance of reporting abnormal preoperative vital signs.

*Rationale*
The purpose of a registered nurse's signing off the chart is to ensure that the safety of the patient has been assessed. Abnormal vital signs identify that priority systems indicate that a stressor or infection is present.

*Classification*
Competency Category: Professional Practice
Taxonomic Level: Critical Thinking

**49. A.** The patient who had the TURP.

*Rationale*
The priority is to assess the potential for bleeding after a TURP because bleeding could quickly compromise the patient' status. In this patient, hemorrhage could become an emergent situation.

*Classification*
Competency Category: Nursing Practice: Health and Wellness
Taxonomic Level: Critical Thinking

**50. B.** Assess his nausea and sleep interferences; call the physiotherapy department to cancel or reschedule his appointment.

*Rationale*
Gathering information regarding possible causes of nausea and sleep problems helps to identify changes and factors that relate to the changes. Modifying the client's schedule helps replan according to his changed state.

*Classification*
Competency Category: Nursing Practice: Health and Wellness
Taxonomic Level: Critical Thinking

**51. A.** Knowing the organizational structure and the lines of communication for the new position.

*Rationale*
The nurse's responsibility is to ensure understanding of lines of communication for safe provision of care and to ensure accountability.

*Classification*
Competency Category: Nursing Practice: Health and Wellness
Taxonomic Level: Knowledge/Comprehension

**52. A.** Giving your opinion and identifying the nurses who have the reduced workload.

*Rationale*
Responses should not be based solely on opinions but should have some factual basis and some suggestions for resolving the issue.

*Classification*
Competency Category: Nurse–Person Relationship
Taxonomic Level: Critical Thinking

**53. B.** Equal sharing of time for discussion of problems so there is mutuality in the relationship.

*Rationale*
With a therapeutic relationship, there needs to be a client-centred approach, with the focus being on the client. A social relationship involves more equal sharing of concerns.

*Classification*
Competency Category: Nurse–Person Relationship
Taxonomic Level: Application

**54. B.** "What ways have you used to help reduce stress and help you cope with significant events in your life?"

*Rationale*
Helping the patient identify stress reduction methods that have been effective and ways to cope with stress help to identify her strengths. This provides the nurse with the best information to assist the client in coping with stress.

*Classification*
Competency Category: Nursing Practice: Health and Wellness
Taxonomic Level: Critical Thinking

**55. B.** Suggest that she inform and discuss with her doctor how traditional therapies could be integrated into her plan of care.

*Rationale*
Respecting the patient's choice is an important ethical principle. Ensuring the safety of the combination of treatments is also part of a nurse's responsibilities.

*Classification*
Competency Category: Nursing Practice: Health and Wellness
Taxonomic Level: Application

**56. A.** Involving her in the development of the teaching plan and encouraging her to question and actively participate.

*Rationale*
Considering the developmental needs of teens is important. Actively involving them in the teaching usually results in better understanding and compliance with the plan of care.

*Classification*
Competency Category: Nursing Practice: Health and Wellness
Taxonomic Level: Application

**57. A.** Reinforce the reason he is taking the medication. Respect his decision if he still refuses the medication and chart his refusal.

*Rationale*
The patient needs to understand the importance of extra fluid removal and how it helps to control blood pressure. The nurse needs to be respectful that he still has a choice in whether he takes the medication.

*Classification*
Competency Category: Nursing Practice: Health and Wellness
Taxonomic Level: Application

**58. B.** Inspect and palpate the lower abdomen; if it is distended and uncomfortable, insert a straight catheter.

*Rationale*
Conservative measures have been unsuccessful. Eight hours after surgery is enough time for bladder tonus return, so assessment of a distended bladder and catheterization would be appropriate.

*Classification*
Competency Category: Nursing Practice: Alterations in Health
Taxonomic Level: Application

**59. B.** Explain the importance of the Heparin in resolving the thrombosis and examine ways that her baby could room in with assistance from her mother.

*Rationale*
Explanation of the importance of the Heparin drip in resolving her problem and while also addressing and responding to her concerns regarding her newborn reflects a response to the client's psychosocial needs as well as her physical needs.

*Classification*
Competency Category: Nursing Practice: Alterations in Health
Taxonomic Level: Critical Thinking

**60. C.** Letting her decide which nursing measures are most important and implementing these measures.

*Rationale*
The nurse has a professional responsibility to share her expertise and explain the reason for nursing measures. The patient also needs to be informed of the rationale of these measures.

*Classification*
Competency Category: Nursing Practice: Alterations in Health
Taxonomic Level: Application

**61. B.** Individualize the care plan according to your evaluation and document care measures and the patient's response.

*Rationale*
Updating and individualizing the care plan is important. Follow-through with documentation is also important after measures have been implemented.

*Classification*
Competency Category: Nursing Practice: Alterations in Health
Taxonomic Level: Application

**62. C.** Perform passive range of motion exercises on the left side and turn the patient from the supine to the right lateral position every 2 hours.

*Rationale*
Prevention of complications, including muscle atrophy, contractures, and pressure ulcers, is a very important goal during the initial stages to enhance tertiary prevention.

*Classification*
Competency Category: Nursing Practice: Alterations in Health
Taxonomic Level: Knowledge/Comprehension

**63. B.** Provide lumbar support when in the supine position, offer her a back rub, and check regarding the possibility of heat treatments to relieve the pain

*Rationale*
It is important to respect her decision and to try other supportive measures to alleviate the pain.

*Classification*
Competency Category: Nursing Practice: Alterations in Health
Taxonomic Level: Application

**64. C.** Physiotherapist and occupational therapist.

*Rationale*
Recognition of her needs and the expertise of these two team members will contribute to the client's rehabilitation.

*Classification*
Competency Category: Nurse–Person Relationship
Taxonomic Level: Knowledge/Comprehension

**65. D.** Sharing assessment information and information on the patient's capability and level of participation in meeting activities of daily living.

*Rationale*
Sharing assessment findings and relevant information helps prepare other health team members and helps coordinate the team efforts, which is one of the nurse's primary roles in relation to the health team.

*Classification*
Competency Category: Nursing Practice: Alterations in Health
Taxonomic Level: Critical Thinking

**66. B.** "We will begin exercises and turning now and start getting you up walking after your condition has stabilized."

*Rationale*
Assisting in outlining the goals of the rehabilitation process assists the patient to know that the process has started and has been individualized to her capabilities.

*Classification*
Competency Category: Nursing Practice: Alterations in Health
Taxonomic Level: Critical Thinking

**67. C.** Checking access to the home with a walker, access and safety measures in the bathroom, and access to food preparation in the kitchen and ensuring safety in her sleeping environment.

*Rationale*
Safety and access in the client's home are important to assess before her discharge to ensure that she can manage at home.

*Classification*
Competency Category: Nursing Practice: Alterations in Health
Taxonomic Level: Critical Thinking

**68. Answers:**

- Thrombosis.
- Embolism.

*Rationale*
You should tell her that either one of these conditions can cause a temporary neurologic deficit that resolves without permanent damage. A hemorrhage will cause more permanent effects.

*Classification*
Competency Category: Nursing Practice: Alterations in Health
Taxonomic Level: Knowledge/Comprehension

**69. Answer:** This was a blessing that the symptoms resolved completely, but it could be a warning of a permanent ischemic cerebrovascular accident (CVA).

*Rationale*
This response acknowledges support of spiritual preferences and practices but also alerts the daughter to the possibility of a permanent CVA.

*Classification*
Competency Category: Nursing Practice: Health and Wellness
Taxonomic Level: Critical Thinking

**70. Answer:** They should avoid smoking, diabetes, high cholesterol, hypertension, obesity, a high-stress lifestyle, and inactivity or lack of exercise.

*Rationale*
Smoking, diabetes, high cholesterol, hypertension, obesity, living a high-stress lifestyle, and being inactive are all factors that contribute to CVAs. Most laypeople identify a CVA as a stroke. As a result, much marketing has focused on stroke prevention.

*Classification*
Competency Category: Nursing Practice: Health and Wellness
Taxonomic Level: Critical Thinking

**71. Answer:** Antiplatelet medication is given to prevent platelet aggregation and lessen the incidence of clot formation.

*Rationale*
Ticlopidine (Ticlid) is an antiplatelet medication used to prevent platelet aggregation and is given during the early onset of a CVA with the goal of reducing clot formation and subsequent damage that can result.

*Classification*
Competency Category: Nursing Practice: Health and Wellness
Taxonomic Level: Critical Thinking

**72. Answer:**

Thrombolytic enzymes are given to cause lysis of thrombosis of embolus.
TPA must be given within 3 hours to restore blood flow and save brain tissue.

*Rationale*
Thrombolytic enzymes are given to cause lysis of thrombosis of embolus. TPA must be given within 3 hours to restore blood flow and save brain tissue.

*Classification*
Competency Category: Nursing Practice: Alterations in Health
Taxonomic Level: Knowledge/Comprehension

**73. Answer:** Level of consciousness and orientation, airway patency, pupil responses, swallowing capability, vital signs, and comparison of sensory and motor responses on the affected and unaffected sides.

*Rationale*
The answers provided are all priority assessments that a nurse must complete when caring for a client initially presenting with a CVA.

*Classification*
Competency Category: Nursing Practice: Alterations in Health
Taxonomic Level: Application

**74. B.** "I give my child NSAIDs only when she is having pain."

*Rationale*
NSAIDs are taken one to four times a day by children with juvenile arthritis and are given to control pain and inflammation as well as malaise and irritability. NSAIDS should be given even when the child is pain free because the antiinflammatory properties of the drugs are key to preventing pain.

*Classification*
Competency Category: Nursing Practice: Health and Wellness
Taxonomic Level: Critical Thinking

**75. D.** Daily range of motion exercises are required to support joint mobility.

*Rationale*
Daily range of motion exercises are required to help children with juvenile arthritis strengthen their muscles and use their joints to their full range of motion. Children should be encouraged to participate in as much of their own care as possible to keep their joints fluid. Excessive exercise, as evidenced by running, jumping, and so on, should be discouraged because it puts an excessive amount of pressure on the joints.

*Classification*
Competency Category: Nursing Practice: Health and Wellness
Taxonomic Level: Critical Thinking

**76. B.** Weighing the diaper before and after micturition.

*Rationale*
Weighing the diaper before applying to the newborn, infant, or toddler and then weighing it after micturition helps evaluate the urine output. The weight is marked directly on the diaper before applying it on the newborn, infant, or toddler, and then the difference between the wet diaper and the dry one will give you the amount of urine.1 g = 1 mL, so amounts may be recorded in millilitres.

*Classification*
Competency Category: Nursing Practice: Health and Wellness
Taxonomic Level: Critical Thinking

**77. B.** It is inherited as an autosomal recessive trait.

*Rationale*
Cystic fibrosis is an inherited autosomal recessive trait. This disease does not occur unless two genes for the disease are present. The gender of the child is unimportant in terms of inheritance, and the disease is not curable.

*Classification*
Competency Category: Nursing Practice: Alterations in Health
Taxonomic Level: Knowledge/Comprehension

**78. A.** Meningitis.

*Rationale*
Head trauma and fractures place an individual at high risk for meningitis. A patient who is febrile with increasing drowsiness should be investigated for post-traumatic meningitis.

*Classification*
Competency Category: Nursing Practice: Alterations in Health
Taxonomic Level: Application

**79. C.** VIII

*Rationale*
Cranial nerve VIII (the acoustic nerve) measures equilibrium and hearing. Hearing would be assessed by asking the child to repeat a whispered word.

*Classification*
Competency Category: Nursing Practice: Health and Wellness
Taxonomic Level: Knowledge/Comprehension

**80. A.** Ruptured appendix.

*Rationale*
When a child with severe right lower quadrant pain has a sudden relief of pain, a ruptured appendix should be suspected.

*Classification*
Competency Category: Nursing Practice: Alterations in Health
Taxonomic Level: Critical Thinking

**81. A.** Preparation for emergency surgery.

*Rationale*
Preparing for emergency surgery is the priority at this point. Antibiotic therapy would be initiated after surgery in addition to addressing pain control and dietary revision.

*Classification*
Competency Category: Nursing Practice: Alterations in Health
Taxonomic Level: Critical Thinking

**82. A.** Decreased renal output.

*Rationale*
Gentamicin sulfate is an antibiotic that can cause ototoxicity and nephrotoxicity. Therefore, a decrease in renal output would be concerning.

*Classification*
Competency Category: Nursing Practice: Alterations in Health
Taxonomic Level: Application

**83. A.** Allergies.

*Rationale*

In children, many symptoms of allergies are often vague and general. They revolve around frequent cold-like symptoms, allergic rhinitis, and pruritus. These symptoms are distracting to children and can affect their ability to concentrate in school. The "itching all the time" descriptor lends itself to allergies and histamine release rather than the other three choices.

*Classification*
Competency Category: Nursing Practice: Alterations in Health
Taxonomic Level: Application

**84. C.** Third degree.

*Rationale*

Third-degree burns are burns of full thickness involving the epidermis, dermis, and underlying tissue. Nerve endings are destroyed, which would explain why the child is not experiencing pain.

*Classification*
Competency Category: Nursing Practice. Alterations in Health
Taxonomic Level: Application

**85. D.** Impaired skin integrity.

*Rationale*

Impaired skin integrity is the priority in the situation of the burned child because of the fluid and electrolyte loss and a high risk for infection.

*Classification*
Competency Category: Nursing Practice: Alterations in Health
Taxonomic Level: Application

**86. B.** Airway obstruction.

*Rationale*

Airway obstruction is the priority because of mucosal edema, impaired ciliary action, and bronchospasm. Additionally, there could be soft tissue damage and swelling around the neck, mouth, and nose that could result in airway obstruction.

*Classification*
Competency Category: Nursing Practice: Alterations in Health
Taxonomic Level: Critical Thinking

**87. C.** As soon as the patient is warmed.

*Rationale*
You cannot determine the neural or hemodynamic status of the child until the child is warmed.

*Classification*
Competency Category: Nursing Practice: Alterations in Health
Taxonomic Level: Application

**88. C.** Repeatedly using the same site is less painful.

*Rationale*
Repeatedly injecting in the same site causes scar tissue (lipohypertrophy) to form, and little or no pain is felt with subsequent injections. It also decreases insulin absorption. Scarring is more likely to occur with same-site injection than with rotating injection sites.

*Classification*
Competency Category: Nursing Practice: Health and Wellness
Taxonomic Level: Critical Thinking

**89. B.** Preschool or toddler (age 2–5 years).

*Rationale*
Children in this age group are in Piaget's preoperational stage of cognitive development and relate pain as punishment for past behaviour. A priority nursing action is to provide reassurance.

*Classification*
Competency Category: Nurse–Person Relationship
Taxonomic Level: Knowledge/Comprehension

**90. C.** Droplet precautions.

*Rationale*
Droplet precautions are used for serious illnesses transmitted by large particle droplets. Standard precautions are used for all patients. Airborne precautions are used for suspected illnesses transmitted by airborne nuclei. Contact precautions are used for serious illnesses that are easily transmitted by direct patient contact or by contact with items in the patient's environment.

*Classification*
Competency Category: Nursing Practice: Alterations in Health
Taxonomic Level: Knowledge/Comprehension

**91. D.** Contact precautions.

*Rationale*
Contact precautions are used for serious illnesses that are easily transmitted by direct patient contact or by contact with items in the patient's environment. Standard precautions are used for all patients. Airborne precautions are used for suspected illness

transmitted by airborne nuclei. Droplet precautions are used for serious illness transmitted by large particle droplets.

*Classification*
Competency Category: Nursing Practice: Alterations in Health
Taxonomic Level: Application

**92. D.** Offering milkshakes and cream soups.

*Rationale*
Children can drink more of a clear fluid than thick fluids because thicker fluids are more filling and less easily absorbed. Small glasses are essential because using large glasses may overwhelm the child. Ice chips, popsicles, and gelatine are all considered fluids and will help increase fluid intake for this child.

*Classification*
Competency Category: Nursing Practice: Health and Wellness
Taxonomic Level: Application

**93. D.** "If discontinued, Ritalin must be tapered off slowly."

*Rationale*
Ritalin must never be stopped abruptly and requires tapering of the dosage as directed by a physician. Parents who see an improvement in the child may believe the child no longer needs to take the medication, so this information is very important.

*Classification*
Competency Category: Nursing Practice: Health and Wellness
Taxonomic Level: Critical Thinking

**94. B.** Sickle cell anemia.

*Rationale*
Sickle cell anemia occurs almost exclusively in people of African descent. The typical presentation is a protruding abdomen from the enlarged spleen and liver and yellow sclera from chronic destruction of the sickled cells.

*Classification*
Competency Category: Nursing Practice: Alterations in Health
Taxonomic Level: Application

**95. C.** Moving his toy box across the room.

*Rationale*
Autistic children react with overresponsiveness to minor changes in their environment. Therefore, moving the child's toy box would potentially be most upsetting to him.

*Classification*
Competency Category: Nurse–Person Relationship
Taxonomic Level: Critical Thinking

**96. A.** "I understand you want me to keep this a secret, but there is a legal obligation for health care providers to report suspected or real abuse."

*Rationale*
The nurse has a legal responsibility to report incidents or suspicions of abuse.

*Classification*
Competency Category: Professional Practice
Taxonomic Level: Critical Thinking

**97. A.** "I am bound by confidentiality not to tell anyone about your visit."

*Rationale*
In Canada, a 16-year-old client is old enough to make an informed decision and consent to engaging in sexual activity. The nurse is bound by confidentiality and cannot by law tell the client's mother about her request for condoms.

*Classification*
Competency Category: Professional Practice
Taxonomic Level: Critical Thinking

**98. Answer:** *Escherichia coli*.

*Rationale*
*Escherichia coli* is a gram-negative pathogen that is commonly spread through stool.

*Classification*
Competency Category: Nursing Practice: Alterations in Health
Taxonomic Level: Knowledge/Comprehension

**99. Answers:**

- Tell the individual that she is breaching confidentiality.
- Tell her to stop talking about the client.

*Rationale*
Nurses must intervene if another member of the health care delivery system fails to maintain his or her duty of confidentiality.

*Classification*
Competency Category: Professional Practice
Taxonomic Level: Critical Thinking

**100. Answers:**

- Offering an explanation of all medical procedure before the procedure occurs to give the child a sense of control.
- Allowing choices when acceptable and appropriate (e.g., choices related to food and toys but not medications and bedtime).
- Addressing regressive behaviours to channel self-expression to acceptable behaviours such as shouting "ouch" or "that hurts" instead of hitting, kicking, or biting.

*Rationale*
All of these steps will offer a sense of autonomy for chronically ill school-age children.

*Classification*
Competency Category: Nurse–Person Relationship
Taxonomic Level: Critical Thinking

**101. B.** At 15 to 60 days after conception.

*Rationale*
A teratogen is any insult that causes abnormal fetal growth or development. Known human teratogens include drugs and chemicals, infections, exposure to radiation, and maternal conditions such as diabetes mellitus and phenylketonuria. A teratogen has the greatest effect on the organs and parts of an embryo during its periods of rapid growth and differentiation, specifically from days 15 to 60.

*Classification*
Competency Category: Nursing Practice: Health and Wellness
Taxonomic Level: Knowledge/Comprehension

**102. C.** Folic acid.

*Rationale*
Proper closure of the neural tube is required for normal formation of the spinal cord, and the neural tube begins to close within the first month of pregnancy. Neural tube defects (malformations of the spinal cord) are more common in infants of women with poor folic acid intake. All women capable of becoming pregnant are advised to consume 0.4 mg/day of folic acid.

*Classification*
Competency Category: Nursing Practice: Alteration in Health
Taxonomic Level: Knowledge/Comprehension

**103. D.** "Supplements may be necessary to meet recommended amounts of vitamins and minerals."

*Rationale*
Some women habitually consume diets that are deficient and may be unable to change this intake during pregnancy. It appears that Norma's lack of appetite and her expressed concern indicate that she may have a diet that is deficient. Multivitamin supplements are recommended during pregnancy to ensure adequate intake of vitamins and minerals.

*Classification*
Competency Category: Nursing Practice: Alterations in Health
Taxonomic Level: Application

**104. A.** "Yes. Carbon monoxide binds with the red blood cells, reducing the amount of oxygen they can carry to the baby."

*Rationale*
Carbon monoxide in the smoke binds with the red blood cells, reducing the amount of oxygen they can carry to the baby.

*Classification*
Competency Category: Nursing Practice: Alterations in Health
Taxonomic Level: Knowledge/Comprehension

**105. A.** Amenorrhea.

*Rationale*
Presumptive signs of pregnancy, including amenorrhea, are changes felt by women at 10 weeks gestational age.

*Classification*
Competency Category: Nursing Practice: Health and Wellness
Taxonomic Level: Application

**106. D.** "They enhance movement of blood through intervillous spaces."

*Rationale*
Braxton Hicks contractions are purposive in that they facilitate the movement of blood throughout the intervillous spaces.

*Classification*
Competency Category: Nursing Practice: Health and Wellness
Taxonomic Level: Knowledge/Comprehension

**107. B.** Nausea.

*Rationale*
Nausea is considered to be a common discomfort of pregnancy rather than a warning sign that needs immediate attention.

*Classification*
Competency Category: Nursing Practice: Alterations in Health
Taxonomic Level: Application

**108. D.** "Eat dry, starchy foods upon awakening."

*Rationale*
Eating dry, starchy foods upon awakening in the morning and at other times may alleviate nausea and vomiting.

*Classification*
Competency Category: Nursing Practice: Alterations in Health
Taxonomic Level: Application

**109. C.** "You are experiencing the results of increased blood supply; one of the pregnancy hormones, estrogen, causes them."

*Rationale*
The upper respiratory tract becomes more vascular in response to elevated levels of estrogen, leading to congestion and stuffiness, nosebleeds, changes in the voice, and a marked inflammatory response.

*Classification*
Competency Category: Nursing Practice: Health and Wellness
Taxonomic Level: Critical Thinking

**110. B.** Serious and requires intervention.

*Rationale*
The incidence of stillbirth increases significantly after 41 weeks gestation, and a fetal movement count is a valuable method of monitoring the condition of the fetus. These data present a very low number of fetal movements in a 24-hour period. Decreases in fetal oxygenation are linked to decreases in gross fetal body movements. A count of fewer than three fetal movements within 1 hour warrants further evaluation by nonstress test, contraction stress test, or biophysical profile.

*Classification*
Competency Category: Nursing Practice: Alterations in Health
Taxonomic Level: Application

**111. C.** "The contractions in my uterus are 3 minutes apart and last 2 minutes each."

*Rationale*
True labour is defined as the onset of regular uterine contractions that increase in frequency, intensity, and duration.

*Classification*
Competency Category: Nursing Practice: Alterations in Health
Taxonomic Level: Critical Thinking

**112. D.** A primigravida at 38 weeks gestation with ruptured membranes, 90-second contractions every 2 minutes, and a pronounced "bloody show."

*Rationale*
This client has a term pregnancy and established in labour, as indicated by frequent, regular, and lengthy contractions. The presence of a pronounced bloody show is indicative of cervical dilatation and effacement. Vaginal examination is indicated to assess the progress of labour.

*Classification*
Competency Category: Nursing Practice: Alterations in Health
Taxonomic Level: Critical Thinking

**113. B.** November 8, 2008.

*Rationale*
Nägele's rule is commonly used to calculate the EDC from the LMP. The equation is to add 7 days to the LMP and count forward 9 calendar months.

*Classification*
Competency Category: Nursing Practice: Health and Wellness
Taxonomic Level: Application

**114. A.** Blended family.

*Rationale*
This is a family formed as the result of divorce and remarriage; it consists of unrelated family members who have joined together to create a new household.

*Classification*
Competency Category: Nursing Practice: Health and Wellness
Taxonomic Level: Application

**115. A.** A fundal height of 27 cm at 32 weeks gestation.

*Rationale*
Optimal fetal growth and development during pregnancy are assessed with a fundal height measurement. Fundal height, measured in centimetres, should equal gestational weeks throughout the pregnancy (e.g., fundal height of 27 cm should occur at 27 weeks gestation). A fundal height of 27 cm at 32 weeks gestation is a very ominous finding that requires immediate attention and investigation.

*Classification*
Competency Category: Nursing Practice: Alterations in Health
Taxonomic Level: Critical Thinking

**116. D.** Instruct her to continue counting for 1 more hour and call back with the results.

*Rationale*
Instruct the woman to continue counting for 1 more hour and call back with the results. The woman should feel 10 movements within 2 hours. If she does not feel further movement in the next hour, she should come in for further assessment.

*Classification*
Competency Category: Nursing Practice: Alterations in Health
Taxonomic Level: Critical Thinking

**117. C.** Stillbirth.

*Rationale*
A fundal height of 30 cm at this point in pregnancy in addition to decreased fetal activity could indicate still birth.

*Classification*
Competency Category: Nursing Practice: Alterations in Health
Taxonomic Level: Critical Thinking

**118. C.** Create a safe and secure atmosphere.

*Rationale*
Marie-Claire has been violated. It is important for the nurse to immediately attend to her basic needs of feeling safe and secure.

*Classification*
Competency Category: Nurse–Person Relationship
Taxonomic Level: Critical Thinking

**119. B.** Increased number of partners increases the risk of gonorrhea.

*Rationale*
The risk of gonorrheal infection increases with an increased number of sexual partners.

*Classification*
Competency Category: Nursing Practice: Alterations in Health
Taxonomic Level: Application

**120. C.** To increase maternal and paternal role attainment.

*Rationale*
Maternal and paternal role attainment is the process by which parents learn behaviours and become comfortable with their identities as parents. The nurse in this situation can role model handling the infant and assessing the baby, with which the parents also need to become comfortable.

*Classification*
Competency Category: Nursing Practice: Health and Wellness
Taxonomic Level: Application

**121. Answer:** Learning the mother's history so as to be aware of a predisposition to a hemorrhage; assessing for firmness of the fundus; assessing for possible sources of bleeding from the cervix, vagina, and perineum; making sure the placenta is intact; checking vital signs that are reliable indicators of shock; and assessing for bladder distension (which can displace the uterus and prevent it from contracting).

*Rationale*
The incidence of postpartum hemorrhage is 4% before 24 hours postpartum and 1% after 24 hours postpartum.

*Classification*
Competency Category: Nursing Practice: Health and Wellness
Taxonomic Level: Critical Thinking

**122. Answers:**

* Time of onset: Less than 24 hours.
* Uterine atony (large baby, multiparity, multiples, precipitous labour, or hydramnios).
* Lacerations of cervix and vagina (malpresentation, forceps-assisted births, vacuum-assisted births, or trauma during birth).
* Pelvic hematoma.
* Placenta problems.
* Retained placental fragments.
* Prolonged labour.
* Oxytocin induction.

*Rationale*
The primary causes of an early postpartum hemorrhage are related to the uterus' not being able to contract from atony, placental fragments, overstretching of the muscle from prolonged labour or oxytocin induction, and lacerations or trauma to the perineum (including the cervix and vagina).

*Classification*
Competency Category: Nursing Practice: Alterations in Health
Taxonomic Level: Critical Thinking

**123. D.** Making observations.

*Rationale*
In this scenario, Rosalind has provided direct feedback as an observation to Stuart and the group. She is not mirroring his behaviour and is not seeking clarification or an explanation of his behaviour. She has not put forward an open-ended question. Making direct observations and providing feedback in this manner are useful in demonstrating attention and concern for group members as and provide an external vantage point on behaviours exhibited in a group setting. Although such a statement makes a space for later clarification, this statement itself if not a statement of clarification; it is simply an observation.

*Classification*
Competency Category: Nurse–Person Relationship
Taxonomic Level: Critical Thinking

**124. C.** "I invite you to briefly summarize your point, Shannon, so that we can hear from others."

*Rationale*
Inviting Shannon to summarize assists her in refocusing and making her point and acknowledges that others require time for the group as well. Ignoring the behaviour does not facilitate group communication and process. The other answers are judgmental and focus more on the nurse's opinions than the group process.

*Classification*
Competency Category: Nurse–Person Relationship
Taxonomic Level: Critical Thinking

**125. B.** Abuse and neglect.

*Rationale*
Role confusion and poor self-concept are often consequences of abusive and neglectful situations and environments. This confusion can lead to boundary blurring. Healthy boundaries evolve when families provide limits, attention, direction, and support.

*Classification*
Competency Category: Nursing Practice: Alterations in Health
Taxonomic Level: Critical Thinking

**126. C.** Severe.

*Rationale*
People with severe anxiety are unable to solve their problems and may have a poor grasp of the happen-ings in their environment. Marcie's described somatic symptoms are usually present. Mild anxiety is less uncomfortable, and some individuals experiencing mild anxiety may even find their perform-ance enhanced. Some difficulty with problem solving and decision making is usually present in people with mild anxiety. When experiencing panic, individuals typically experience markedly disturbed behaviour and may lose touch with reality.

*Classification*
Competency Category: Nursing Practice: Alterations in Health
Taxonomic Level: Application

**127. B.** Somatisation.

*Rationale*
Marcie has several physical symptoms associated with severe anxiety. Emotional conflict and anxiety may be experienced through physical symptoms and is referred to as somatisation. Anger, crying, laughter, and physical or verbal abuse are often referred to as "acting-out behaviours." Withdrawing energy from the environment that is refocused on the self in response to anxiety is known as withdrawal and is a common reaction to anxiety, although it is not exhibited in this case. After anxiety is identified and needs contributing to the anxiety are met, the process is referred to as "problem solving."

*Classification*
Competency Category: Nursing Practice: Alterations in Health
Taxonomic Level: Knowledge/Comprehension

**128. D.** "There is nothing physically wrong with you. You need to stop breathing so rapidly."

*Rationale*
With this response, the nurse would be addressing Marcie's hyperventilation and other somatic symptoms rather than Marcie's feelings about the accident.

*Classification*
Competency Category: Nursing Practice: Alterations in Health
Taxonomic Level: Critical Thinking

**129. D.** "Many people who have been in your situa-tion experience similar emotions and behaviours."

*Rationale*
Providing reassurance that anger and depression are normal responses to trauma is one way a nurse assists the client in dealing with the difficult feelings of a trauma. The other options are clichés and do not address the client's feelings.

*Classification*
Competency Category: Nursing Practice: Alterations in Health
Taxonomic Level: Critical Thinking

**130. B.** Flashbacks, recurring dreams, and numbness.

*Rationale*
Recurring dreams about the event or flashbacks to the event are hallmark symptoms of PTSD that distinguish it from other disorders. People with PTSD may feel a general sense of numbness and estrangement from others. Emotional reactions such as guilt, denial of the event, anger, humiliation, and fatigue are all normal experiences to traumatic events but are not consistent with PTSD.

*Classification*
Competency Category: Nursing Practice: Alterations in Health
Taxonomic Level: Critical Thinking

**131. B.** Exploring the meaning of the traumatic event with Randy.

*Rationale*
Clients with PTSD need support in examining the meaning of the traumatic event. Without this meaning making, symptoms may worsen, and the client may become depressed or engage in self-destructive behaviours (commonly substance abuse). No matter how much time passes, without exploring the meaning of the event, the client will not heal from the trauma. Behavioural techniques such as relaxation therapy may help decrease the client's anxiety and induce sleep. Antianxiety agents or antidepressants may be cautiously used to avoid dependence; sleep medication is rarely appropriate for longer term treatment, however. Unless the client also has an eating disorder or a nutritional problem, a special diet is not indicated.

*Classification*
Competency Category: Nursing Practice: Alterations in Health
Taxonomic Level: Application

**132. C.** Phase 3, the honeymoon phase.

*Rationale*
The phase of the cycle of violence that Isabella's situation exemplifies is the honeymoon phase, in which, after a violent episode, the abuser expresses remorse and pledges that he or she will change. The abused partner is flooded with good will and good feelings and believes that these good feelings will persist.

*Classification*
Competency Category: Nursing Practice: Alterations in Health
Taxonomic Level: Knowledge/Comprehension

**133. C.** Carry the number of the distress centre and have the address of the nearest safe house for women.

*Rationale*
The best alternative will be for Isabella to have some resources to access when she is ready and able to address the situation.

*Classification*
Competency Category: Nursing Practice: Alterations in Health
Taxonomic Level: Application

**134. D.** The therapeutic environment is structured so that stressors are used as opportunities for assessment and learning.

*Rationale*
The therapeutic milieu includes the psychiatric unit and community around the client. There are inherent stressors and triggers within this environment that are relevant to the role of therapy. Being treated on a psychiatric inpatient unit is not all about care and comfort; sometimes the learning and growth that must happen create some points of discomfort, and these stressors can be opportunities for learning. Still, the learning should not be punitive, and the environment should be managed in such a way as to be safe and structured for assessment and learning.

*Classification*
Competency Category: Nursing Practice: Health and Wellness
Taxonomic Level: Application

**135. C.** Determine if Howard is experiencing abuse or neglect.

*Rationale*
Initial observation of the symptoms (dehydration, bruising, and poor hygiene) indicates possible abuse or neglect, which should be immediately assessed or reported. The nurse would then proceed with the history, determine medication use, and take a social history.

*Classification*
Competency Category: Nursing Practice: Alterations in Health
Taxonomic Level: Application

**136. B.** Often masked by aggressive behaviours.

*Rationale*
Depression in adolescents is often masked by anger or aggressive behaviours. Symptoms are usually different from adults in that adolescents exhibit intense mood swings.

*Classification*
Competency Category: Nursing Practice: Alterations in Health
Taxonomic Level: Application

**137. C.** Immediate problems, as perceived by the client, with the short-term goal of problem solving.

*Rationale*
Focusing on the immediate problem and short-term goals to solve that problem are the priorities of nurses dealing with crisis intervention work. Delving into the complete history is not the priority because it takes time away from resolving the immediate crisis. The client's role in the problem is not the goal of this sort of intervention but rather longer term therapy that would hopefully prevent future crises, as would assisting the client to identify what sort of patterns exist in his or her problems.

*Classification*
Competency Category: Nurse–Person Relationship
Taxonomic Level: Application

**138. C.** Remaining focused on the immediate problem.

*Rationale*
In a crisis situation, it is important for the health care professional to help the client focus on the most important issue so that some immediate solutions can be put into place to help decrease the immediate stress.

*Classification*
Competency Category: Nursing Practice: Alterations in Health
Taxonomic Level: Application

**139. B.** "I understand that you are angry, but I must be able to see you at all times to make sure you are safe."

*Rationale*
It is important to acknowledge the client's feelings and allow her to know the rationale of your actions. The nurse is demonstrating respect for the client's feelings while still ensuring her safety.

*Classification*
Competency Category: Nurse–Person Relationship
Taxonomic Level: Application

**140. B.** Create an opportunity for Bill to talk about his experience, ask how he has coped thus far, and explore enhanced coping skills.

*Rationale*
It is important for Bill to begin to explore his feelings and identify how he could enhance his coping skills. He needs to be an active participant in his care, and in identifying his strengths, he can take further control of his life.

*Classification*
Competency Category: Nursing Practice: Alterations in Health
Taxonomic Level: Application

**141. Answer:** Hypertensive crisis (related to interactions).

*Rationale*
MAOIs inhibit the breakdown of tyramine in the body. If foods high in tyramine or sympathetomimetic drugs are consumed at the same time as an MAOI, the potential result is a dangerously high blood pressure.

*Classification*
Competency Category: Nursing Practice: Alterations in Health
Taxonomic Level: Critical Thinking

**142. Answer:** Chocolate, cheese, and wine.

*Rationale*
Any food that has been fermented contains tyramine.

*Classification*
Competency Category: Nursing Practice: Alterations in Health
Taxonomic Level: Knowledge/Comprehension

**143. Answer:** Inattention, short attention span, impulsivity, and hyperactivity.

*Rationale*
ADHD appears before age 7 years and lasts for at least 6 months with symptoms that are more frequent and severe (disabling usual functioning) than typical attention and behavioural concerns for children of the same age.

*Classification*
Competency Category: Nursing Practice: Alterations in Health
Taxonomic Level: Application

# ▶ Self-Analysis for Chapter 8

Comprehensive Practice Exam I

123 Multiple-choice questions × 1 point each = /123 points
+
15 Short answer questions for a total of 30 points = /30 points

***Total Comprehensive Practice Exam I review
questions = /153 points***

Comprehensive Practice Exam II

126 Multiple-choice questions × 1 point each = /126 points
+
17 Short answer questions for a total of 35 points = /35 points

***Total Comprehensive Practice Exam II review
questions = /161 points***